MANAGEMENT OF VASCULAR SURGICAL PROBLEMS

MANAGEMENT OF VASCULAR SURGICAL PROBLEMS

W. Andrew Dale, M.D., F.A.C.S.

Clinical Professor of Surgery
Vanderbilt University School of Medicine
Nashville, Tennessee

McGRAW-HILL BOOK COMPANY

New York St. Louis San Francisco Auckland Bogotá Guatemala
Hamburg Johannesburg Lisbon London Madrid Mexico Montreal New Delhi
Panama Paris San Juan São Paulo Singapore Sydney Tokyo Toronto

This book was set in Times Roman by University Graphics, Inc.; the editors were Robert E. McGrath and Steven Tenney; the production supervisor was Avé McCracken. The cover was designed by Edward R. Schultheis.
Halliday Lithograph Corporation was printer and binder.

Notice

Medicine is an ever-changing science. As new research and clinical experience broaden our knowledge, changes in treatment and drug therapy are required. The editors and the publisher of this work have checked with sources believed to be reliable in their efforts to provide drug dosage schedules that are complete and in accord with the standards accepted at the time of publication. However, readers are advised to check the product information sheet included in the package of each drug they plan to administer to be certain that the information contained in these schedules is accurate and that changes have not been made in the recommended dose or in the contraindications for administration. This recommendation is of particular importance in connection with new or infrequently used drugs.

MANAGEMENT OF VASCULAR SURGICAL PROBLEMS

1234567890HALHAL898765

ISBN 0-07-044999-6

Library of Congress Cataloging in Publication Data

Dale, W. Andrew (William Andrew), date.
Management of vascular sugical problems.

Each chapter is followed by invited commentary.
Includes bibliographies and index.
1. Blood-vessels—Surgery—Complications and sequelae. I. Title. [DNLM: 1. Vascular Sugery. WG 170 D139m]
RD598.5.D35 1985 617′.413 85-134
ISBN 0-07-044999-6

DEDICATED TO MY GREAT TEACHERS

Henry R. (Red) Sanders, 8th grade teacher (later football Coach of the Year at U.C.L.A.), inspiring leader of young men, who put spectacles on me at age 12, saying "That kid can't be as dumb as he acts; he can't see!"

Richard M. Yankee, Headmaster, Darlington School, Rome, Georgia, A modern Mr. Chips, who introduced me to the world of men: "I have never met a bad boy, but there are some whom I have not yet understood."

Samuel B. Knight, Ph.D. Professor of Chemistry, Davidson College, changed the boredom of school work into the adventure of learning and the pleasure of understanding: "You must all do well so that I will know that you understand my teaching."

Barney Brooks, M.D. Chairman, Department of Surgery, Vanderbilt University, martinet, teacher and proponent of the Grail of Surgery: "There is no place for second best."

Earle B. Mahoney, M.D. Professor of Surgery, University of Rochester, physiologic surgeon, inspiring teacher and friend: "We must find a better way."

Corinne Howell Dale, beautiful in stature, lovely in spirit, courageous, my best friend and dear wife for 40 years: "I will go with you."

CONTENTS

INVITED COMMENTATORS

JOHN J. BERGAN, M.D.
Magerstadt Professor of Surgery
Chief, Division of Vascular Surgery
Northwestern University
Chicago, Illinois

F. WILLIAM BLAISDELL, M.D.
Professor and Chairman
Department of Surgery
University of California, Davis
Sacramento, California

ROBERT M. BLUMENBERG, M.D.
Assistant Clinical Professor of Surgery
Albany Medical College
Schenectady, New York

ALLAN D. CALLOW, M.D.
Chairman of the Board
Senior Vascular Surgeon
Tufts University
Boston, Massachusetts

JOHN E. CONNOLLY, M.D.
Professor of Surgery
Chief, Vascular Service
University of California at Irvine
Irvine, California

JOHN J. CRANLEY, JR., M.D.
Clinical Professor of Surgery
University of Cincinnati
Cincinnati, Ohio

E. STANLEY CRAWFORD, M.D.
Professor of Surgery
Baylor College of Medicine
Houston, Texas

HERBERT DARDIK, M.D.
Associate Clinical Professor of Surgery
University of Medicine and Dentistry of New Jersey
Newark, New Jersey

RICHARD H. DEAN, M.D.
Professor of Surgery
Head, Division of Vascular Surgery
Vanderbilt University School of Medicine
Nashville, Tennessee

DOMINIC A. DeLAURENTIS, M.D.
Professor of Surgery
University of Pennsylvania School of Medicine
Philadelphia, Pennsylvania

JAMES A. DeWEESE, M.D.
Chairman
Division of Cardiothroacic Surgery
University of Rochester Medical Center
Rochester, New York

WILLIAM H. EDWARDS, M.D.
Clinical Professor of Surgery
Vanderbilt University School of Medicine
Nashville, Tennessee

W. STERLING EDWARDS, M.D.
Professor and Chairman
Department of Surgery
University of New Mexico
Albuquerque, New Mexico

CALVIN B. ERNST, M.D.
Professor of Surgery
Johns Hopkins University
School of Medicine
Chairman, Section Surgical Sciences
Francis Scott Key Medical Center
Baltimore, Maryland

THOMAS J. FOGARTY, M.D.
Chief, Cardiovascular Surgery
Sequoia Hospital
Redwood City, California

JERRY GOLDSTONE, M.D.
Professor of Surgery
University of California
San Francisco, California

JACKSON HARRIS, M.D.
Associate Clinical Professor of Vanderbilt University School of Medicine
Nashville, Tennessee

ROBERT W. HOBSON II, M.D.
Department of Surgery
Chief, Section Vascular Surgery
University of Medicine and Dentistry of New Jersey
Newark, New Jersey

GEORGE JOHNSON, JR., M.D.
Professor of Surgery
Chairman, Division of Vascular Surgery
University of North Carolina
Chapel Hill, North Carolina

JOHN A. MANNICK, M.D.
Moseley Professor of Surgery
Harvard Medical School
Brigham and Women's Hospital
Boston, Massachusetts

WESLEY S. MOORE, M.D.
Professor of Surgery
Chief, Section of Vascular Surgery
University of California
Los Angeles, California

JOSEPH L. MULHERIN, JR., M.D.
Assistant Clinical Professor of Surgery
Vanderbilt University School of Medicine
Nashville, Tennessee

JOHN OCHSNER, M.D.
Chairman
Department of Surgery
Ochsner Clinic
New Orleans, Louisiana

MALCOLM O. PERRY, M.D.
Professor of Surgery
Cornell University Medical College
New York, New York

NORMAN M. RICH, M.D.
Professor and Chairman
Department of Surgery
Uniformed Services University of the Health Sciences
Bethesda, Maryland

CHARLES G. ROB, M.D.
Professor of Surgery
Uniformed Services University of the Health Sciences
Bethesda, Maryland

DAVID B. ROOS, M.D.
Assistant Clinical Professor of Surgery
University of Colorado
Denver, Colorado

RONALD J. STONEY, M.D.
Professor of Surgery
University of California
San Francisco, California

D. EUGENE STRANDNESS JR., M.D.
Professor of Surgery
University of Washington
Seattle, Washington

GEZA de TAKATS, M.D.
Professor of Surgery, Emeritus
University of Illinois College of Medicine at Chicago
Rush-Presbyterian-St. Luke's Medical Center
Chicago, Illinois

JESSE E. THOMPSON, M.D.
Chairman
Department of Surgery
Baylor University Medical Center
Dallas, Texas

FRANK J. VEITH, M.D.
Professor of Surgery
Chairman, Division of Vascular Surgery
Albert Einstein College of Medicine—Montefiore Hospital
New York, New York

JAMES S. T. YAO, M.D.
Professor of Surgery
Director Blood Flow Laboratory
Northwestern University Medical School
Chicago, Illinois

PREFACE

The National Conference on Arterial Occlusive Disease, the first of its kind, attracted 462 vascular surgeons to Nashville in November 1970. The resultant book (*Management of Arterial Occlusive Disease,* Year Book Publishers, Chicago, 1971) is now out of print. Updating the chapters composed by many authors would be difficult or impossible. The format of this present volume written by a single author was therefore chosen in the belief that practical experience added to the results of others may prove worthwhile to students of vascular surgery.

The planned injection of personal conclusions, to say nothing of philosophy, is intentional, to avoid the monotonous style forced upon writers by the editors of American surgical journals, who insist upon uniformity at whatever cost of interest and understanding. My editor at McGraw-Hill, Robert McGrath, himself a classicist, has tolerated this aberration.

These chapters are not encyclopedic either in the subjects chosen or their discussion. They are intended to be practical, to examine all sides of controversial topics and recommend a choice, or at least an approach to a decision. In each instance, for better or worse, there is a recommendation for action.

In order to balance any tendency toward authoritarianism a recognized expert has been invited to add a commentary to each chapter. Each was asked to focus upon points of disagreement or omissions. All agreed, for which I thank them.

Appreciation is expressed to my friend and coworker, Elizabeth Maney, who has tirelessly placed the corrected text on the word processor, as well as to editors Robert McGrath and Steven Tenney and their associates at McGraw-Hill for their advice and cooperation.

Now, having grasped the proverbial "tiger by the tail" for two years, the result is released. The tiger and I are too exhausted to pursue the matter further.

W. Andrew Dale
312 Lynwood Blvd.
Nashville, Tennessee, 37205

MANAGEMENT OF VASCULAR SURGICAL PROBLEMS

1 THE SURGEON

The only total "human activity" is senior command in combat, according to one modern historian, because it requires equal exercise of the intellectual, physical, and moral faculties simultaneously.[1] While I admire that approach to history as well as the author's elegant style, the attributes of physical and moral activity are dubious in the military officer. The description better fits the surgeon. Surgeons' tasks are difficult; their knowledge and skill may be insufficient, but they must decide, commit, put in the reserves—in short, be responsible. The surgeon is a captain. What are the characteristics of this Galahad to which we aspire?

KNOWLEDGE

The intellect of our paragon, dependent more upon genes than environment, is God- (or parent-) given, the base upon which education and experience act. Intelligence is prized: actually it is less important than motivation and courage. The first lesson learned in medical school is that everyone is "smart." Intelligence alone is not enough. Motivation and prowess (the medieval concept of courage and accomplishment) are vital.

Continuing education has two sources. First is the critical analysis of one's own experience as well as that of others. Second is the pursuit of the accumulated knowledge recorded in books and journals. Neither alone is adequate. Reading without experience is a sterile exercise, but proceeding without books is to sail an uncharted sea. It has been said that President Franklin Roosevelt read few books, relying for information upon conversation.[2] That may suffice for a politician but not for a surgeon. Osmosis is insufficient; learning is hard work.

PHYSICAL ATTRIBUTES

In some quarters a bumbling, labored approach to a surgical operation is acceptable so long as the operator is knowledgeable—and especially if the operator can lecture while bumbling. We all recall instances when a resident was technically superior to the chief. In a sense that is proper—the next generation should be better. On the other hand the student does deserve an expert teacher. The master should know the trade. Aspiring students who lack dexterity should be shifted to a more suitable field.

The reverse of the coin is the overachiever—Mack the Knife—in whom technical skill exceeds judgment. Citing low risk as a surgical indication, the overachiever "operates upon x-rays" rather than for a clinical syndrome. Thereafter assistants are sent to care for the patient while this overachiever whets the blade for the next. Mack the Knife views an operation as the only answer and fights a rearguard action against nonsurgical alternatives. This is self-serving. Despite the surgeon's technical skill, every patient does not "deserve" an operation.

Stamina is the other physical necessity for the surgeon. The body and its resources must be capable of finishing long, tedious procedures and thereafter be capable of spending further time correcting complications or accepting a new emergency without rest. Some days have no end.

SPIRITUAL AND EMOTIONAL CHARACTERISTICS

Life is a struggle where courage and determination are more decisive than are intellect or sensibility. The surgeon requires the resolution to overcome difficult situations, to guide the team through adverse circumstances, and to instill in them the will to follow a calm, strong lead to a successful conclusion. The surgical suite, like the battlefield or the sports arena, requires a captain rather than a prima donna.

More precious than technical skill, which a teenager may acquire, more difficult than knowledge, which is available to all, the most prized attribute of the surgeon is judgment—the ultimate tribute. Judgment has been defined as "the ability to think of many matters at once in their interdependence, their related importance and their consequences."[1]

Judgment must be diligently sought and carefully nurtured by examination of the alternatives prior to execution, along with criticism of the result. Judgment benefits from knowledge of the applicable facts as well as from a correct assessment of the situation. Nothing is more important than a background of vicissitudes (whose origins have been studied) along with success (where luck has been assigned a proper role). Critical recollection of past experiences allows a realistic projection of the probable outcome of the alternatives.

Consequences must be projected. When the decision is difficult and there is likelihood of error, the surgeon must choose the course of action which is safer for the patient. Thus, one removes the appendix if there is serious doubt, repairs an aortic aneurysm when pain suggests perforation, and performs fasciotomy if there is a question of compartmental pressure. Errors will be made but their results should be minimized.

With the exception of the hermit-scholar, most surgeons find an urge to transmit their knowledge—in short, to teach at one or another level, with or without a title. This characteristic perpetuates the profession, ensuring that each generation stands on the shoulders of its predecessors.

THE SURGEON AS A SEMISCIENTIST

Some of us would like to be scientists. We are not, for the technique and judgment that are necessary in surgical practice are often nearer art than science. Further, ethical conduct rules out prospective double-blind studies of every question. We are semiscientists, often facing what may be called the Arrowsmith dilemma. You may recall that Sinclair Lewis in his 1926 novel *Arrowsmith* presented the conflict between science and humanitarianism in terms of whether a supposedly effective new vaccine should be supplied to everyone during a developing epidemic or whether a prospective controlled study should be done to discover the facts.

Fortunately, with increasing knowledge among laypersons there are now more opportunities for controlled research under the doctrine of informed consent. Surgeons must look more for such answers and less for opinions which reflect bias rather than critical experience.

RELATION TO THE PATIENT

Professionalism traditionally suggests more than a contractual relationship, the performance of a service for pay, and a disinterest in the client's welfare beyond the problem at hand. It implies trust deserved by integrity, respect earned by competence, and the empathy which mature self-love extends to the patient and family. The age-old golden rule does apply to the surgeon-patient relationship.

REFERENCES

1 Tuchman BW: *Practicing History.* Ballantine, New York, 1982.
2 Manchester W: *The Glory and the Dream.* Bantam, New York, 1975.

2 THE EVOLUTION OF VASCULAR SURGERY

To understand a science it is necessary to know its history.

Auguste Comte (1798–1857)

An age-old dream of the human race has been the replacement of worn parts of the body, repairs to prolong life and function, even a magical fountain of youth!

Modern vascular surgery has fulfilled some of those visions, and its future promises even more. Today's high road of achievement was built upon the unmarked trails of the past not only by imagination and courage but also with toil and tears. This history deserves some attention.

Several important developments form the foundation for the present practice of vascular surgery. These are briefly summarized from my detailed presentations in 1974[1] and 1978[2] along with some previously unpublished notes and recollections from those times.

VASCULAR ANASTOMOSIS

The early lateral arterial repair by Hallowell of England in 1759[3] (Figure 2-1) occurred in an age when violence and warfare made bloodshed commonplace, when the average life span in France was 22 years and investigative science was hardly known. It was little noted nor long remembered.

Over a century later a number of surgeons began to perform animal experiments (Figure 2-2).[4] Dorfler is credited with the description of an all layer intima-to-intima anastomosis in 1899.[5] An experimental as well as master clinical surgeon, the legendary John B. Murphy of Chicago, "the stormy petrel of surgery," in 1897 first successfully rejoined the human femoral artery by invagination of the proximal into the distal end (Figure 2-3).[6]

To Alexis Carrel must be awarded the chief distinction among the pioneers for his continuing animal studies of all types of venous and arterial anastomoses and transplants (including transplantation of the head of a dog 50 years ahead of the later Russian report[7]) which culminated in the Nobel prize for 1912[8] (Figure 2-4). Whether his collaborator, Charles C. Guthrie, should have been a joint recipient is still debated.[9,10] It was recently remarked that Guthrie "enjoyed a sabbatical year off and missed the Nobel Prize!"[11]

BLOOD TRANSFUSION

Blood transfusion had been sporadically attempted for centuries, but it required Landsteiner's discovery of the blood groups in 1900 in Vienna to allow it to be done safely. Its practical use in the United States progressed at once and even surpassed that in Europe. Alton Ochsner recalled how, in 1923, transfusion was in disrepute in Zurich because of its 60 percent mortality rate. Their *biologische probe* test consisted of giving 25 cc of whole blood to the patient, and if the patient survived the main transfusion would be given! Ochsner was allowed to treat an exsanguinated criminal, shot through the femoral artery, because "if he died it would be all right as

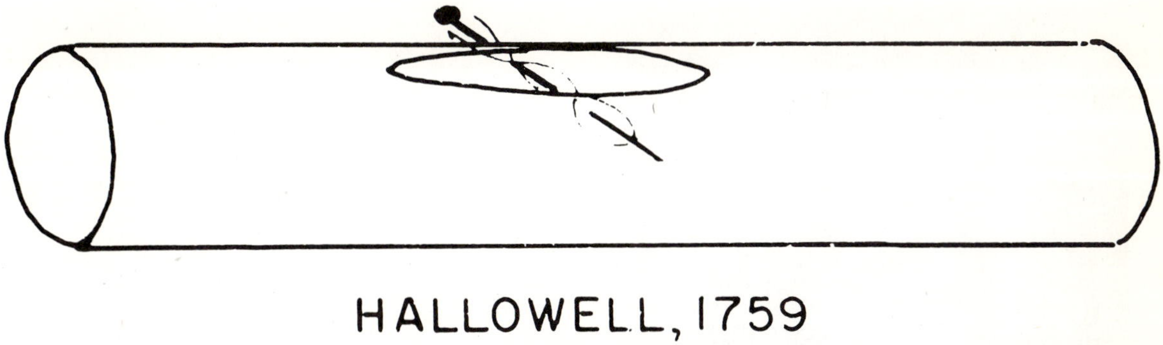

FIGURE 2-1 Hallowell's lateral arterial repair by tightening of a thread about the ends of a pin passed through the edges of the artery was at the time an ingenious if unusual method which had no future.

they were anxious to get rid of him anyway!" He did survive and the young surgeon was then allowed to type and transfuse a leading banker, who also did well.[12] These cases altered their practice of blood transfusion.

ANGIOGRAPHY

The development of angiography began approximately three months after Roentgen's discovery of the x-ray in 1896, when Haschek and Lindenthal injected a mixture of radiopaque material into the arteries of an amputated arm and demonstrated its radiopacity on an exposed film.[13] Sicard and Forestier first reported its use in a live person in France when they injected poppy-seed oil (Lipiodol) into the antecubital vein and observed its passage toward the lungs fluoroscopically.[14] In the following year, 1924, Barney Brooks initiated clinical angiography by injecting

FIGURE 2-2 Jaboulay's all layer interrupted mattress suture anastomosis was performed in the dog as the "proper" method of joining arteries in 1896. It represents a long-ago effort of the great French school of surgeons, who produced repeated advances in vascular surgery over a period of 50 years.

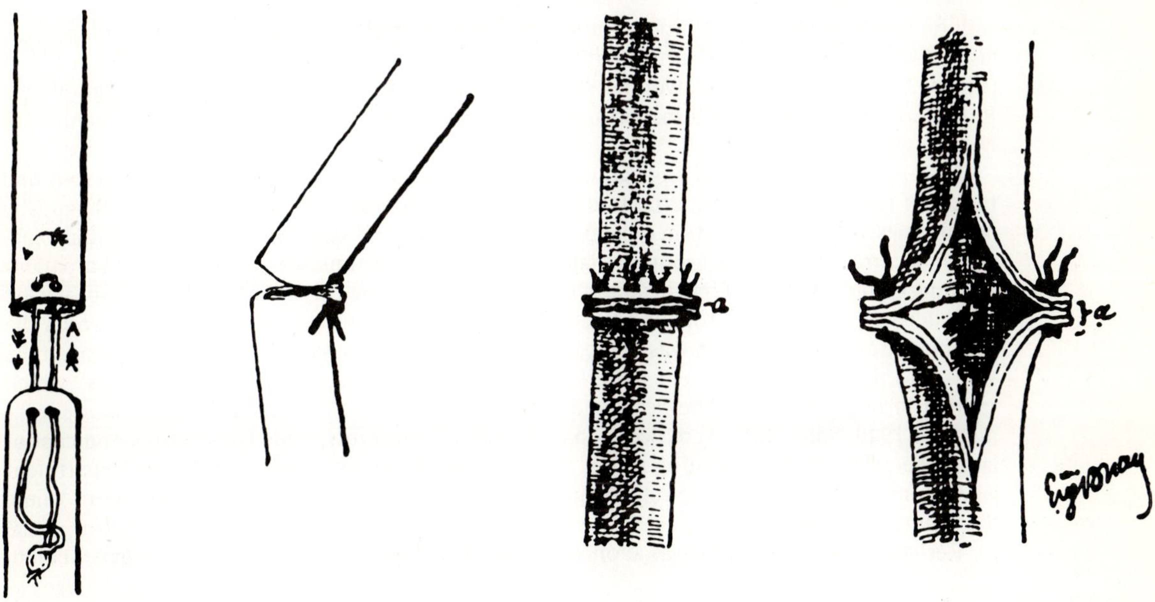

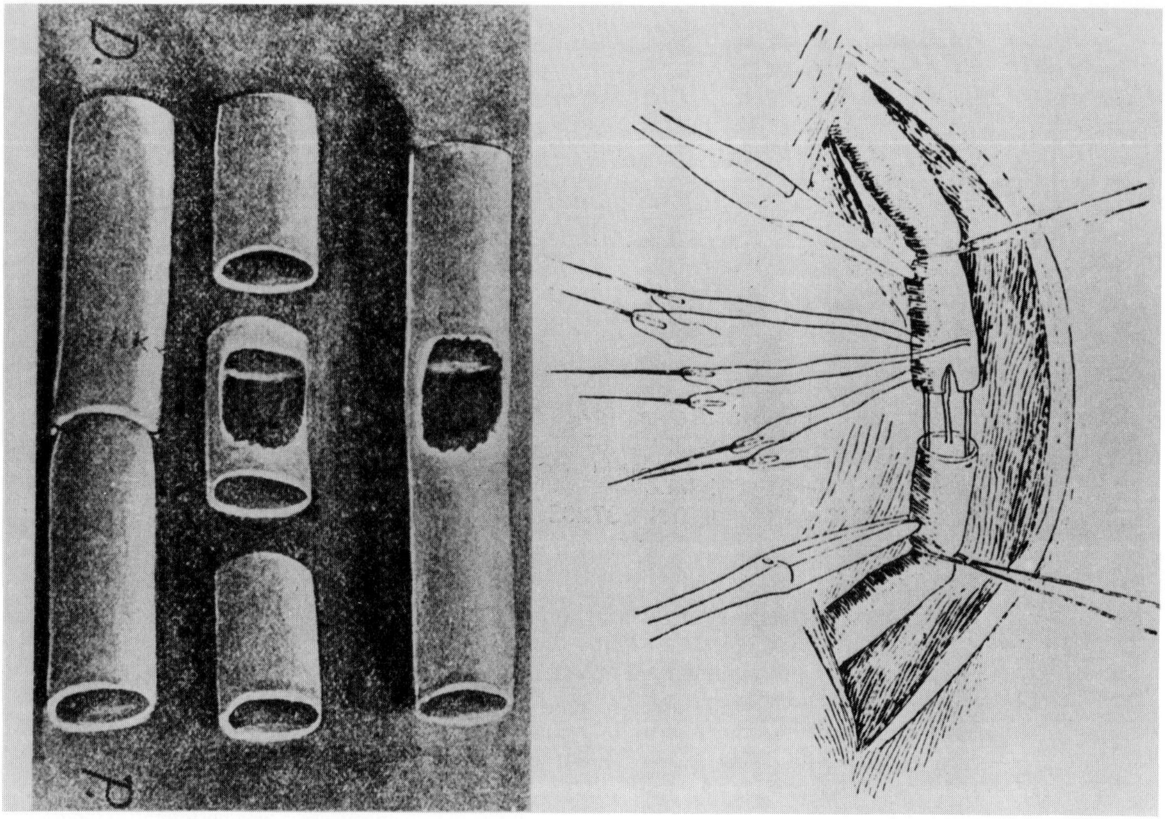

FIGURE 2-3 In 1897 the Chicago surgeon John B. Murphy first anastomosed a human artery by invaginating the proximal into the distal femoral segment to repair an injury.

sodium iodide to study the femoropopliteal arterial system (Figure 2-5).[15] Further developments largely occurred outside the United States, such as cerebral angiography by Egas Moniz in 1927[16] (Figure 2-6) (he later, in 1949, won the Nobel prize for prefrontal lobotomy) and aortography by Reynaldo dos Santos in 1929 in Portugal.[17] But there was a long delay before these techniques became widely accepted.

The appearance of clinical angiography in the United States was delayed until the 1950s due to fear of injection of any material into an artery, to failure to appreciate its clinical diagnostic possibilities, and to the cessation of laboratory efforts during World War II. My own initial experience occurred as one of a group of eight physicians and technicians who supported a patient standing before a series of films in a rack, each film dropping by gravity into a radiation-protected box after its exposure. My role was to stand upon a ladder to support one arm into which the forcible intravenous injection was made, thus ensuring rapid passage of the material through the veins into the heart. The patient remarked loudly upon "the purple and yellow flames" which spurted through her head. The heart and great vessels were well delineated by this crude technique in 1949. Soon there were occasional femoral arteriograms made by exposing and cannulating the artery in the operating room, transporting the patient to the Radiology Department where films were made, thence returning up the elevator to the awaiting operating room where the wound was closed.

Resistance to angiography was at once encountered. Following presentation of a patient along

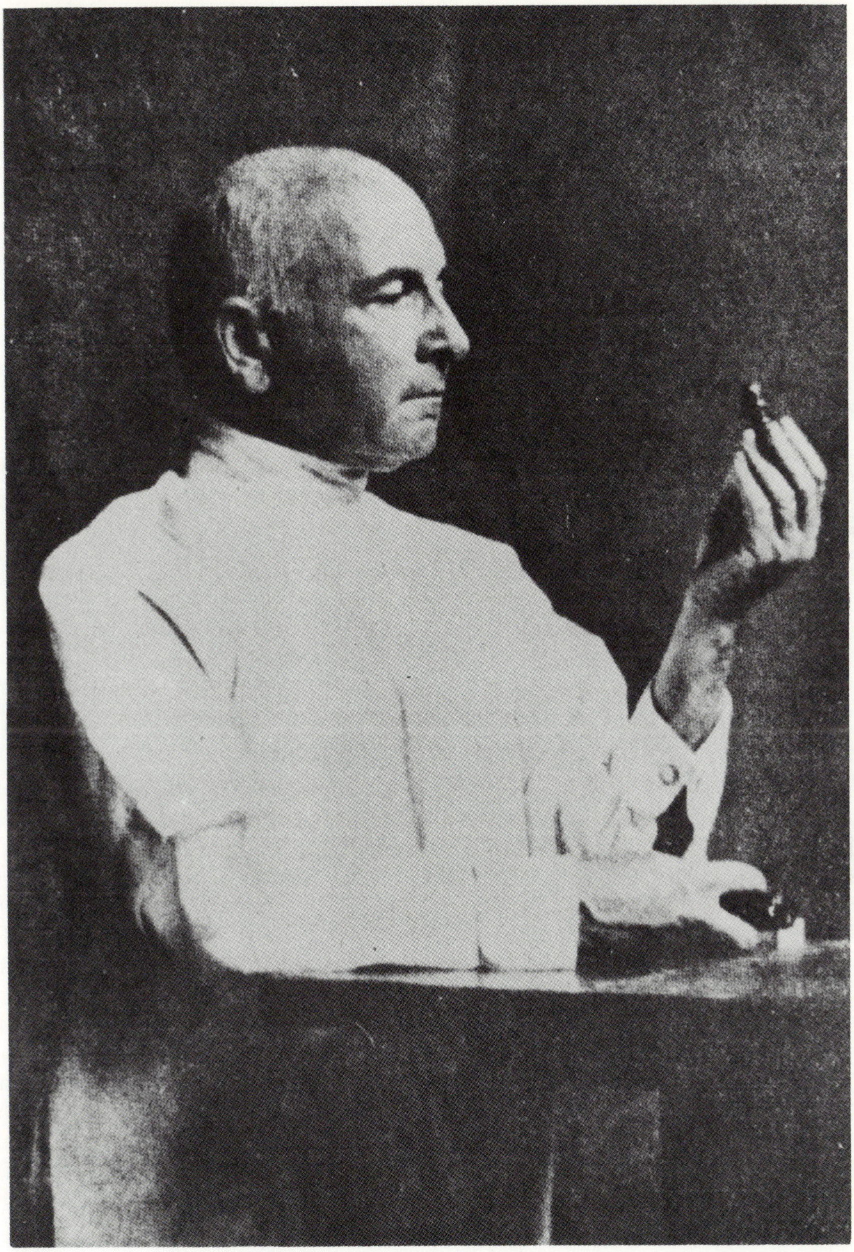

FIGURE 2-4 Alexis Carrel, eccentric mystic, performed all the modern vascular procedures in the experimental laboratory more than half a century ago, for which he was awarded the Nobel prize in 1912.

with his femoral arteriogram, there was a stern warning from a respected senior surgeon, himself a surgical pioneer, that such was dangerous and could lead to loss of limb. As late as 1958, when I moved to a new locale in Nashville, the head of the Radiology Department answered my query

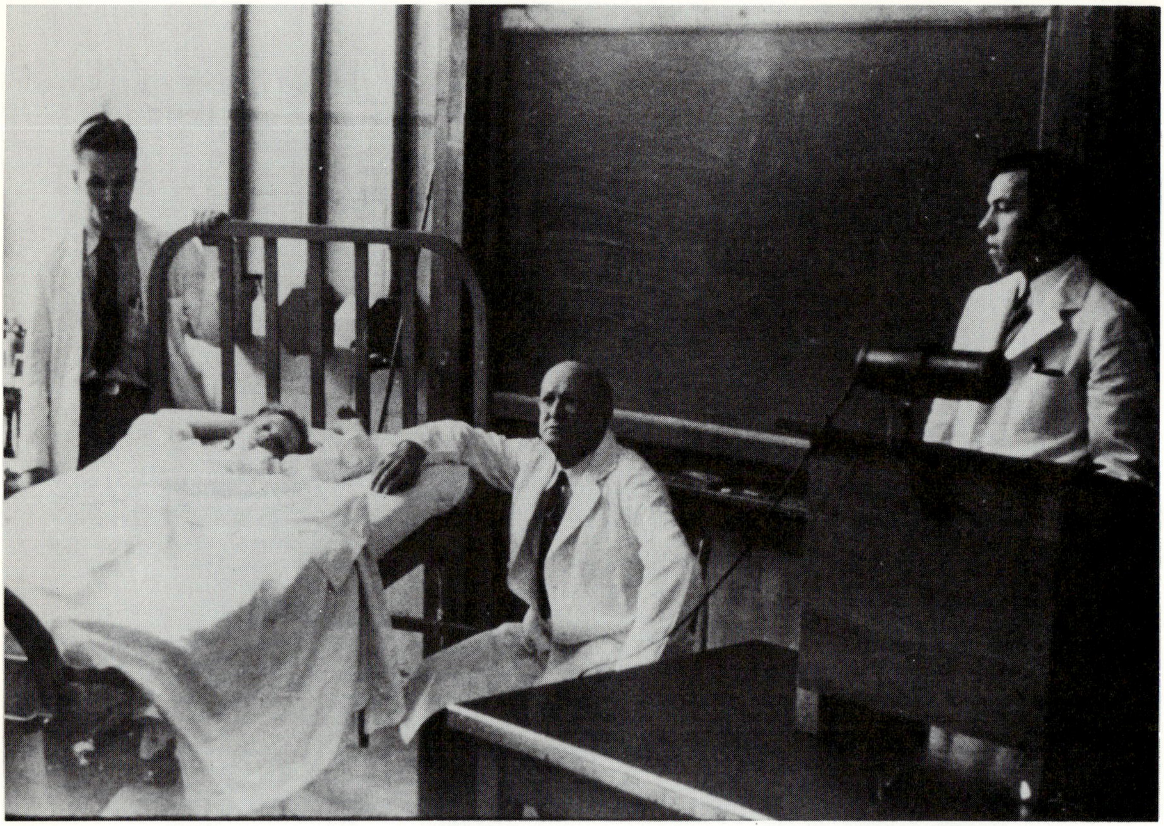

FIGURE 2-5 Barney Brooks insisted upon bedside teaching rather than formal lectures and conferences. Here he discusses a clinical problem for students of my class at Vanderbilt in 1943. Perhaps this was taken at the memorable session when he began at 8:00 A.M. and finished at 12:25 P.M., with the students and resident staff completely collapsed by that time.

regarding angiographic facilities with a curt negative, since there had recently occurred a tragic instance of transverse myelitis with paraplegia following a translumbar aortogram.

The toxicity of the early radiopaque materials was corrected, and techniques became standardized with resultant safety as well as the provision of accurate vascular delineation for the vascular surgeon. With care and use of appropriate methods I have not had limb loss nor death due to angiography during my thirty-odd years of vascular experience.

HEPARIN

In 1916 W. H. Howell reported discovery of the anticoagulant heparin, but because of impurities, it remained too toxic for clinical use for twenty-odd years.[18]

In 1940 a purified form of heparin was administered intravenously by Gordon Murray of Toronto during and after embolectomy and as prophylaxis as well as treatment of venous thromboembolism.[19] My own advocacy of intravenous heparin shortly thereafter was not widely accepted. Usage of heparin in North America lagged considerably behind the experience of the Scandinavians, and it was only in the 1970s that this outstanding drug gained wide acceptance as a relatively safe and useful anticoagulant for both arterial and venous problems.

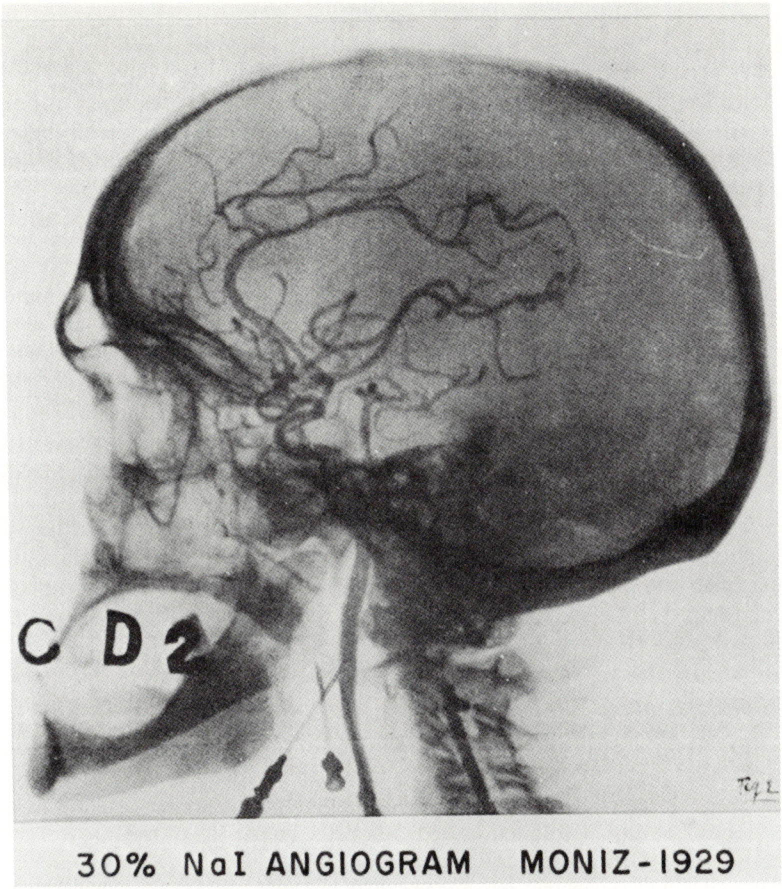

FIGURE 2-6 Over 50 years ago Egas Moniz published this cerebral angiogram.

EXPERIMENTAL LABORATORY

The urgent need for arterial replacements and the aggressive nature of surgeons has sometimes led to human usage prior to detailed laboratory investigation. This has not been totally without benefit. since more than one significant development has resulted from a courageous clinical effort undertaken with little or no experimental background. Thus, the French vascular surgeons in the late 1940s and 1950s reported one after another well-conceived and executed "first" and usually bypassed a slower laboratory effort. Kunlin's femoropopliteal vein bypass in 1948,[20] Jacques Oudot's first aortic resection and graft in 1950,[21] and Charles Dubost's initial replacement of aortic aneurysm in 1951[22] are worthy examples of bold clinical advances with little or no experimental preparation.

It should also be recognized that animal studies did not predict the eventual failure of both the homologous arterial graft[23] and the heterologous bovine graft.[24] This recognition of late complications depended upon long-term follow-ups in human patients.

On the other hand, experimental conditions usually allowed controlled conditions not possible in clinical usage. The much better patency rates of autogenous veins versus synthetic grafts to replace the canine femoral artery predicted the preferable graft for small human arteries, as well as indicating that a variety of materials were suitable for large aortic replacements.[25,26]

Another sometimes-overlooked dividend of the experimental laboratory and its controlled experiments has been the training of young surgeons in the development of not only technical surgical skills but also an understanding of the difference between clinical impressions and the actual facts. The generation of North American surgeons who developed the field of vascular surgery almost all benefited by such laboratory experience.

VASCULAR GRAFTS

The brilliant promise of the early years of the twentieth century failed to materialize because surgical technique had too far outstripped methods of diagnosis and of support. A long period of dormancy followed. Actually there were, during this time, occasional successful grafting operations—such as Gluck's in 1898,[27] Goyanes' vein grafts for popliteal aneurysm in Madrid in 1906 (Figure 2-7),[28] Erich Lexer's vein replacement of an axillary aneurysm in Königsberg in 1906,[29] and J. Hogarth Pringle's two vein grafts for popliteal aneurysm in Glasgow in 1913.[30] The surgical world, however, ignored these scattered successes and instead applauded the widespread development of extirpative techniques.

After World War II, accumulated knowledge exploded in a Renaissance for vascular surgery, as imaginative and bold young surgeons seized new knowledge in animal laboratories and translated it at once into patient care in wards and operating rooms. Thereafter the rapid expansion of vascular surgery in only a few years is staggering in relation to its slow progress for all of previous history.

Homologous Artery Grafts

An urgent need for a graft to replace the aorta occurred in the mid-1940s when diagnostic techniques indicated that aortic problems were correctable by surgery once the chest and abdomen could be entered with relative ease and safety. The first answer to this need was the homologous artery, a solution which within a decade led into the cul de sac of difficulty of procurement and later degeneration of the graft.[23]

Earlier attempts to preserve arteries for later transplantation date back to Carrel, with later occasional efforts by others such as Blakemore and Lord[31] and Hufnagel.[32] Robert Gross of Boston first correlated his own experiments with earlier ones and organized a clinical artery bank. In 1949 he reported 15 successful homologous arterial grafts used for coarctation of the aorta and the tetralogy of Fallot.[33]

A variety of techniques for preservation of arteries from young persons dying of trauma or of nonmalignant disease developed, and by the mid-1950s most large hospitals throughout North America maintained artery banks where sterile, frozen arterial grafts were constantly maintained.

The homologous artery bank in Rochester was promoted by W. J. Merle Scott, who headed the Department of Surgery at the University of Rochester in the 1950s; the organization and work were largely done by James A. DeWeese, later to become an internationally known cardiovascular surgeon, and by Frank Bauer, who continued on to a fine career in general surgery in Little Rock. The rest of us benefited from their often late-at-night procurements of arteries for the bank (Figure 2-8).

Increasing experience, however, indicated that although homologous arterial replacements of the aorta were satisfactory, the incidence of degenerative changes with thrombosis, aneurysm formation, and other problems was too high to be generally acceptable in the peripheral arterial system. By 1959 there were several large series attesting to these problems, including our own experience of eight severe late complications among 90 homologous arterial grafts.[23]

These intrinsic problems, along with the difficulties in procurement of homologous arteries, forced them into a role of historic interest after about 15 years of widespread use.

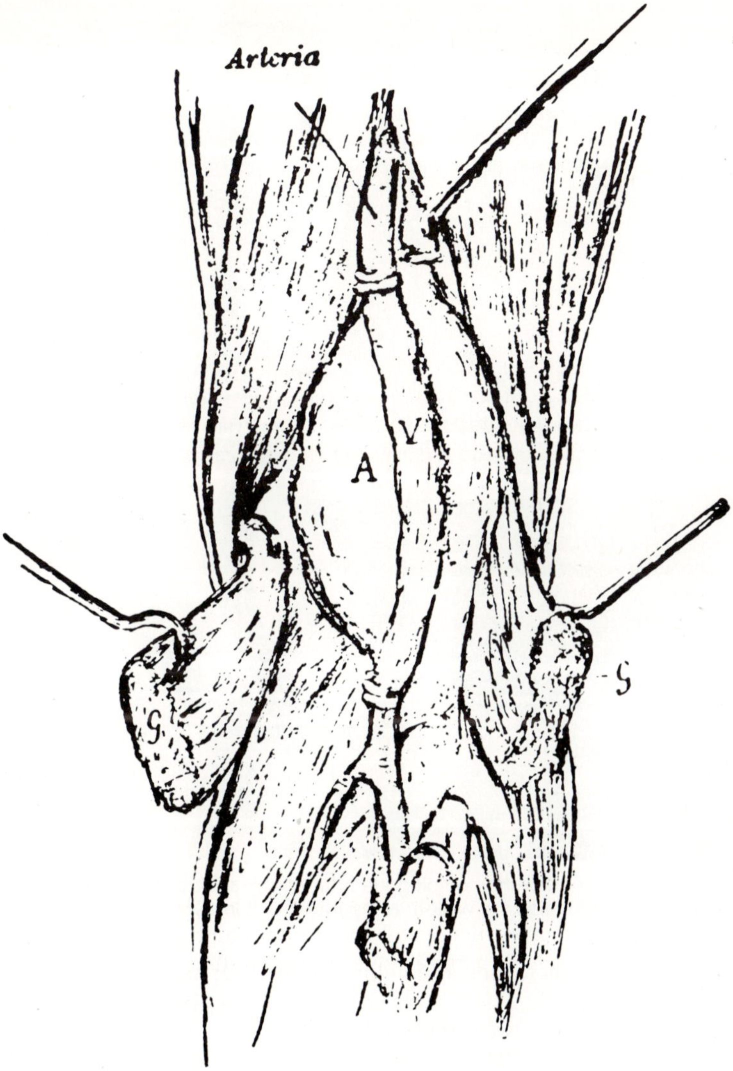

Goyanes - Madrid - 1906

FIGURE 2-7 This original drawing demonstrates an interpolated venous bypass around a popliteal aneurysm.

Autogenous Vein Grafts

The idea of the autogenous vein graft, essentially lying dormant for several decades, was revived by Jean Kunlin's femoropopliteal bypass technique in France in 1948,[34] was popularized by Robert Linton in the United States,[35] and was confirmed in trauma situations by its successful use during the Korean War.[36] There did remain a considerable bias opposing vein grafts in the 1950s.

During the war years the Surgical Experimental Laboratory at Rochester had become dormant, its space largely empty and its budget nonexistent. This situation forced me to work in the

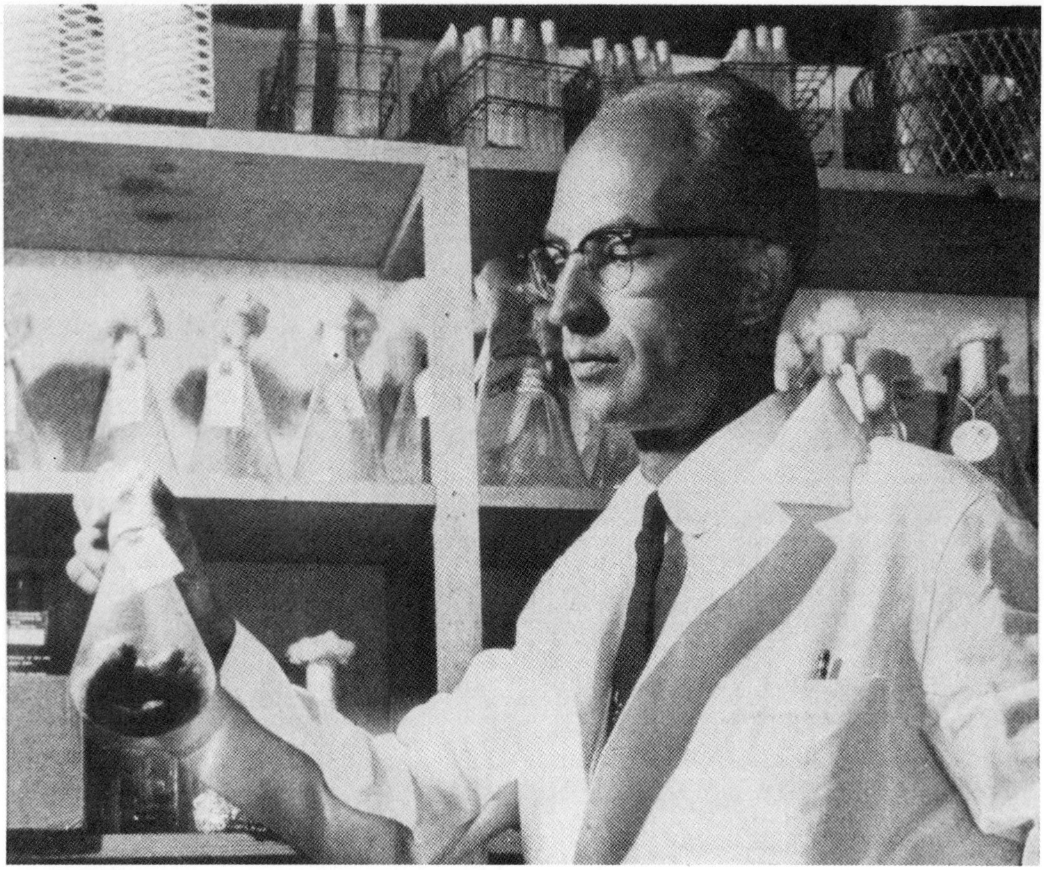

FIGURE 2-8 This photograph of the homologous artery bank at Strong Memorial Hospital, Rochester, New York, shows the author inside the walk-in refrigerated unit in 1955.

Department of Physiology there, first as a volunteer and later as Assistant Professor, in an effort to learn experimental methods. Three years later my studies of pulmonary atelectasis under the supervision of Hermann Rahn were interrupted when Merle Scott suggested that I move two floors down and attempt to revitalize the Surgical Experimental Laboratory as Director—a big title with no equipment or money!

Sporadic attempts at arterial replacement by tubes had occurred, so we at once agreed that the main thrust of study should be in the vascular field and specifically aimed at arterial replacement. A number of materials were used as grafts to replace the canine aorta, but it was soon realized that this was not a difficult test, so the model was shifted to bypass of the dog's femoral artery. George Mavor came over from Aberdeen in Scotland, and Jim DeWeese joined the group, adding development of the extracorporeal cardiac pump to the program (Figure 2-9). Earle Mahoney provided steady encouragement and wise advice.

All the then available materials were tried—homologous arteries, autogenous veins, Ivalon, nylon, Teflon, and Dacron as they became available. Many were hand-sewn from sheets into tubes. The ends were often fused with the actual heat cautery. Teflon tubes which arrived brown with coating impurities were boiled for a week beneath a hood in concentrated sulfuric acid to produce gleaming white tubes (Figure 2-10).

It became increasingly apparent to us that autogenous veins and homologous arteries had

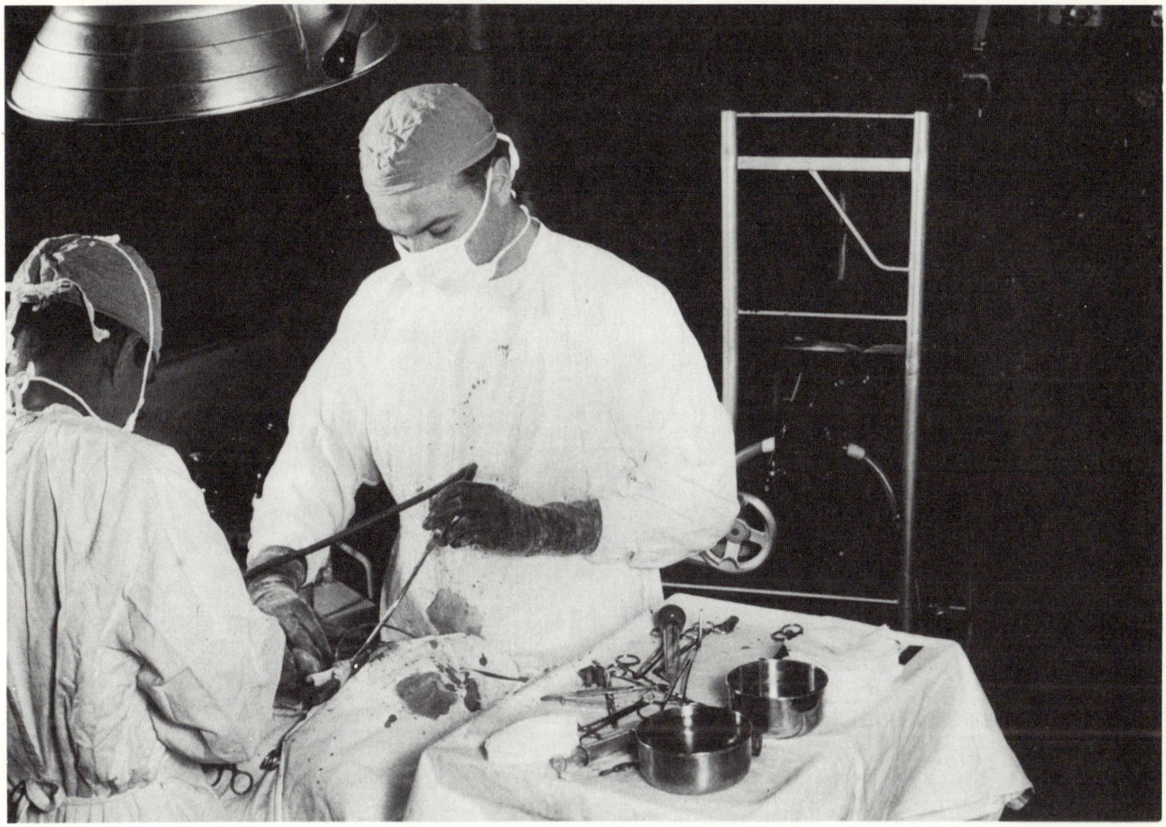

FIGURE 2-9 James A. DeWeese using an extracorporeal pump in the experimental laboratory at Rochester in 1954.

considerably higher patency rates in the dog's femoral artery position than did any synthetic. Homologous arteries, doing well in the dog, began to be clinically suspect, first in terms of difficulties with procurement and with maintenance of the artery bank, but of more importance in terms of the increasing numbers of aneurysm and of degeneration. Thus the autogenous vein appeared to be the best replacement for medium and small arteries.

My first clinical use of an autogenous saphenous vein instead of a homologous artery as a femoropopliteal graft occurred in 1957 when it was used in a 77-year-old man who was the grandfather of my secretary. Happily, it remained patent until his passing 14 years later.

There did remain a considerable bias against the vein graft well into the 1960s. For example, the Motion Picture Committee of the American College of Surgeons in 1959 refused to approve the film *Autogenous Vein Graft for Femoral-popliteal Arterial Occlusion* because it was believed to be a procedure of no merit! In the same year there was the threat of litigation on the same grounds.

The present acceptance of the autogenous vein graft by all vascular surgeons requires no further comment.

Synthetic Grafts

Solution of the long-recognized problem of arterial replacement by nonbiologic grafts began in 1952.

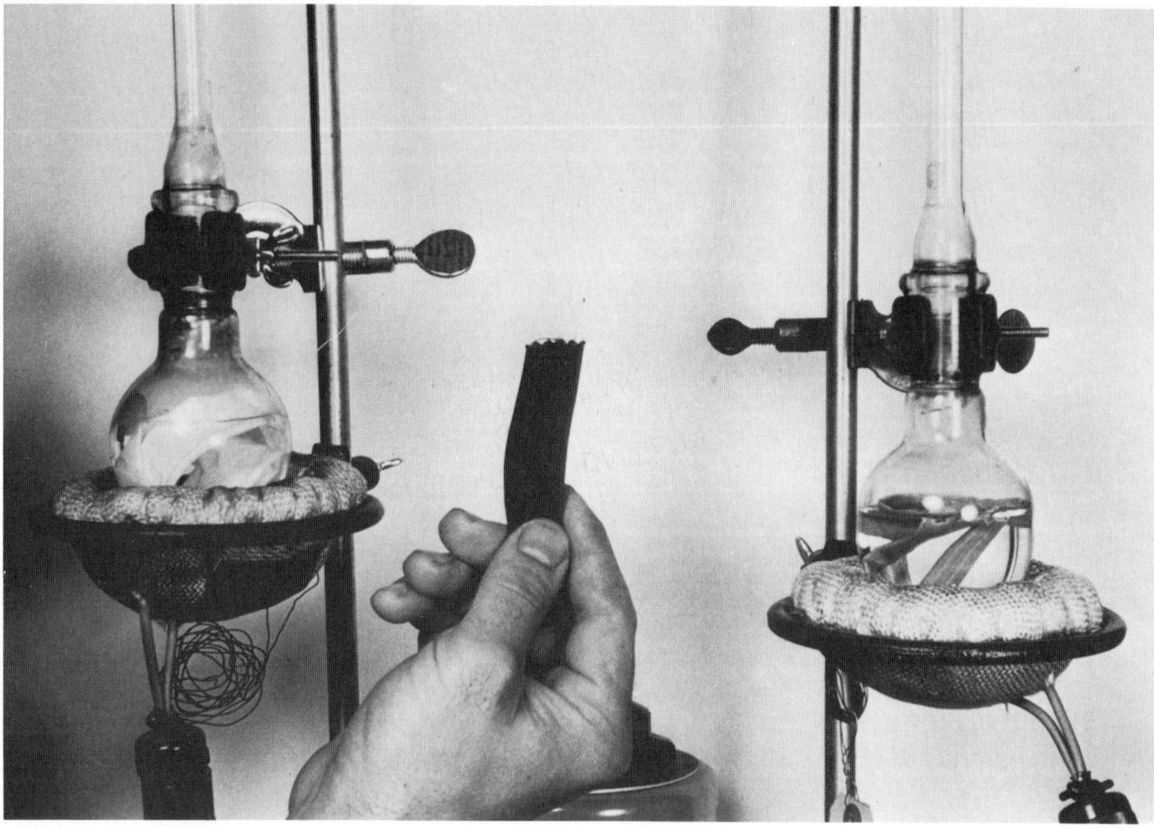

FIGURE 2-10 In the early 1960s Teflon tubes were heavily coated with a brown contaminant, probably grease. The grafts were cleaned by boiling in concentrated sulfuric acid beneath a hood for a week. At *center* is the original tubular graft, at *right* the partial clearing of the discoloration, and at *left* the final white appearance.

Throughout many years a variety of materials had been tried as artificial replacements for arteries, with repeated failures due to thrombosis or to hemorrhage from the junction of the graft with the host vessel. Thus, Tuffier in World War I used paraffin-lined silver tubes,[37] Murray and Jones failed with glass ones,[38] and Blakemore's Vitallium tubes thrombosed,[39] as did Moore's polyethylene tubes.[40] Hollow, nonporous tubes thus uniformly failed.

It remained for Voorhees, Jaretski, and Blakemore to take the giant step that opened the door. Having noted that a silk suture projecting into a dog's cardiac lumen became covered with a thin tissue, they postulated that the interior of a cloth tube might be similarly covered while its interstices became blocked with fibrin and platelets. In 1952 they announced their success in using tubes of vinyon-N to replace the aorta in dogs (Figure 2-11).[41] This justifiably renowned research soon led to intense investigation of many porous synthetic materials and triggered the explosive development of modern vascular surgery.

The Society for Vascular Surgery soon recognized the chaotic situation and appointed a committee to investigate then available synthetic materials, which were vinyon-N, nylon, Orlon, Dacron, Teflon, Ivalon, Fortisan, and steel. The committee report by Oscar Creech, Ralph Deterling, Sterling Edwards, Ormand Julian, Robert Linton, and Harris Shumacker was formally presented in June 1955 following a survey of the members of that society.[42] The committee recog-

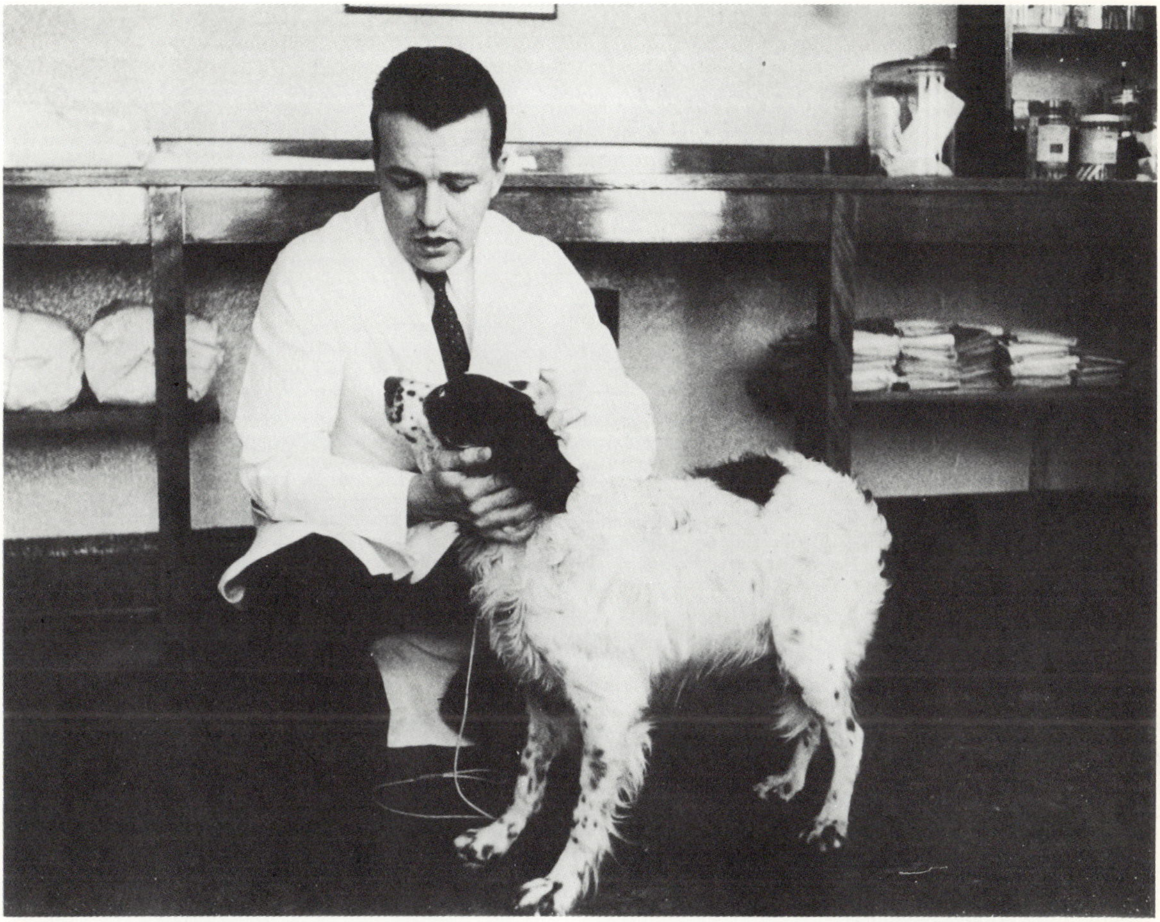

FIGURE 2-11 Arthur Voorhees' seminal discovery of the synthetic graft in 1951 triggered the explosive development of vascular surgery. Here in 1958 he addresses a dog carrying an implant of vinyon-N $7\frac{1}{2}$ years after it was placed in the abdominal aorta.

nized the preliminary nature of its report and pointed out that the large diameter of the aorta and its blood velocity allowed a variety of materials to be satisfactorily placed there, but agreed that no currently available prosthetic met suitable criteria for peripheral small vessel replacement, although the better ones were Dacron and Teflon. The Society for Vascular Surgery then wisely chose to encourage the free development of grafts and did not attempt authoritarian control.

Bovine Grafts

Another line of investigation was reopened in 1956 when Norman Rosenberg reported a new chemical modification of the bovine arterial graft (henceforth called heterograft). By ficin enzymatic digestion the process removed other tissue, leaving a pure collagen tube, which was then tanned (Figure 2-12).[43]

Heterografts functioned well in many instances, but as time passed it became apparent that the incidence of aneurysmal degeneration was approximately 4 percent, that infections of such grafts were apt to result in catastrophic hemorrhage, and that secondary operations were difficult.

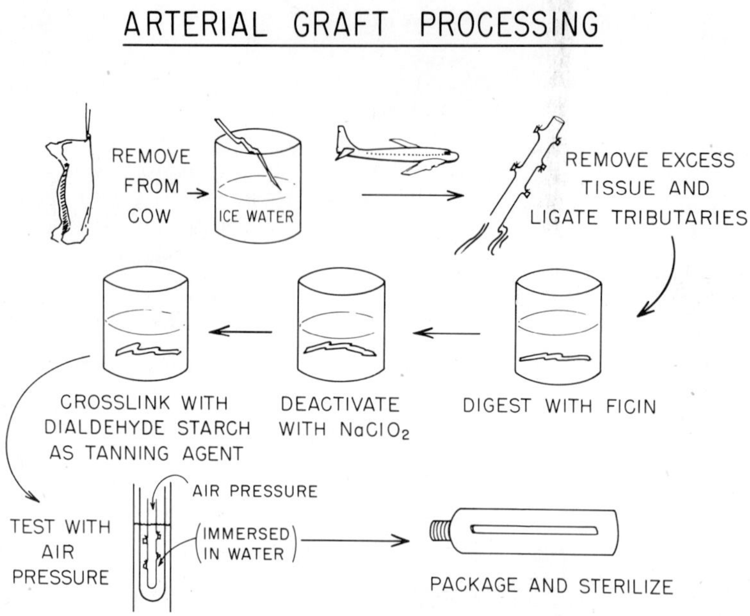

FIGURE 2-12 The bovine heterograft required a complicated processing mechanism whereby the carotid arteries removed from cows in Chicago were shipped by air to New Jersey, where they were processed with ficin obtained from the wild fig tree of the upper Amazon valley in Brazil. *(Reprinted courtesy of Surgery 1976, 80:711.)*

These objections, combined with the problems of the heterografts' cost and availability, placed them at a considerable disadvantage when compared to synthetic tubes. We reported these results in 1976 along with the results of a national questionnaire which indicated general agreement; thus, the modern effort at peripheral arterial replacement with heterografts ended.[24]

FOGARTY BALLOON CATHETER

The creative genius of Tom Fogarty emerged in his teens when he developed and patented a modification of the carburetor of a motor scooter. Somewhat later, while a junior surgical resident working in the laboratory of John J. Cranley in Cincinnati, Fogarty developed and presented to his chief the balloon catheter which thereafter has borne his name.[44] Overnight it revolutionized the management of arterial embolism. It would be difficult to estimate how many lives and limbs this relatively simple device has saved. It is also interesting to speculate upon why it was not developed earlier, in view of the commonly used Foley urinary catheter.

The evolution of modern vascular surgery is suggested by Figure 2-13. The twisting paths from the past, beginning as unmarked trails in a jungle of ignorance, leading past many false sidetracks built with imagination and courage but also with toil and tears, emerge upon the plateau of today, a broad, illuminated avenue teeming with surgical travelers.

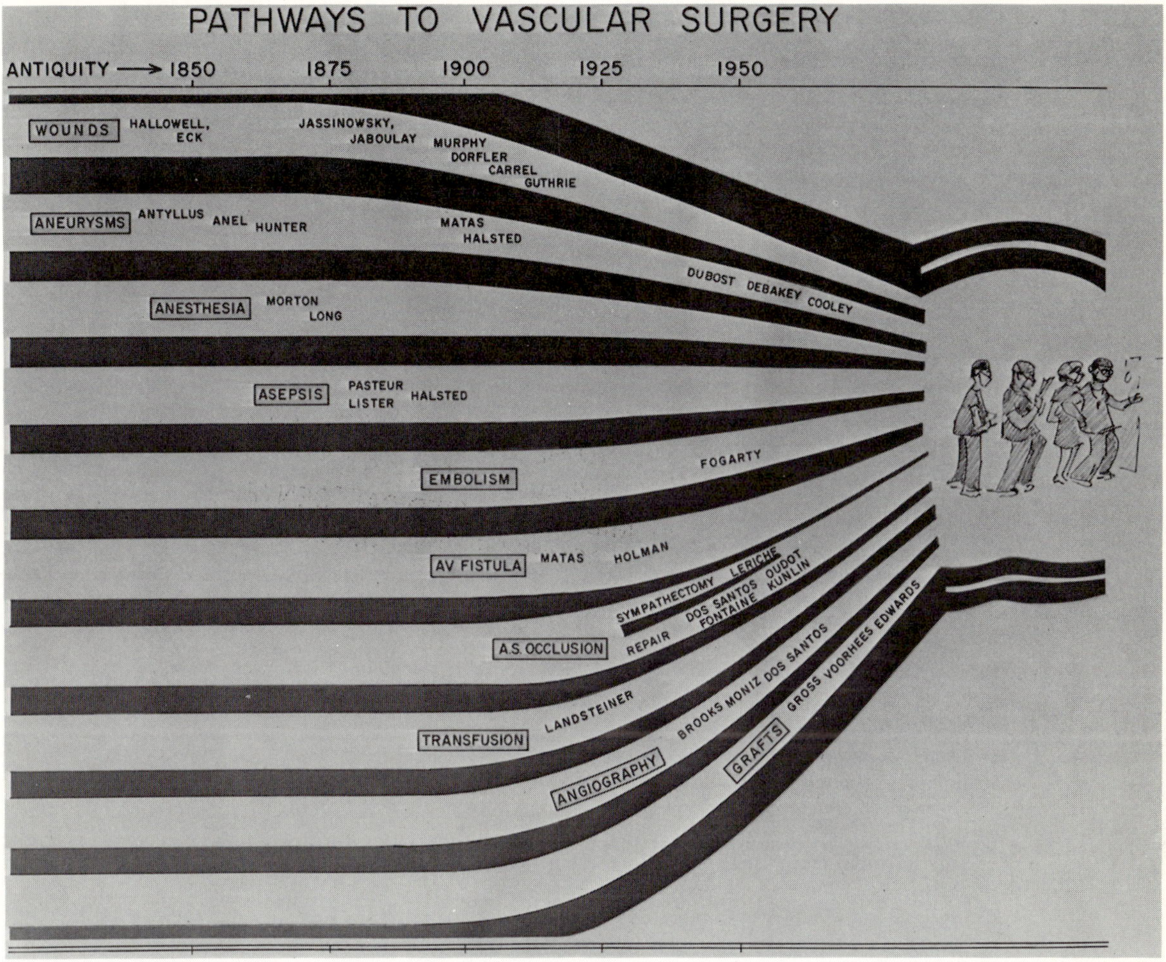

FIGURE 2-13 The many pathways which led to modern vascular surgery.[1] *(Reprinted courtesy of Surgery 1974, 76:849.)*

REFERENCES

1 Dale WA: The beginnings of vascular surgery. *Surgery* 1974, 76:849.

2 Dale WA: Arterial grafts: 1900–1978, in Dardik H (ed): *Graft Materials in Vascular Surgery.* Symposia Specialists, Miami, 1978, p. 3.

3 Eastcott HHG: *Arterial Surgery.* JB Lippincott, Philadelphia, 1969, p 235.

4 Jaboulay M, Briau E: Recherches expérimentales sur la suture et la greffe arterielle. *Lyon Med* 1896, 81:97.

5 Dorfler J: Uber arteriennaht. *Beitr Klin Chir* 1899, 25:781.

6 Murphy JB: Resection of arteries and veins injured in continuing end-to-end suture experimental and clinical research. *Med Rec* 1897, 51:73.

7 Edwards WS, Edwards PD: *Alexis Carrel: Visionary Surgeon.* Charles C Thomas, Springfield, Illinois, 1974.

8 Schück H, Sohlman R, Osterling A, Liljestrand G, Westgren A, Siegbahn M, Schou A, Stahle NK: *Nobel, the man and his prizes.* University of Oklahoma, Norman, 1951, p 256.
9 Carrel A, Guthrie CC: Results of biterminal transplantation of veins. *Am J Med Sci* 1906, 132:415.
10 Carrel A, Guthrie CC: Uniterminal and biterminal venous transplantation. *Surg Gynecol Obstet* 1906, 2:266.
11 Harris J: Presidential Address, Nashville Surgical Society, November 1982.
12 Ochsner A: Personal Letter, 1974.
13 Haschek E, Lindenthal OT: Ein Beitrag zur praktischen Verwerthung der Photographie nach Rontgen. *Wien Klin Wochenschr* 1896, 9:63.
14 Sicard JA, Forestier G: Injections intra-vasculaires d'huile iodee sous controle radiologigue. *C R Soc Biol* (Paris) 1923, 88:1200.
15 Brooks B: Injection of sodium iodide. *JAMA* 1924, 128:1016.
16 Moniz E: L'encephalographique arterielle; son importance dans la localization des tumeurs cérébrales. *Rev Neurol* (Paris) 1927, 2:172.
17 dos Santos R, Lanas A, Pereirgi CJ: L'arteriographie des membres de l'aorte et ses branches abdominales. *Bull Soc Nat Chir* 1929, 55:587.
18 Howell WH: Two new factors in blood coagulation—heparin and proantithrombin *Am J Physiol* 1918, 47:328.
19 Murray G: Heparin in surgical treatment of blood vessels *Arch Surg* 1940, 40:307.
20 Kunlin J: Treatment of arterial ischemia by long vein grafts. *Rev Chir* 1951, 70:206.
21 Oudot J: La greffe vasculaire dans les thromboses du carrefour aortique. *Presse Med* 1951, 59:234.
22 Dubost C, Allary M, Oeconomos NA: Propos de traitement des aneurysmes de l'aorte ablauon de l'aneurysme. Retablissement de la continuité. *Mem Acad Chir* (Paris) 1951, 77:381.
23 DeWeese JA, Woods WD, Dale WA: Failure of homografts as arterial replacements. *Surgery* 1959, 46:565.
24 Dale WA, Lewis MR: Further experiences with bovine arterial grafts. *Surgery* 1976, 80:711.
25 Dale WA, DeWeese JA, Scott WJM: Autogenous venous shunt grafts: Rationale and report of 31 for atherosclerosis. *Surgery* 1959, 46:145.
26 Dale WA, Mavor GE: Peripheral vascular grafts, experimental comparison of autogenous veins, homologous arteries and synthetic tubes. *Br J Surg* 1959, 46:20.
27 Gluck T: Die moderne chirurgie des circulation sapparates. *Berl Klin* 1898, 70:1.
28 Goyanes J: Neuvos trabajos de chirurgia vascular: Substiucion plastica de las arterias por las venas, o arterioplastia venosa, aplicado, como neuvo metodo, al traitamiento de los aneurismas. *El Sig Med* 1906, 53:561.
29 Lexer E: Die ideale operation des arteriellen und des arteriellvenosen aneurysma. *Arch Klin Chir* 1907, 83:45.
30 Pringle JH: Two cases of vein grafting for the maintenance of direct arterial circulation. *Lancet* 1913, 1:1795.
31 Blakemore AH, Lord JW, Stefko PL: The severed primary artery in the war wounded. *Surgery* 1942, 12:488.
32 Hufnagel CA: Permanent intubation of the thoracic aorta. *Arch Surg* 1947, 54:382.
33 Gross RE, Bill AH, Pierce EC: Methods for presentation and transplantation of arterial grafts: Observations on arterial grafts in dogs. *Surg Gynecol Obstet* 1949, 88:689.
34 Kunlin J: Le traitement de l'arterite obliterante par la greffe veineuse. *Arch Mal Coeur* 1949, 42:371.
35 Linton RR: Some practical considerations in the surgery of blood vessel grafts. *Surgery* 1955, 38:817.
36 Hughes CW: Arterial repair during the Korean War. *Ann Surg* 1958, 147:555.
37 Tuffier T: L'intubation arterielle. *Bull Acad Natl Med* (Paris) 1915, 74:455.
38 Murray G, Jones JM: Prevention of acute failure of circulation following injuries to large arteries; Experiments with glass cannulae kept patent by administration of heparin. *Br Med J* 1940, 2:6.
39 Blakemore AH, Lord JW: A non-suture method of blood vessel anastomosis: Experimental and clinical study. *JAMA* 1945, 127:585.
40 Moore HD: Replacement of blood vessels by polyethylene tubes. *Surg Gynecol Obstet* 1950, 91:593.
41 Voorhees AB, Jaretski A, Blakemore AH: The use of tubes constructed from vinyon-N cloth in bridging arterial defects. *Ann Surg* 1952, 135:332.
42 Creech O, Deterling RA, Edwards S, Julian OC, Linton RR, Shumacker H Jr: Report of the vascular society's committee on vascular prostheses. *Surgery* 1957, 41:62.

43 Rosenberg N: The bovine arterial graft and its several applications. *Surg Gynecol Obstet* 1976, 142:104.
44 Fogarty T: Personal Conversation, 1980.

Invited Commentary

Jackson Harris, M.D.
Nashville, Tennessee

The historical evolution of vascular surgery would be incomplete without reference to the ongoing disagreement concerning the relative contributions of Charles Guthrie and Alexis Carrel.

The long hiatus between their experimental work in 1904–1906 and its clinical applications beginning in the 1940s is clearly explained by Dr. Dale's exposition of the stepwise progression of the necessary ancillary discoveries, i.e., transfusions, angiography, heparin, antibiotics, and grafting materials.

The remarkable achievements of these two disparate investigators, Carrel and Guthrie, were the result of a relatively short collaboration in Chicago: from the fall of 1904 until the spring of 1906. Twenty-one papers were published, in spite of Guthrie's absence from February to December 1905 on a sabbatical to Missouri. Guthrie was senior author of 11 papers, Carrel of 10.

Guthrie was methodical and quiet, Carrel critical and enthusiastic. Their work was composed primarily of various kinds of blood vessel anastomoses and organ transplantations. Guthrie was a superb technician and, although Carrel's previous anastomoses had frequently thrombosed, following their collaboration they began to have spectacular success. Guthrie suggested using Dorfler's technique of through-and-through sutures of all layers rather than the adventitia-to-adventitia anastomosis that Carrel had previously used. They developed the triangulation technique.

Carrel was nominated for the Nobel prize by Dr. Karl Beck, with whom he had visited in Chicago and who considered Carrel somewhat of a protégé. Beck, like Carrel, was a European by birth, whereas Guthrie was a typical American farm boy. Additionally, Guthrie was absent from Chicago on sabbatical leave when the prestigious Society of Clinical Surgery visited the laboratory. Present were Matas, Cushing, Crowell, Lecant, J.B. Murphy, Crile, and others.

Dr. Guthrie's book, *Blood Vessel Surgery and Its Applications,* is a classic volume for any vascular surgeon's library. Ironically, it was published in 1912, the year that Alexis Carrel received the Nobel prize in physiology and medicine for his transfusions, successful suturing of blood vessels, and transplantation of organs in experimental animals.

Both Samuel Harbison and J. R. D. M. Saunders have published brief papers suggesting Guthrie did not receive full credit for his work with Carrel. L. G. Walker, Jr., and Serge J. Dos are equally committed to Carrel's preeminence.

Dr. Dale makes a common error in crediting Carrel with the successful transplantation of a dog's head. This was actually done by Guthrie two years after they had gone their separate ways.

3 MANAGEMENT OF PROBLEMS COMMON TO VASCULAR SURGERY

Problems which are common to a variety of vascular patients are discussed in this chapter, with further details in some of the later sections.

DIAGNOSTIC STUDIES

A reasonably firm diagnosis can be obtained by listening to the account of symptoms and examining the patient. From this clinical appraisal may be determined the type and extent of studies needed to delineate the lesions anatomically.

Noninvasive Studies

Sometimes additional information may be obtained by noninvasive laboratory techniques, but these are more useful as scouting tests, particularly upon nonhospitalized patients. The late E. J. (Jack) Wylie's perceptive comments about overuse of such tests are pertinent: "I am concerned about the spreading fallacy that non-invasive testing is an essential component of the clinical evaluation."[1] Noninvasive laboratory tests have not quite fulfilled their early promise. Many physicians have been encouraged to order them rather than to listen to and examine the patient.

Noninvasive studies are now so numerous and complex that an in-depth discussion lies outside the realm of this book: indeed their discussion already occupies chapters and books. They have value (1) as scouting studies for outpatients, (2) as simple follow-up procedures in the recovery room and office, and (3) as sources of adjunctive information to the clinical history, examination, and angiograms, which they have not yet replaced.

Angiography

Examination of arteries and veins by a variety of angiographic techniques has become a safe and accurate procedure. Its importance in management warrants brief discussion of several points.

First is the necessity for cooperation between the angiographer and clinician so that the proper method is used and the examination provides the information needed. This should be controlled by the responsible vascular surgeon. Angiograms ordered by nonsurgeons often are not properly directed, or complete, and require additional or repetitive studies. Thus, the patient with an aortic aneurysm and carotid bruits requires visualization of the vessels in the neck as well as the visceral vessels and the pelvic and leg arteries. The information may be obtained by two different studies or, better, by a single planned procedure.

Second, angiography should be conducted at the proper time in relation to other procedures.

It may be necessary to delay it temporarily because of a renal problem or to allow improvement in the pulmonary situation. On the other hand an operation for acute femoral arterial embolism should not be delayed to study an asymptomatic carotid bruit.

Third, cooperation between the radiologist and surgeon is necessary to promote efficient intraoperative angiography as well as percutaneous transluminal angioplasty when indicated.

Finally there is the availability of angiographic services for emergency patients as well as for in-hospital complications. An efficient and readily available angiographic service on a 24-hour daily basis is an absolute necessity for a first-rate vascular surgical unit. Economics as well as medical needs suggest operation soon after angiography, even though an occasional instance of renal toxicity may occur. Proper hydration prior to angiography reduces the risk, as does limitation of the injected contrast material. Delay in operation until the renal status is clear is recommended for (1) known renal insufficiency, (2) serious cardiac disease, and (3) advanced age.[2]

DRUGS

Vasodilator drugs have been tested widely in obstructive arterial disease and have demonstrated no benefit—to the extent that they face withdrawal from the United States market in the absence of proof of efficacy. The already wide dilatation of the available vascular bed in ischemic tissue due to the products of anaerobic glycolysis makes it unlikely that further dilatation can be produced.

There are two indications for vasodilator drugs. First are young females with nonorganic vasospastic leg syndromes. Second are cases where the drugs may demonstrate to the patient the interest and concern of the surgeon preoperatively—the "art" may be useful when science is lacking or is not accepted.

The *prostaglandins* have both vasodilating effects and inhibiting effects on platelet aggregation. Recent blind controlled studies, however, have failed to corroborate the early hopes of their usefulness in peripheral arterial disease.[3]

Pentoxifylline, which reverses the impaired flexibility of the red cell associated with obstructive arterial disease, has recently been reported to improve the walking distance of claudicators, associated with improvement of the muscle Po_2.

Despite the widely recognized inconsistencies in treadmill walking tests noted by Zarin[4] and by Szilagyi,[5] the accumulating favorable reports from Europe[6,7] have been affirmed by the multicenter, double-blind, placebo-controlled study of 128 patients by Porter's group, indicating the usefulness of pentoxifylline.[8] This drug does therefore appear to be useful and is the first thus classified by the U.S. Federal Drug Administration.

STABILIZATION OF EXISTENT DISEASE

It is perhaps trite to recognize the necessity to correct lesions of the important functional systems, to stabilize early renal failure, to correct anemia and blood volume deficits, and to provide for the insulin needs of the diabetic. Essential to this is cooperation with consultants in these fields. Low morbidity and mortality following vascular reconstructions are aided considerably by insistence upon preoperative consultation with a surgically oriented internist, who may advise delay of a surgical procedure or even prohibition of it while at the same time providing guidance in the management of problems in the preoperative and postoperative periods. Subspecialists in cardiology, pulmonary medicine, infectious diseases, or diabetes occasionally provide aid in a critical situation, but their narrow views limit their overall usefulness and often result in multiple consultants. My experience leads to the conclusion that management by such a "committee" is less worthwhile to ultimate success than is a surgically oriented general internist—if one can be found.

TRANSFUSIONS

Recently there has developed in some quarters the opinion that correction of blood volume and anemia preoperatively is not always necessary, particularly in view of the risk of posttransfusion hepatitis. It came as a considerable surprise to me to learn from the 1980 review of Aach and Kahn that posttransfusion hepatitis occurs in 7 percent of recipients (rather than the 0.1 percent usually quoted).[9] This incidence of posttransfusion anicteric hepatitis is based upon two different elevations of serum alanine aminotransferase.

One way to avoid the risk of hepatitis for the elective patient is to use the patient's own previously stored blood, which can be kept for as long as 2 years. The administrative mechanism and the cost of storage at present prevent general adoption of this method, but it is useful for selected patients.

The issue of operating upon a patient known to be anemic was addressed by Hiram Polk, who stated that "large defects in red cell mass occurring over a long period are well tolerated" and that "if one could ascertain that no unforeseen blood losses nor inadvertent hypoxia would occur, a patient could expect to safely undergo an elective operation with a distinctly low hemoglobin concentration."[10] The risk of an unexpected event is greater than the hazard of transfusion for most vascular patients. Thus the patient who without an operation might be allowed to rebuild the red cell mass spontaneously would require correction of the anemia prior to an operation upon the cardiovascular system. Certainly the patient is in a better position to withstand the stress of acute blood loss if preoperative transfusions have provided a normal red cell mass and blood volume. Further, the risk of transfusion is less when the patient is alert and oriented than when blood is administered during the course of general anesthesia.

Autotransfusion is another useful alternative. Analysis of its cost indicates a balance at two units of reinfused red cells. It therefore is not ordinarily worthwhile for femoral nor carotid procedures, but it is for aortic reconstructions. Our earlier bad experiences with autotransfusion, reported in 1974,[11] have not recurred with the use of the modern cell-saver device.

Diabetes

Arteriosclerotic problems occur earlier and in a more severe form but are not qualitatively different in diabetics. These patients require metabolic control, but their lesions have the same indications for surgical repair as do those of nondiabetics.

Diabetic patients are often fat, and this makes wound management more difficult, but as Polk noted, "the well controlled diabetic is probably not more prone to infection than other individuals of similar age and illness."[12] My analysis of 139 limbs facing early loss because of intractable pain and/or tissue necrosis showed an insignificant difference in the salvage rate for diabetics as compared with the others.[13]

The importance of detailed care of the extremities of such patients is documented by the heating pad burn shown in Figure 3-1. Loss of sensation made the patient unaware of the lesion, and it was discovered only after the fact.

WHICH OPERATIVE LESION SHOULD BE CORRECTED FIRST?

Arteriosclerosis is a widespread degenerative process, although its stenoses and occlusions are segmental. When one artery is diseased, it is likely that similar lesions are present elsewhere, so preoperative evaluation of all vessels is necessary. Aneurysms are frequently multiple, so the presence of one indicates a search for others. Lesions in the neck vessels supplying the brain are similarly common and require evaluation, as do those of the coronary arterial system.

In Table 3-1 are listed six commonly observed situations where one operation must be done prior to another. Sometimes it is possible to perform two reconstructions (such as carotid and coronary revascularizations) at the same session.

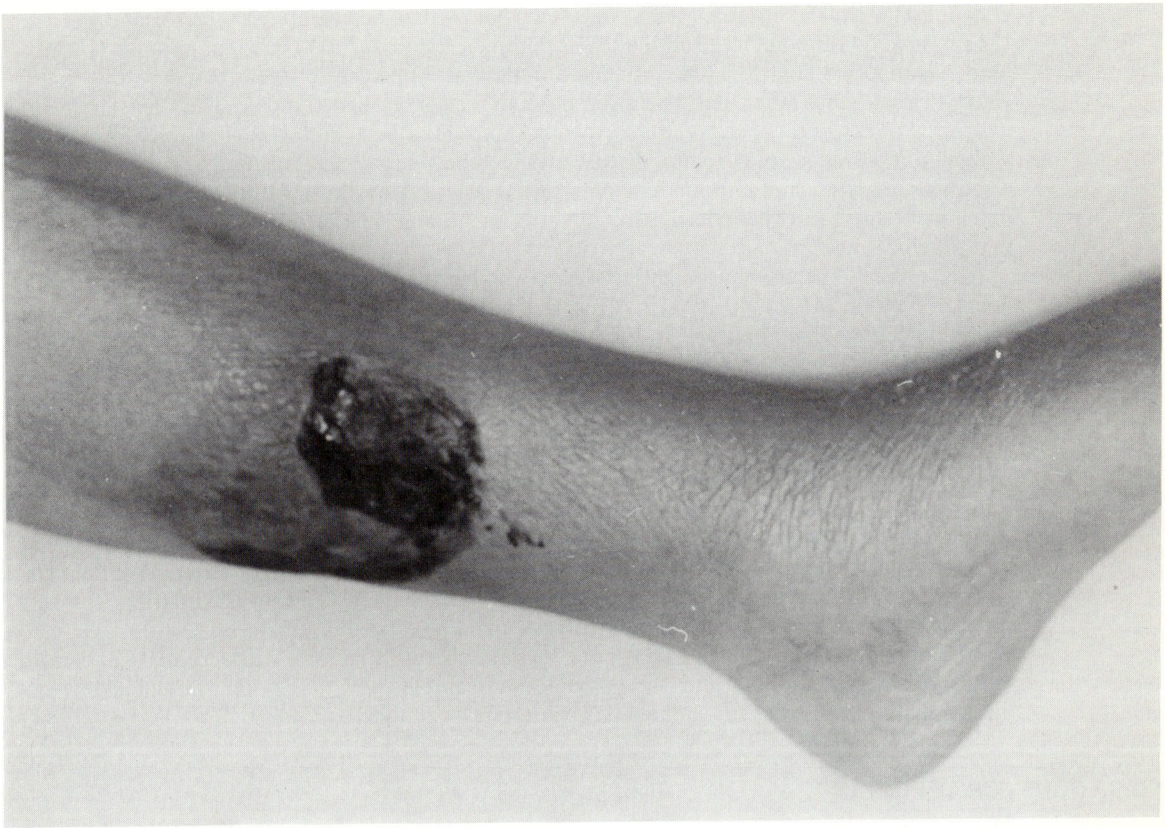

FIGURE 3-1 Third-degree burn of the ankle of a diabetic whose lack of sensation failed to warn him of the effect of the ill-advised use of a heating pad.

Recently Lawrie and Morris discussed the increased risk of coronary artery bypass surgery when there is associated carotid disease along with the lower mortality when both arteries are simultaneously repaired.[14] Others have confirmed this, including Emery and associates, who in 1983 on the basis of a 42-patient series without deaths recommended simultaneous coronary bypass and carotid thromboendarterectomy for both symptomatic and asymptomatic lesions.[15] This sophisticated approach requires proper monitoring as well as a double team of experienced surgeons and is certainly not for the beginner in a small facility, where an unduly prolonged procedure or excessive blood loss may result in excessive risk.

It has been proposed that the coronary arteries should always be evaluated prior to another vascular procedure. Earlier hopes that stress testing would be critical have not been realized.[16] The next step of coronary arteriography for every patient facing aortic surgical reconstruction has been investigated at the Cleveland Clinic. Norman Hertzer in 1983 reviewed the results of the first 400 patients who had routine coronary angiograms prior to aortic surgery and concluded that "most patients with severe CAD [coronary artery disease] could be identified . . . by

TABLE 3-1 RELATIVE ORDER OF PRIORITY OF ARTERIAL LESIONS FOR OPERATION

1	Urgent carotid
2	Threatening coronary
3	"Salvage" aorta-femoral-popliteal
4	Elective coronary
5	Stable aorta-femoral-popliteal
6	Asymptomatic carotid

conventional clinical criteria." This suggested that cardiac angiography be performed only for clear indications and not as a routine.[17] The completed study of 1000 vascular patients in Cleveland was reported later in 1984, with the finding that 30 percent of them had severe coronary artery disease which warranted operation prior to the contemplated repair. The Cleveland Clinic's stated policy of preoperative study then became (1) catheterization angiography for patients with clinical evidence of coronary disease and (2) noninvasive tests such as screening by stress electrocardiography and radionuclide myocardial scanning for those without cardiac symptoms or signs.[18] Another experienced vascular surgeon, Stanley Crawford, has agreed with such individualization.[19]

There has also been extensive discussion of whether the patient with a completely asymptomatic carotid stenosis should have that repaired prior to an aortic repair because of the risk of stroke during the operation and in the immediate postoperative period. Several studies of this problem have now essentially laid that fear to rest. Treiman and associates showed that there was no correlation of the four strokes which occurred in patients who had either a bruit or cerebral vascular symptoms among 516 patients having aortic surgery.[20] Carney and others with Roberts studied 248 aortic operations and also concluded that an asymptomatic bruit was not associated with increased risk of postoperative stroke, since the four who had strokes did not have bruits to suggest study or repair of the carotid artery.[21]

With these considerations in mind, the priorities shown in Table 3-1 have evolved. The threatening coronary category includes patients with crescendo angina and those with tight stenosis of the left main coronary artery, as opposed to patients whose cardiac situation is judged stable enough to allow some other necessary repair to be carried out first.

Patients undergoing repeated transient cerebral ischemic attacks or with a quite tight carotid stenosis or in whom one carotid is already blocked completely with the other threatened by stenosis may be classified as threatening and require priority for that reason.

INDICATIONS FOR OPERATION

The indications for an operation or for some other form of treatment are derived from the overall clinical situation and are not primarily based upon angiography. Arteriograms serve as a map to aid the proper placement of incisions and the optimal methods of reconstruction and are not primary indicators for operation.

The Everest Syndrome

There is in some quarters an inclination to "operate upon x-rays" showing stenoses and occlusions which are clinically asymptomatic or insignificant. This is an example of the "Everest Syndrome" (derived from the answer of George Mallory to why he wished to climb Mount Everest—"because it is there"). The late Alfred Blalock expressed an opinion of this rationale to his surgical resident when he remarked, "You don't have to operate on every patient before he dies!"

It may be argued that the presence of renal arterial stenosis in a patient requiring aortic replacement is an indication for a concomitant bypass to the renal artery even though there is no hypertension or renal failure. Such procedures are possible technically, demonstrate the skill of the surgeon, and often may be conducted without great risk. On the other hand they lead to unneeded or unnecessarily complicated operations and to a misunderstanding of the role of surgical treatment. Low surgical morbidity and mortality are not indications for an operation.

Vascular reconstructions are palliative procedures for a disease process which is inexorably progressive and often unpredictable. The optimal plan for surgical reconstruction lies somewhere between doing too little and doing too much. Most patients with combined aortic and femoropopliteal disease do perfectly well with an aortobifemoral bypass without concomitant femoropopliteal grafts. Occasionally there are those who require both; 10 to 15 percent need a secondary femoropopliteal bypass after a successful aortobifemoral operation. Rarely is it needed at the same time.

INFORMED CONSENT

Specific permission by a patient who understands the planned procedure, and to at least some extent its hazards, for the performance of an operative procedure has become increasingly important to the surgeon as well as to the hospital and its trustees. The manner in which this informed consent is obtained will vary from one surgeon to another.

Most patients and their families appreciate a factual description of the problem along with its contemplated correction and possible variations. Diagrammatic explanations are well received, and factual descriptions of approximate statistics of the expected results and complications reflect an open explanation and invite appropriate questions. This important responsibility should not be delegated to an assistant or to paramedical personnel, since that dilutes the relationship and casts some doubt upon the concept of truly informed consent between the surgeon and the individual patient. At the time of the conversation it is appropriate to make a note in the patient's record and obtain the patient's signature on the form (for whatever that form is worth).

An interesting and perhaps better variation is the procedure of one leading institution, in which the surgeon's note summarizing the preoperative conversation has replaced the usual consent form, which in any controversy is usually repudiated by the patient as erroneous or misunderstood.

It is sometimes believed that the signature of the spouse or near relative makes that of the patient unnecessary. If there is physical inability to understand and sign, this may be the best that is available, but a secondary consent is better avoided (or added to that of the patient). A minor child's consent signature is proper for a teenager, along with that of a parent.

Finally it should be noted that a person may not be judged incompetent by physicians or by relatives, such decision being reserved for the courts of law.

ANESTHESIA

A first-rate anesthesia team is today a sine qua non for good results in complicated vascular surgery problems, not only to provide the anesthetic, but also to monitor patients, to support the function of their major organ systems, and to correct physiologic derangements as they occur.*

For operations on vessels in the extremities, some form of conduction anesthetic—epidural, spinal (subdural), or peripheral nerve block—is preferable to a general anesthetic, since safe doses of regional anesthetics cause virtually no depression of cardiac, pulmonary, renal, hepatic, or endocrine function. The risk of acute hypotension is low when an expert places the agent and supports the patient's circulation with adequate hydration, proper positioning, and the timely use of vasopressors such as phenylephrine. Spinal anesthesia below T6 has minimal effects on ventilation and on gas exchange, except in very obese patients or in patients with bronchitis.[22]

Regional anesthesia is especially advantageous for vascular surgery on the extremities for several types of patients who remain conscious but sedated during the procedure; patients with angina may notice chest pain and may be treated appropriately with intravenous phenylephrine and trinitroglycerine during surgery; patients with carotid or vertebral lesions may show signs of cerebral ischemia during regional anesthesia, and appropriate treatment to increase cerebral blood flow and mean arterial pressure may quickly reverse cerebral ischemia; diabetics who

*Appreciation is expressed to Thomas Caldwell, M.D., who supervised this section on anesthesia.

become hypoglycemic will show decreased consciousness and may be treated with intravenous glucose during surgery. Many patients, particularly the elderly, appear less depressed or disoriented following surgery under regional anesthesia.

Regional blocks are only relatively contraindicated in heparinized patients. Wust in Germany has performed over 3000 vascular procedures under epidural anesthesia in patients on prophylactic heparin without causing an epidural hematoma.[23] Here we have frequently performed vascular procedures under spinal anesthesia in patients with prothrombin times 35/15 or partial thromboplastin times 55/35 without difficulty. It is a matter of judgment whether the risk of hematoma is outweighed by the risks from a general anesthetic in an individual patient.

The safety of epidural or subdural anesthesia during major vascular procedures during which general heparinization is used is attested by the 100 cases reported by Cunningham, Egan, and Inahara[24] and the 756 patients of Cioroiu, Baron, and LaRaja.[25] Our own experiences over the past 25 years confirm these reports, and such anesthetics are used for most limb procedures.

General endotracheal anesthesia is preferable to regional anesthesia in patients who are uncooperative or extremely anxious and who might require heavy sedation during regional anesthesia, since that can lead to hypoxemia. For example, the use of local anesthesia to allow placement of an inferior vena caval filter may be dangerous because of both hypoxemia and the inability to control a panicky patient. General anesthesia allows better oxygenation, prevents uncooperative motions, and minimizes the risk of air embolism. The anesthesiologist can also reduce pulmonary vascular resistance and support right ventricular function by administering sodium bicarbonate, isoproterenol, trinitroglycerine, and if necessary, epinephrine. General anesthesia also seems preferable to regional anesthesia for carotid endarterectomy, since the management of the airway in a patient having a transient ischemic attack during operation may be quite difficult.[26]

In the past decade significant advances have occurred in the management of patients requiring general anesthesia for major vascular procedures such as renal and aortic reconstructions. These major operations can be done with relative safety even in patients with angina decubitus or compensated congestive heart failure. With the Swan-Ganz catheter monitoring pulmonary artery wedge pressures and cardiac output, such patients can be given large fluid and solute loads to minimize cardiac output and renal function without risking pulmonary edema, providing wedge pressures are low. Dopamine, 2 micrograms per kilogram per minute, helps maximize renal blood flow and urine output.[27]

Patients with either poor left ventricular function or angina can be protected from the myocardial ischemia that accompanies the increase in afterload during aortic cross-clamping; an infusion of sodium nitroprusside at 15 to 40 micrograms per minute can eliminate myocardial ischemia.[28]

Other advances have made perioperative myocardial infarction less likely in the patient with ischemic heart disease. Monitoring the V_5 lead of the electrocardiograph intraoperatively can detect left ventricular ischemia that does not appear in the limb leads. Sudden increases in pulmonary artery diastolic pressure may indicate global myocardial ischemia in patients with coronary artery disease. Myocardial ischemia during general anesthesia can be treated with intravenous trinitroglycerine, as shown by Kaplan, Dunbar, and Jones.[29]

Slow heart rates which increase coronary artery blood flow by lengthening diastole can be achieved with the use of large doses of fentanyl, 25 to 75 micrograms per kilogram. Aortic diastolic pressures can be maintained at satisfactory levels by the infusion of phenylephrine.

Improvements in intraoperative ventilatory management of patients should not be overlooked, since many patients with arterial disease have obstructive pulmonary disease due to smoking. Preoperative steroids may lessen the incidence of bronchospasm, cimetidine and diphenhydramine can be used to block histamine receptors, isoetharine preferentially stimulates bronchial beta-2 receptors and reduces bronchospasm, and intravenous aminophylline is useful to treat bronchospasm during general anesthesia.

Some vascular procedures should be performed with local or regional anesthesia in the intensive care unit, for example, femoral embolectomy in a patient with a recent myocardial infarction. The inconvenience of the surgical procedure may be outweighed by the advantage of not having to move a critically ill patient who requires infusions of catechols, vasodilators, or antiarrhythmics. Another advantage is the availability of the team of cardiologists and intensive care nursing staff to manage acute arrhythmias or cardiac arrest.

PREVENTION OF INFECTION

Infection is the bête noire of the vascular surgeon, since it immediately threatens the vascular repair either by hemorrhage or by thrombosis and often threatens life itself. Proper preparation of the patient—of the skin area through which the procedure is conducted—and the assurance of sterile equipment form the basic elements of prophylaxis. To these must be added a refined technique of dissection and wound closure, during which infinite attention must be paid to hemostasis for the prevention of seromas and hematomas, which are exceptionally good culture media for the inevitable bacterial contamination.

Local Skin Care

Bacteria thrive in moisture. Ischemic toe and foot skin should be kept dry. The old practice of soaking toes in various solutions may lead to skin maceration, open lesions, and spreading infection. If there is undrained pus, it should be released with a knife and not by soaking.

Toe separation by placement of cotton gauze sponges between the digits allows air to circulate and sweat to evaporate.

Adhesive should be avoided for fear of tearing the skin. Similarly, heating pads are dangerous because they may burn tissues whose sensory nerves are deficient. Figure 3-1 demonstrates a burn due to this.

Continued pressure to ischemic areas with decreased sensation may cause skin necrosis, often the trigger event leading to later amputation. Ever-present vigilance is necessary to prevent pressure.

Skin Preparation

Washing with a povidone-iodine preparation twice daily should begin 72 to 48 hours preoperatively. The same is used in the operating room. The effectiveness of this, contrasted with a hexachlorophene-alcohol preparation, was demonstrated in our study where the infection rate of 2.8 percent among 394 patients prepared with povidone-iodine contrasted sharply with the 10.3 percent infection rate among 68 patients receiving hexachlorophene-ethanol skin preparation.[30,31]

The removal of hair from the operative site has long been performed with a razor—a straight one in the past, a disposable safety type today. From time to time this procedure has been questioned. It probably persists only because of tradition. Hairs are smooth shafts without pits and can be more readily sterilized than can skin. Relatively hairless areas such as the upper abdomen of the female actually require no depilation.

Investigators such as Alexander and associates present evidence that close clipping is less harmful than is shaving. Among 1013 patients undergoing elective operations they found that the infection rate was 1.8 percent following hair clipping immediately prior to operation (and 4 percent when clipping was done the previous evening) versus 6.4 percent following use of a razor in the morning (and 5.2 percent when the razor was used the previous evening).[32] These results are more favorable toward clipping than are those of Cruse and Foord, who reported 2.3 percent infection after shaving versus 1.7 percent after clipping among 18,090 clean cases. The 0.9 percent infection rate among patients who had no hair removed is even better.[33]

The reader may wish to pursue this further via the referenced articles and their discussions.

It appears that shaving should be superseded by either clipping or a chemical depilatory.[34] However, it does take time to change established ways.

During the immediate preoperative preparation the skin may be scrubbed, but it cannot be rendered absolutely sterile.[35] Neither gloved hands, instruments, nor grafts should be allowed to touch the skin. The fact that violations of this are not often followed by infections attests to the effective defenses of the tissues rather than to invalidity of the principle. Isolating sterile adherent plastic is a worthwhile protection.

Antibiotics

Some disillusionment with antibiotic prophylaxis occurred in the past because of its incorrect usage, whereby blood levels of the appropriate agent were not provided until after termination of the procedure. Recognition of the importance of achieving proper serum and tissue levels prior to any operative manipulation and maintaining them throughout the procedure allows early termination of antibiotic administration in the immediate postoperative period so that potential side effects can be avoided.

Documentation of our study of antibiotic prophylaxis is detailed in Chapter 24. In brief, the patient receives 1 g of cefazolin intravenously 15 to 20 minutes prior to the incision. This is followed by similar doses at 6-hour intervals for four doses.[30]

Whether to irrigate the peritoneal cavity and/or wounds with any of several antibiotic or antiseptic agents is a complex problem whose answer remains controversial. I irrigate a contaminated wound with 1 g of cefoxitin in 1000 mL of saline. There is no reason for this in clean vascular procedures. Povidone-iodine solution is contraindicated as dangerous and without virtue. The interested reader may pursue this controversy further in the writing of Rodeheaver[36] and of Zamora and Feldtman.[37]

ATRAUMATIC TECHNIQUE

Considerable lip service is paid to the concept of delicate tissue technique. Yet poorly vascularized fat is repeatedly picked up with toothed forceps rather than with a towel clip, which can be placed once and used for traction.

Controlled studies have demonstrated that wounds made with a knife heal and resist infection better than do those made with an electric cautery. Thus Wangensteen's team at Minnesota reported that a standard bacterial inoculation produced 100 percent infection in electroknife wounds versus 30 percent in those made with a scalpel.[38] Tissue damage by such methods invites infection and to at least some extent explains the (usually unspoken) fact that some surgeons have higher infection rates than others.

Of even more importance are serum, lymph, and blood, which act as foreign bodies within closed wounds. Minute final hemostasis, with suction drainage as needed, should be backed up by closure of the wound as walls being placed in apposition rather than by overloading it with excessive suture material, much of which serves no function.

Sutures

A monofilament synthetic suture such as polypropylene may be a bit more difficult to use because of kinking and its tendency to untie but is safer than are multifilament synthetics, silk, or cotton in terms of infection. Sharp's group has documented the virtue of polypropylene in terms of infection. They studied 16 different sutures in mice exposed to staphylococcus and *Escherichia coli.* The monofilament synthetic proved superior to multifilament and absorbable sutures.[39]

One can easily solve the slippage problem by throwing three ties initially, then passing one end back through the tissue and tying back onto the remaining end with three more throws. This completely eliminates untying of the knot. This is seen in the inferior angle of the wound in

Figure 3-2 and is useful wherever a polypropylene suture is placed, whether it be in a vascular anastomosis or to close an abdominal wound. Despite occasional lugubrious statements regarding the deficits of the monofilament suture, it has largely replaced all others for vascular reconstruction.

Polypropylene is equally useful for the abdominal wall closure, where it may be placed as a continuous suture with the end tied back on at each extremity of the incision and in the center, where the two sutures join at the conclusion (Figure 3-2). For the past four years I have used 0 polypropylene as a continuous suture, placing each bite 15 to 20 mm away from the cut edge to ensure a large bite of tissue, thus closing the entire peritoneal and fascial layer as one, then allowing the fat to fall together about a suction drain in the subcutaneous tissue, and following this by mattress sutures in the skin (Figure 3-3).

This efficient and functional abdominal wall closure is different from the small-bite, interrupted suture technique used in the past but has served well in terms of good closure without dehiscence or hernia. Only four problems have occurred during a four-year experience with this continuous closure. One patient on the fourth postoperative night required secondary closure after the polypropylene sutures joined in the center of the wound untied, not having been passed back through the tissue and retied. A second problem occurred when the beginning of the suture line inferiorly did not include the posterior peritoneum and thus allowed a fluid leak. On the fifth day this was explored and reclosed. Two ventral hernias have occurred. Thus the continuous one-layer monofilament closure has proven to be quick and sure. The recent reports of Knight and Griffen[40] and of Richards' group[41] confirm these findings.

A suture should never be handled or crushed by a metal instrument. Failures of polypropylene because of such damage reflect upon the operator, not the suture (Figure 3-4).

The French Suture for Vascular Anastomosis The vein or synthetic graft mounted on the Huang vein holder is held by the assistant 2 or 3 cm away from the arteriotomy in the host vessel. The 6-0 polypropylene suture is then passed from outside into the graft lumen and then from

FIGURE 3-2 One-layer continuous closure of the abdominal wall using continuous 0 polypropylene suture. At each end three throws are placed; the suture is carried back through the tissue and the short end is tied back on with another three throws to prevent slipping.

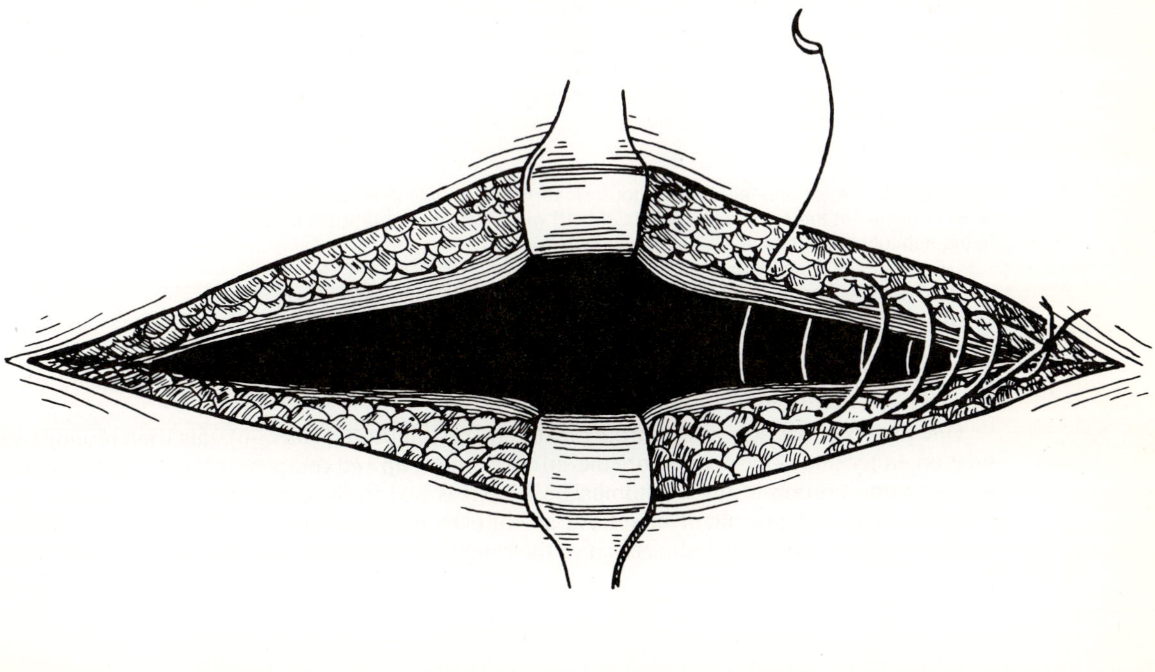

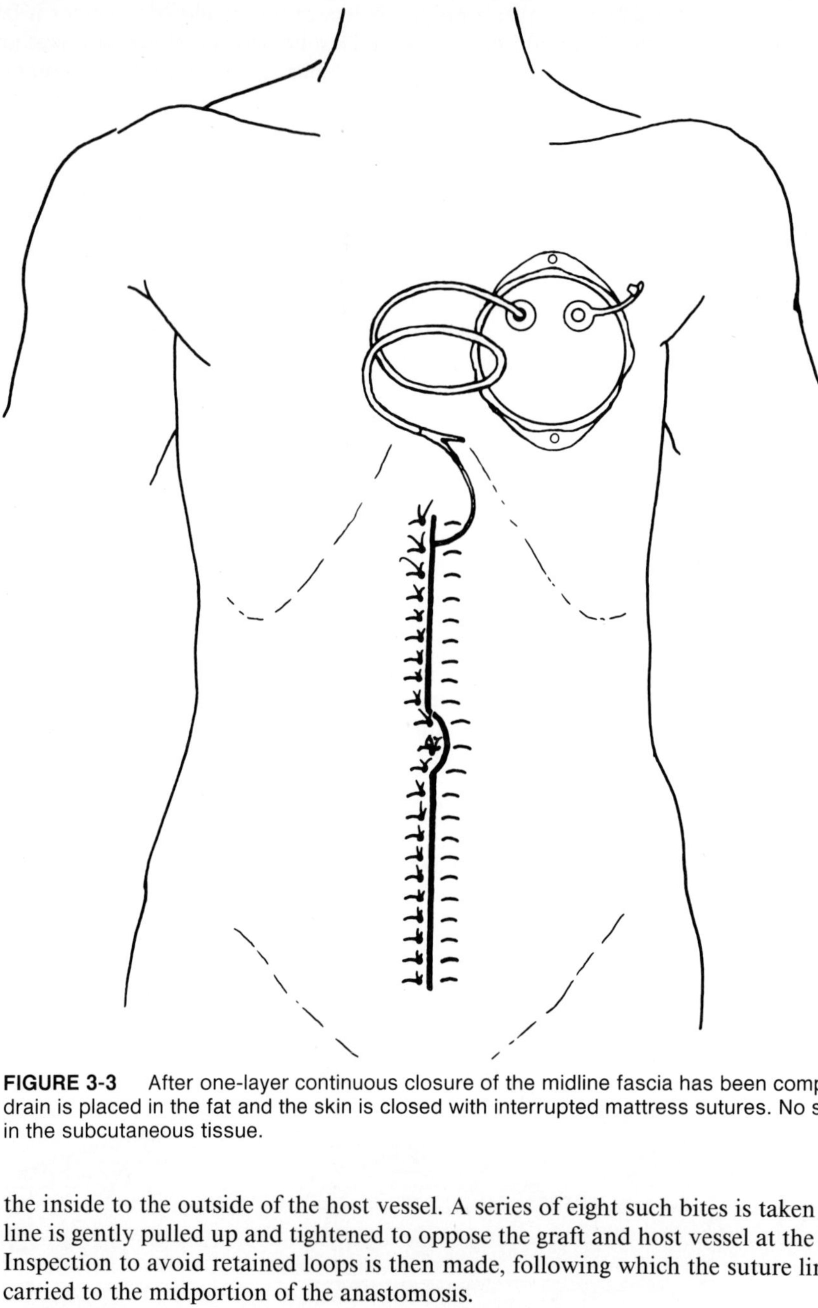

FIGURE 3-3 After one-layer continuous closure of the midline fascia has been completed, a suction drain is placed in the fat and the skin is closed with interrupted mattress sutures. No sutures are placed in the subcutaneous tissue.

the inside to the outside of the host vessel. A series of eight such bites is taken before the suture line is gently pulled up and tightened to oppose the graft and host vessel at the heel (Figure 3-5). Inspection to avoid retained loops is then made, following which the suture line on each side is carried to the midportion of the anastomosis.

One then begins a new suture at the toe of the anastomosis (Figure 3-6), this time placing two bites on either side of the apex before the suture is pulled up and completing the suture line down to the central portion of the anastomosis, where it is tied to the other end. The technique not only allows careful placement of sutures at both the heel and toe but also does away with a weakening knot at the end and places it in the central portion of the anastomosis, where there is

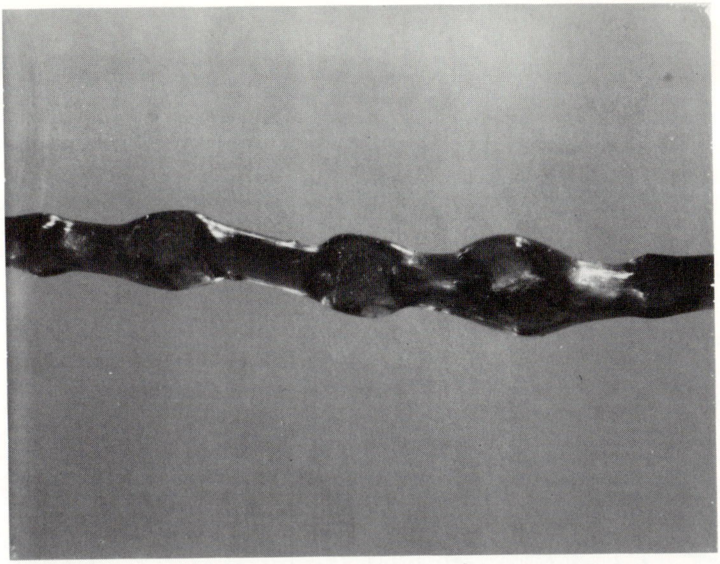

FIGURE 3-4 Damaged and deformed polypropylene suture resulting from clamping with a steel instrument.

more room for error. It allows clear visualization and accurate bites and generally ends the problems of leaks.

This technique has become routine for all difficult or deep anastomoses, with entire satisfaction. When this technique was recently described,[42] a letter to the authors in England procured the information that it was learned from Professor Corbier in Marseille, France. I have not yet

FIGURE 3-5 Beginning the "French connection" anastomotic suture using continuous 6-0 polypropylene to perform an end-to-side anastomosis to a small distal artery. Four sutures are placed down the side toward the heel of the anastomosis, as shown, and then another four are placed on the near side before any are pulled up.

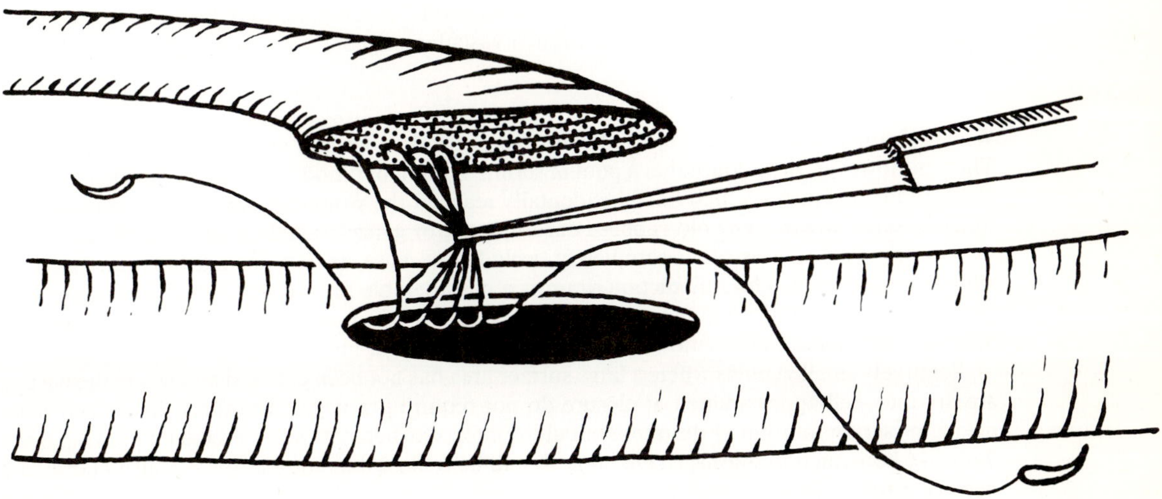

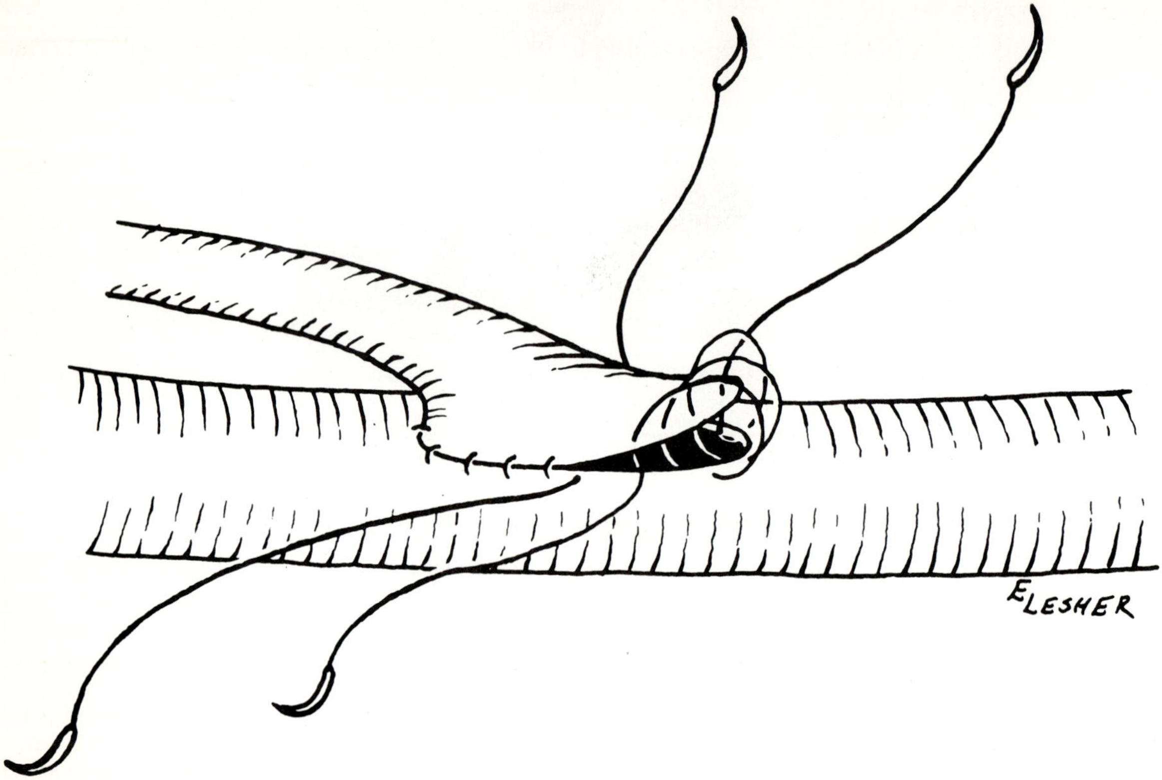

FIGURE 3-6 Finishing the "French connection" vascular anastomosis. The heel sutures have been pulled up firmly. The toe sutures are placed loosely before the final tightening. This technique allows clear visualization of the most difficult portion of the suture line at the toe and heel.

learned whether the latter originated this or adopted it from someone else, but I have taken the liberty of naming the technique the "French connection," bearing in mind the many outstanding achievements of a long line of eminent French vascular surgeons.[43]

DRAINS

Wound drainage has been a subject of controversy for decades and very likely will continue so. There is, however, little doubt that a pool of serum, lymph, or blood serves as an excellent culture medium for organisms which have incidentally reached the wound or which may be passersby from the bloodstream. The old rubber Penrose drain, or gauze-stuffed cigarette drain, served as an overflow vent; it was often completely occluded because its exit opening was too small to allow egress of fluid. The soft suction drain is a considerable improvement; the amount of serosanguineous material removed in a 24-hour period is often astonishing. Fear that a suction drain properly placed and removed early will cause a wound infection is unreal.

Relatively small wounds where a large surface area has not been exposed and where the tissues are dry and well-approximated at closure do not require drainage. Secondary dissections with oozing of serum and blood despite meticulous efforts at hemostasis heal better following brief 24- to 48-hour suction drainage. The tube should be removed as soon as the 8-hour volume has become 5 mL or less.

Intraabdominal drains have no usefulness following clean vascular surgery.

ANTICOAGULANTS

Details of the pharmacokinetics of the complex of polysaccharides which constitute heparin are beyond the scope of discussion here. A few brief summarizing statements do allow some degree of rational management in clinical practice.

The coagulation cascade comprises a series of linked proteolytic reactions which ultimately lead to the generation of thrombin and the formation of a fibrin clot. Heparin rapidly catalyzes the antithrombin fixation of thrombin, thus effectively stopping the clotting mechanism.[44]

In America the sodium salt of heparin is measured in U.S.P. units, with considerable variation in potency from one batch to another. Laboratory tests generally reflect the anticoagulant effects of heparin rather than its actual blood level.

While the plasma activated partial thromboplastic time (APTT) is the most precise and predictive test available, the whole blood partial thromboplastic time (WBPTT) is considerably more economical with little sacrifice of precision.

Heparin also increases the electronegative potential of the vascular wall. It is rapidly retrieved from the blood by the endothelial cells along with those of the reticuloendothelial system and macrophages, in which it is stored and thereafter slowly released. The half-life of heparin is about 90 minutes.

Intraoperative heparinization during temporary interruption of the circulation has become widespread in vascular surgery, with a few outstanding exceptions. Robert Linton of Boston predicted this to me in 1962, and despite early fears that heparinization would lead to increased bleeding, such did not occur and patency rates immediately began to improve. Subsequently, the standard (if empirical) administration of 5000 U.S.P. units of aqueous heparin prior to clamping any vessel has been followed. Recently the anticoagulant has been injected intraarterially just proximal to the intended site of clamping because of the evidence that intraarterial heparin is at once stored in the endothelium, where it produces an electronegative effect and repels thrombosis.[45]

Following removal of the vascular clamps, a period of time often serves to allow graft and anastomotic bleeding to subside, but reversal by protamine sulfate is often necessary. Protamine has the disadvantage of sometimes producing pulmonary hypertension and congestion with systemic hypotension; its introduction should therefore be slow, in increments, and observed for this possibility. Three intravenous injections of 25 mg each at 5-minute intervals represent a well-tried regimen for reversing the heparin effect.

POSTOPERATIVE MONITORING

A knowledgeable around-the-clock team in the intensive care unit is basic to good results after reconstructive vascular surgery. With few exceptions every vascular surgery patient requires an initial postoperative period there.

The early detection of complications in the form of bleeding or thrombosis, cardiac rhythm problems, and pulmonary changes often allows their correction prior to irreversible damage.

Frequent assessment of patency of the vascular reconstruction by hourly examination for neurologic changes after carotid procedures and for proper perfusion of the foot and toes after aortoiliac and femoropopliteal operations must be routine. Examination of the peripheral pulses by the fingers and by the Doppler instrument are the usual methods. The advice of Reginald Smithwick 25 years ago should be recalled: "It is unfortunate but true that medical students, interns and even residents of considerable experience are quite inaccurate about their evaluation of peripheral pulses. The most common error is feeling pulses which are not present."[46] A practical plan for the bedside attendants is to notify a responsible surgeon—resident or attending surgeon—if the temperature or color of the foot decreases or if previously palpated pulses disappear.

POSTOPERATIVE ACTIVITY

Twenty years of experience (1950–1970) with a variety of anastomoses in dogs in the experimental laboratory clearly indicated to me that postoperative bleeding due to activity was unlikely unless infection occurred. The activity of vascular patients has therefore never been limited for fear of anastomotic disruption and, in the absence of some specific contraindication, early activity has been encouraged.

The multiple benefits of early ambulation have been apparent since the early 1940s.[47] There is, however, one supposed benefit which is probably only wishful thought, namely the prevention of deep venous thrombosis and pulmonary embolism. I have doubted this widely held belief since observing long ago that tuberculosis patients confined to bed rest rarely developed thromboembolism, probably because the chronic disease process did not trigger the coagulation process. Of course, venous thromboembolism is often associated with trauma and disease processes which force rest and cessation of activity, but that is a different matter from a direct causation. There is no direct evidence to support the concept that early ambulation lowers the incidence of venous thromboembolism.

SMOKING

Sieffert, Keown, and Moore demonstrated major endothelial damage in rats exposed repeatedly to tobacco smoke.[48] The ill effects of tobacco are widely accepted as detrimental to patients with arterial disease (to say nothing of its pulmonary cancer–producing effects).*

In a retrospective analysis of 217 patients those who smoked more than five cigarettes daily were "three times more likely to occlude an aorta-femoral graft and four times more likely to thrombose a femoral-popliteal vein graft than those who smoked less than five a day or none."[50]

Unfortunately no one has yet been able to devise any certain or easy method to stop the tobacco habit. Tapering is always doomed to failure; the only hope for successful cessation is the "cold turkey" method, which is difficult and for a time produces quite unpleasant physiologic withdrawal reactions.

My approach to this consists of a 10-minute conversation with the patient and spouse based on the following points. First, the physiologic effects of tobacco smoking are explained in lay terms. Second is a frank statement of the dangers of continuation. Third, it is recommended that the patient recognize tobacco as a poison, the use of which must absolutely cease forever upon the day of the vascular operation. Fourth, it is pointed out that only the patient can make the change and that the spouse must not enter into either the decision or the process of elimination, since that usually produces friction without real help. Fifth, the difficulties of withdrawal and the temptation to revert to tobacco use are explained. Finally, it is recognized that smoking is not a moral or ethical problem but a physical one and that the patient's decision to stop will be fully supported but that if she or he continues, it will in no way disrupt the patient-physician relationship because of feelings of rejection or anger.

Approximately 50 percent of patients thus advised have ceased smoking. One who did not and who finally lost both lower extremities following a number of vascular procedures is shown in Figure 3-7. Another well-remembered failure was an intelligent male who had five successful revascularizations of the lower extremity. He continued smoking, saying, "Why should I stop when you can fix the artery if it gets into trouble?" He died of acute myocardial infarction at age 42.

*Roger M. Greenhalgh has recently provided a well-written and easily understood summary of current information concerning smoking.[49]

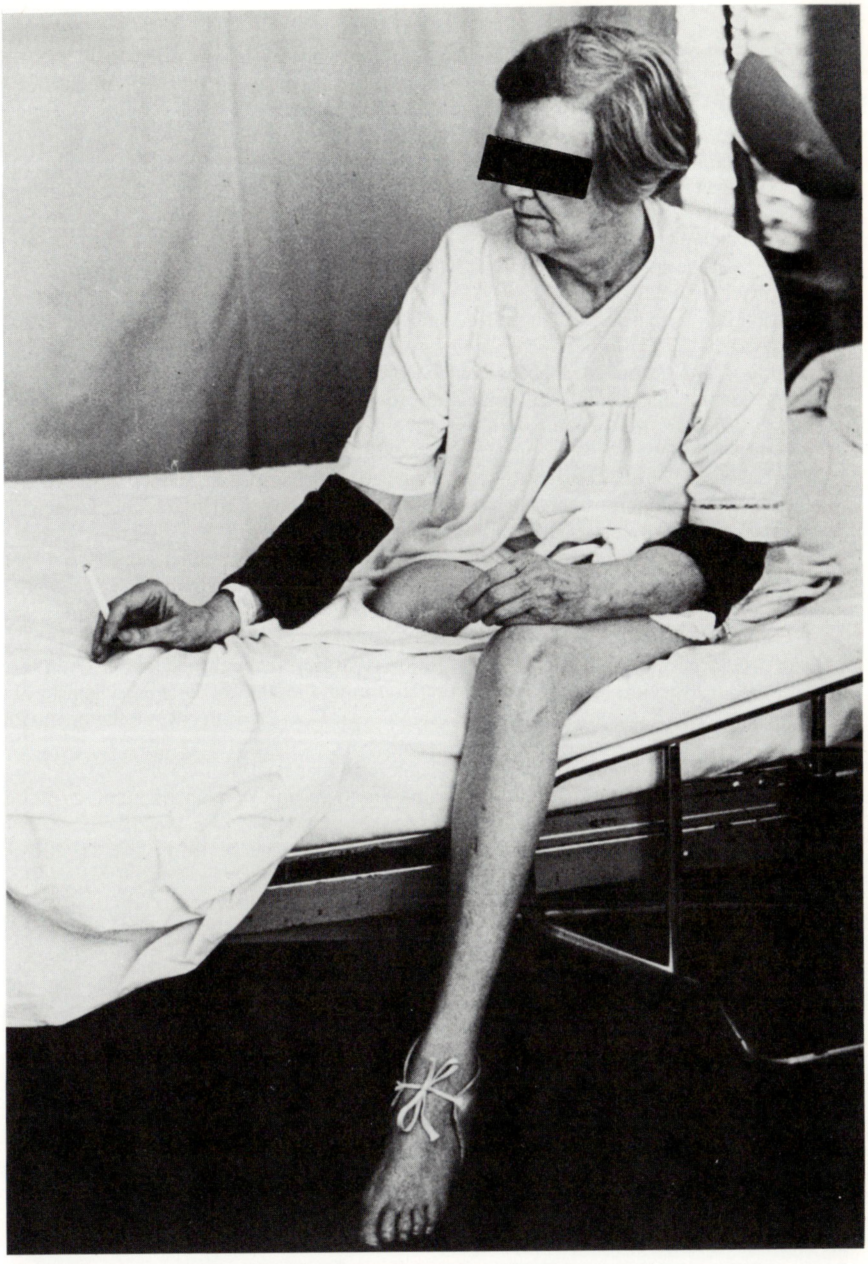

FIGURE 3-7 A patient awaiting the second lower-extremity amputation for continuing severe arterial disease with repeated occlusion of bypass grafts. She was unable to quit smoking.

REFERENCES

1 Wylie EJ: Presidential address. Vascular surgery: reflections of past three decades. *Surgery* 1980, 88:743.

2 Martin-Paredero V, Dixon SM, Baker J, Takiff H, Gomes AS, Pais SO, Machleder HI, Busuttil RW, Moore WS: Scheduling of operations after major angiography: Risk of renal dysfunction. *J Cardiovasc Surg* 1983, 24:370.

3 Schuler JJ, Flanigan DP, Holcroft JW, Ursprung JJ, Mohrland JS, Pyke J: The efficacy of prostaglandin E-1 (PGE-1) in the treatment of lower extremity ischemic ulcers secondary to peripheral vascular occlusive disease (PVOD): Results of a prospective, randomized, double blind, multicenter clinical trial. *J Vasc Surg* 1984, 1:160.

4 Zarin SK: Discussion of Porter JM, Baur GM: Pharmacologic treatment of intermittent claudication. *Surgery* 1982, 92:970.

5 Szilagyi DE: Discussion of Porter JM, Baur GM: Pharmacologic treatment of intermittent claudication. *Surgery* 1982, 92:970.

6 De Pierri T, Guerrini M: Placebo controlled double blind study with pentoxifylline of walking performance in patients with intermittent claudication. *Angiology* 1983, 34:40.

7 Ehrly AM: The effect of pentoxifylline on the deformability of erythrocytes and on the muscular oxygen pressure in patients with chronic arterial disease. *Med* 1979, 10:331.

8 Porter JM, Cutler BS, Lee BY, Reich T, Reichle FA, Scogin JT, Strandness DE: Pentoxifylline efficacy in the treatment of intermittent claudication: Multicenter controlled double-blind trial with objective assessment of chronic occlusive arterial disease patients. *Am Heart J* 1982, 104:66.

9 Aach RD, Kahn RA: Post-transfusion hepatitis—Current perspectives. *Ann Intern Med* 1980, 91:539.

10 Polk HC Jr: Principles of preoperative preparation of the surgical patient, in Sabiston DC (ed): *Textbook of Surgery: The Biological Basis of Modern Surgical Practice.* 12th ed. WB Saunders, Philadelphia, 1981, p 118.

11 Duncan SE, Edwards WH, Dale WA: Caution regarding autotransfusion. *Surgery* 1974, 76:1024.

12 Polk HC Jr: Principles of preoperative preparation of the surgical patient, in Sabiston DC (ed): *Textbook of Surgery: The Biological Basis of Modern Surgical Practice.* 12th ed. WB Saunders, Philadelphia, 1981, p 121.

13 Dale WA: Salvage of the arteriosclerotic leg by vascular repair. *Ann Surg* 1967, 165:844.

14 Lawrie GM, Morris GC: Combined coronary and carotid revascularization, in Cohn L (ed): *Modern Techniques in Surgery: Cardiothoracic Surgery.* Futura, New York, 1980, p 1.

15 Emery RW, Cohn LH, Whittemore AD, Mannick JA, Couch NP, Collins JJ: Coexistent carotid and coronary artery disease. *Arch Surg* 1983, 118:1035.

16 Gage AA, Bhayana JN, Balu V, Hook N: Assessment of cardiac risk in surgical patients. *Arch Surg* 1977, 112:1488.

17 Hertzer N: Myocardial ischemia. *Surgery* 1983, 93:97.

18 Hertzer N, Beven E, Young J, O'Hara P, Ruschhaupt W, Graor R, Dewolfe V, Maljovec L: Coronary artery disease in peripheral vascular patients: A classification of 1000 coronary angiograms and results of surgical management. *Ann Surg* 1984, 199:233.

19 Crawford S: Introduction to symposium: Prevention of complications of abdominal aortic reconstruction. *Surgery* 1983, 93:91.

20 Treiman RL, Foran RF, Cohen JL, Levin PM, Cossman DV: Carotid bruit: A follow-up report on its significance in patients undergoing an abdominal aortic operation. *Arch Surg* 1979, 14:1138.

21 Carney WI Jr, Stewart WB, DePinto DJ, Mucha SJ, Roberts B: Carotid bruit as a risk factor in aortoiliac reconstruction. *Surgery* 1977, 81:567.

22 Greene NM: *Physiology of Spinal Anesthesia.* Williams & Wilkins, Baltimore, 1981, pp 149, 164.

23 Wust *Anesthesiology News* 1982, 8:1.

24 Cunningham FO, Egan JM, Inahara T: Continuous epidural anesthesia in abdominal vascular surgery. *Am J Surg* 1980, 139:624.

25 Cioroiu M, Baron HC, LaRaja RD: Continuous epidural anesthesia in the heparinized vascular surgical patient: A retrospective review of 756 patients.

26 Dritz RA: Extracranial carotid artery surgery, in Ream AK, Fogdall RK (eds); *Acute Cardiovascular Management.* JB Lippincott, Philadelphia, 1982, p 762.

27 Hilberman M: The kidneys: Function, failure and protection in the perioperative period, in Ream AK, Fogdall RK (eds): *Acute Cardiovascular Management.* JB Lippincott, Philadelphia, 1982, p 818.

28 Attia RR, Murphy JD, Snider M, Lappas DG, Darling RC, Lowenstein E: Myocardial ischemia due to infrarenal aortic cross-clamping during aortic surgery in patients with severe coronary artery disease. *Circulation* 1976, 53:961.
29 Kaplan JA, Dunbar RW, Jones EL: Nitroglycerine infusion during coronary artery surgery. *Anesthesiology* 1976, 45:14.
30 Kaiser AB, Clayson KR, Mulherin JL, Roach AB, Allen TR, Edwards WH, Dale WA: Antibiotic prophylaxis in vascular surgery. *Ann Surg* 1978, 188:283.
31 Dale WA, Kaiser AB: Prevention of infection in vascular surgery, in Karran S (ed): *Controversies in Surgical Sepsis.* Praeger Special Studies, New York, 1980, p 275.
32 Alexander JW, Fischer JE, Boyajian M, Palmquist J, Morris MJ: The influence of hair removal methods on wound infections. *Arch Surg* 1983, 118:341.
33 Cruse PJE, Foord R: A five year prospective study of 23,649 surgical wounds. *Arch Surg* 1973, 1007:206.
34 Seropian R, Reynolds RM: Wound infections after preoperative depilatory versus razor preparation. *Am J Surg* 1971, 121:251.
35 Geelhoed G, Sharpe K: The rationale and ritual of preoperative skin preparation. *Contemporary Surg* 1983, 23:31.
36 Rodeheaver G, Bellamy W, Kody M, Spatafora G, Fitton L, Leyden K, Edlich R: Bactericidal activity and toxicity of iodine containing solutions in wounds. *Arch Surg* 1982, 117:181.
37 Zamora JL, Feldtman RW: Letter. *Arch Surg* 1983, 118:367.
38 Madden JE, Edlich RF, Custer JR, Panek PH, Thul J, Wangensteen OH: Studies in the management of the contaminated wound IV. Resistance to infection of surgical wounds made by knife, electrosurgery, and laser. *Am J Surg* 1970, 119:222.
39 Sharp WV, Beldon TA, King PH, Teague PC: Suture resistance to infection. *Surgery* 1982, 91:61.
40 Knight C, Griffen F: Abdominal wound closure with a continuous monofilament polypropylene suture: Experience with 1,000 cases. *Arch Surg* 1983, 118:1305.
41 Richards PC, Balch CM, Aldrete JS: A randomized prospective study of 571 patients comparing continuous vs. interrupted suture techniques. *Ann Surg* 1983, 197:238.
42 McCollum CN, Kester RC: A sliding suture technique for inaccessible arterial anastomoses. *Surg Gynecol Obstet* 1982, 153:970.
43 Dale WA: The beginnings of vascular surgery. *Surgery* 1974, 76:849.
44 Rosenberg RD, Rosenberg JS: The anticoagulant function of heparin. *Drug Ther Bull* Sept 1979.
45 Estes JW: Heparin in clinical practice. *Drug Ther Bull* Sept 1979.
46 Smithwick RH: Lumbar sympathectomy in treatment of obliterative vascular disease of lower extremities. *Surgery* 1957, 42:415.
47 Brieger GH: Early ambulation: A study in the history of surgery. *Ann Surg* 1983, 197:443.
48 Sieffert GF, Keown K, Moore WS: Pathologic effect of tobacco smoke inhalation on arterial intima. *Surg Forum* 1981, 32:333.
49 Greenhalgh RM: *Smoking and Arterial Occlusion.* Pitman Medical, Bath, England, 1981.
50 Myers KA, King RB, Scott DF, Johnson N, Morris PJ: The effect of smoking on the late patency of arterial reconstruction in the legs. *Br J Surg* 1978, 65:267.

Invited Commentary

Malcolm O. Perry, M.D.
New York

There is appropriate emphasis upon the importance of clinical evaluation in establishing the diagnosis of vascular occlusive disease, particularly in the extremities. One can make this diagnosis firmly in most patients by obtaining an accurate history and performing a thorough physical examination. In patients with cerebrovascular insufficiency and symptoms suggestive of visceral arterial disease more sophisticated tests are required, but when the extremities are the major focus of the disease, the clinical diagnosis is usually straightforward and often quite simple.

Noninvasive tests are always supplementary in these situations, and on no occasion are they a substitute for the history and physical examination. Tests of segmental blood pressures, exercise tolerance, and ankle-brachial indices and similar tests are useful in following up a patient and in determining if recurrent disease is developing. Recent studies suggest that the newer techniques of evaluating the carotid bifurcation (B-mode echosonography and sound spectrum analysis) are especially helpful in ascertaining if significant narrowing is present. In fact, some studies suggest that this form of noninvasive testing may be at least as accurate as digital intravenous arteriography.

In most centers vascular surgeons require arteriograms prior to operation in order to plan properly the procedure, even though the diagnosis may have been established on a clinical basis. The vascular surgeon must take primary responsibility for the tests that are performed and for their interpretation. The subtle changes seen on arteriograms may not be appreciated even by the experienced vascular radiologist, who rarely sees the morbid pathology at the operating table and thus may not correctly interpret minor changes on the arteriograms which are consistent markers of atherosclerosis. The vascular surgeon, on the other hand, having correlated the arteriographic findings with the actual pathology hundreds of times, is more likely to make an accurate interpretation of the films. In fact, vascular surgeons are rarely surprised by operative findings. From this experience it is difficult to understand recent reports suggesting that arteriograms are inaccurate; one can only speculate that this alleged inaccuracy is a result of a failure of the vascular surgeon to examine carefully the arteriograms.

The priorities of repair of simultaneous atherosclerotic lesions are discussed in detail; this is an especially important section, since those decisions are never easy to reach. The dilemma of whether to stage or perform simultaneous coronary artery bypass and carotid endarterectomy is a recurring problem. As noted, recent studies by Hertzer and Hollier suggest that a careful clinical evaluation, perhaps supplemented by noninvasive studies such as radionuclide imaging, is a useful method for screening these patients. Most surgeons, as proposed, will operate upon the lesion according to its own merits, thus symptomatic carotid artery lesions and critical stenoses to a dominant hemisphere (especially if contralateral carotid occlusion is present) may require surgery. If such a patient also has unstable angina, simultaneous operations may be considered.

The section dealing with the prevention of infection is timely and very important. Although infections in vascular operations are rare, when they occur they often are life-threatening or can lead to loss of an extremity. The simple measures of local skin care and skin preparation are extremely important. Clearly, shaving and prepping the night before is no longer acceptable, since the incidence of wound infection in clean wounds is unfavorably influenced by such practices. Excessive hair can be removed by clipping prior to the operation if it interferes with the incisions; there is little evidence that shaving is needed.

During the course of the operation it is desirable to cover the skin and the skin edges and especially to avoid laying plastic vascular prostheses on the skin. Contamination of a graft at time of insertion, although uncommon, is clearly a risk.

The use of prophylactic antibiotics is an established procedure in vascular operations, but there is correct emphasis upon the importance of proper blood and tissue levels of the antibiotic. All too often the method of administration of the antibiotic may not take into account the peak blood and tissue levels. If it is to be effective in the operating room, there are certain times during the operation when the vascular surgeon would prefer to have high levels of antibiotics in the blood (such as when preclotting the graft or inserting the graft) and other times when she or he would prefer higher levels in the tissues (such as when opening and closing the groin wounds). The pharmacokinetics of the antibiotics should be well understood, and the method of administration should take these characteristics into account.

4 VASCULAR TRAUMA

Trauma to blood vessels demands immediate treatment, correct judgment, and skill in vascular reconstruction to maintain viability and function. When the vascular injury accompanies nearby bone damage or serious lesions elsewhere, the problems indeed become complex and require triage as well as correct management of the individual lesions. High on the priority list and surpassed only by the need to provide oxygenation and arrest bleeding is ischemia due to an arterial injury.

HISTORICAL BACKGROUND

The control of serious hemorrhage by local pressure, tourniquet, and early amputation dates from antiquity. Wars produced numbers of amputees, and most towns also had one or two such citizens as a result of farm or industrial accidents. During our Civil War early amputation for compound injuries of the extremities produced a lower mortality than did procrastination until sepsis and malnutrition had occurred. Even so, the risk of thigh amputation was 62 percent.[1]

After the bacterial cause of infection was understood, it became possible to ligate a damaged vessel with the hope that distal perfusion would be maintained by the collateral circulation. The policy of ligation of injured arteries was practiced during World Wars I and II but produced a high amputation rate, such as the 73 percent limb loss among 502 World War II injuries documented by DeBakey and Simeone.[2]

Immediate arterial reconstruction was first practiced in the Korean and Vietnam conflicts, with approximately 13 percent of extremities lost to amputation thereafter.[3] As might be expected, an even better salvage rate has been produced in civilian practice, such as the 2 percent amputation rate among 165 patients having vascular repairs reported by Perry, Thal, and Shires.[4]

Today injuries of major vessels have become a frequent problem, not only because of our violent society, but also because improved on-the-scene treatment and rapid transport to definitive care centers mean that many patients who would formerly have died undergo treatment. The majority of such wounds are gunshot-inflicted; some are knife wounds, and a few follow blunt trauma (55, 36, and 9 percent in Perry's series of 665 cases).[5] Most vascular injuries now can be repaired by one or another method.

Illustrative Case

The thigh of a 36-year-old male was crushed by a truck bumper against the fender of another vehicle. He was transported by helicopter to our tertiary care center.

There was a massive blowout of the soft tissues of the midthigh, along with shredding of 3 inches of both the superficial femoral artery and the vein and a compound comminuted fracture of the femur (Figure 4-1).

The foot was cold, pale, and pulseless. A femoral arteriogram showed cessation of arterial flow at the site of the injury without collateralization. Nerve function was normal.

FIGURE 4-1 Compound comminuted femoral fracture. Radiographic contrast material outlines a few collaterals of the severed and occluded superficial femoral artery.

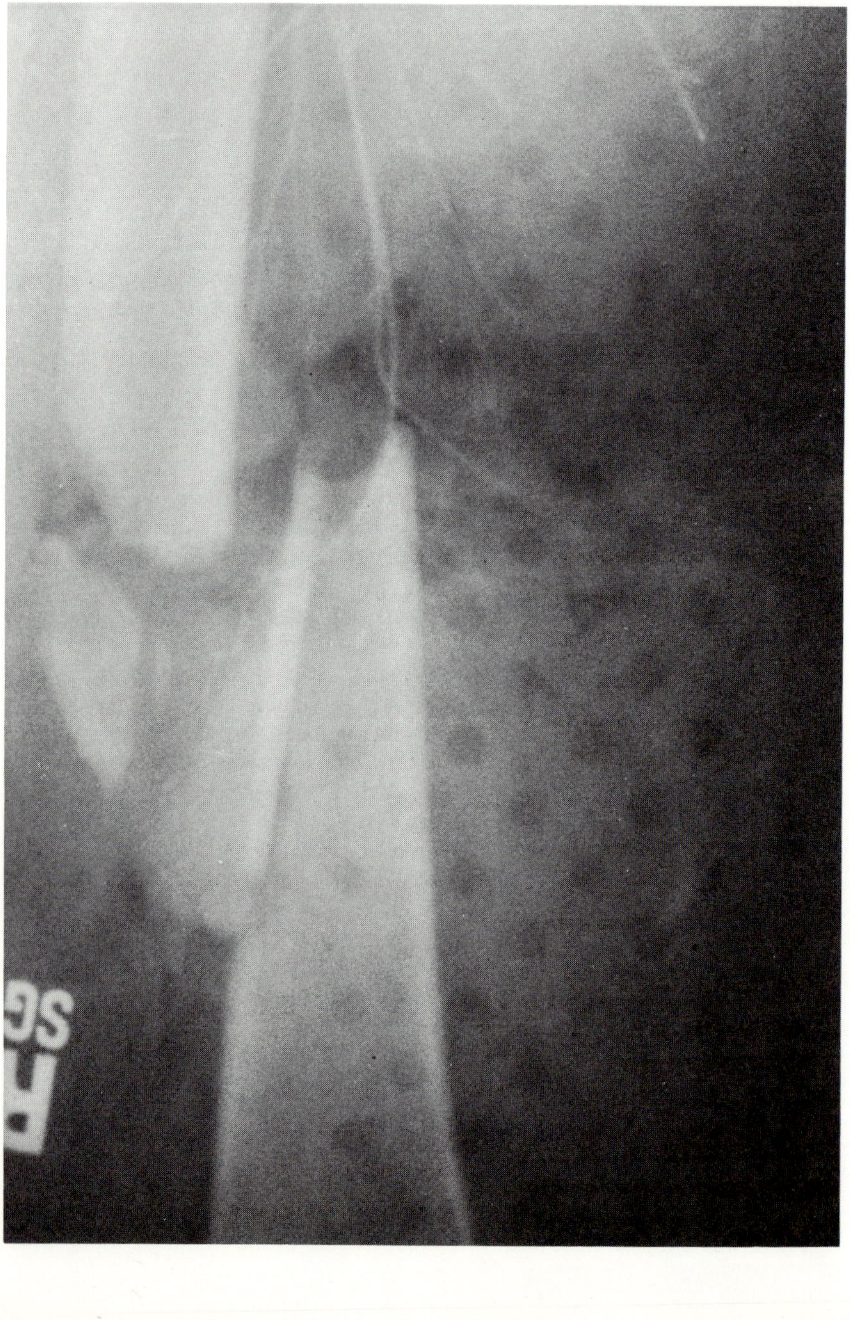

Initially steel plates were placed through a clean lateral incision to fix the femoral fracture. Debridement of the macerated tissues of the medial thigh was quickly performed.

The damaged portion of the femoral artery was removed, and the normal vessel ends were split to allow interposition of the ipsilateral saphenous vein, which had meanwhile been removed from the calf below the knee. A similar vein graft was used to repair the superficial femoral vein (Figure 4-2). Both grafts now lay completely exposed, so the quadratus muscle was pulled over them with absorbable sutures. The remainder of the wound was packed open with vaseline gauze (Figure 4-3). The foot was now pink and warm, and pulses were palpable.

Postoperatively some edema of the foot and ankle persisted. Split-thickness skin grafts were placed on the wound. All dressings were performed in the sterile environment of the operating room. The main wound healed well, but a posterior sinus drained for several months.

Seven months later a phlebogram showed that the venous reconstruction had failed. The foot pulses have persisted, so no arteriogram has been done.

Comment Immediate transportation and revascularization were fortunately available for this battlefield-type injury. Spontaneous thrombosis of the vessels had prevented excessive blood loss, and the young, otherwise healthy patient arrived in good condition. Bone stabilization was discussed, considering whether balanced traction or rigid fixation should be placed through an elective clean incision. The severe comminution ruled against intramedullary nailing. It was decided to allow ischemia to persist long enough to apply rigid plates to provide bone stabilization; this was achieved in 45 minutes.

It may also be remarked that the orthopedic surgeon was chosen because of knowledge of his ability to manage the fracture without delay or "fiddling about." There is no place in such circumstances of ischemia for a slow, inefficient operator. Wide debridement delayed the repair another 15 minutes. Thus 60 minutes after starting, the bone was fixed, the wound was cleaned up, and the vascular repair was begun.

Ideally, the vein graft should have come from the normal contralateral limb, but the patient's position made removal of this vein awkward, so the ipsilateral saphenous vein below the knee was quickly removed and prepared. The artery was reconstructed first, to relieve the acute ischemia, and a similar venous repair followed.

The large wound was packed open, with split graft coverage planned for 5 to 7 days later; muscle was pulled over the grafts as a protective layer.

No wound exposure was allowed in the patient's room for fear of contamination and infection by hospital organisms. The first dressing was done in the operating room 5 days later. The wound was granulating well without clinical evidence of infection, so immediate split-thickness skin grafting was performed.

Finally may be considered whether immediate primary amputation would have been a better alternative. The remarkable presence of a normal nerve supply encouraged reconstructive efforts.

The hospital cost of $56,775.70 is large but must be measured against the function and independence of a courageous young man, who 14 months later walked upon a functional limb. Some edema persists.

CLINICAL DIAGNOSIS

When an injury is followed by bleeding with pain, dysesthesia, and loss of motor function along with the signs of ischemia—coolness, pallor, and loss of pulses—it is obvious that a vascular obstruction is present. Lesser injuries, including lacerations, contusions, and those with prompt perfusion by collateral circulation are more difficult to detect.

Important arterial lesions which need repair may be masked by palpable distal pulses, since pulse pressure waves may be transmitted through clots and internal flaps even though little or no actual blood flow is present.[5] Drapanas and his New Orleans associates palpated distal pulses in 22 percent of 128 patients with arterial injuries.[6] An arteriogram usually reveals the lesion,

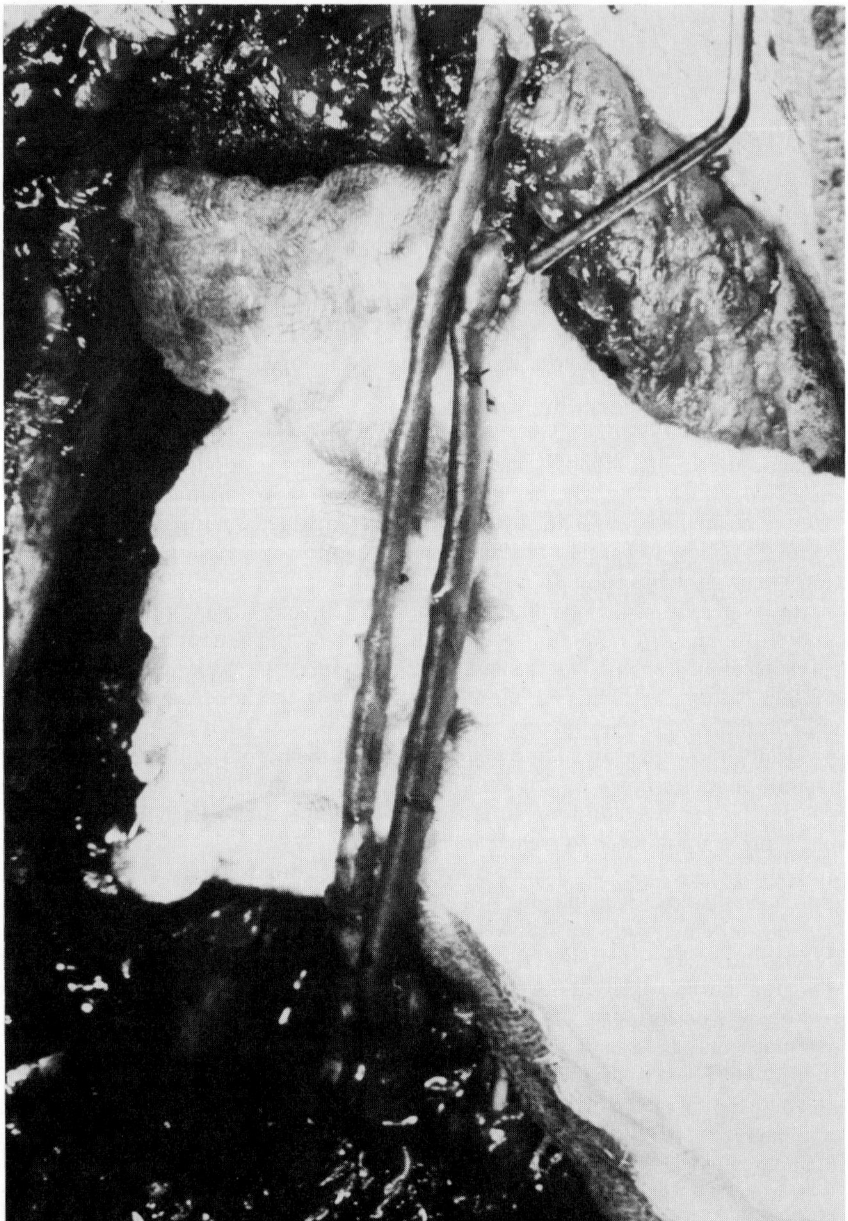

FIGURE 4-2 Interpolated autogenous saphenous vein grafts reconstituted both the femoral artery and the vein.

but a few pass that test also and later appear as fistulas or aneurysms. A policy of suspicion is mandatory.

Minimal signs of ischemia with absent pulses, especially if the arterial injury is not at once apparent, may initially be attributed to spasm and suggest a delay in operation. The Vietnam rule of Rich, Collins, and Hobson is pertinent here—"spasm should be spelled C-L-O-T."[7]

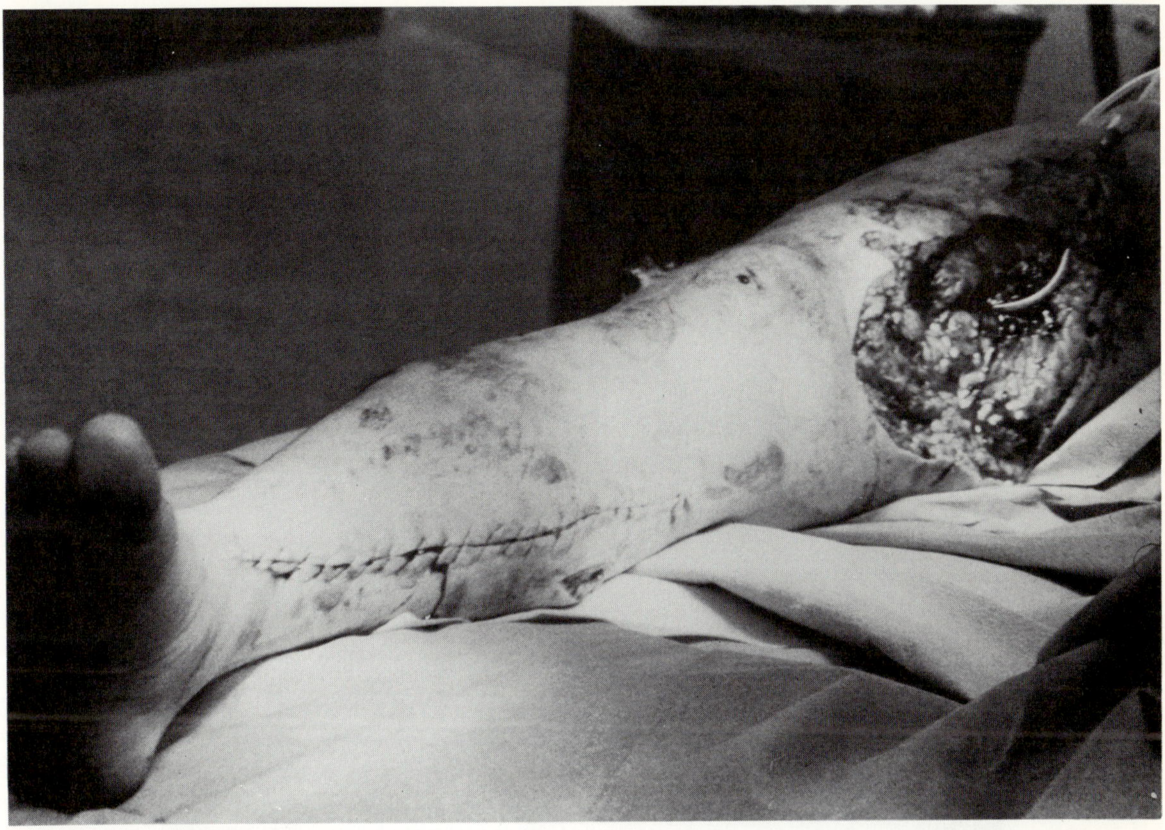

FIGURE 4-3 At the operation's conclusion, viable muscle was sutured over the interpolated grafts and the wound was packed open. The calf incision indicates the site of removal of the saphenous vein.

ANGIOGRAPHY

The role of arteriograms in determining vascular damage and its location unfortunately depends to some extent upon its availability. A first-rate vascular center should offer this capability day and night, 8760 hours yearly, yet the same can hardly be expected of a 50-bed community hospital. Whatever the availability, it would be used to the fullest extent. Thus, in a vascular center an angiogram is indicated for any suspicion of an arterial injury; even in overt cases it should be obtained quickly while the surgical team is being assembled in the operating room. In a small hospital its lack may necessitate the patient's transfer to a more fully equipped facility.

It may be argued that angiography is unnecessary and wastes time for some clear-cut injuries.[8] It does, however, document the location and extent of the lesion and may serve to modify the surgical procedure.

Illustrative Case

H. G., a 60-year-old male, had a 4-hour-old undermined dirty wound of the medial knee region with considerable skin avulsion. No pulses were palpable in the foot, which was cool and ischemic although retaining sensation and motor power.

A femoral arteriogram showed a 2-cm occlusion of the popliteal artery just above the knee joint (Figure 4-4).

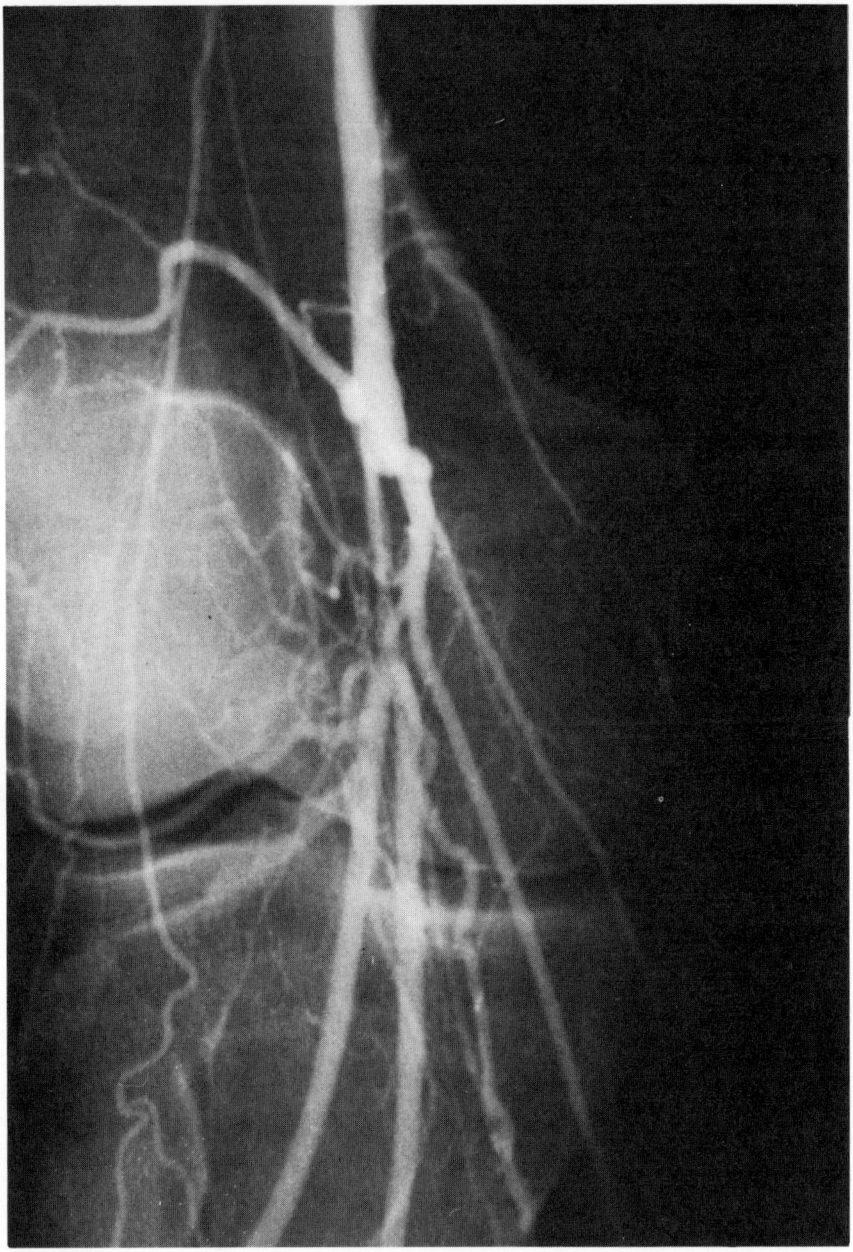

FIGURE 4-4 Chronic occlusion of a popliteal artery in a patient with severe soft tissue injury medially was explored and repaired via a posterior approach through clean tissue.

Through a posterior approach to the popliteal space, a local thromboendarterectomy of an atherosclerotic plaque was performed, followed by a patch graft closure, using a vein from the dorsal wrist. After these wounds were closed, the medial wound was completely debrided and closed using split-thickness skin grafts.

Uneventful healing with continued revascularization of the foot followed.

Comment The preoperative arteriogram indicating a short occlusion suggested a chronic atherosclerotic process, but the occlusion was in an unusual position and could have been due to an intimal flap or an arterial contusion due to the trauma. The issue was settled by immediate exploration through a clean wound with appropriate revascularization, following which the main wound was widely debrided and closed. The arteriogram allowed preoperative decision as to the proper positioning, approach, and procedure.

Another patient transferred with hemostats "upon the brachial artery" had a normal arteriogram just prior to exploration. The clamps were removed from muscle bleeders, and the wound was debrided and closed without the extensive exploration which might have been needed otherwise.

Sometimes the abnormality seen by angiography appears trival or minor. This only reflects minimal leakage of contrast material and should not encourage a nonoperative strategy.

Angiography should be available and should be used for (1) overt arterial injury, (2) ischemia denoted by the absence of pulses or coolness, (3) fractures or wounds which common sense indicates may have caused an arterial lesion, and (4) stab or gunshot wounds near a major vessel, especially by multiple pellets of shot. If the question seriously arises, an arteriogram should be done.

Computerized tomography (CT scan) is especially useful for patients with multiple injuries due to trauma. Visceral organ injuries and hematomas are well seen. A negative scan, however, does not contraindicate an exploration which is otherwise indicated.

OPERATIVE MANAGEMENT

Heparin

If systemic heparinization appears safe in view of the overall evaluation of other injuries, it should be instituted immediately to prevent distal thrombosis, particularly of the small branch arteries and collateral veins. Heparin solution should also be injected through the damaged artery once that is isolated, to be certain that there is an adequate concentration in the ischemic extremity.

Extent of the Repair

It is often tempting to perform a limited local procedure to reconstruct a laterally damaged artery or make an end-to-end anastomosis of an artery which is torn across. Experience, however, indicates that the vessel is usually damaged considerably beyond the apparent gross evidence, as a result of stretching and contusion by the external wounding object or bone or other structure. Several centimeters of artery should be excluded or resected to place the interpolated or bypass graft well away from the injured portion of the vessel. It is far better to place a graft that is too long than to place one that is too short.

Two recent cases demonstrated the point. The first patient's popliteal artery, damaged by dislocation of the knee, had elsewhere been bypassed with a vein graft, with immediate thrombosis. A new and longer bypass performed 9 hours after injury has remained patent.*

The other patient, with contusion and thrombosis of the brachial artery due to a hockey stick injury, also had repair by an interpolated vein graft (Figure 4-5). Despite various maneuvers this failed, doubtless due to failure to bypass all the damaged artery (Figures 4-6, 4-7). Later secondary repair was unnecessary since the collateral circulation provided a perfectly functional extremity.

*Dr. Joseph L. Mulherin performed the second procedure.

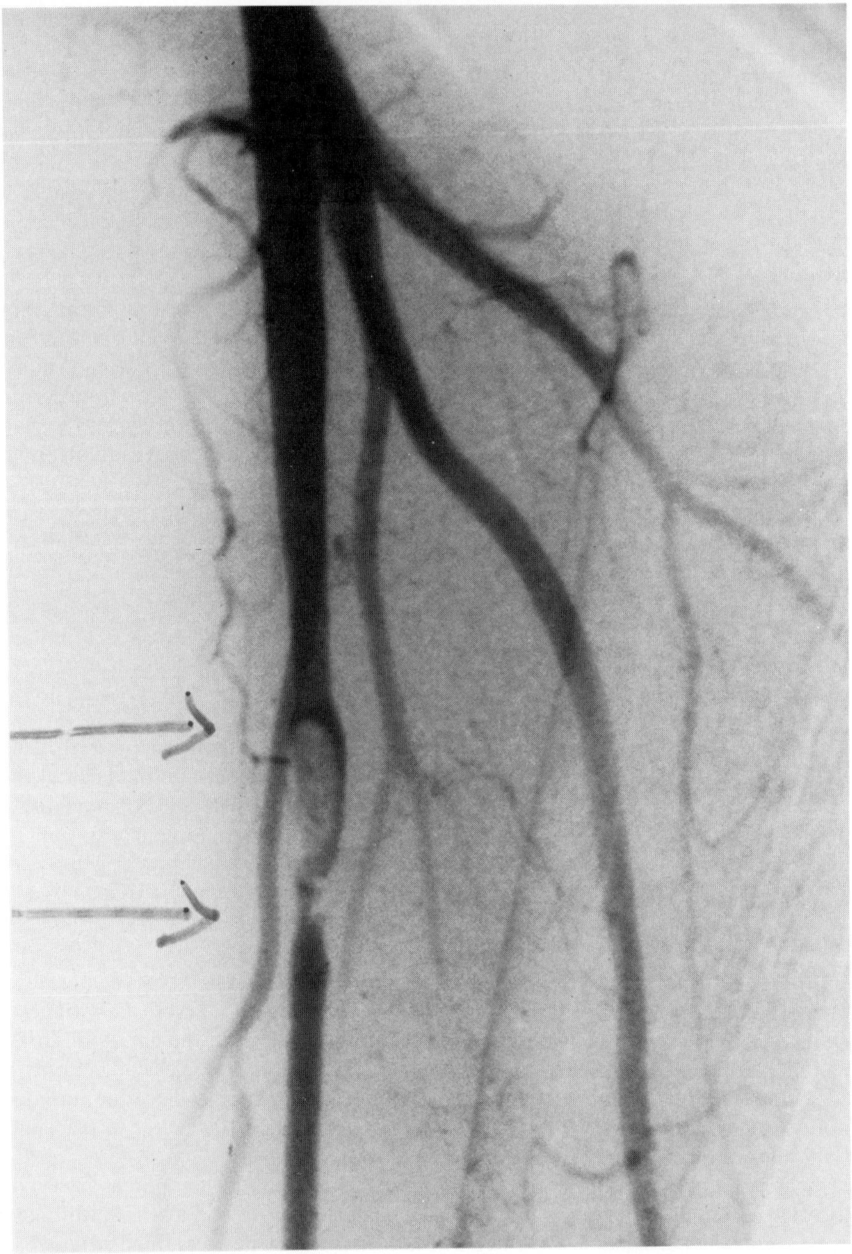

FIGURE 4-5 A hockey stick blunt injury of the brachial artery with intraluminal thrombus and distal disruption.

Vein Repairs

The possibility of reconstructing large veins has not been recognized until recently. Just as the Korean War of the 1950s led to a policy of direct arterial repair, the Vietnam conflict provided the first large experience with successful venous repair.[9] In 1976 Rich, Hobson, Collins, and

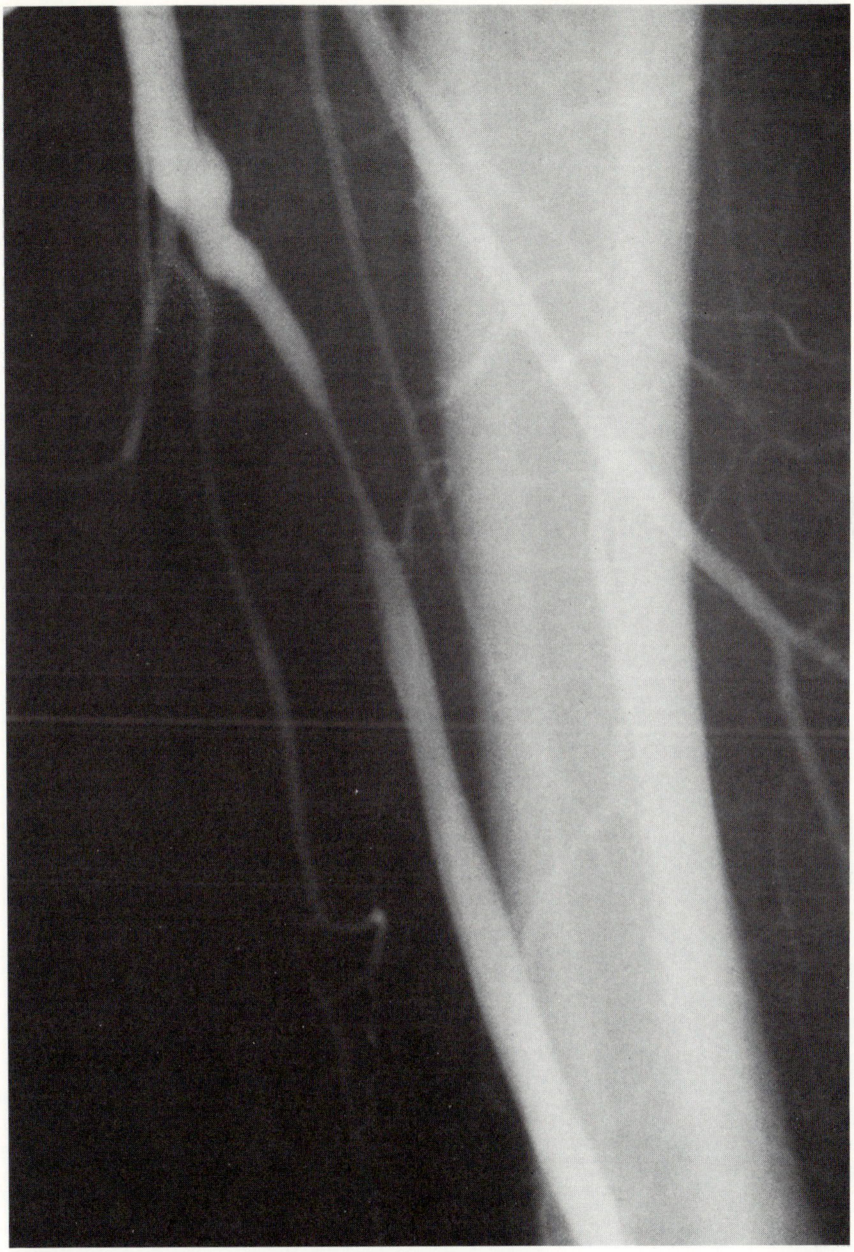

FIGURE 4-6 Following autogenous vein repair, a completion arteriogram showed stenosis beyond the distal anastomosis. This was treated by passing a Fogarty catheter, and later a dilator.

Andersen reported the long-term results of 110 popliteal vein injuries. Half were ligated, with 51 percent showing later edema, and half were repaired, with 13 percent later edema.[10]

Small veins and the tributaries of large ones may be ligated with impunity because of the extensive venous collateralization which is present throughout the body. In general, this includes

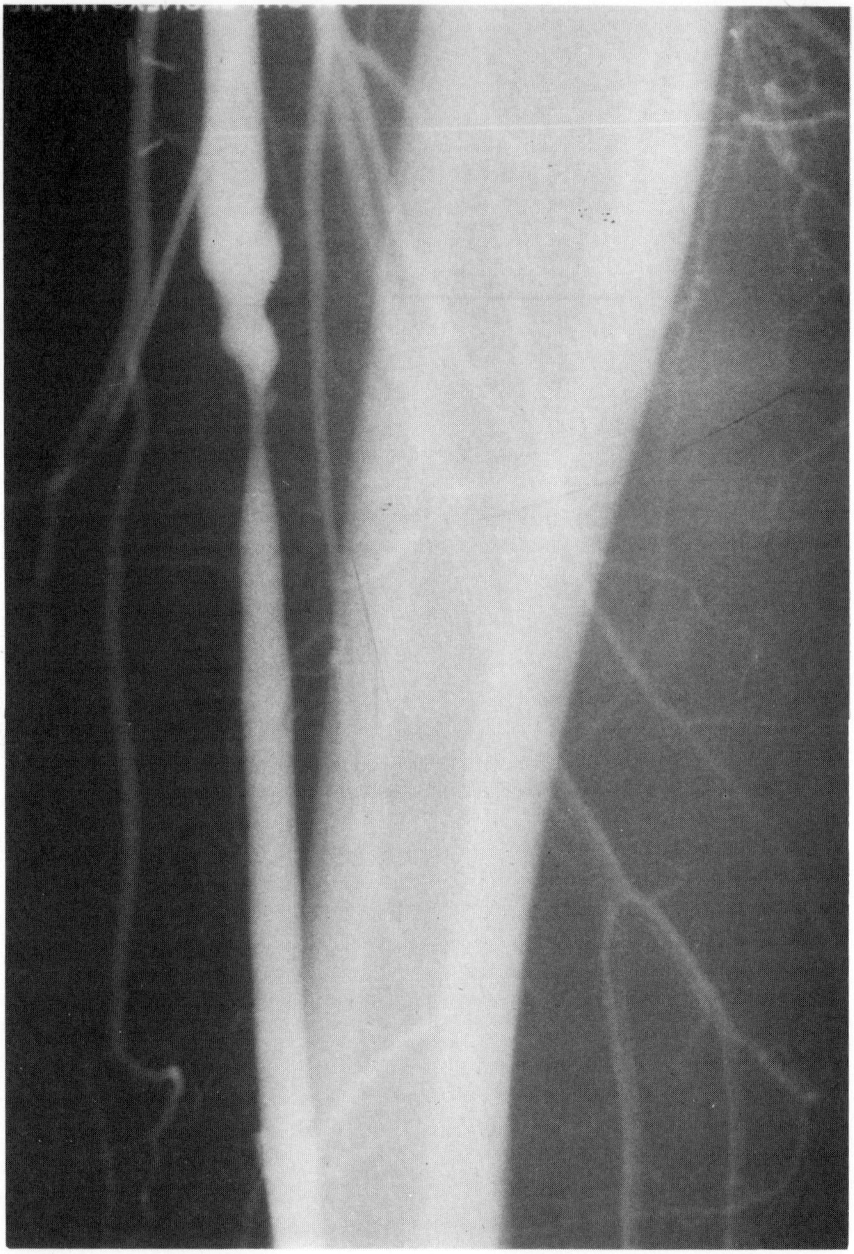

FIGURE 4-7 A completion arteriogram following Fogarty catheterization and dilatation showed another area of distal stenosis, which was again treated by Fogarty catheterization and instrumental dilation. Despite these efforts the pulses disappeared on the fourth day. The arm maintained viability and usefulness via collateral circulation.

venous injuries below the level of the elbow and knee, where there are multiple venous channels to return blood. When there is an injury of a major vein proximal to these levels, repair should be done even if this requires a vein graft.

When a vein graft is necessary, it should be obtained from the contralateral extremity or from an arm vein, so as not to destroy additional veins of the involved extremity. This advice was disregarded in the first illustrative case in this chapter because of the special circumstance of positioning.

The expected patency rate of venous reconstruction for trauma is not known[11] because few of these patients have had phlebograms performed later after the reconstruction. Some patients who show failed anastomoses by phlebography have not shown edema clinically, as a result of abundant collateral circulation. Thus the patient described on pages 39–41 had only a little edema, yet the phlebogram made 7 months later failed to visualize patency of the interpolated graft.

Arteriovenous fistulization to increase the blood flow and pressure within a venous anastomosis or graft may be considered for a clean elective case but because of the danger of infection, has no place in the repair of vascular trauma.

Whether an external compression boot is better[9] than elastic bandage upon the extremity, or indeed whether either improves patency results, is unknown.

Choice of Graft Material

An autogenous vein is the preferable material for an arterial or a venous graft, since the patient's own tissue has the considerable advantage of resistance to infection. This can be obtained not only from the saphenous vein of the thigh or the lower leg but also from the arm veins. The vein graft should ordinarily not be taken from the extremity which has been injured.

If the wound containing an autogenous vein graft should become infected, it should be managed by wide opening to allow immediate drainage and thereby prevent extension of infection to the graft and its suture lines. An autogenous vein graft usually will remain patent throughout the period of granulation or at worst will thrombose, whereas a synthetic graft usually requires removal from an infected wound. Hemorrhage due to infection of a vein graft is unusual.

The Surgical Approach

A correct anatomic approach should be made to the injured vessel regardless of wounds of entry or exit. Early proximal and distal control of the vessels is essential so that vascular clamps may be used to provide temporary closure during the repair.

If bony or other injuries are present, their immediate or later repair should be considered in planning incisions. Thus, tendons near the knee should not be severed if a later arthroplasty is probable. To allow for possible infection and/or the necessity for later removal, bone plates should be placed away from an arterial graft rather than through the same incision.

Skeletal Fixation

When fracture of a long bone accompanies a serious arterial injury, its immediate stabilization—either by skeletal traction or by internal or external fixation—must be accomplished at once.

Skeletal traction has the advantage of simplicity. Foreign objects are not placed within the wound, and it may be the only fixation method available if there is considerable comminution of the fragments and/or loss of tissue.[12] Some fear has been expressed in the past about pulling a vascular anastomosis apart, but this is largely theoretical. In both clinical and laboratory studies strong degrees of skeletal traction have been tolerated without disruption of a vascular suture line. Eighteen kilograms of skeletal traction have been used experimentally without anastomotic difficulty, whereas only four to seven kilograms are usually necessary for a patient.[13,14]

The advantage of immediate stabilization of the fracture by internal fixation prior to the arterial repair is considerable if the stabilization can be carried out expeditiously by an experienced orthopedic surgeon working under ideal conditions. Internal or external fixation can be accomplished without unduly prolonging the ischemia time and is more effective than is skeletal traction.[12]

Soft Tissue Management

Contused, torn, and contaminated skin, fat, and muscle should be removed with a knife and scissors to rid the wound of necrotic tissue, to decrease bacterial contamination, and to provide viable surfaces for immediate healing without infection. This may involve removal of large masses of muscle. The hazard of infection is too great, however, to permit damaged muscle to be left in situ with the hope that it will be revascularized. If the muscle tissue is questionable, it should be removed from the wound, even though this leaves a defect and perhaps an extremity without flexion or extension.

Some type of soft tissue covering should be provided for a necessary arterial repair, whether this be a suture line or a graft. Often this can be obtained by swinging a flap of viable muscle or creating a subcutaneous tissue-skin flap for coverage while leaving the majority of the wound open for drainage.

Wound Dressings

Exposure of a wound which has been recently debrided and packed without primary closure should be done with considerable caution to prevent contamination by hospital organisms. The surgeon should be reluctant to open the wound in the following few days in the patient's room, even while wearing a mask and using gloves. The operating room is a better place, particularly if a secondary closure is in order. Dressing changes should not be delegated far down the line of experience in the early postoperative days. Although the responsible nurse may be quite competent to change the dressing, her multiple duties may cause delegation of the task to a technician or, at worst, to some family member. The surgeon has a considerable personal responsibility to provide the best possible dressing conditions, and in some situations this may require frequent trips to the operating room.

Fasciotomy

Most surgeons do not perform fasciotomy early enough or often enough. Decompression of the fascial spaces may not be invariably necessary but should be considered, particularly as time passes since the onset of ischemia.

Fasciotomy may be conducted through several separated skin incisions or through a completely open one, in which case some type of secondary closure may later be necessary. Most fasciotomies should be done through small skin incisions, using the scissors to open the fascia longitudinally.[15]

LATE COMPLICATIONS

The incidence of infections varies with the extent of wounding and the time interval prior to definitive treatment. Their management is no different from similar problems in elective vascular surgery except as modified by other concomitant injuries.

Arteriovenous fistulas and false aneurysms may be recognized in a few days or many years after the initial injury.[16] They require angiography and definitive surgical treatment at an early elective time.

Late stenosis of a vascular repair, or even complete occlusion, may also later require a definitive reconstruction.

SPECIFIC INJURIES

No attempt will be made herein to detail all the exposures needed for deep hidden vessels such as the intrahepatic portion of the inferior vena cava and the portal vein, the great vessels at the root of the neck, or the cephalad portion of the carotid and vertebral arteries. All these require planning and technical skill in an emergency which is not commonly met. Lights, retractors, and multiple hands are basic to good exposure, which in turn allows proper vascular control and reconstruction. Sometimes the best assistance is derived from a quick trip to the library to review the pertinent anatomy.

Finally, it should be remarked that seemingly uncontrollable bleeding can occasionally be stopped by tight packing with delayed removal. Large packs or towels are not *desirable* intracavitary objects but may allow salvage until their removal at a later time.

Cervical Wounds

It has been stated that wounds extending through the platysma require surgical exploration.[17] Further to be noted is the need for angiography for most neck wounds, and particularly those at the base and near the head, because of inaccessibility to the usual surgical exploration.

An exception to the general policy of immediate arterial repair is carotid injury with a fixed neurologic deficit. Reconstruction in this situation may lead to bleeding into a cerebral infarct. Ligation of the carotid artery is indicated.[18]

Catheter and needle injuries of the brachial and femoral artery have become increasingly common with the advent of frequent catheter studies by cardiologists. Early local repair by suture or venous patch graft is preferable to allowing an injury to persist in the hope that collaterals will perfuse the extremity. The latter policy too often leads to a viable limb with dysfunction that later necessitates a bypass.

Abdominal Wounds

Abdominal wounds are best explored via a long midline incision. Requeana, Cherekuri, and Lerner have recently provided a rational and methodical plan for such injuries[19] which, if more aggressive than customary, is worthy of consideration, since it is designed to salvage types of patients who have previously bled to death despite operation.

In brief, they perform the usual exploration for patients who respond well to blood replacement. Those who do not stabilize after rapid transfusion are assumed to have continued bleeding, which can be temporarily controlled by passing a large Fogarty catheter upward from an insertion into a femoral artery to a proximal aortic position just above the diaphragm, where the balloon is distended. After the abdomen is opened, the source of hemorrhage may be identified and repaired or ligated. If some bleeding persists despite this aortic control, there is a presumption of venous bleeding from the vena cava or the portal or mesenteric veins, which can be temporarily controlled by an intracaval balloon catheter or by direct pressure. Sometimes a tube placed through the right atrium into the inferior vena cava, with tourniquet isolation of the retrohepatic portion of the cava, may be needed. Reflection of the viscera to the right or left to allow a retroperitoneal approach may be useful.

An aortic injury may require replacement with a synthetic graft. If there is associated injury of the intestine, the likelihood of graft infection is so great that the aorta should be closed by oversewing of the cut ends and revascularization should be achieved by an extraanatomic axillobifemoral graft.

Inferior vena caval injuries should usually be repaired rather than ligated, since the latter treatment may result in chronic lower-extremity complications. A lateral venous patch graft may be used as well as the side of a loop of intestine.[20] Attempts to use the saphenous vein as an interposed graft of the inferior vena cava usually fail because of the disproportion in size. A spiral vein graft takes too long to prepare. The matter is not well-established, but success using an externally stented polytetrafluoroethylene (PTFE) graft suggests it may be the material of choice, provided there is no contamination with intestinal content.[21]

REFERENCES

1 Dale WA: *The Yellow Rose of Texas.* (To be published.)
2 DeBakey ME, Simeone FA: Battle injuries of arteries in World War II: An analysis of 2,471 cases. *Ann Surg* 1946, 123:534.
3 Rich NM, Collins GJ, Hobson RW: Venous injuries of the extremities: Combined arterial and venous injuries, in Hobson RW (ed): *Venous Trauma, Pathophysiology Diagnosis and Surgical Management,* Futura, Mount Kisco, New York, 1983.
4 Perry MO, Thal ER, Shires GT: Management of arterial injuries. *Ann Surg* 1971; 173:403.
5 Perry MO: Vascular trauma, in Moore WS (ed): *Vascular Surgery, A Comprehensive Review.* Grune & Stratton, New York, 1983.
6 Drapanas T, Hewitt RL, Weichert RF III, Smith AD: Civilian vascular injuries: A critical appraisal of three decades of management. *Ann Surg* 1970, 172:351.
7 Rich NM, Collins GJ, Hobson RW: Venous injuries of the extremities (Chapter 6), in Hobson RW (ed): *Venous Trauma, Pathophysiology, Diagnosis and Surgical Management.* Futura, Mount Kisco, New York, 1983.
8 Birnstingl M: *Vascular Surgery.* JB Lippincott, Philadelphia, 1973, p 336.
9 Hobson RW, Rich NM: Introduction—Initial care of the vascular injury (Chapter 1), in Hobson RW (ed): *Venous Trauma, Pathophysiology, Diagnosis and Surgical Management.* Futura, Mount Kisco, New York, 1983.
10 Rich NM, Hobson RW, Collins GL Jr, Andersen CA: The effect of acute popliteal venous interruption. *Ann Surg* 1976, 183:365.
11 Hiratzka LF, Wright CB: Experimental and clinical results of grafts in the venous system: A current review. *J Surg Res* (in press).
12 Viola AR, Gossling HR, Buckham CA: Femoral shaft fractures with associated arterial injuries. *Orthop Rev* 1981, 10:99.
13 Connolly J: Management of fractures associated with arterial injuries. *Am J Surg* 1970, 120:331.
14 Rosental JJ, Gaspar MR, Gjerdrum TC, Newman J: Vascular injuries associated with fractures of the femur. *Arch Surg* 1975, 110:494.
15 Patman RD: Fasciotomy: Indications and technique (Chapter 50), in Rutherford E (ed): *Vascular Surgery.* WB Saunders, Philadelphia, 1977.
16 Rich NM, Hobson RW, Collins GJ Jr: Traumatic arteriovenous fistulas and false aneurysms: A review of 558 lesions. *Surgery* 1975, 78:817.
17 Perry MO: , in Moore WS (ed): *Vascular Surgery: A Comprehensive Review.* Grune & Stratton, New York, 1983, p 674.
18 Rosenwasser R, Delgado T, Bucheit W: Cerebrovascular complication of closed neck and head trauma: Injuries to the carotid artery, *Surg Rounds* June 1983, p 56.
19 Requeana R, Cherekuri R, Lerner R: A logical approach in the management of intraabdominal vascular surgery. *Contemp Surg* 1983, 23:31.
20 Dale WA, Lewis MR: Lateral patch grafts. *Surg* 1965, 57:36.
21 Dale WA, Harris J, Terry RB: PTFE reconstruction of inferior vena cava. *Surg* 1984, 95:625.

Invited Commentary

Norman M. Rich, M.D.
Bethesda, Maryland

Throughout recorded history there have been few days when there was not a war going on somewhere in the world. Successful gambles in difficult situations often lead to standard surgical procedures. Successful results under the less-than-ideal conditions of warfare, in particular, have stimulated additional efforts and successes in civilian experiences.

It is ironic that many of the principles used today in the repair of injured arteries and veins were discovered at the turn of the twentieth century. Carrel's 1912 Nobel prize in medicine applauded his discoveries in experimental vascular surgery. During World War I and World War II, however, in the absence of antibiotics and without the development of blood banks, ligation of both arteries and veins was acceptable in managing the majority of vascular injuries. During the Korean War it was demonstrated for the first time that successful results could be obtained by reconstructive vascular surgery. This experience has been rapidly transferred to civilian trauma centers. The experience with 456 vascular injuries in 1 year at the Ben Taub General Hospital in Houston provides an appropriate reference.[1]

Increasing numbers of diagnostic and therapeutic procedures also contribute to the larger number of vascular injuries.[2]

Amputation rates, as the author states, represent a definitive measure of whether or not the vascular repair has contributed to salvage of an extremity. Unfortunately, there are some extremities which remain essentially functionally useless even though there is tissue viability.

A number of controversial points have been discussed. One is the role of routine angiography. Not enough prospective studies have been done to provide a clear answer. The "road map" is helpful in identifying vascular injuries.

Stabilization of concomitant fractures is another area of controversy where civilian and military experiences have differed. External immobilization has been preferred by the military, while many civilian centers have continued to use internal fixation devices successfully.

Soft tissue management is often a particular challenge. Muscle flaps and temporary biologic dressings may be needed.

The role of fasciotomy is not clear. Some believe that fasciotomy should never be done. A majority opinion is that appropriate fasciotomy is mandatory.

There are specific challenges associated with injuries to arteries and veins in various locations of the anatomy. The management of carotid arterial injuries remains a major area of discussion. Except in patients with profound coma or massive fixed neurologic deficit, many surgeons are attempting to repair the carotid artery, especially in patients who have a minor neurologic deficit.

The arteriovenous fistula remains one of the most fascinating changes associated with injured arteries and veins. Approximately 7 percent of vascular injuries later produce arteriovenous fistulas or false aneurysms.

The long-term follow-up of patients who have sustained vascular trauma has not been documented appropriately to date. The true magnitude of the results of these injuries will be greater than anticipated. Careful follow-up and long-term documentation will be required.

COMMENTARY REFERENCES

1 Feliciano DV, Bitondo CG, Mattox KL, Burch JM, Jordan GL Jr, DeBakey ME: Civilian trauma in the 1980's: A one year experience with 456 vascular and cardiac injuries. *Ann Surg* 1984, 199:717.

2 Youkey JR, Claggett GP, Rich NM, Jaffin JH, Cohen AJ, Brigham RB, Orecchia PM, Salander JM: Vascular trauma secondary to diagnostic and therapeutic procedures: 1974–1982. *Am J Surg* 1983, 146:788.

3 Rich NM, Spencer FC: *Vascular Trauma.* WB Saunders, Philadelphia, 1978.

4 Perry MO: *The Management of Acute Vascular Injuries.* Williams & Wilkins, Baltimore, 1981.

5 Hobson RW II, Rich NM, Wright CB: *Venous Trauma: Pathophysiology Diagnosis and Surgical Management.* Futura, Mount Kisco, New York, 1983.

5 ACUTE PERIPHERAL ARTERIAL ISCHEMIA

Sudden failure of the main arterial blood supply to a limb stops tissue perfusion and threatens its loss by gangrenous necrosis unless an adequate collateral circulation is immediately available. In addition to the threatened loss of limb, there is often a continuing threat to life itself, since most of these patients also have heart disease or widespread peripheral arteriosclerosis as well as diabetes or other lesions. The combination of acute ischemia with underlying chronic cardiovascular disease accounts for the considerable morbidity and mortality of ischemia.

My interest in arterial embolism dates back to at least 1958,[1] when three cases of aortic saddle embolism were successfully treated. Later the frequent occurrence of acute thrombosis, which often mimicked embolism, was recognized.[2]

The results of 140 consecutive, personally managed cases of acute ischemia of the lower extremity were reviewed in preparing this chapter. Excluded were patients whose history was longer than 5 days, those with late occlusion of a previous arterial repair, and instances of trauma. Each patient presented with a serious problem of acute ischemia which threatened ultimate loss of tissue. They are not patients whose claudication worsened or who insidiously developed a gangrenous toe or skin area. Table 5-1 summarizes the overall results in terms of salvage of life and limb.

From this experience and from the reports of others have evolved the principles of management which are presented here. These stress correct diagnosis and selection of the optimal surgical procedure for most patients, with nonoperative treatment in certain situations.

The overall plan of management is summarized in Table 5-2, which emphasizes initial measures designed (1) to prevent further thrombosis, (2) to make a correct diagnosis of the cause and extent of the vascular occlusion, and (3) to determine the need, timing, and type of operation.

PREVENTION OF FURTHER CLOTTING

Since distal thrombosis with occlusion of small arteries is likely to foil efforts at salvage, the clotting mechanism should be controlled at once by intravenous administration of 5000 U.S.P. units of aqueous sodium heparin. This effective anticoagulant is safe; the referring physician should be requested to give the initial dose in the office or in the emergency room without delay. Angiography and/or operation need not be delayed by the presence of heparin, since its action can readily be reversed by protamine sulfate, although this is not usually necessary. The patients in this series received at least a single initial intravenous dose of heparin without complications.

TABLE 5-1 140 ACUTE PERIPHERAL ISCHEMIAS

	No.	Limb salvage	Mortality
71 embolisms			
Aortic	6	2	3 (50%)
Iliac and femoral	37	30	3 (8%)
Popliteal	19	12	1 (5%)
Subclavian, axillary, brachial	9	8	1 (11%)
Total	71	52 (73%)	8 (11%)
69 acute thromboses			
Aortic	3	3	0 (0%)
Iliac and femoral	38	25	1 (3%)
Popliteal	28	27	1 (4%)
Total	69	45 (65%)	1 (3%)
Overall		69%	7.7%

DIAGNOSIS

The causes of sudden arterial occlusion are legion. Fairbairn, Juergens, and Spittell listed over 50 of these, to which the reader is referred for completeness.[3] Many of the causes are rare or involve small vessels rather than major arteries. A simpler classification is shown in Table 5-3.

The onset of acute peripheral arterial occlusion may be acutely painful, yet in many patients there is the gradual development of symptoms over a period of several hours. Others are awakened by a cold and painful foot. Variations in the mode of onset are due to differences in the available collateral circulation, cardiac output, and the extent of distal occlusive disease.

The physical signs of complete occlusion center upon absence of peripheral pulses with associated loss of color and decreased skin temperature. Sensory and motor function fail in varying degrees; these phenomena suggest nonviability. Swelling is not a part of early arterial occlusion but instead suggests venous blockage.

Improvement may occur if an embolus fragments or moves distally, but the improvement in symptoms which sometimes happens soon after occlusion usually parallels the opening of collaterals and does not go on to complete relief. When antispasmodics and vasodilator drugs are administered about this time, they often receive credit for improvement and falsely promise complete relief.

Arterial embolism usually follows a cardiac arrhythmia or infarction, although many other

TABLE 5-2 MANAGEMENT OF ACUTE ISCHEMIA OF THE LEG

1 *Prevent further clotting;* use heparin intravenously.

2 *Make a differential diagnosis from* history, examination, pulses, Doppler, electrocardiogram, and angiography *of* arterial embolism, acute thrombosis, atherosclerotic artery, atherosclerotic aneurysm, dissecting aneurysm, or phlegmasia cerulea dolens

3 *Compensate other lesions* without undue delay of operation.

4 *Avoid delay* for vasodilators, sympathetic blocks, or unnecessary lab work.

5 *Operate* with proper timing
on the correct site
with restoration of blood flow (embolectomy, arterial repair, venous thrombectomy)
and proof of distal patency (pulses, angiogram).

TABLE 5-3 DIFFERENTIAL DIAGNOSIS OF THE ACUTELY ISCHEMIC LEG

Lesion	History	Examination	Angiogram
1 Acute thrombosis (*a*) Atherosclerotic artery	Sudden appearance, mimicking embolism, but without cardiac lesion or arrhythmia	Paleness, no edema; tenderness; slight peripheral sensory deficiency occurring soon	Tapering to obstruction; other arterial irregularities
(*b*) Aneurysm	Previous mass in femoral or popliteal region	Possible femoral or popliteal mass	Possible calcified wall
(*c*) Dissecting aneurysm	Chest or abdominal pain	Same as history	Wide mediastinum; double lumen on aortogram
(*d*) Previous repair	Operation	Scars	Nonpatent repair
2 Embolism	Cardiac lesion or arrhythmia	Same as history	Nontapering occlusion of artery, without other arterial irregularities
3 Phlegmasia cerulea dolens	Occurrence with or without previous thrombophlebitis	Marked edema; cyanosis; diminished or absent pulses	Normal artery

causes are known. Indeed, one young patient lost both feet after two embolic episodes whose origin has never been determined despite repeated examinations and angiographies. However, if there is neither arrhythmia nor myocardial infarction, the diagnosis of peripheral arterial embolism must be suspect and acute thrombosis considered.

On the other hand, while the presence of an arrhythmia at once suggests embolism, the possibility of acute arterial thrombosis should be remembered, since it too is likely to occur in people with cardiac problems. It may be an initial episode but often is preceded by lesser arterial symptoms and is often associated with chronic arteriosclerosis on other vessels.

The frequency of acute arterial thrombosis has not been widely recognized, and many such episodes are still erroneously thought to be emboli. Humphries' enormous study of almost 2000 legs revealed that acute thromboses occurred suddenly in 11 percent of patients with previous aortoiliac atherosclerosis and in 31 percent of those with chiefly femoropopliteal disease.[4] Undoubtedly, many minor instances of acute occlusion are overlooked, with only major ones detected. Thus, Wessler found a correct diagnosis of acute occlusion in 94 percent if fresh clot was over 10 cm long but in only 10 percent if the clot was less than 5 cm long.[5] Acute atherosclerotic thrombosis of arteries is common and should be suspected frequently.

Angiography may not always be needed, particularly in clear-cut arterial embolism, but is so often helpful and safe that it should invariably be considered. We do not insist upon angiography prior to aortic embolectomy or when early postoperative thrombosis has blocked a graft in the recovery room, but most other patients require such diagnostic study. Either a direct needle puncture or a retrograde catheter can be used to place the contrast material to outline the lesion and its extent and, of greater importance, to ascertain the patency of the distal arterial bed. Absence of a developed collateral circulation makes this last impossible in most cases of embolism and necessitates angiography after the clot is removed.

While emboli usually lodge at arterial bifurcations, where the vessel narrows, and acute thrombosis mostly occurs elsewhere, both may be followed by proximal (as well as distal) clotting, which confuses the issue. A variety of angiographic patterns occur. Some contrast material often passes alongside the proximal portion of the thrombus (Figure 5-1), but a sharp transverse

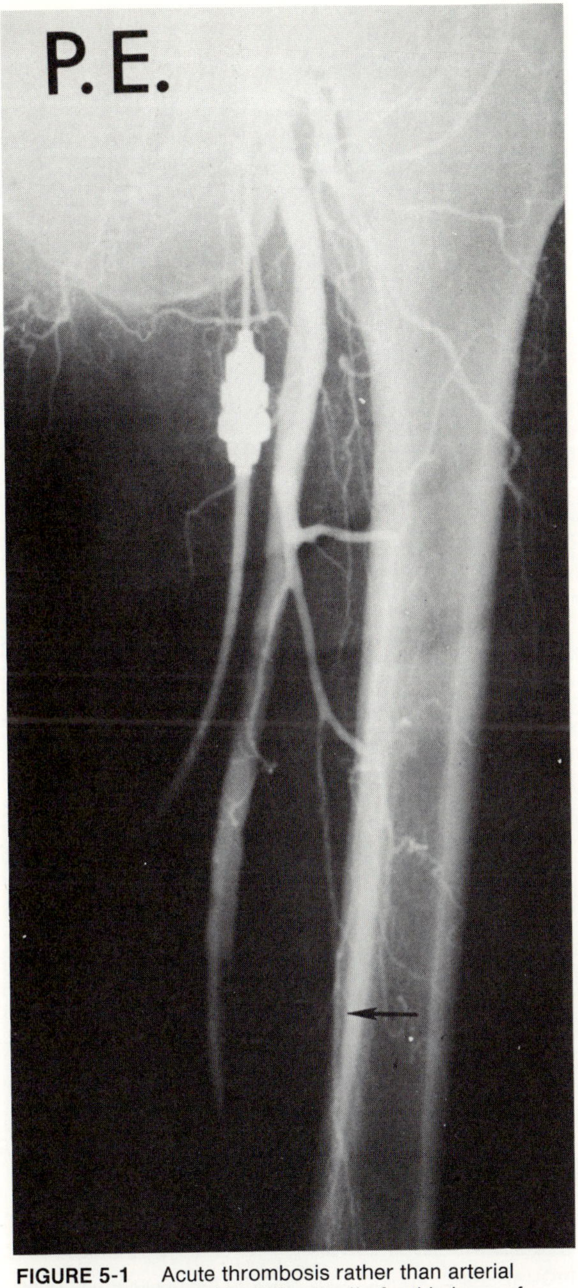

FIGURE 5-1 Acute thrombosis rather than arterial embolism, suggested by "ghosting" of a thin layer of radiopaque material alongside the thrombus in the femoral artery.

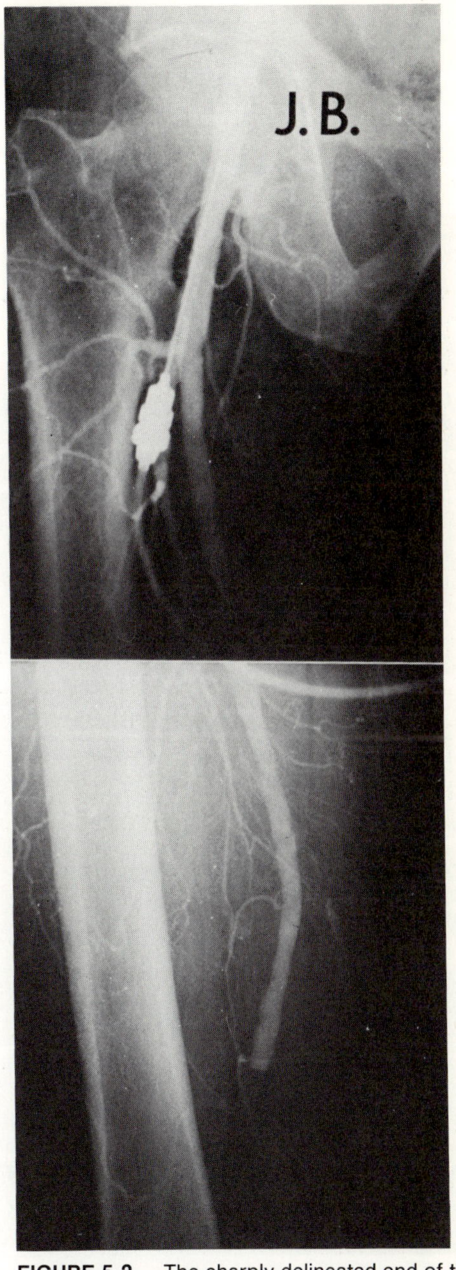

FIGURE 5-2 The sharply delineated end of the column of radiopaque material in this femoral artery suggested embolism, although the actual lesion was acute arterial thrombosis.

cutoff at the thrombus without proximal tapering may also be seen (Figure 5-2). Embolism usually shows a sharp distal end of the contrast medium, and the arterial wall is often smooth and lacking irregularities which would indicate arteriosclerosis (Figure 5-3). Differentiation at the

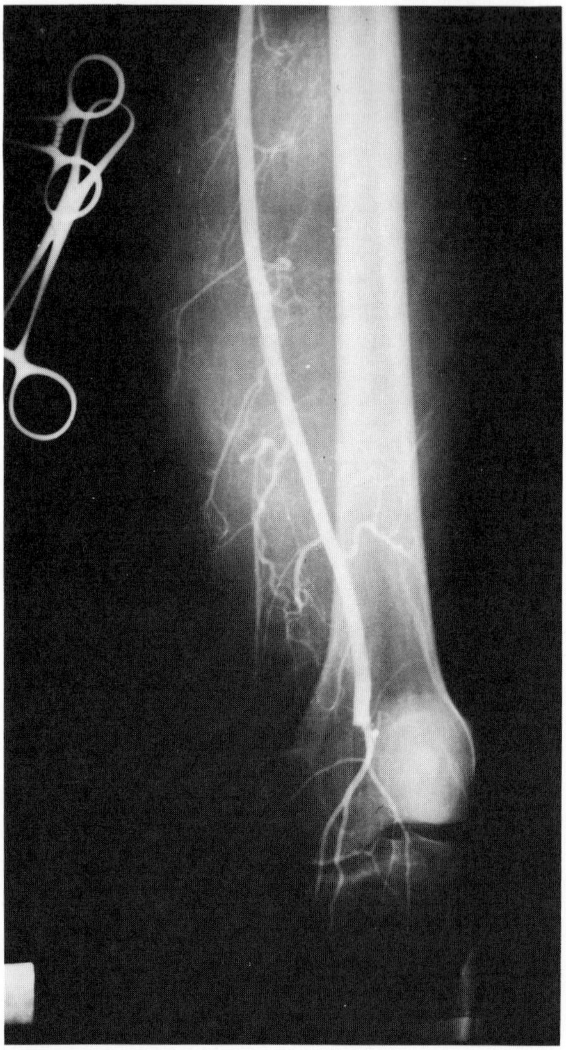

FIGURE 5-3 The sharply squared end of the column of radiopaque material just proximal to the popliteal birfurcation indicates embolism.

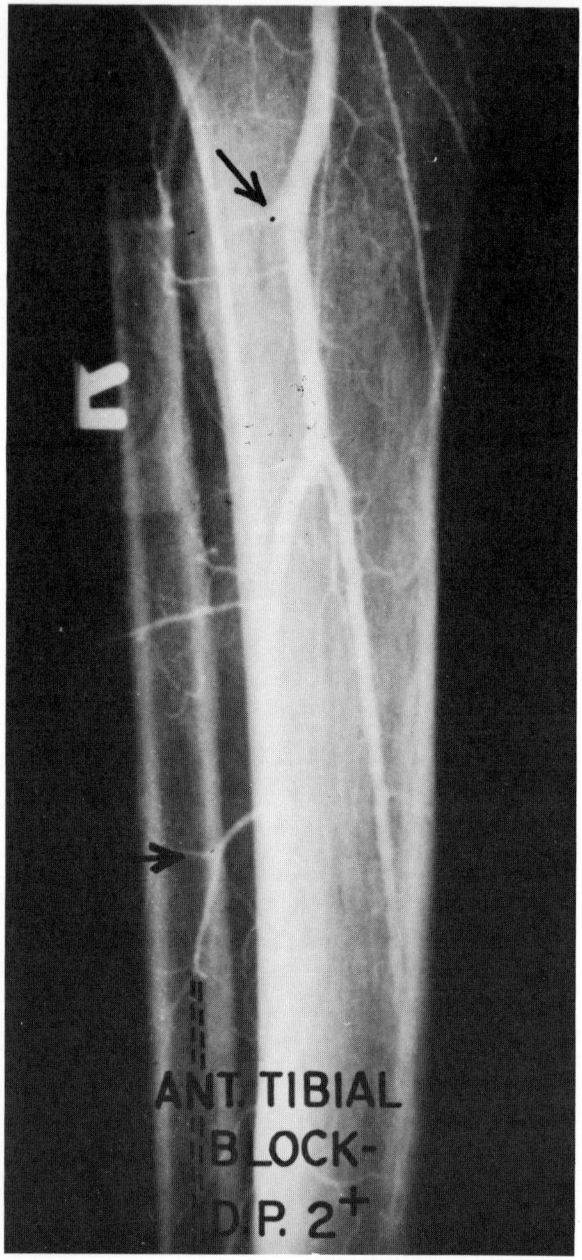

FIGURE 5-4 Angiography showed the occluded anterior tibial artery with distal collateral reconstruction, which allowed the dorsalis pedis pulse to be palpable.

distal femoral and popliteal level is especially difficult, but correlation of history with the arteriogram usually leads to a correct diagnosis.

Angiography also delineates the site and extent of occlusion. For example, Figure 5-4 shows acute thrombosis of the anterior tibial artery in a patient whose palpable popliteal and dorsalis pedis pulses made localization of the site impossible until the film showed anterior tibial occlusion (and presumable dorsalis pedis pulse reconstitution via collaterals).

The cause of severe ischemia of the foot in the presence of a strong popliteal pulse was demonstrated to be emboli in both the main calf vessels (Figure 5-5), and angiography indicated that popliteal arteriotomy was the correct method of revascularization (Figure 5-6).

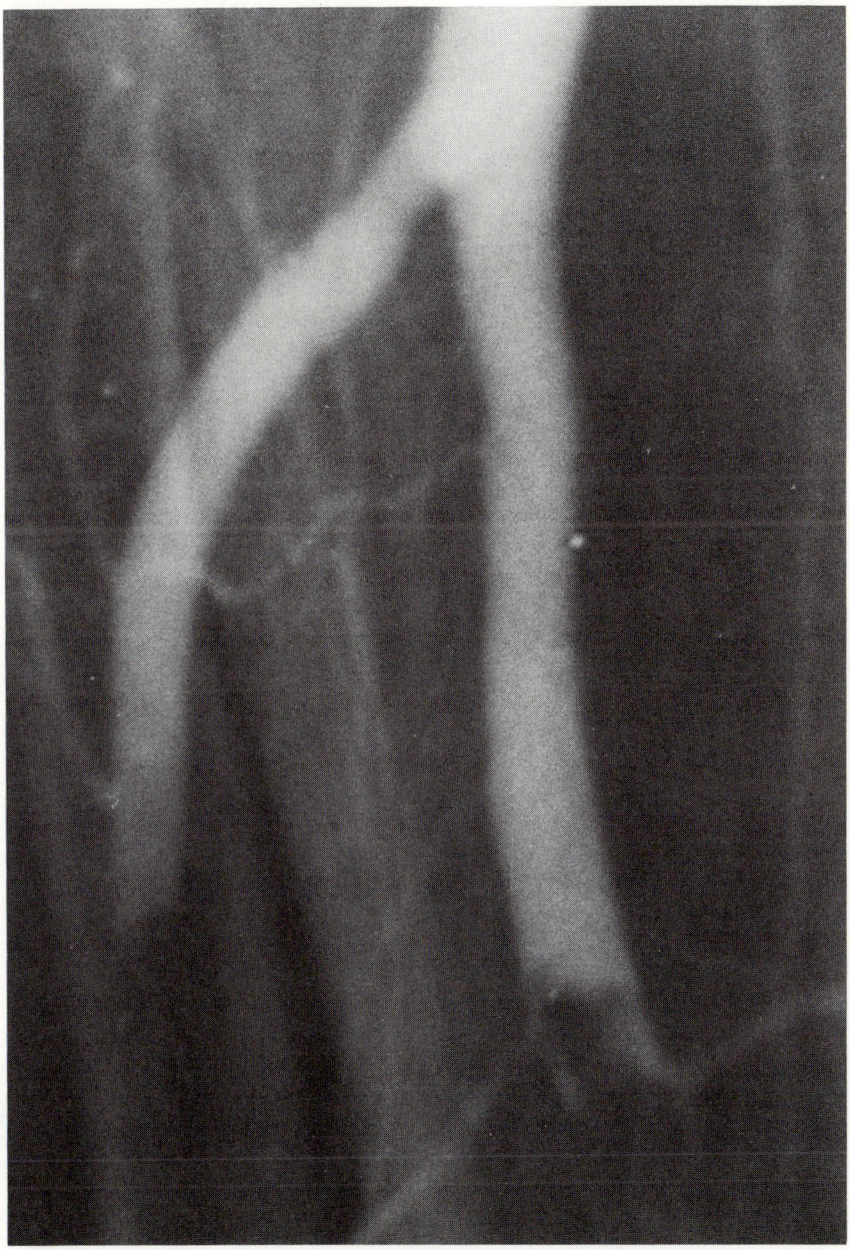

FIGURE 5-5 Emboli were present in both branches of the popliteal artery.

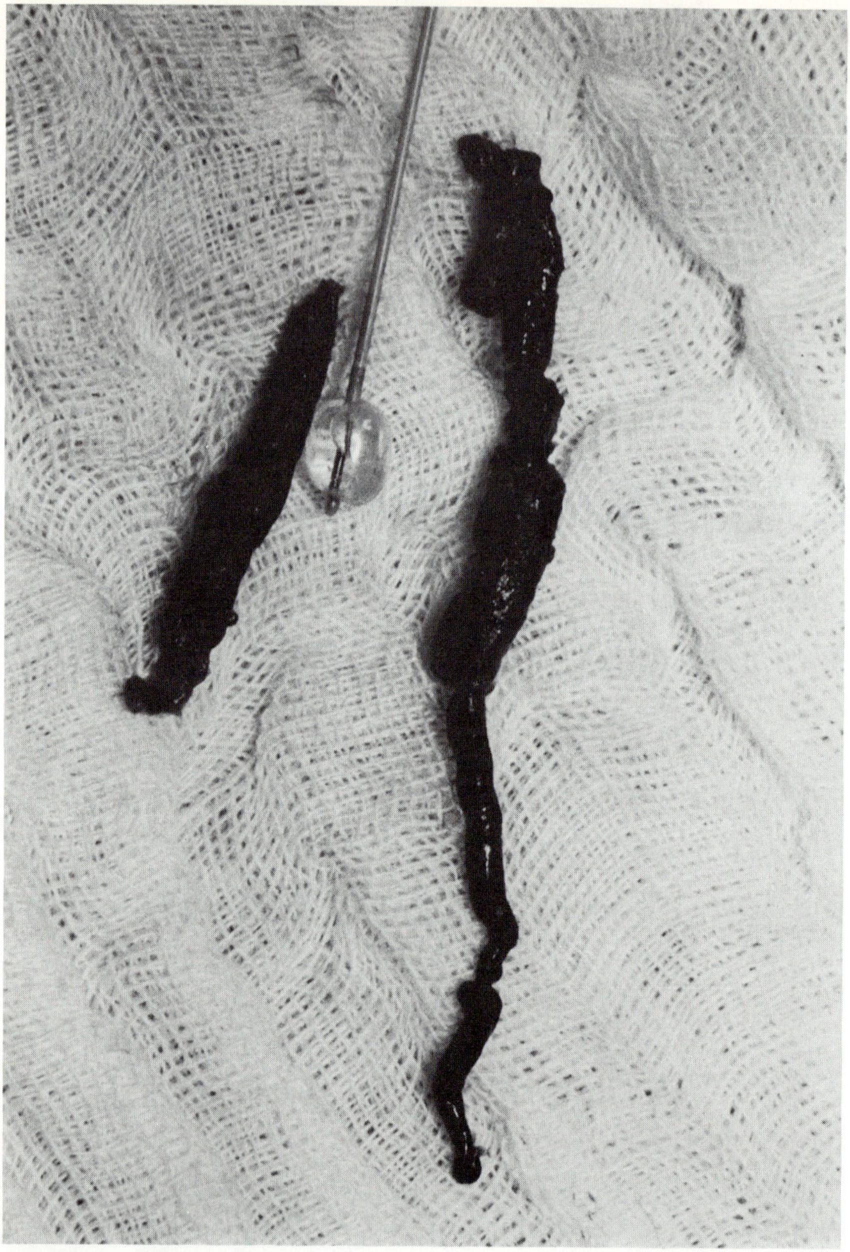

FIGURE 5-6 The emboli were successfully removed by a Fogarty catheter placed through the popliteal arteriotomy.

PREOPERATIVE PREPARATION

It is commonly stated that correctable lesions such as diabetes, heart failure, and pulmonary and renal problems should be compensated prior to operation. Long ago it seemed to me that this policy often led to needless delay of revascularization, which in this series has been aggressively pursued, using local or spinal block anesthesia without waiting for a work-up or for correction of deficits. If the ischemia is relieved, there is then time for the other lesions to be treated. The overall mortality rate of 7 percent supports this aggressive approach. This policy of immediate surgery parallels the policy of urgent operation for ruptured aneurysm, which replaced the old program of stabilization prior to operation.

Particularly to be avoided is delay to determine the effect of vasodilator drugs, sympathetic blocks, and such measures which are not helpful and which cause needless delay.

IMMEDIATE OPERATION

Early surgical correction is needed for (1) arterial occlusion of any cause where the distal tissues are clearly becoming nonviable, (2) early postoperative occlusions, and (3) most arterial emboli, even with viable distal tissue.

The elapsed time is of much less importance than is evaluation of the physical signs of nonviability. Differences in cardiac output, in collateral circulation, and in the metabolic need of the distal tissue make the time lapse between arterial occlusion and final tissue death variable. Coolness and pallor of the distal tissues do not indicate nonviability, but loss of sensation and of motor power do indicate this. Unless ischemia has persisted to the stage of final gangrene (none in this series), an immediate effort should be made to revascularize the distal tissues, either by embolectomy or by some form of arterial repair.

Levin and Giordano discussed the results of embolectomies delayed for 2 days to 7 weeks, finding a 12 percent mortality rate and 71 percent limb salvage rate among 241 patients,[6] thus documenting the concept of success even in late cases.

Delayed revascularization occasionally leads to the reabsorption syndrome in which the metabolic products of tissue degeneration are swept back into the body by revascularization of an extremity. Severe or fatal renal damage may occur. In North America early access to medical care and prompt transportation when needed have largely prevented the necessity for immediate amputation.

If the extremity is not viable either originally or after an attempt at revascularization, it should be removed without delay.

Illustrative Case

An 84-year-old female with atrial fibrillation was transferred with a 4-day history of the slow development of a cold, mottled lower extremity without pulses. Blood derangements included blood urea nitrogen (BUN) 32, total bilirubin 1.6, and calcium 8.1.

Immediate femoral embolectomy was performed under spinal anesthesia. The femoropopliteal arterial tree was cleared down to run off into the peroneal artery, but there was no filling of its other branches. On the following day the restored pulses had completely disappeared and edema had occurred. Immediate midthigh amputation was performed. She survived.

Comment The limb was initially believed to be salvageable but in grave danger; immediate amputation was indicated by the secondary thrombosis. This case represents a close judgment call.

CORRECT OPERATION

Simple thrombectomy alone is insufficient for acute thrombosis in an atherosclerotic artery. A more extensive procedure, usually a bypass graft, is necessary. Unless the arterial configuration is changed to allow rapid flow under high pressure through a vessel not lined with fresh thrombus, there is apt to be failure which anticoagulation will not remedy. It therefore is usually necessary to bypass the thrombosed vessel completely. Additionally, the host artery may require ligation proximal to the distal anastomosis to prevent embolism or extension of thrombosis.

Embolectomy

TABLE 5-4 ESSENTIALS OF EMBOLECTOMY

1. Heparinize immediately.
2. Open the artery without clamping.
3. Pass a Fogarty catheter via an artery outside the chest or abdomen.
4. Prove distal patency by palpable pulses or an arteriogram.
5. Close with a patch graft if needed.

In this series 73 percent of 71 limbs were saved. Invariably the embolus could be removed, so the cause of failure was distal small vessel occlusion which defied opening by the Fogarty catheter.

The essentials of embolectomy are outlined in Table 5-4. These procedures were usually performed with spinal or local anesthesia, and the deaths (11 percent mortality) were due to complicating problems rather than to the embolectomy itself. No patients were found to be too ill to undergo embolectomy.

Wide preparation and draping were done to allow secondary incisions when needed. The artery was not clamped prior to embolectomy, to avoid fragmentation of the clot. Fogarty catheterization usually removed the clot easily. Sometimes secondary distal arteriotomy was needed. Distal patency was proved by palpation of pulses or by angiography. Mere back bleeding from the arteriotomy was not accepted as proof of distal patency. The popliteal artery in Figure 5-7 bled from the distal end. Completion angiography (Figure 5-8) showed the remaining clot, which was removed with the Fogarty catheter.

The discovery of thrombosis rather than embolism is a signal to change the procedure to a bypass because the results of simple thrombectomy alone are poor and thrombectomy alone usually results in failure due to rethrombosis. One such patient referred after operation elsewhere and rethrombosis did well after a lumbar sympathectomy, but this is unusual.

Illustrative Case A 61-year-old male was admitted with a cool, painful foot 2 days following unsuccessful thrombectomy of a thrombosed popliteal aneurysm. Angiography showed the femoral and popliteal arteries to be completely blocked with a patent profunda femoris. Nothing was visible below the knee. Intravenous heparin was administered, and a lumbar sympathectomy was done. Ischemia slowly improved and he was discharged walking well.

The contralateral popliteal aneurysm recognized at admission was successfully bypassed with a vein graft 7 months later.

Comment Heparin and sympathectomy were preferred to secondary exploration of the calf vessels because of the fear of damage to collaterals and failure of vascular reconstruction, which would probably lead to loss of the limb.

Operations for Acute Arterial Thrombosis

The limb salvage rate of acute thrombosis was 69 percent. This reflects the known high risk of acute thrombotic episodes,[7] which is one of the chief reasons for elective repair prior to such.

There were eight acutely thrombosed popliteal aneurysms requiring bypass. Five bypasses were successful in saving the foot and leg. Graft length ranged from the ones where thrombosis was limited to the aneurysm itself (Figure 5-9) to long vein grafts from the common femoral artery to the popliteal vessel below the knee in cases where proximal femoral extension of thrombosis had occurred (Figure 5-10). The thrombosed aneurysm was invariably left in situ with its distal end tied in continuity to prevent extension of thrombosis. The medial approach described by Sterling Edwards[8] is the simplest one.

An unusual case of dissecting iliac aneurysm with popliteal embolism was treated.

Illustrative Case A 54-year-old male had a 60-hour history of slowly increasing ischemia of the leg and thigh with loss of all pulses. A dissecting aneurysm of the left iliac artery was treated by resection and Dacron tube grafting (Figure 5-11). Foot pulses did not return. An operative arteriogram disclosed a popliteal embolus, which was removed, with return of the foot pulses. Postoperative pulmonary thromboembolism was managed by anticoagulant therapy. He suddenly died at home 44 days after operation.

Comment Dissecting aneurysm of the iliac artery is an unusual event causing acute ischemia of the lower extremity. The unexpected distal popliteal embolus formation was disclosed by the completion angiogram.

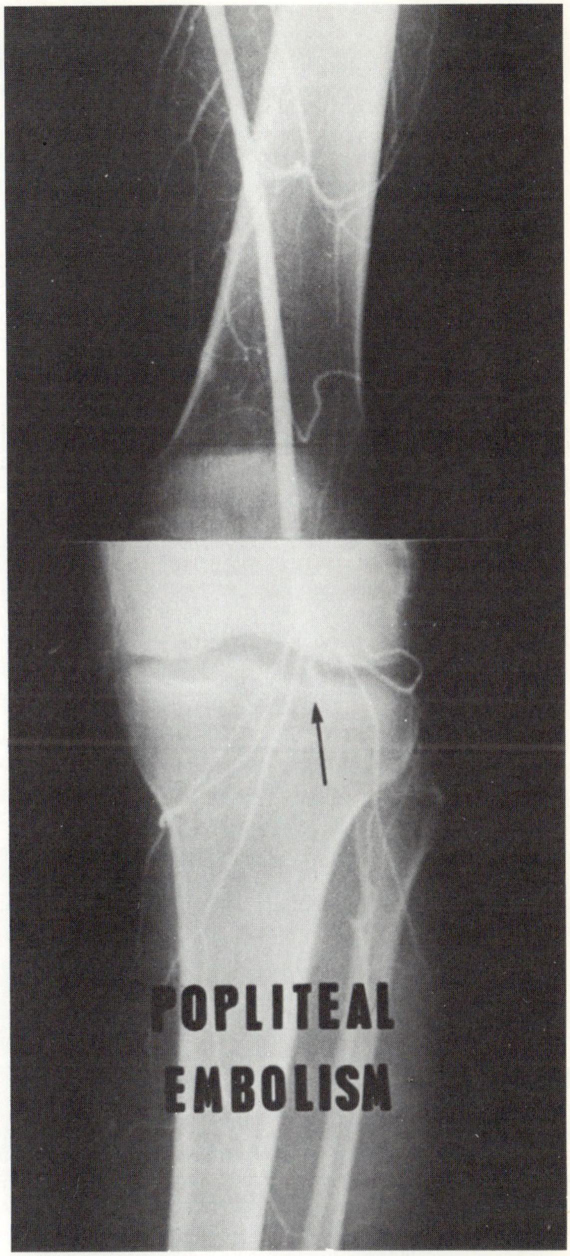

FIGURE 5-7 Preoperative angiography explained the severe ischemia of the foot and the presence of a strong popliteal pulse because both the tibial-peroneal and the anterior tibial arteries were blocked by emboli.

Heparin as Primary Treatment

It has been proposed that the policy of immediate surgical revascularization for acute ischemia be changed to heparinization because of the high risk of operation. Blaisdell, Steele, and Allen in 1978 cited an average mortality in excess of 25 percent from collected reports, which they believed was due to the systemic resorption of toxic metabolites flushed out by revascularization of the limb. They advocated heparinization with early amputation of nonviable extremities and achieved an overall 7 percent mortality rate.[9]

The recent improved statistics of early operative management of embolism summarized in Table 5-5 are well below the high risk figures of earlier years. The results of our policy of early operation are comparable to the Blaisdell series, especially if it be recognized that they did not differentiate the higher-risk embolisms from the lower-risk acute thromboses. These data suggest continuation of the policy of most surgeons of early operation for acute arterial embolism.

On the other hand there are the patients with acute thrombosis whose limbs are viable (although ischemic), for whom operation may be delayed. Immediate operation for these patients has several disadvantages. First is the uncertainty as to whether further thrombosis will occur, either distally or proximally, which might occlude an anastomosis. Second is the desirability of allowing collaterals to develop as fully as possible prior to a reconstructive operation. Third is

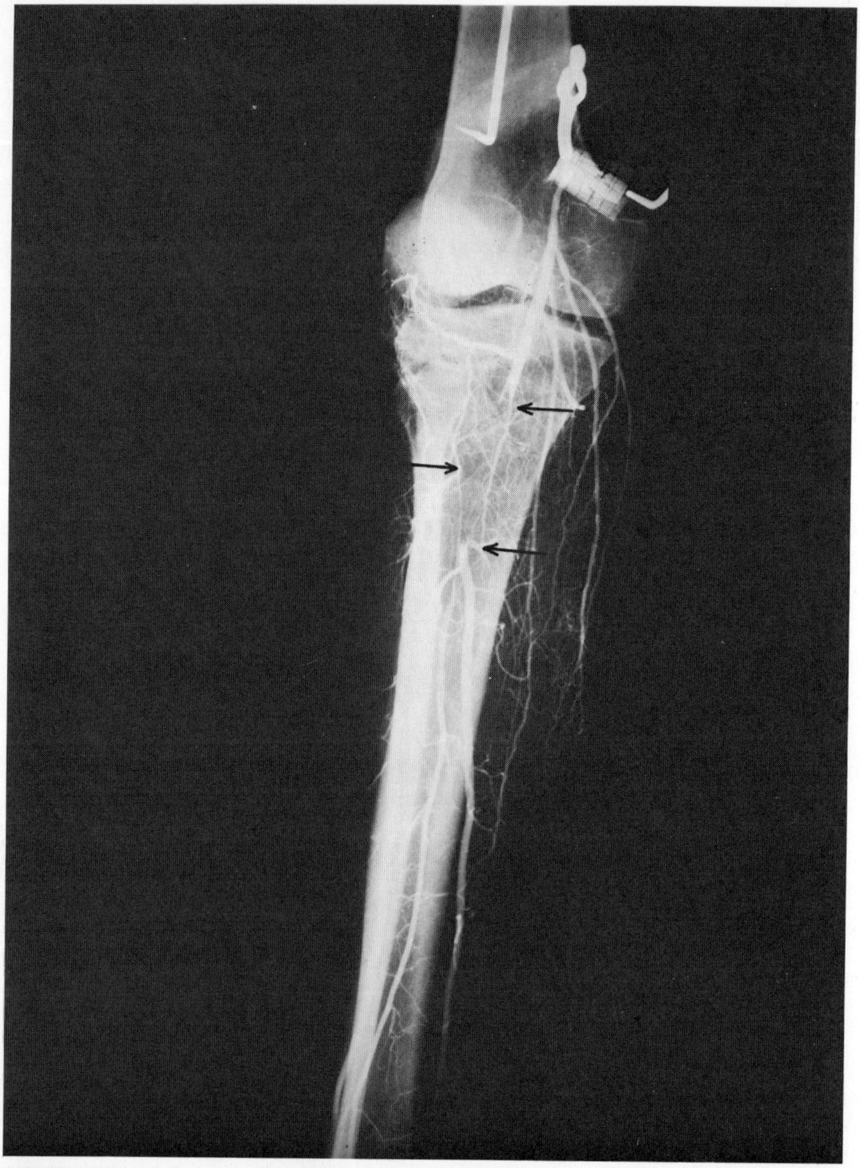

FIGURE 5-8 Following apparently successful removal of a clot by a femoral arteriotomy just above the knee, there was good back bleeding. A completion arteriogram, however, disclosed continued occlusion of the tibial-peroneal trunk and the anterior tibial artery. Fogarty catheter removal of these was successful.

the need to compensate reversible associated disease processes prior to a major grafting procedure. Fourth is the importance of detailed angiographic mapping, not always available in its most sophisticated form in an emergency. Last is the desirability of performing major surgery electively rather than with a partial team assembled from the personnel available at whatever odd hour the event occurs. The sum of these reasons persuades me as well as others to delay reconstruction for acute arterial thrombosis when the distal tissues are viable.

Couch, Wheeler, Hyatt, Crane, Edwards, and Warren in 1967 reported a 75 percent femoro-

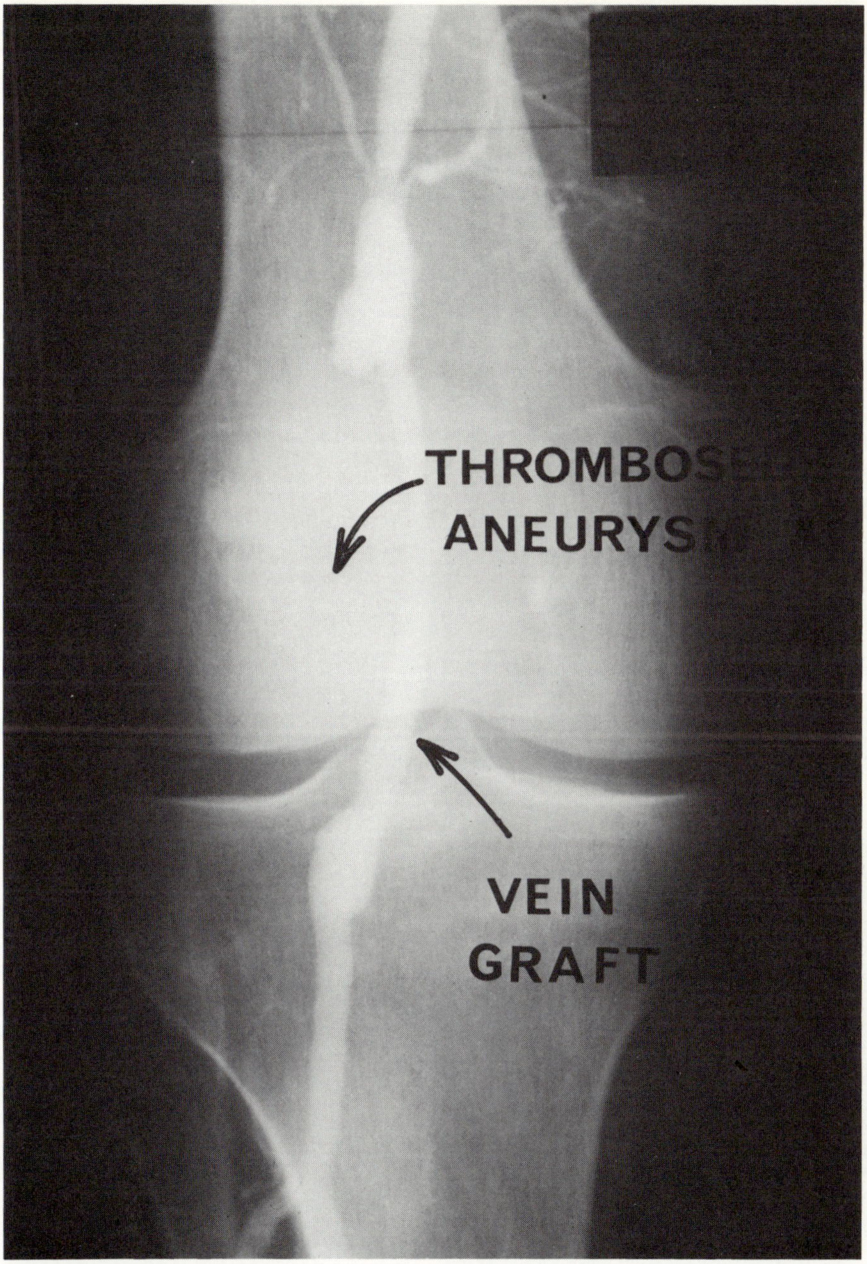

FIGURE 5-9 The preoperative diagnosis of popliteal embolism associated with atrial fibrillation was changed to acute thrombosis of popliteal aneurysm by operative exploration. Revascularization by a bypass vein graft was successful.

popliteal graft failure rate among 19 patients having onset of symptoms within 3 weeks and suggested delayed vascular repair when possible.[10] Humphries stated that "if the leg can survive the first few hours, it can probably survive the first few days" and described "fewer immediate operations for acute occlusions."[4]

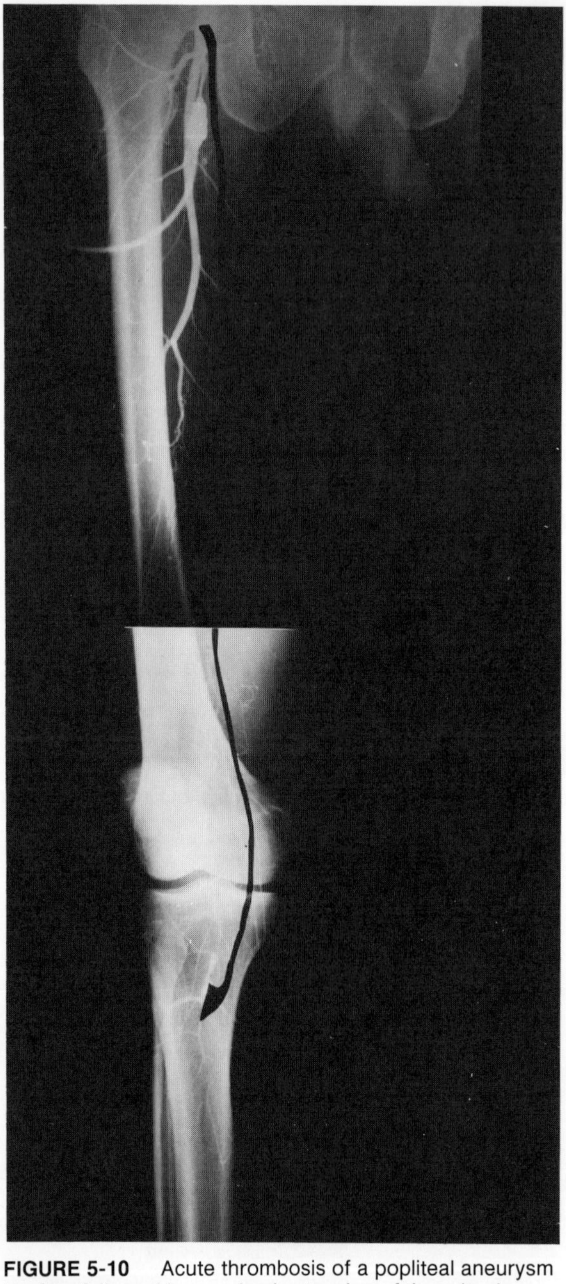

FIGURE 5-10 Acute thrombosis of a popliteal aneurysm is often followed by proximal extension of thrombosis, which necessitates the long autogenous venous bypass graft.

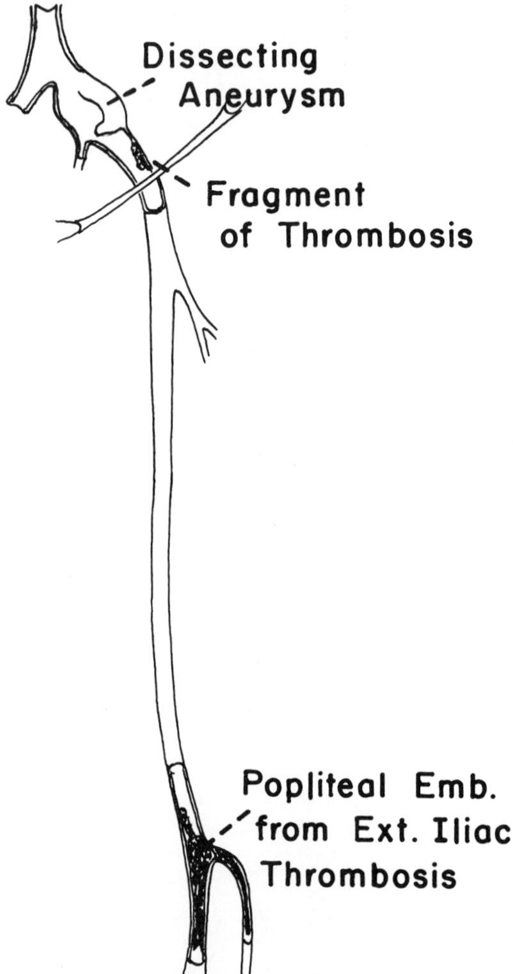

FIGURE 5-11 A dissecting aneurysm of the left common iliac artery was repaired with a Dacron tube. Completion angiography disclosed an unsuspected secondary embolism at the popliteal bifurcation. Direct popliteal embolectomy by Fogarty catheter was successful.

The principle of delayed reconstruction for acute thrombosis with viable distal tissue fits well with a program of heparinization for control of further clotting, so aqueous heparin was admin-

TABLE 5-5 RECENT REPORTS OF ARTERIAL EMBOLISM

Author	Year	Number of episodes	Number of patients	Limb salvage, %	Mortality, %
Green[12]	1975	166	149	86.5	22
Hight[13]	1976	152	124	78	29.8
Blaisdell[9]*	1978	58	54	74	7.5
Fogarty[14]	1978	395	360	94	15
Plecha[15]	1978	NA†	63	97	24
Santiani[16]	1978	135	122	81	10.6
Elliott[7]	1980	215	NA†	85	3
Lorentzen[17]	1980	152	130	77	14
Silvers[18]	1980	141	106	86.5	21.7
Caruana[19]	1981	67	61	75	11.4
Kendrick[20]	1981	121	90	71	18
Abbott[21]	1982	NA†	313	86	25
Sheiner[22]	1982	148	134	87	20
Present series	1983	71	65	73	11

*No differentiation between acute thrombosis and embolism.
†Not available.

istered by intravenous drip in doses of 5000 to 10,000 U.S.P. units initially, followed by the intravenous infusion of 1000 to 1200 U.S.P. units hourly thereafter.

The 13 patients with acute thrombosis who were treated primarily by intravenous heparin are summarized in Table 5-6. All their extremities remained viable. Eight had later arterial reconstruction; of these three failed and required later amputation. Two others had sympathectomy, and two had no operation. There was no loss of limb or life due to anticoagulant per se.

Two patients bled. A 71-year-old male leaked from a known abdominal aortic aneurysm. It was successfully removed and replaced with a graft. A 77-year-old male, whose extremity was in traction for fracture, had urinary bleeding, which required cessation of heparin. His leg remained viable (Figure 5-12).

Illustrative Case An 83-year old woman had a 6-hour episode of acute ischemia, overlaid upon a history of previous severe claudication. Despite coolness, pallor, and pain, the sensation was intact and tissues were viable. Intravenous heparinization was given for 5 days, following which a crossover femorofemoral heterograft was placed to bypass an iliac occlusion and revascularize the lower extremity. This allowed walking without claudication.

Comment Heparin controlled the thrombosis. A simple extraabdominal operation revascularized the leg.

Another situation for heparin treatment arises when there is a nonvascular contraindication to surgery. The patient in Figure 5-11 was in traction for a fracture when he developed distal popliteal thrombosis, which was successfully treated by heparin for 9 days.

Three cases in Table 5-6 emphasize that distal occlusion beyond the knee or elbow usually will not cause loss of limb, because of the development of collateral circulation. The results of a direct surgical attack upon small distal vessels are less satisfactory, and a policy of nonoperative management is usually best. Sometimes rest pain becomes progressive and forces operation (as in case 6). Certainly it is now feasible to place bypass grafts to the arteries of the ankle and foot.

The Role of Venous Thrombectomy

Enthusiasm for immediate removal of clots from veins has diminished considerably in recent years as it has become recognized that most patients respond as well to nonoperative measures

TABLE 5-6 ACUTE ARTERIAL THROMBOSES WITH PRIMARY HEPARIN TREATMENT

Patient	Age	Sex	Artery occluded	Days of heparin	Other procedures	Result
1 J.T.	71	M	Superficial femoral	4	Resection and graft of bleeding abdominal aneurysm	Good
2 G.V.	83	F	Iliac	5	Femorofemoral crossover	Good
3 O.R.	59	M	Superficial femoral	6	Later femoropopliteal graft	Good
4 M.G.	84	M	Superficial femoral	5	Later deep femoral thrombectomy (failure of femoropopliteal graft)	Above-knee amputation
5 J.G.	61	M	Popliteal (aneurysm)	3	Thrombectomy elsewhere; later sympathectomy	Good
6 V.W.	76	F	Anterior tibial	*	Later femoropopliteal graft (failed)	Above-knee amputation
7 J.T.	77	M	Popliteal	9	Traction (bled)	Good
8 P.P.	61	M	Anterior tibial	9	No operation	Good
9 W.H.	66	M	2 tibials	6	Later sympathectomy	Good
10 A.T.	84	M	Femoral	1	Femoral thrombectomy	Above-knee amputation
11 W.S.	53	M	Popliteal (aneurysm)	6	Femoropopliteal graft	Good
12 J.S.	74	M	Popliteal	4	Femoropopliteal graft	Above-knee amputation
13 A.M.	49	F	Iliac	10	Femorofemoral graft	Good

*Unknown.

based upon intravenous heparinization and elevation. Further, the late results in terms of leg edema and the postphlebitic syndrome are as good with heparin as with venous thrombectomy.

In 1975 we reported upon 159 episodes of venous thrombosis in 133 patients and proposed that the indications for venous thrombectomy be restricted to extremities with severe arterial ischemia associated with venous thrombosis.[11] We still follow this policy. However, if there is necessity for immediate relief of ischemia along with massive venous thrombosis, a venous thrombectomy is faster than the slow resolution achieved with heparin.

LATE ANTICOAGULATION

Whether lifetime drug therapy by warfarin is useful remains speculative and outside our scope. When we studied this problem 25 years ago,[1] it appeared that the evidence slightly favored warfarin therapy over no drug treatment. Since then it has become generally believed that such is helpful. Yet the facts from a properly designed double-blind long-term study are not available. Warfarin therapy has risks; the decision should be individualized.

CONCLUSIONS

The following principles of management have evolved from study of my own patients and the reports of others. First, differentiation between embolism and acute thrombosis is often difficult and requires operation or autopsy for accurate determination. Second, clinical evaluation should be complemented by angiography to allow optimal etiologic and anatomic diagnosis, proper tim-

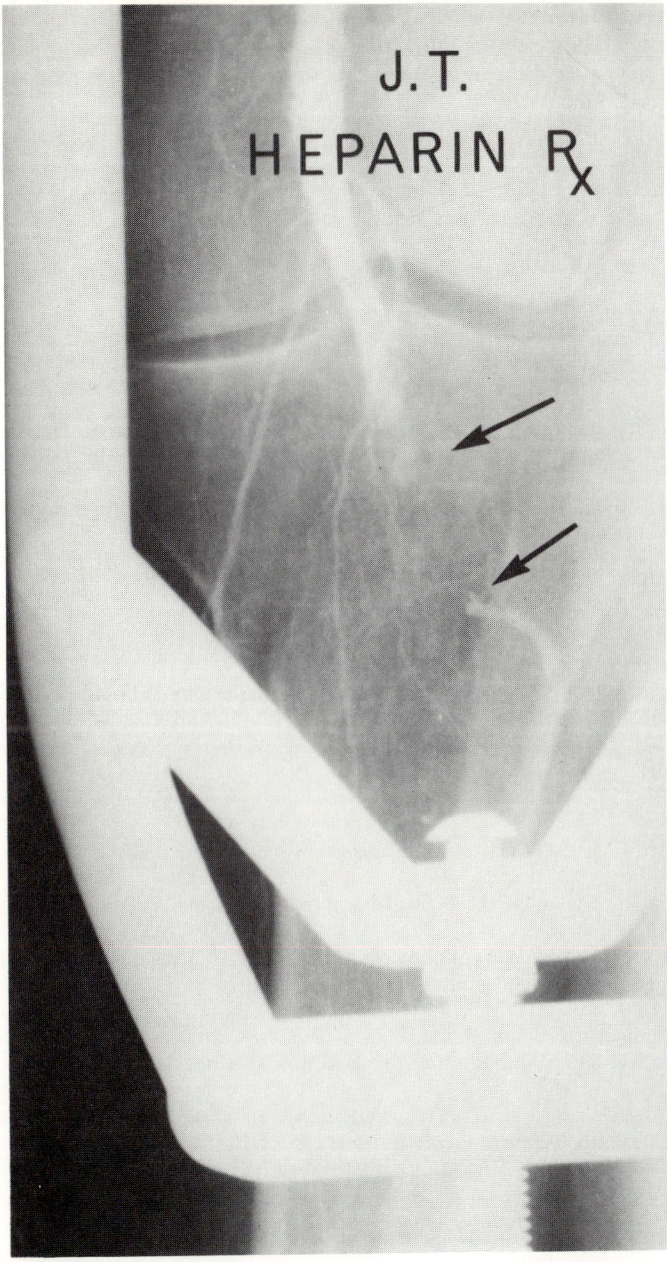

FIGURE 5-12 Arteriography disclosed acute thrombosis of the distal popliteal artery in the limb being held in traction for a femoral fracture. Heparin here was successful, although hematuria required premature termination.

ing of operation, and correct choice of operation. Third, immediate heparinization is harmless and probably aids in preventing propagation of distal thrombosis. It is not a suitable substitute for a needed operation. Fourth, long-continued heparin (instead of operation), recently advocated by some, does not produce better results than those presented here (7.7 percent overall mortality and 69 percent limb salvage). It is, however, useful for recent acute thrombosis with a viable limb to allow stabilization, compensation of other lesions, and complete angiographic study. Thirteen (19 percent) of the 69 acute thrombosis patients were thus managed, all but three having delayed arterial reconstruction. Fifth, thrombectomy alone is not sufficient for acute atherosclerotic thrombosis. A bypassing graft or thromboendarterectomy is necessary. Sixth, completion angiography is harmless, can be done easily, and discloses unsuspected remaining lesions, which can be immediately corrected. Finally, embolism is more dangerous than acute thrombosis, probably because of more serious accompanying cardiac lesions.

REFERENCES

1 Dale WA, Mahoney EB: Aortic saddle embolism. *Arch Surg* 1958, 76:930.
2 Dale WA: Differential management of acute peripheral ischemia. *J Vasc Surg* 1984, 1:269.
3 Fairbairn JF II, Juergens JL, Spittell JA: *Peripheral Vascular Disease.* WB Saunders, Philadelphia, 1972, 255.
4 Humphries AW: The relation of the natural history of arteriosclerosis to surgical management (Chapter 5), in Dale WA (ed): *Management of Arterial Occlusive Disease.* Year Book Medical Publishers, Chicago, 1971.
5 Wessler S, Sheps SG, Gilber M, Sheps MC: Studies in peripheral arterial occlusive disease. III Acute arterial occlusion. *Circulation* 1958, 17:512.
6 Levin BH, Giordano JM: Delayed arterial embolectomy. *Surg Gynecol Obstet* 1982, 155:549.
7 Elliott JP Jr, Hageman JH, Szilagyi E, Ramakrishnan V, Bravo JJ, Smith RF: Arterial embolization: Problems of source, multiplicity. *Surgery* 1980, 88:833.
8 Edwards WS: Arterial occlusions due to popliteal aneurysm, in Dale WA (ed): *Management of Arterial Occlusive Disease.* Year Book Publishers, Chicago, 1971, p 227.
9 Blaisdell FW, Steele M, Allen RE: Management of acute lower extremity arterial ischemia due to embolism and thrombosis. *Surgery* 1978, 84:822.
10 Couch NP, Wheeler HB, Hyatt DF, Crane C, Edwards EE, Warren R: Factors influencing limb survival after femoropopliteal reconstruction. *Arch Surg* 1967, 95:163.
11 Hume, M, Dale WA, Salzman EW: A spectrum of viewpoints on managing thromboembolism. *Contemp Surg* 1975, 6:82.
12 Green RM, DeWeese JA, Rob CG: Arterial embolectomy before and after the Fogarty catheter. *Surgery* 1975, 77:24.
13 Hight DW, Tilney NL, Couch NP: Changing clinical trends in patients with peripheral arterial emboli. *Surgery* 1976, 79:171.
14 Fogarty TH: Discussion of Blaisdell WF, Steele M, Allen RE: Management of acute lower extremity arterial ischemia due to embolism and thrombosis. *Surgery* 1978, 84:832.
15 Plecha FR: Discussion of Blaisdell WF, Steele M, Allen RE: Management of acute lower extremity arterial ischemia due to embolism and thrombosis. *Surgery* 1978, 84:832.
16 Santiani B, Gross WS, Evans WE: Improved limb salvage after arterial embolectomy. *Ann Surg* 1978, 188:153
17 Lorentzen JE, Rider OC, Hansen JH: Peripheral arterial embolism. A follow-up of 130 consecutive patients submitted to embolectomy. *Acta Chir Scand* 1980, 501:111.
18 Silvers LW, Royster TS, Mulcare RJ: Peripheral arterial emboli and factors in their recurrence rate. *Ann Surg* 1980, 92:232.
19 Caruana JA, Gutierrez IA, Andersen MN, Gage AA: Factors that affect the outcome of peripheral arterial embolization. *Arch Surg* 1981, 116:423.
20 Kendrick J, Thompson BW, Read RC, Campbell GS, Walls RC, Casali RE: Arterial embolectomy in the legs. Results in a referral hospital. *Am J Surg* 1981, 142:729.
21 Abbott WM, Maloney RD, McCabe CC, Lee CE, Wirthlin LS: Arterial embolism: A 44 year perspective. *Am J Surg* 1982, 143:460.
22 Sheiner NM, Zeltzer J, MacIntosh E: Arterial embolectomy in the modern era. *Can J Surg* 1982, 25:373.

Invited Commentary

F. William Blaisdell, M.D.
Sacramento, California

These recommendations for the management of acute arterial ischemia should be reviewed carefully by anyone dealing with this disease, since the results are better than any other large surgical series reported in the literature.

The key to the success is related to the liberal use of heparin preoperatively, operatively, and postoperatively, as the cause of death in most surgical series is related to thromboembolic complications (Table 5-A).

I favor a more conservative approach than is described for most instances of arterial ischemia, but I would suggest that this series is different. Most of my experience has been in large municipal or teaching hospitals, which deal with less affluent patients, who tend to present late with advanced symptoms. My experience is colored by a 1969 review of our experience with advanced arterial ischemia, in which the mortality rate was 80 percent.[1]

It is my contention that if the patient is seen in the first few hours following acute arterial occlusion, surgical treatment combined with heparin may well be the treatment of choice and result in the least morbidity. However, once 6 or 8 hours of severe ischemia have passed, there is inevitably loss of viability of much of the skeletal muscle. Reperfusion of large amounts of dead muscle releases toxic tissue-breakdown products and results in a hypercoagulable state. This, I believe, is the factor responsible not only for the respiratory distress syndrome, but for acute myocardial infarction, renal failure, venous thrombosis, and risk of subsequent pulmonary macroembolism. Certainly, when the limb has advanced to the point where it is blue and mottled, the muscle is firm, and the limb is anesthetic, attempts at reperfusion will result in mortality rates of 50 percent or more. Conservative management, consisting of anticoagulation or immediate amputation, is the treatment of choice in these instances.

My argument for a conservative initial approach to acute limb ischemia is as follows: If after 6 or 8 hours of ischemia the limb is still viable, the viability will be enhanced by appropriate anticoagulation. This will prevent propagation of a thrombus, further improve collateral flow, result in lysis of any clots present in small vessels, and result in a progressive improvement of the viability of the limb. If the limb has been profoundly ischemic for more than 6 or 8 hours, immediate reperfusion of the limb by surgical treatment will run the risk of significant mortality during the attempt to salvage the limb. When the choice becomes life or limb, orientation toward preserving life is most appropriate.

Our conservatively managed series resulted in a mortality rate of 7.5 percent.[2] This result has been difficult to match in the surgical series which was reviewed so well by Dr. Dale, in which the average mortality remains 20 to 25 percent. I would acknowledge, however, that his surgical series provides results similar to our conservatively managed group.

TABLE 5-A ARTERIAL EMBOLECTOMY (669 CASES)

Cause of death	Percent
Cardiopulmonary	53
Pulmonary embolism	11
Stroke	8
Renal	4
Mesenteric infarct	2
Recurrent emboli	4
Sepsis	5
Other	12

Source: Blaisdell FW et al: Management of acute lower extremity arterial ischemia due to embolism and thrombosis. *Surgery* 1978; 84:822.

I do not agree with the author's conclusion that arterial thrombosis carries less risk than embolism; it would be my contention that it is similar or even worse, provided the severity of the ischemia is the same. I would acknowledge that in our nonoperative series it was difficult to sort out acute embolism from thrombosis. However, in our series we tabulated the severity of the ischemia so that it would be compared with that of others. The primary reason why thrombosis is less dangerous than embolism is that thrombotic states usually are preceded by marked atherosclerotic narrowing and stimulation of collateral. But given the same degree of ischemia, the mortality following reperfusion in embolism and thrombosis should be similar. However, the operation required to treat thrombosis is more complex than embolic extraction.

I would like to point out that the only perfect results in Dr. Dale's series were the 13 cases he managed with heparin therapy alone. All of those patients survived, and all of the limbs did well, permitting elective surgery to be carried out at a later date. Since even with arteriography it is difficult to differentiate acute thrombosis from acute embolism until after the fact, I would suggest that had Dr. Dale not operated on any patient, he might well have had the best series and the only perfect results in the literature.

As regards simultaneous venous thrombectomy, I have attempted this and found that while adequately clearing the vein of a clot, large amounts of blood are usually lost. Complete venous thrombectomy associated with advanced arterial ischemia requires that at least 3 to 4 units of blood be sacrificed. All too often, follow-up phlebography reveals recurrence of the venous thrombosis. For that reason, we have abandoned simultaneous venous thrombectomy except for instances of phlegmasia cerulea dolens.

COMMENTARY REFERENCES

1 Stallone RJ, Blaisdell FW: *Surgery* 1969, 65:207.
2 Blaisdell FW, Steele M, Allen RE: Management of acute lower extremity arterial ischemia due to embolism and thrombosis. *Surgery* 1978, 84:822.

6 ABDOMINAL AORTIC ANEURYSMS

The treatment of abdominal aortic aneurysms has now evolved to the modern low-risk procedure, so today an infrarenal aortic aneurysm should usually be treated by reconstructive grafting.

In the distant past various forms of compression aimed at producing internal thrombosis (Figure 6-1) salvaged occasional patients,[1] as did internal wiring with electrocoagulation.[2] The latter was the best available method until 1951, when Charles Dubost of Paris reported the successful replacement of an abdominal aortic aneurysm with a homologous aortic graft.[3]

CURRENT MORTALITY RATES

During the ensuing thirty-odd years the hazards of aneurysmectomy and graft replacement have diminished as the procedure has become standardized. The risk of nonoperative management now far exceeds that of surgical grafting for most patients. As stated by Crawford, "the natural course of this disease . . . progresses to rupture and death in about half of the patients within a year of diagnosis and in 91% . . . within five years."[4] Furthermore, the long-term survival curves for patients treated by grafting versus patients treated without surgery clearly recommend surgical relief (Figure 6-2).

Surgical mortality rates of 3 to 5 percent are now commonplace. Some large series, such as the 517 cases reported by Darling and Brewster,[5] had a 1.7 percent death rate in the decade ending in 1980, while Mannick in that year noted a 0.9 percent mortality rate during the previous 7 years.[6]

The hazards of rupture, with an immediate severe increase in mortality due to hemorrhage, shock, and organ failure, strongly suggest that all aneurysms should be removed unless there is a real contraindication in one of the important functional systems. An aneurysm is therefore usually an indication for operation, whatever its size.

SMALL ANEURYSMS

In the 1970s there was still doubt that patients harboring small aneurysms should have an operation. Standardization of technique with a resultant low risk of operation now indicates that even small aneurysms should be removed.

Reports of rupture of 18 percent of aneurysms smaller than 5 cm by Darling[7] and of rupture of 31 percent of those less than 6 cm by Szilagyi,[8] along with others, indicate the significant risk of rupture even in small aneurysms. The threatening, deep, punched-out ulcer 1 cm wide in the anterior wall of a 5-cm aneurysm which was recently resected electively (Figure 6-3) shows how a weak area at any point may go on to rupture.

Another argument for removal of a small aneurysm is the relative simplicity with which this

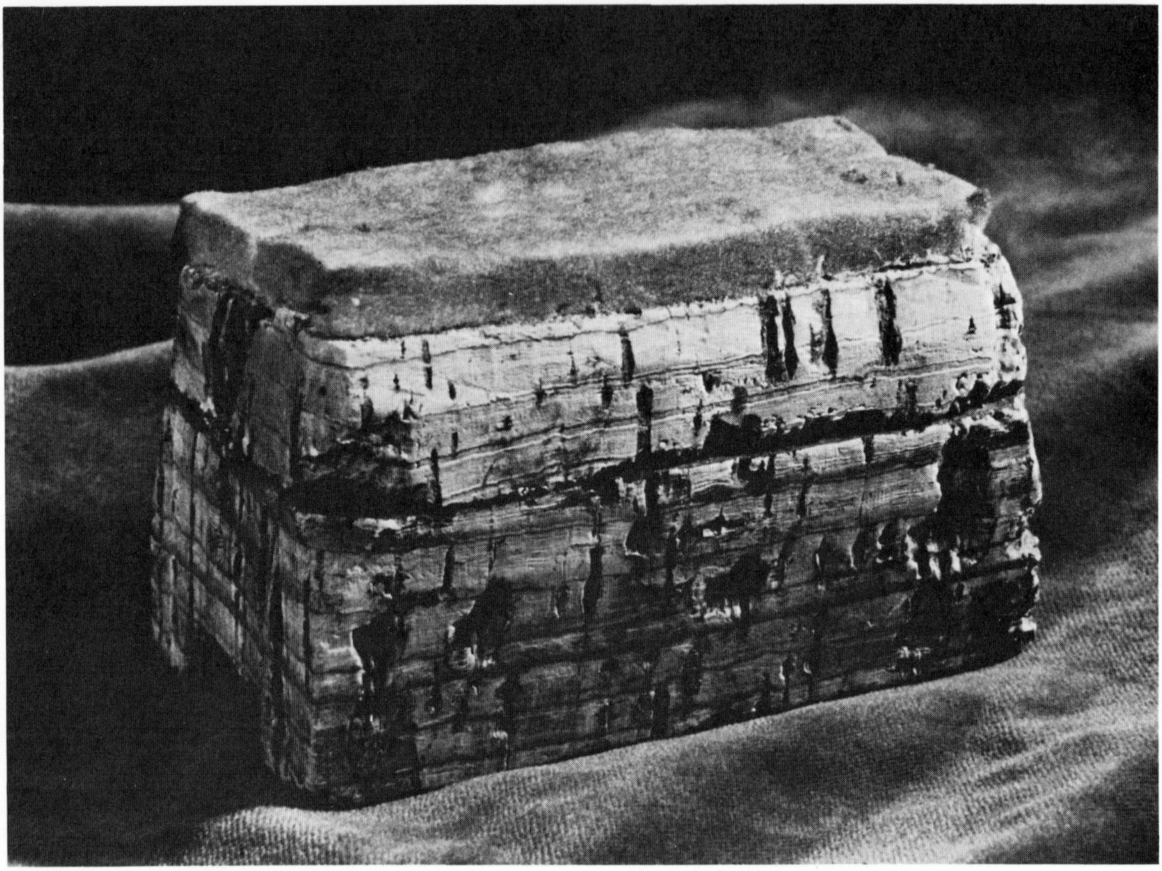

FIGURE 6-1 Syme's compressor, made of cork, with padding glued on top. The undersurface is hollowed out to allow it to override the peripheral arterial aneurysm during the time of pressure designed to produce thrombosis. The device resides in the museum of the Royal College of Surgeons in London.

can be done so that a minimum morbidity and mortality is expected. Figure 6-4 illustrates the shortest graft personally placed in an aorta, which could not quite be anastomosed primarily following complete removal of a small aneurysm.

Eugene Bernstein and I discussed the pros and cons of operating upon small aortic aneurysms in 1976,[9] finding agreement that "good risk patients should have elective resection . . . regardless of the size of the aneurysm."[9,10] Patients with small asymptomatic aneurysms who have significant problems in the cardiac, pulmonary, or renal system may be better treated without operation unless symptoms occur. Only a few fall into this latter category of patients whose functional problems cannot be corrected sufficiently to allow operation.

Peripheral embolism may result from an otherwise asymptomatic aortic aneurysm.[11] Small aneurysms are no exception and may create a situation where repetitive peripheral embolism requires decision for or against removal of an otherwise relatively unimportant enlargement of the aorta. In this case the resection really is required for the ulcerative lesion which releases the clots. Figure 6-5 demonstrates such a patient, whose severe cardiac disease at age 80 indicated a nonoperative course. Fortunately, a single shower of peripheral emboli did not recur.

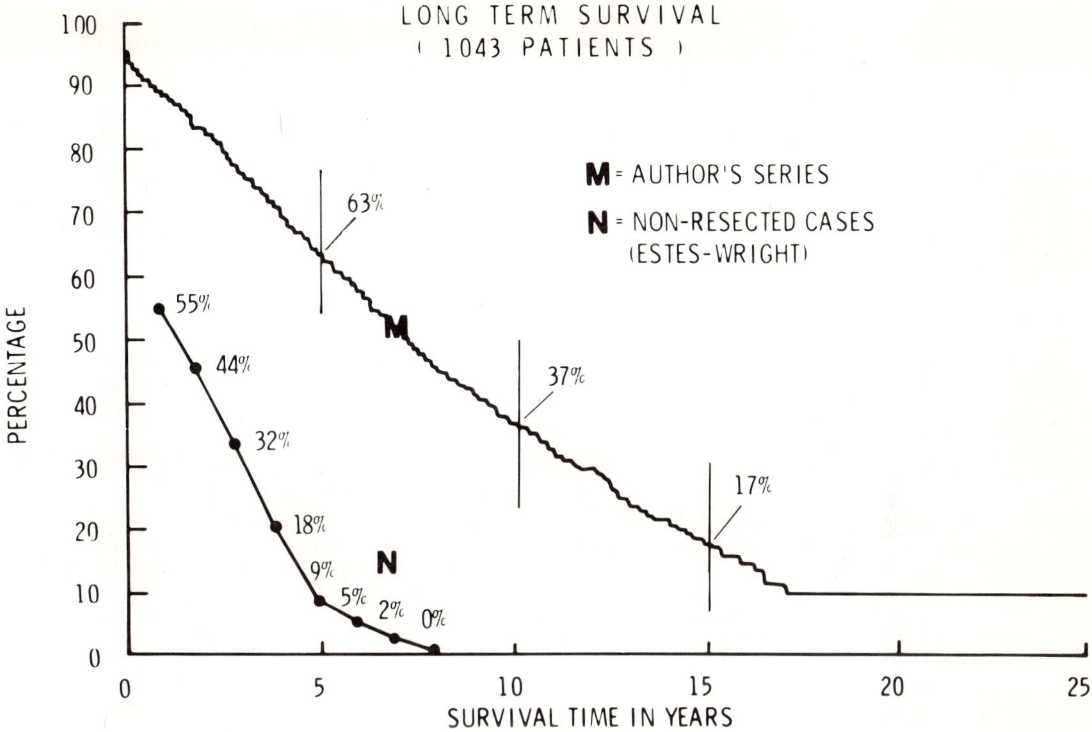

FIGURE 6-2 Long-term survival in treated versus untreated abdominal aortic aneurysms. (Reprinted courtesy of Crawford ES, Stowe C, in Moore WS (ed): *Vascular Surgery.* Grune & Stratton, New York, 1983.)

CONTRAINDICATIONS

Complicating problems may require correction prior to operation or, if uncorrectable, may increase the risk to an unacceptable level. Chronologic age per se is not a contraindication, since the body which has already passed beyond the average life span has proved itself superior to the average.

Uncompensated functional lesions such as advanced obstructive pulmonary disease, delicately balanced cardiac compensation, renal failure, and advanced liver disease may be noncorrectable. Obesity must be added to this list, as well as malignant tumors.

Local conditions such as colostomy or chronic furunculosis invite infection. Retroperitoneal fibrosis increases the technical difficulty, as does a horseshoe kidney, and suggests consideration of the increased risk as well as of a different operative approach.

Proximal extension of the aneurysm to involve the renal and other visceral arteries requires a larger procedure and increases the risk.

Noncooperation by the patient or family places the surgeon in an uncomfortable and compromised situation and may warn of later difficulty if an unexpected complication occurs during or after the operation. This last category also includes the few patients who refuse to allow complete control of the situation by the surgeon by stipulating against the use of blood products or other materials. Recognizably, some aneurysms do not require transfusion; the real objection is denial of the surgeon's total responsibility for care.

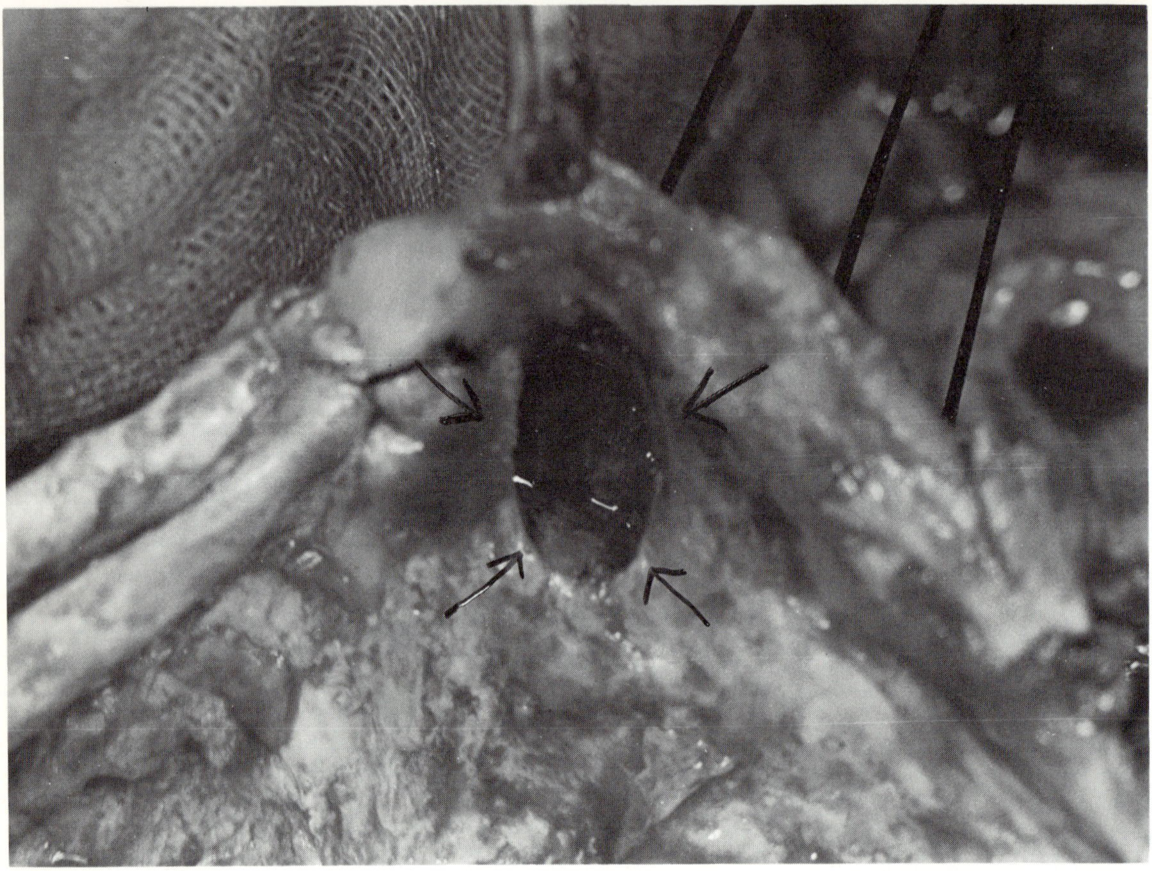

FIGURE 6-3 Anterior view of opened aneurysmal sac, with arrows delineating edges of the 1-cm-deep ulceration which was threatening early perforation.

PREOPERATIVE STUDY

In Table 6-1 are summarized the several laboratory tests which are usually performed after a careful history and physical examination are completed. These are relatively straightforward and require no particular comment. It is often helpful to the laboratory to have the request for blood typing and screening for antibodies as soon as possible, so difficult blood matching will not become a problem in the late afternoon or night before the scheduled operation. A myriad of additional studies may sometimes be needed, such as pulmonary function studies upon elderly patients and particularly those who are long-term smokers. Further renal evaluation may be needed for some.

The indications for cardiac stress testing and coronary arteriograms have been previously discussed in Chapter 3 and will not be repeated. In brief, such cardiac evaluation is indicated by the clinical situation and is not uniformly required for all patients with aneurysms.

Preliminary Aortography

From time to time the routine performance of aortography prior to resection of abdominal aortic aneurysms has been questioned on the basis of its failure to influence the plan of management or operative procedure, its slight risk, and its excessive cost. Rutherford has stated that "aorto-

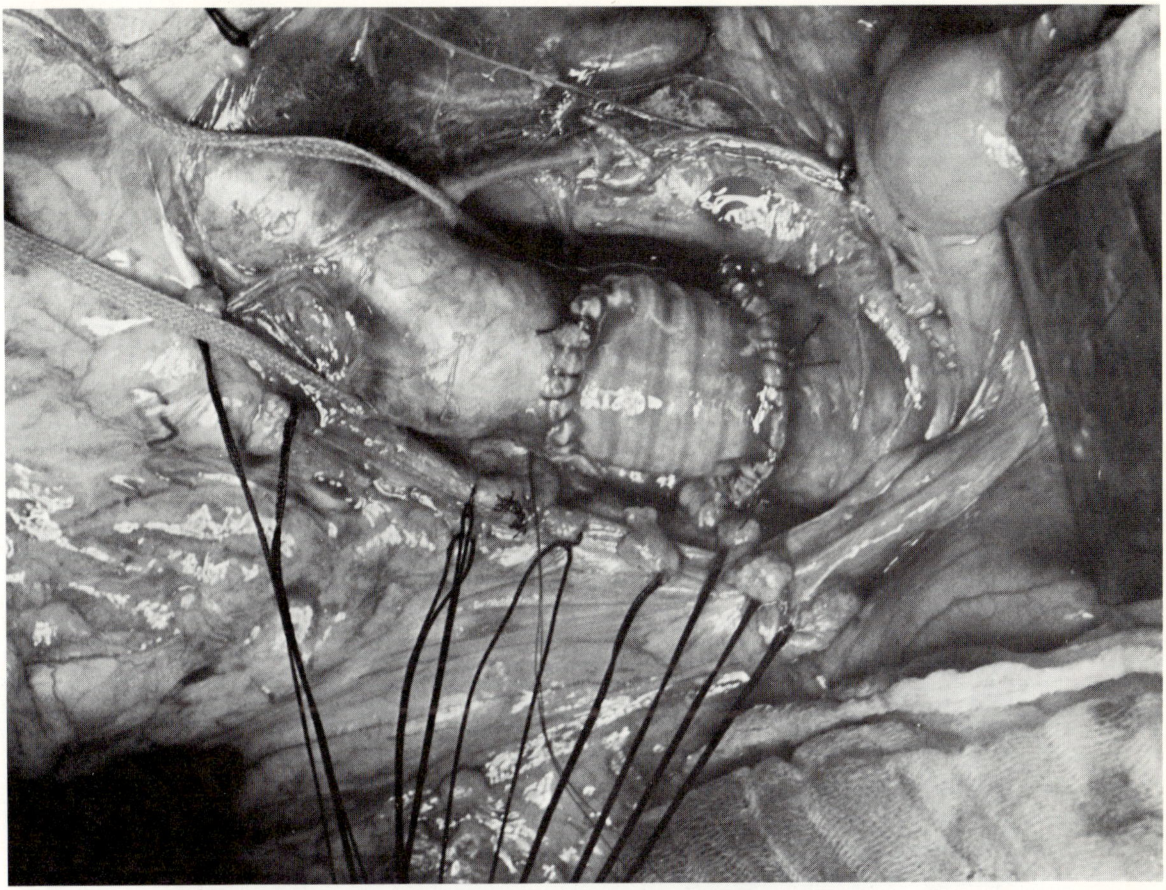

FIGURE 6-4 This small aneurysm was replaced by a short tube graft, since the ends of the resected aorta would not quite come together.

grams . . . now are requested only for specific indications" and relies upon Doppler ultrasound evaluation of the distal arteries, and excretory urography for the presence of horseshoe kidney.[12] Couch and his associates in Boston retrospectively analyzed 110 of their patients and surveyed the pertinent literature in 1983. The morbidity and mortality of aortography was zero. About seven nonhelpful aortograms were performed for each one that caused a change in the plan of management. They concluded that preliminary aortography could be reasonably limited to patients in whom it was indicated by clinical features such as hypertension, impaired renal function, abnormal femoral pulses, suspected mesenteric ischemia, and suspected suprarenal extension of the aneurysm.[13]

A number of objections may be raised to this oversimplified concept. The value of preoperative angiography does not lie in determining the size of the aneurysm, since interior clot usually makes that inaccurate, but rather in determining the origins and functions of the visceral arteries, the proximal extension of the aneurysm, the presence of other aneurysms or of occlusions in the iliac and femoral arteries, and the occasional presence of an anomaly such as a horseshoe kidney. This information should supplement, rather than compete with, noninvasive studies and intraoperative evaluation, which alone may be unreliable. A policy of no angiography represents a "desert island" concept, where there is limitation due to the absence of tools and resources.

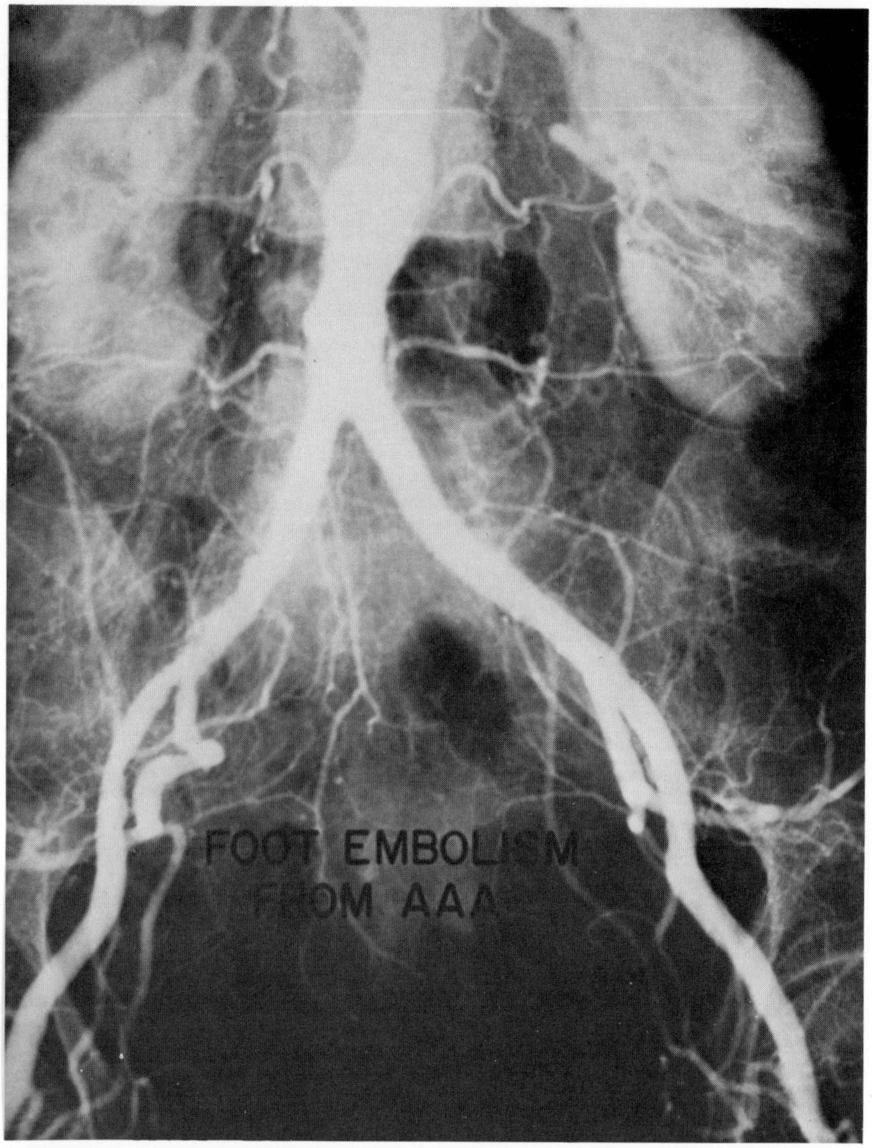

FIGURE 6-5 Small aneurysmal dilatation of the aorta associated with a single shower of emboli to both feet. Because of the overall risk a nonoperative course was elected, and no further embolism occurred throughout the remaining life of this 80-year-old man.

Properly conducted angiography is a low-risk procedure. Robicsek recorded 1700 translumbar aortograms without significant complications or deaths.[14] There has not been loss of limb or life due to it in my personal experience during the past 30 years. Large collected series also reflect few problems (Table 6-2). Bauer and associates noted that angiography "had substantial influence upon management decisions and performance of surgery in 75% of 100 abdominal aortic aneurysms."[15]

There are no facts to determine the cost of angiographic-supported surgery versus that without it. Certainly the cost of angiography is small compared with the overall cost of treatment and surgery, or the high costs that could result if a complication should occur due to failure to appreciate an anomaly. These considerations lead to rejection of a nonangiographic preoperative evaluation as a retrogressive step and to the belief that aortography should be done.

TABLE 6-1 LAB TESTS FOR ABDOMINAL AORTIC ANEURYSMS

1. Complete blood count, hematocrit
2. Prothrombin time, partial thromboplastin time, platelets, bleeding time
3. Blood type, antibody screen
4. Electrolytes, blood urea nitrogen, creatinine, fasting blood sugar
5. Liver function
   - Serum glutamic oxaloacetic transaminase
   - Alkaline phosphatase
   - Bilirubin
6. Urinalysis
7. Chest x-ray
8. Electrocardiogram

Ultrasound

Ultrasound helps determine the size of an aneurysm. It is a screening test which is useful in the initial diagnosis of an aneurysm and in following changes in its size if it is to be managed without operation.[16] It is not useful for aneurysms which lie within the thorax.

CT Scan

Computerized tomography (CT) scans are useful in searching for intrathoracic aneurysms, the extent of thoracoabdominal aneurysms, for sealed-off hematomas and for studying grafts after operations. Most patients do not need CT scans.

OPERATIVE MANAGEMENT

A number of factors may be identified as important in the reduction of risk. Let us briefly examine some of these.

Monitor Lines Monitor lines cause little or no delay at the start of the procedure when placed by experienced attendants. Placement may be done in a preparation room prior to induction of anesthesia. A peripheral arterial line, indwelling bladder catheter, and nasogastric tube ordinarily are placed, along with a Swan-Ganz pulmonary artery catheter in some instances to allow accurate assessment of the cardiac situation. Problems with acute renal failure often encountered during the late 1950s and early 1960s were finally recognized as due to inadequate fluid replacement and at present are of historic interest only.

Incision and Exposure Exposure is the sine qua non for an efficient and safe operation, yet how often does one find a surgeon struggling with a restricted field, lacking sufficient help, and

TABLE 6-2 RISK FROM AORTOGRAMS

Source	Ref	Number	Complications, %	Mortality, %
Robiscek 1978	14	1,700 translumbar	0	0
Szilagyi 1977	35	9,438 translumbar	0.2	0.1
(collected)		21,324 catheter	1.2	0.07
Hessell 1981	36	83,068 transfemoral	1.7	0.03
(collected)		4,590 transaxillary	3.3	0.09
		4,118 translumbar	2.9	0.05

handicapped by lack of suitable retractors? Not only must the surgeon bring personal skill and knowledge to the operation, but also the team must be proficient and experienced in their supporting roles. Vascular operations are now beyond the capacity of one specialist with a pickup team; they require skilled and experienced people at all positions. There is a large difference between the hospital where occasional such cases occur and the center where multiple vascular procedures are performed daily with low attendant risks.

The traditional approach to an abdominal aortic aneurysm has been via a long midline incision. The alternative approach of a high bucket handle incision places the center of exposure considerably nearer the proximal aortic neck and allows wider exposure in the vicinity of the renal arteries (Figure 6-6). This transverse incision is particularly useful for large, difficult aneurysms.[17] Contrary to expectation, it is possible to retract the inferior abdominal flap sufficiently to allow distal iliac anastomoses without any particular problem.

A less useful approach is the modern version of the extraperitoneal approach originally described by Sir Astley Cooper 150 years ago. In 1963 Rob advocated a high left oblique incision;[18] this was later modified by Shumacher[19] and by Williams and associates.[20] While these exposures do not traverse the peritoneal cavity, they both require extensive and vigorous retraction. They are best left to their advocates.

FIGURE 6-6 A bucket handle transverse incision centers considerably higher than does the usual longitudinal incision, allowing easier access to the neck of the large aneurysm and to the renal arteries. (Courtesy *Surg Gynecol Obstet* 1968, 126:1321.)

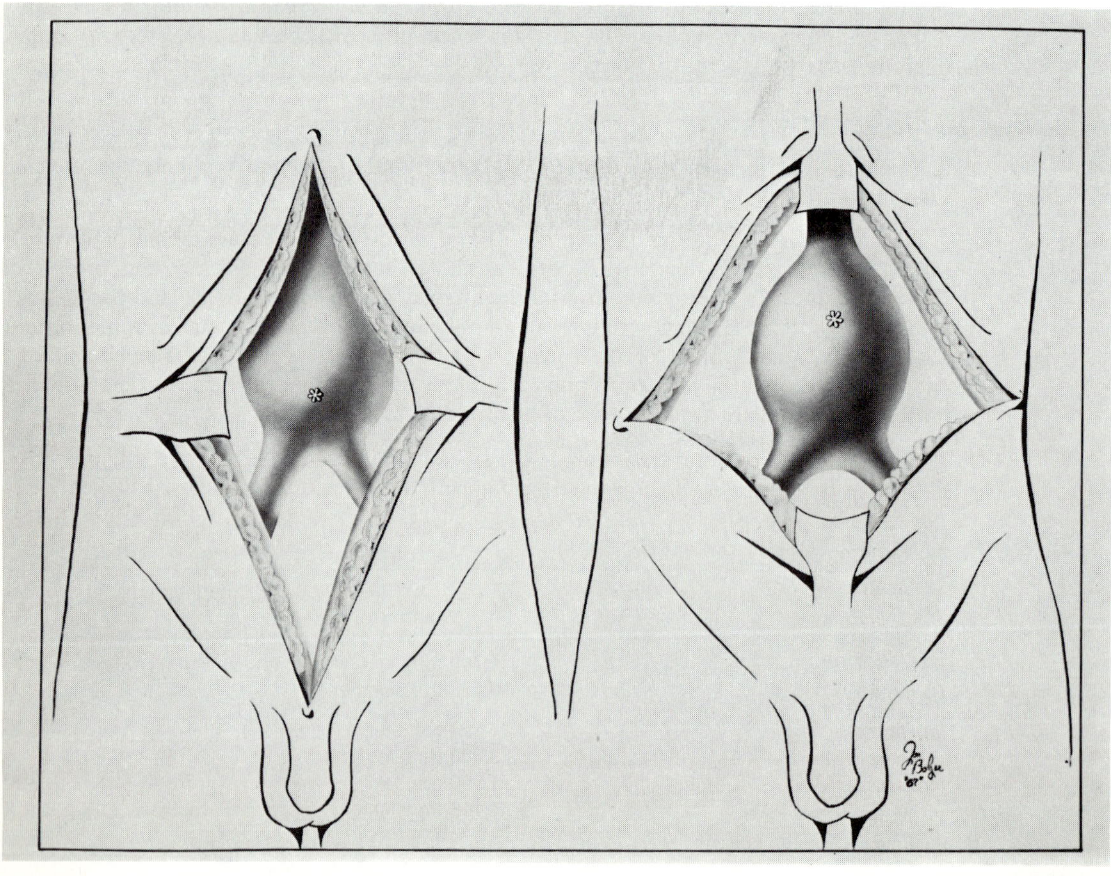

Overall simplification of the operative technique not only reduces blood loss but also produces an efficient procedure which minimizes anesthesia time. A long midline exposure may quickly be accomplished without extensive use of the electrocautery or placement of many ligatures if the lower part of the incision is deepened through the fat and fascia to the peritoneum, to enable two fingers to be placed inside the peritoneal cavity. With the abdominal wall thus elevated, it is a simple matter to open the incision widely, place one or two clamps on each side, and rapidly explore the viscera. Moist sponges on the wound edges during this brief period allow oozing to stop, so only one or two spurting vessels require control.

An efficient operator thereafter opens the posterior peritoneum, releases the duodenum to the right, and identifies the crossing left renal vein superiorly. If the inferior mesenteric vein hampers the exposure, it is at once divided.

There is little need for further dissection. Vascular clamps may be placed proximally on the aorta and distally on the iliac vessels without any effort to encircle the vessels. This avoids injury to the veins which lie posteriorly. Some surgeons prefer to place the distal clamps first, with the belief that this prevents distal embolization and "trash foot." Embolization is also prevented by flushing from both ends of the vessel prior to final closure of the graft.

The aneurysm is opened anteriorly without further dissection. Its walls may be held apart by clamps, by suture-ligatures, or by an indwelling spring retractor. The back-bleeding lumbar vessels are suture-ligated, and the inferior mesenteric opening is controlled from within (and not tied off at a distance).

The chief difference in technique when the aneurysm has ruptured is connected with the necessity to control the aorta quickly. Several techniques of transthoracic exposure for temporary aortic control and of high intraabdominal control have been described. It is simpler, and therefore more effective, to open the abdomen quickly and place a "T"-shaped "occluder" across the suprarenal aorta (Figure 6-7) to stop all flow briefly until the proximal neck can be located and clamped.

Inlaying the Graft Inlaying the graft allows deep bites to be placed from inside the proximal neck of the clamped aorta. There is no attempt to cut across the posterior portion of the aorta (Figure 6-8).

Tube Replacement Instead of a "Y" graft, tube replacement is feasible for more than 50 percent of abdominal aortic aneurysms. Some aneurysmal dilatation of the iliac arteries may be accepted and left in place, since continuing dilatation and rupture there is unusual. An experienced surgeon considers tube grafting as the standard, with bifurcation grafting as a sometimes necessary variation.

Graft Material Material for the aortic reconstruction is not critical. Blood loss may be minimized by use of a woven graft or a preclotted knit Dacron graft or one of the newly available albuminized or collagenized knit grafts. The newer polytetrafluoroethylene (PTFE) graft is another choice. Long ago it was recognized that many different materials will serve as an aortic replacement; the surgeon should use the most readily available and easily used material.

Continuous Monofilament Polypropylene Suture This suture has generally replaced interrupted techniques, which are unnecessarily cumbersome and time-consuming. Multifilament sutures are more likely to harbor organisms. The chief criticism of the monofilament suture has been that it occasionally breaks, but if the surgical team avoids holding the suture with steel instruments, that problem is solved.

Plication of the Aneurysmal Sac Folding the aneurysmal sac over the completed graft aids hemostasis (Figure 6-9).

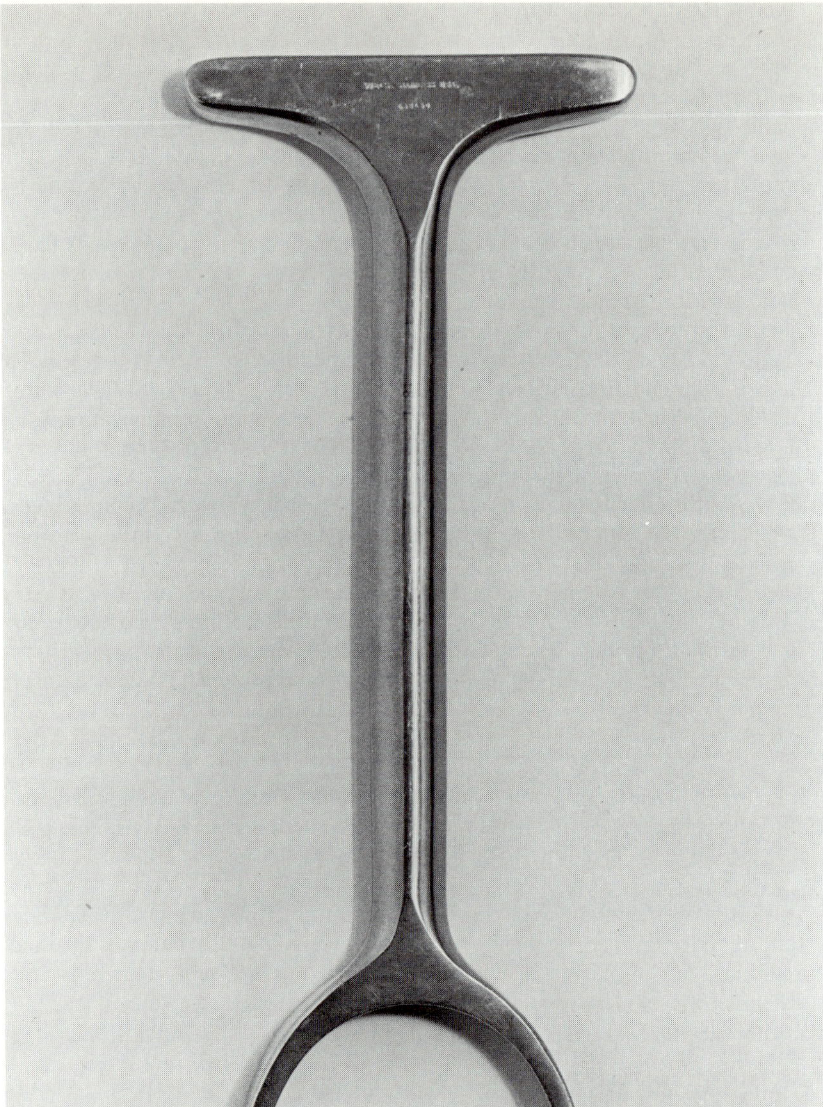

FIGURE 6-7 An aortic compressor to occlude the aorta against the underlying vertebral bodies, for temporary control of a ruptured abdominal aortic aneurysm or to allow access to the renal arteries.

Autotransfusion Returning the patient's own red cells reduces the need for bank blood, with its attendant risks of hepatitis and transfusion reactions. This also allows proper flushing of the anastomoses and graft prior to their final closure.

Temporary Gastrostomy This precaution is worthwhile for selected poor-risk patients, who are thereby relieved of the necessity for a nasogastric tube, which lies within the nasopharynx and may provoke pulmonary problems. A self-sealing Witzel's or Stamm's gastrostomy should

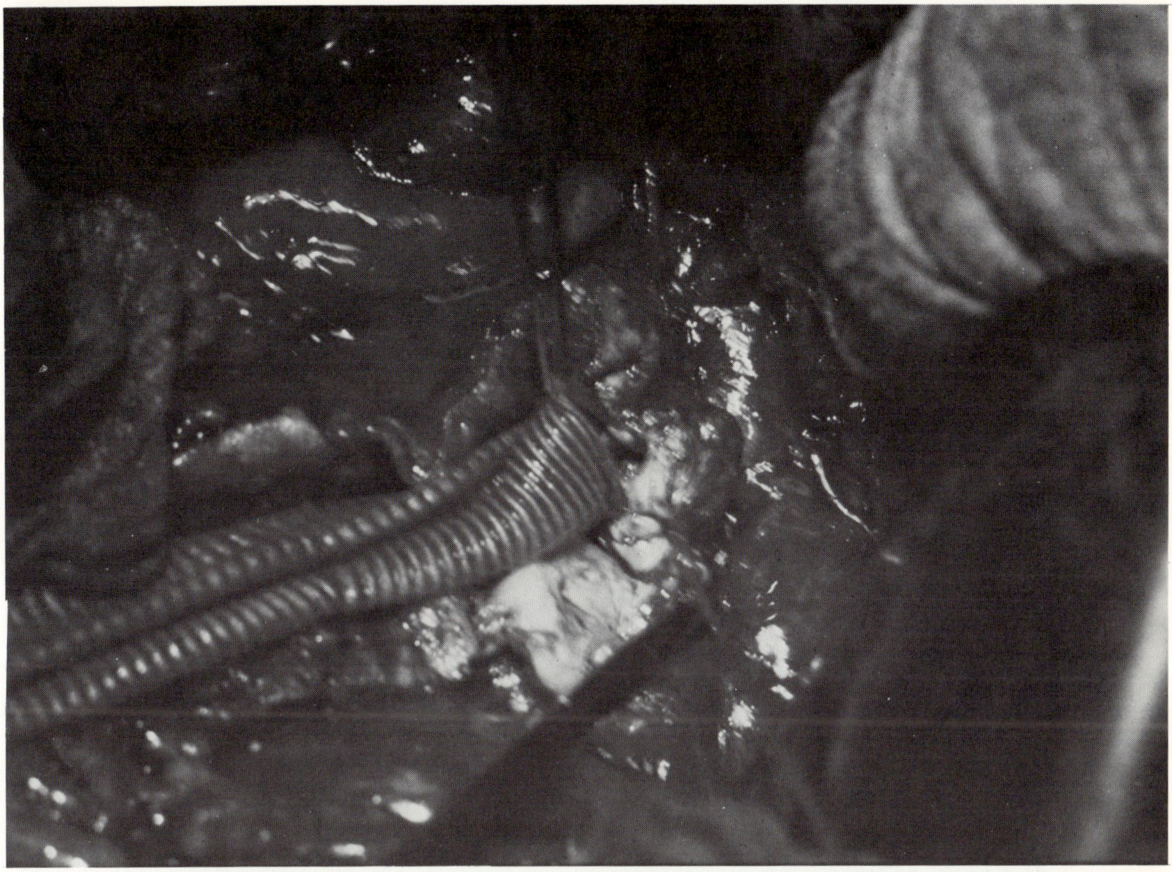

FIGURE 6-8 Beginning the posterior continuous suture line of an inlaid woven Dacron bifurcation graft.

be sutured to the parietal peritoneum in the left upper quadrant of the abdomen just prior to its closure. The only complication of 34 of these done personally was bleeding from the gastric stab wound in one patient. Electrocautery opening has since replaced the knife stab which led to that.

The Intensive Care Unit The ICU, with its experienced team and readily available consultants, is listed last but certainly makes a vast contribution to the lower mortality rate following resection of aortic aneurysms.

RUPTURED ANEURYSMS

A patient harboring an abdominal aortic aneurysm who develops abdominal, flank, or back pain must at once be considered to have a *threatening, if not already ruptured, aneurysm,* whether or not there be another lesion which may cause abdominal pain. Gallstones, kidney stones, intraabdominal adhesions, diverticulitis, and other entities do of course cause pain, but the burden of proof lies upon the clinician who ascribes pain to a nonaneurysmal source under such circumstances. Early surgical exploration without delay to obtain complicated visceral x-rays or other studies should be the order of the day.

Such threatening aneurysms (i.e., pain without local or systemic evidence of blood loss)

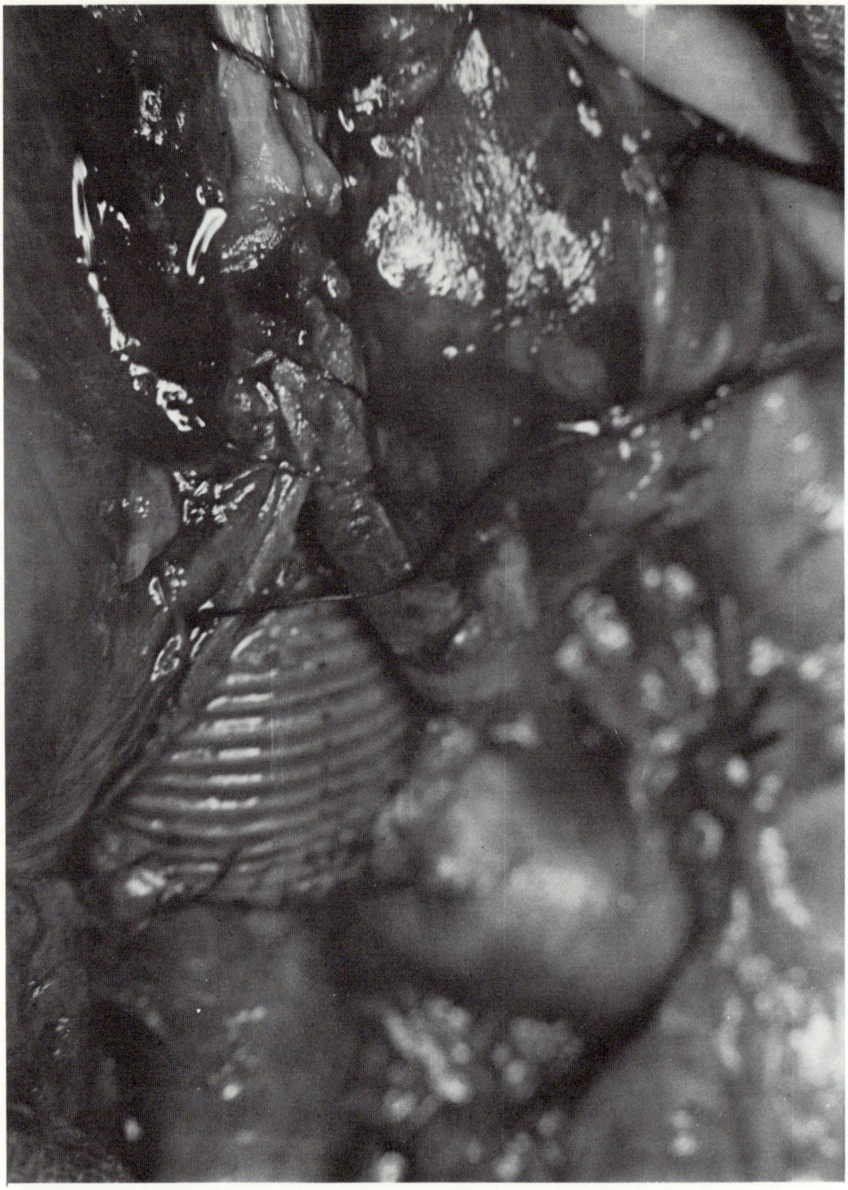

FIGURE 6-9 After placement of the inlay tube graft the original aneurysmal sac is plicated snugly about the graft with continuous 0-0 Dexon suture.

should be operated upon as a semiemergency within 12 to 24 hours. They may be repaired at the end of the day's schedule or, if seen late at night, at the beginning of the next day, if at all possible, since procedures done with the regular team in a methodical way fare better than do middle-of-the-night emergencies. As Emerick Szilagyi has stated, "An elective operation has a better prospect for freedom from complications."[21]

Illustrative Case

A 59-year-old female with abdominal pain was admitted with a palpable aortic aneurysm. There was a history of a previous operation for intestinal obstruction due to intraabdominal adhesions. The initial examiner believed the pain was probably due to partial small-bowel obstruction. The aneurysm was moderately tender to direct palpation, so the patient was operated upon immediately.

There was a 1-cm-deep cavitary lesion on the anterior surface of the aneurysm, where impending rupture was threatening (Figure 6-3). A tube graft was placed, and the patient had an uneventful postoperative course.

Comment The recommendation of delay relies on the opinion that pain is not due to a demonstrable aneurysm. Delay in surgical treatment is dangerous.

Ruptured Aortic Aneurysm A ruptured aneurysm with bleeding is a completely different matter and requires the earliest possible operation. Most patients survive for several hours after the initial rupture, since it usually occurs retroperitoneally (commonly on the left). A hematoma develops and a tamponade is life-saving for several hours. Rapid transport to a vascular center during this interval often allows salvage.

Telephone notification of such a patient should lead to advice for immediate transfer to the tertiary care center, without any delay for laboratory work or for extensive supportive treatment to stabilize the patient. An estimate is made of the arrival time, and the treatment team is notified. Thus, the patient is greeted in the emergency room by a responsible surgical team member, who at once decides whether a few minutes may be allowed for blood to be drawn there or whether direct admission to the operating room is necessary.

The surgical team is already present in either event and regardless of the hour. The patient's clothes are often not removed, blood is often obtained in the operating room, the admitting officer is fended away, and an immediate laparotomy is done to control the aortic hemorrhage. This policy of urgency requires some indoctrination of personnel in the emergency room as well as in the surgical unit. It does save lives and the paperwork can be done later.

Some years ago it was feared that this policy of calling in the anesthesia and surgical team upon notification of the transport of a patient with a ruptured aneurysm would lead to considerable wasted effort, either because many of the patients would be dead upon arrival or because others would be found to have an erroneous diagnosis. This fear has proved to be incorrect. Most of these patients do survive the 60- to 90-minute period of transportation, and instances of death in the ambulance have become uncommon since the surrounding referring physicians (within a 100-mile radius) have recognized the importance of immediate transport without delay for further study (Table 6-3).

The incidence of incorrect diagnosis has been low. There has been an occasional patient with some other type of intraabdominal catastrophe, who has benefited from the immediate operation. For example, a ruptured diverticulum of the transverse colon overlying an intact aortic aneurysm did need operation even though the diagnosis was incorrect. Another patient with a quite pulsatile aorta underlying a mass of pancreatic carcinoma had a biopsy diagnosis made in the middle of the night rather than after a prolonged period of study. There have also been occasional patients whose aneurysms have not been ruptured who have undergone emergency operation with resection and graft.

TABLE 6-3 RUPTURED ABDOMINAL AORTIC ANEURYSMS: LAST 25 PERSONAL CASES

Died in operating room	2	20% mortality
Died in hospital	3	
Survived	20*	80% survival

*One died elsewhere at 2 months of late perinephric abscess with secondary graft infection.

Rupture into the Vena Cava In rare instances an atherosclerotic aortic aneurysm ruptures into the adjacent inferior vena cava, at once creating an arteriovenous fistula. Sudden and often intractable congestive heart failure ensues and cannot be compensated until the fistula is corrected (along with resection of the aneurysm) (Figure 6-10). Johnson and Wood reported five patients operated upon for rupture of an aortic aneurysm into the inferior vena cava. The three deaths were due to cardiac complications. They noted the importance of proximal caval control, either by pressure or by balloon occlusion, to prevent pulmonary embolization of debris through the fistula.[22]

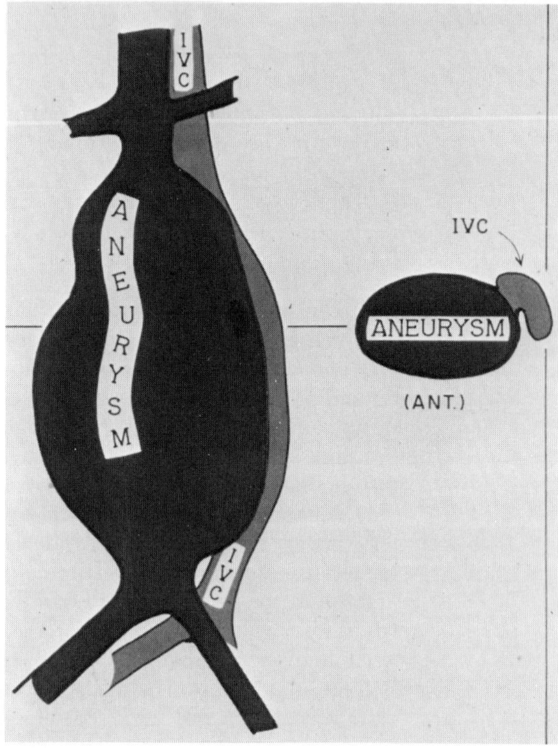

FIGURE 6-10 Spontaneous rupture of an abdominal aortic aneurysm into an anomalous inferior vena cava on the left side. Intractable heart failure required emergency operation.

THORACOABDOMINAL ANEURYSMS

Multiple aneurysms are common, so the discovery of one suggests a search for others. Patients with thoracic aneurysms have a 25 percent incidence of intraabdominal extension, and patients with abdominal aortic aneurysms have an 8 percent incidence of involvement of the proximal visceral vessels.[23]

Replacement of a thoracoabdominal aneurysm is a formidable procedure requiring an experienced surgical team. This includes not only the surgeons but knowledgeable nurses and assisting technicians, anesthesiologists, and an intensive care unit accustomed to dealing promptly with the various postoperative situations which arise quickly and frequently. Prior to accepting responsibility for excision and graft of a thoracoabdominal aneurysm, the team should already have achieved a low morbidity and mortality rate among a variety of ruptured and unruptured infrarenal aortic aneurysms and a virtually 100 percent postoperative graft patency rate.

Clear preoperative angiographic visualization is necessary to avoid surprises at the time of operation. Repetitive studies are sometimes required.

The operation developed by Stanley Crawford has simplified the surgical reconstruction of thoracoabdominal aneurysms and proximal extension of abdominal ones to an acceptable level of risk. It consists of an inlay graft with transplantation of an island of the aortic wall around the cluster of visceral vessels onto the side of the graft so that the number of anastomoses is greatly diminished.[24]

The peritoneal cavity should first be explored against the possibility of some contraindication to continuing the procedure in the form of an unsuspected tumor or other lesion. At the same time the surgeon should explore and expose the aorta and iliac vessels to determine where the distal end of the graft is to be placed. The incision may then be extended into the eighth interspace or higher, depending upon the proximal extent of the thoracic component of the aneurysm. If the diaphragm is incised circumferentially near its attachment to the thoracic wall, its function is better preserved than by a simple radial incision. The electrocautery is useful in hemostasis and in minimizing the time for exposure.

A thoracoabdominal aneurysm is best approached from its left lateral aspect through the peritoneal attachment in the left paracolic gutter so that all the viscera may be rolled anteriorly and to the right, allowing entry into the aneurysmal sac as far posteriorly as possible. The anterior wall of the sac may then be retracted with a series of sutures so that the interior is easily visualized. Internal placement of a self-retaining spring retractor may be helpful. Ordinarily the visceral arteries do not back-bleed sufficiently to warrant the use of multiple indwelling Fogarty catheters for their control, since that is cumbersome and time-consuming.

The inlay graft should be impermeable to blood. Woven Dacron, albuminized Dacron, or completely preclotted knit Dacron should be used, to avoid the excessive blood loss which may occur otherwise (Figure 6-11). The autotransfusion unit is worthwhile.

The inlay graft should be sutured with monofilament carried by a large needle so that sufficiently deep bites of the aortic wall are placed to avoid bleeding from a suture line which has already been covered. Inexperienced surgeons tend to transfer the delicate technique used for a below-knee arterial graft to the repair of aortic aneurysms. The tissue bite should be 6 mm to 1

FIGURE 6-11 This woven Dacron inlay graft reconstructed a thoracoabdominal aneurysm. The tube was attached *(left)* to a short bifurcation graft anastomosed distally to both iliac arteries. The central kinking and depression illustrates the technical error of removing too large an oval segment from the undersurface where the graft was anastomosed about the island containing the visceral vessels. The left renal artery was separately anastomosed. Function was excellent despite the odd appearance of the graft.

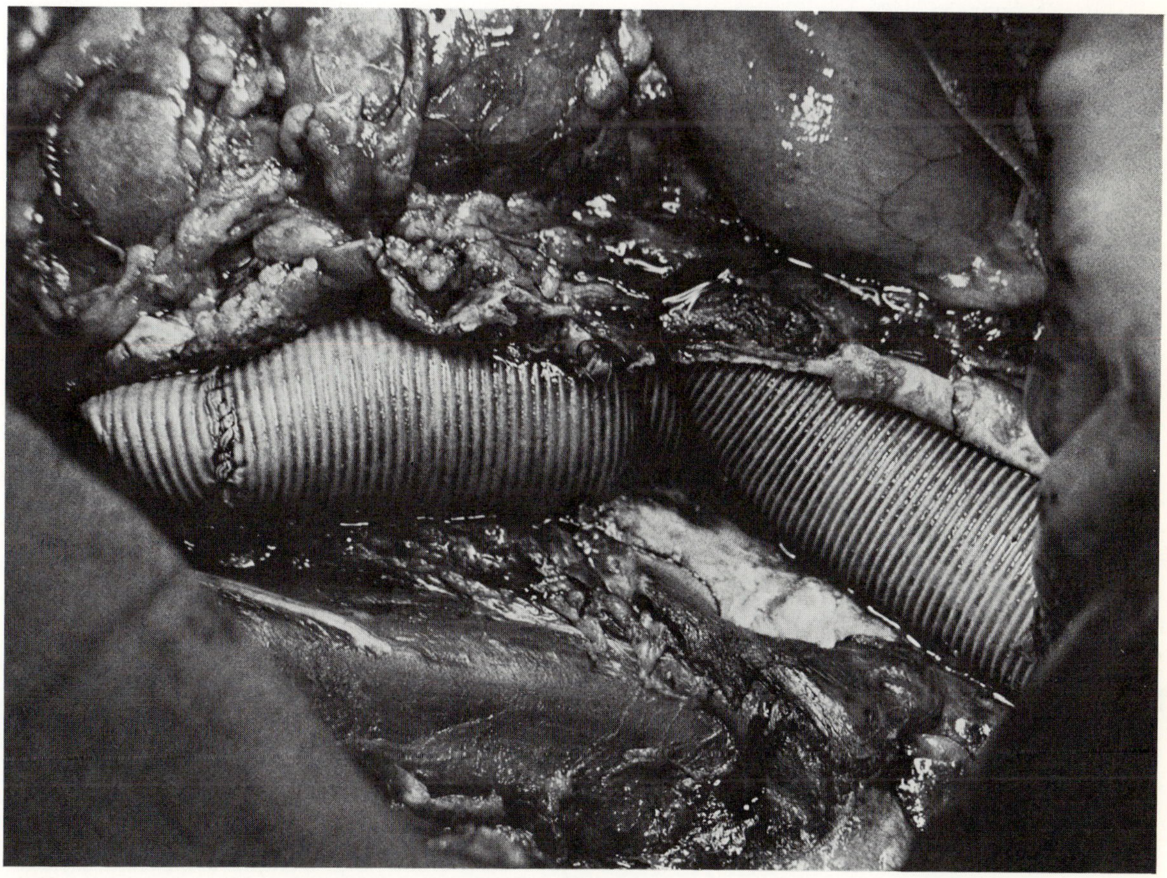

cm to insure holding as well as to buttress the wall of the graft against the wall of the aneurysm and avoid bleeding. Continuous sutures are time-saving as well as hemostatic.

An island containing the visceral vessels may be transferred into an oval cut from the side of the graft. The left renal artery may be too far away, so it may have to be placed separately, in which event considerable care must be taken to ensure that it does not kink the graft or artery. Sometimes a separate graft from the artery to the main graft is needed.

Systemic heparinization may be associated with considerable bleeding; experienced operators often avoid it. A compromise is to inject heparinized solution distally after the main portion of the aneurysm has been opened.

The ischemic time from initial placement of the proximal aortic clamp to its release and resumption of blood flow to the viscera should be the shortest that allows proper suturing, preferably between 30 and 45 minutes. After restoration of blood flow to the viscera, the distal anastomosis to the terminal aorta or to a bifurcation graft going onto either iliac or femoral arteries is done as efficiently as possible.

Hypothermia should be prevented by the use of a warming pad beneath the patient and over the lower legs, the use of warm rather than cold irrigating solution, and a warm temperature in the operating room. Warm saline may be poured into the wound from time to time, but this slows the overall procedure if used excessively.

After completion of the various anastomoses and restoration of flow, the operation should be terminated by rapid closure of the incision, to reduce anesthesia time as much as possible.

The reader interested in details of this procedure may consult Crawford's excellent discussion.[23]

INFLAMMATORY ANEURYSMS

A number of reports have discussed the occasional occurrence of a dense inflammatory reaction about an abdominal aortic aneurysm, which makes the surgical approach difficult or even impossible. No doubt, many of these patients have retroperitoneal fibrosis in one or another form, but this knowledge simply changes the terminology without improving the treatment.

The CT scan will usually suggest the problem but will not allow a preoperative decision on reconstructive grafting, a bypass with internal graft thrombosis, or a nonoperative strategy. Rupture is less likely inside the dense fibrosis, so a retreat may at times be safer than forcing a difficult and dangerous procedure.

Baskerville and associates in 1983 found 15 such among 103 patients by preoperative CT scans,[25] an incidence higher than most. They found resolution over periods up to 18 months and recommend treatment with 5 mg prednisone daily. However, it is not unusual for retroperitoneal fibroses to slowly resolve without any treatment, so their experience does not prove the point.

Savarese, Rosenfeld, and DeLaurentis had 11 such among 240 aneurysms (5 percent). They performed an axillofemoral bypass with internal thrombosis of the aneurysm for the single patient whose aneurysm could not be safely resected.[26]

HORSESHOE KIDNEY

Although horseshoe kidney in combination with abdominal aortic aneurysm is rare (1 in 385 people[27] and 0.5 percent in Crawford's report of 1110 patients[4]), its preoperative recognition is important in terms of proper operative management of the renal arteries, which may be multiple as well as aberrant. The aortographic series ordinarily delineates the vessels along with the fused kidneys and allows proper planning.[28] The need for such recognition is one of the reasons why proposals to omit routine preoperative angiography are poor judgment.

The most common type of horseshoe kidney is associated with a single renal artery on each side and can be managed by elevating the isthmus off the aneurysm to allow the usual inlay of a synthetic graft. If the fused kidney has vessels whose origins arise from the aneurysmal sac, the retroperitoneal approach may be used to allow grafting, with transfer of a portion of the wall containing the vessels to the side of the graft, or more simply, the bottom may be transferred to the anterior surface of the graft as it lies.

Rarely a ruptured aneurysm may be associated with a horseshoe kidney, as occurred in one of our cases. The isthmus of the fused kidneys lay in the retroperitoneal hematoma and was transected during the rapid approach to the aneurysm. Later each edge was oversewn with continuous suture, as the best recovery from the transection.

If abdominal exploration at the time of contemplated aneurysmectomy discloses a horseshoe kidney whose arterial supply has not been properly delineated preoperatively, it may be wise to terminate the operation in order to obtain such information prior to later resection of the aneurysm, since in a minority of instances important renal vessels exit from the aneurysmal sac itself rather than proximal to it. Intraoperative angiography may also be helpful.

CONCOMITANT LESIONS

Lesions not recognized preoperatively may require a variation in the operative plan when discovered after the abdomen is opened.

A mass in any portion of the colon requires particular consideration. Sometimes the differentiation between carcinoma and diverticulitis with inflammation is difficult or impossible without an open biopsy, which would preclude safe aortic grafting. In this situation or where the mass clearly represents cancer, it is often preferable to perform an immediate resection and primary anastomosis of the colon, even though the bowel is unprepared. A second-stage aneurysmectomy may then be performed some days later, but certainly not at the time of an open colon resection. If, on the other hand, the aneurysm is threatening in terms of acute symptoms, it may be advisable to remove it as the primary procedure and preserve the colon procedure for a later date.

Asymptomatic duodenal ulcers discovered at the time of laparotomy ordinarily do not require surgical treatment and are better managed by other methods.

Ovarian tumors can usually be removed by a rapid resection, since no bacterial contamination is to be feared. Uterine masses are better left to a secondary operation.

Renal lesions should have been discovered and evaluated preoperatively. If an unrecognized renal lesion is encountered, there is required a decision as to whether to deal with this primarily or to continue with dissection of the aneurysm and leave the renal lesion for another time, the latter being more usual.

The reason is not clear, but the fact is that acute cholecystitis is a threat to patients who harbor gallstones and undergo nonbiliary procedures.[29] Abdominal exploration just preceding the aortic repair should therefore particularly be directed toward the gallbladder. If one or more calculi are found, the gallbladder should usually be removed prior to final abdominal closure. Since cholecystectomy may scatter bacteria, it is necessary to secure a tight (and usually double-layered) closure of the posterior peritoneum over the aortic graft before excising the gallbladder. Also, if the distal graft limbs lie exposed in the groins, these wounds should be closed prior to removal of the gallbladder.

Although the number of concomitant cholecystectomies cannot be retrieved from the records, I have always followed this plan. No infections have occurred. The only complication was in one patient who bled from the bed of the gallbladder, leading to exploration because it was thought that the graft anastomosis was leaking. Recovery followed.

The recently reported experience of the University of Rochester group, with 42 instances of cholelithiasis among 865 patients with aneurysms, confirms this plan. None of their 18 patients who had aneurysmectomy with concomitant cholecystectomy had a complication, except one with a late graft infection at 26 months. That patient's original procedure was faulty, since the gallbladder was removed before the retroperitoneal tissues were closed. Among the 11 patients having aneurysmectomy without removal of a gallbladder containing stones, there was 1 who developed acute cholecystitis on the third postoperative day and a second who died of biliary sepsis, which began 5 days after the aneurysm operation. This 18 percent early biliary complication rate, along with the benign course of those having concomitant cholecystectomy, constitutes a strong argument for the procedure.[30]

NONRESECTION TREATMENT OF ANEURYSMS

There are occasional patients with large and/or threatening aortic aneurysms who, for one or another reason, are bad risks for the resection and graft operation. These include (1) patients with severe disease of an important functional system (lungs, heart, kidneys, liver), (2) those with intraperitoneal conditions, such as tumor or retroperitoneal fibrosis, which cause severe technical problems, (3) others with conditions likely to cause infection (colostomy, furunculosis), and (4) the extremely obese.

Some method of producing intraaneurysmal thrombosis may be considered as an alternative

FIGURE 6-12 This abdominal aortic aneurysm was palpable and actually larger (by ultrasound) than the aortogram appears to indicate. This 82-year-old male with severe pulmonary disease and compensated heart disease was managed without operation until pain indicated a change in strategy. He did well.

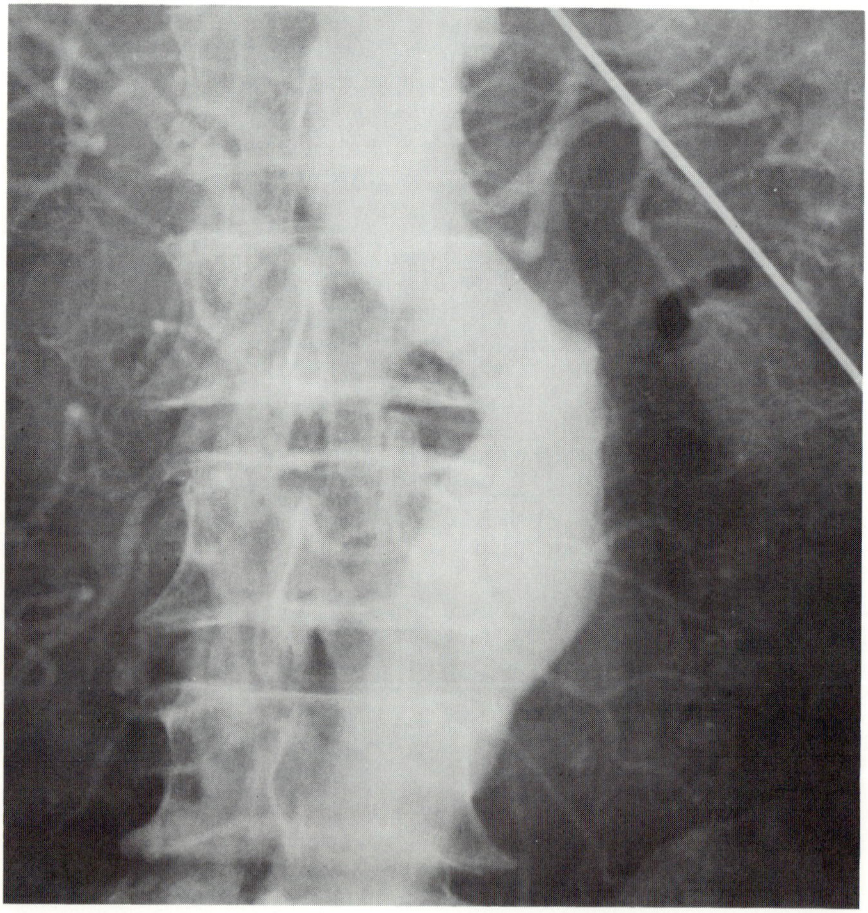

to the usual resection and graft. The old technique of placing coils of steel wire within the sac through small abdominal incisions and heating the wire electrically may be recalled.[31] Eastcott has used this occasionally in recent years.[32]

More recently thrombosis has been produced by placement of occluding balloons within the common iliac arteries, with or without an irritating substance, or by surgical ligation of both iliac arteries via an extraperitoneal approach. Revascularization of the distal body is simultaneously produced by an axillo-bifemoral graft. Karmody and his group in 1983 reported their 5-year experience with 60 such high-risk patients, the 40-day mortality being 7 percent. In addition, 18 thrombectomies in 15 patients were required to reopen bypass grafts. Retrograde thrombosis of the renal arteries did not occur in their series. CT scan was the best method to detect completion of the thrombosis.[33]

No doubt, there is an occasional patient for whom the nonresection procedure may be considered. However, it does require a complicated technique, the risks are still formidable, and the complication rate is high. Further, there has been reported rupture through the neck after intraluminal thrombosis.[34]

My strategy for a small asymptomatic aneurysm in a poor-risk patient continues to be nonoperative, even though a few of these will rupture at home (Figure 6-12). If the aneurysm is threatening by virtue of size or symptoms, it is usually possible to remove it, using all possible support for the deranged functional system or some special bypass technique if there is a local technical problem. There has been no experience in our center with the nonoperative techniques discussed above.

REFERENCES

1 Dale WA: The beginnings of vascular surgery. *Surgery* 1974, 76:849–866.

2 Blakemore AH: Surgical aspects of aneurysm of the aorta. *Trans South Surg Assoc* 1947, 59:27.

3 Dubost C, Allary M, Oeconomos NA: Propos de traitement des aneurysmes de l'aorte ablauon de l'aneurysme. Retablissement de la continuite. *Mem Acad Chir* (Paris) 1951, 77:381.

4 Crawford ES, Stowe C: True aneurysm of the aorta and iliac arteries (Chapter 10), in Moore WS (ed): *Vascular Surgery.* Grune & Stratton, New York, 1983, pp 269–339.

5 Darling RC, Brewster DC: Elective treatment of abdominal aortic aneurysms. *World J Surg* 1980, 4:661–667.

6 Mannick JA: Invited commentary. *World J Surg* 1980, 4:666–667.

7 Darling RC: Ruptured arteriosclerotic abdominal aneurysms. *Am J Surg* 1970, 119:397.

8 Szilagyi DE, Elliott JP, Smith RF: Clinical fate of the patient with asymptomatic abdominal aortic aneurysm unfit for surgical treatment. *Arch Surg* 1972, 104:600.

9 Dale WA: Small aortic aneurysms should be treated by operation, in Varco RL, Delaney JP (eds): *Controversy in Surgery.* WB Saunders, Philadelphia, 1976, pp 261–265.

10 Bernstein EF: Considerations in the management of poor-risk patients with small asymptomatic aneurysms, in Varco RL, Delaney JP (eds): *Controversy in Surgery.* WB Saunders, Philadelphia, 1976, pp 267–275.

11 Lord JW Jr. Giuseppi R, Daliana M, Drago JR, Schwartz AM: Unsuspected abdominal aortic aneurysms as the cause of peripheral arterial disease. *Ann Surg* 1963, 177:767.

12 Rutherford RB: *Vascular Surgery.* WB Saunders, Philadelphia, 1977, p 642.

13 Couch N, O'Mahony J, McIrvine A, Whittemore A, Lombara J, Mannick J: The place of abdominal aortography in abdominal aortic aneurysm resection. *Arch Surg* 1983, 118:1029–1034.

14 Robiscek F: The safety of lumbar aortography. *Surgery* 1978, 83:489–490.

15 Bauer GM, Porter JM, Eidemiller LR, Rosch J, Keller F: The role of arteriography in abdominal aortic aneurysm. *Am J Surg* 1978, 136:184–189.

16 Doust RBC, Cohen HE: Ultrasonic evaluation of abdominal aortic aneurysm (Chapter 76), in Rutherford RB (ed): *Vascular Surgery.* WB Saunders, Philadelphia, 1977, pp 661–672.

17 Dale WA: Transverse incisions for intraabdominal vascular repairs. *Surg Gynecol Obstet* 1968; 126:1321–1324.

18 Rob C: Extraperitoneal approach to the abdominal aorta. *Surgery* 1963, 53:87.

19 Shumacher HB: Discussion of Rob C: Extraperitoneal approach to the abdominal aorta. *Surgery* 1963, 53:87.
20 Williams, GM, Ricotta JJ, Zinner M, Burdick FJ: The extended retroperitoneal approach for treatment of extensive atherosclerosis of the aorta and renal vessels. *Surgery* 1980, 88:846.
21 Szilagyi DE: Personal Letter, 1984.
22 Johnson JN, Wood M: Arteriovenous fistula secondary to rupture of atherosclerotic abdominal aortic aneurysm. *Am J Surg* 1978, 136:171–175.
23 Crawford ES, Stowe C: True Aneurysms of the Aorta and Iliac Arteries, in Moore WS (ed): *Vascular Surgery, a Comprehensive Review.* Grune & Stratton, New York, 1983, pp 305–318.
24 Crawford ES, Snyder DM, Cho GC, Roehm JOF Jr: Progress and treatment of thoracoabdominal aneurysms involving celiac, superior mesenteric and renal arteries. *Ann Surg* 1978, 188:404.
25 Baskerville PA, Blakeney CG, Young AE, Browse NL: The diagnosis and treatment of peri-aortic fibrosis (inflammatory aneurysms). *J Cardiovasc Surg* (Torino) 1983, 24:393.
26 Savarese RP, Rosenfeld JC, DeLaurentis DA: Inflammatory aneurysm. *J Cardiovasc Surg* (Torino) 1983, 24:393.
27 Campbell MF: *Urology.* Vol 2. WB Saunders, Philadelphia, 1970, p 1448.
28 Lobe TE, Martin EW, Cooperman M, Vasko J, Evans WE: Abdominal aortic surgery in the presence of horseshoe kidney. *Ann Surg* 1978, 188:71.
29 Gately JF, Thomas EJ: Acute cholecystitis occurring as a complication of other diseases. *Arch Surg* 1983, 118:1137–1141.
30 Ouriel K, Ricotta JJ, Adams JT, DeWeese JA: Management of cholelithiasis in patients with abdominal aortic aneurysm. *Ann Surg* 1983, 198:717–719.
31 Blakemore AH: Surgical aspects of aneurysm of the aorta. *Trans South Surg Assoc* 1947, 59:27.
32 Eastcott HHG: *Arterial Surgery.* JB Lippincott, Philadelphia, 1969, p 184.
33 Karmody AK, Leather RP, Goldman M, Corson JD, Shaw DM: The current position of nonresective treatment for abdominal aneurysm. *Surgery* 1983, 94:591–597.
34 Kwaan J, Dahl R: Fatal rupture after successful surgical thrombosis of an abdominal aortic aneurysm. *Surgery* 1984, 95:235–237.
35 Szilagyi DE, Smith R, Elliott J, Hageman J: Translumbar aortography: A study of its safety and usefulness. *Arch Surg* 1977, 112:399–408.
36 Hessell SJ, Adams DF, Abrams HL: Complications of angiography. *Diagn Radiol* 1981, 138:273–281.

Invited Commentary

E. Stanley Crawford, M.D.
Houston, Texas

This chapter is a well-organized, clear, and comprehensive discussion of abdominal aortic aneurysms, the problems which they present, and current concepts of therapy. It is based upon an extensive personal experience and a thorough knowledge of that of others, obtained during the entire period during which modern therapy has evolved. The author has contributed significantly to this field in general and to his region in particular. The former is well-known, and the latter is evident from this description of local organization for the proper institutional approach to the treatment of patients with suspected leaking or ruptured aneurysm. It is difficult to add anything of significance; thus, this discussion is an expansion of two points that he has made, i.e., of staged operations and the treatment of inflammatory aneurysms.

STAGED OPERATIONS

The risk of staging operations in patients with aortic aneurysm is frequently greatest when an aneurysm is left for the second operation. The risk is of aneurysm rupture before the second operation is performed. I agree entirely with the author on combining certain operations, such as aneurysm removal and cholecystectomy, and staging others, as in patients with aneurysm and colon lesions that require resection. I feel, as he does, (but more emphatically than he stated) that in patients with aneurysm and cancer of the colon, the aneurysm should be removed first unless the tumor is associated with obstruction or bleeding, because the colon operation can be performed sooner after aneurysmectomy than the aneurysm can be removed after a colon resection. The latter operation is associated with a higher incidence of wound and intraperitoneal infection, which could prolong the interval between operations. There are no palliative methods of treating ruptured aneurysms, whereas if the colon cancer produces obstruction in the early period after aneurysm operation, this can be safely treated by an immediate decompressing transverse colostomy and later colon resection.

INFLAMMATORY ANEURYSM

My concept of the pathogenesis of inflammatory aneurysmal disease is based upon a recent review of the literature and an analysis of 30 patients treated personally. The acute form of the disease or condition appears to have two components: (1) an underlying atherosclerotic infrarenal or more extensive aortic aneurysm, and (2) a superimposed inflammatory reaction that involves the anterior and lateral walls of the aneurysm, contiguous with a similar reaction in the retroperitoneal area to an extent that varies from moderate local extension to involvement of the entire retroperitoneum and lower mediastinal region. This disease is associated with three complications: pain, ureteral obstruction, and aneurysmal rupture. The last-named occurs posterolaterally where the aneurysmal wall is weakest and not involved by the acute inflammatory reaction. These complications were prevented or relieved by graft insertion performed from inside the aneurysm without disturbing the retroperitoneal reaction, with survival in 29 patients. Proximal aortic clamping for operation is performed above the inflammatory reaction, at the infrarenal level, at the diaphragm, or in the thorax. Steroid therapy may immediately relieve pain and systemic symptoms and may ultimately relieve partial ureteral obstruction, but the underlying atherosclerotic aneurysm is uncontrolled and may ultimately rupture. This method of therapy alone is not recommended. Extraanatomic bypass and intraluminal obliteration should also be reserved for the exceptional case because of the relatively high incidence of complications associated with the former part of this procedure.

7 COMPLICATIONS OF AORTIC SURGERY

Besides the usual hazards of any anesthesia and operation, there are several particular postoperative problems which may arise following aortic grafting for aneurysm or occlusive disease.

BLEEDING

Increasing experience has led to the concept that absolute hemostasis is imperative prior to closure. Additional time in the operating room to achieve this is better tolerated than is continued bleeding in the recovery room. The standard of hemostasis believed to be acceptable 10 years ago would be viewed as "too wet to close" today. This elevation of the standard of hemostasis has been associated with a parallel decline in the number of secondary explorations for bleeding. It is also considerably less demanding for the surgeon to spend an additional 30 to 45 minutes in the operating room than to arise that night for a secondary laparotomy.

Nevertheless, bleeding in the postoperative period does necessitate an early decision regarding return to the operating room or transfusion to await spontaneous cessation. The problem is particularly troublesome if the patient is believed to have a blood dyscrasia, in which case efforts to correct the situation may be in order prior to secondary laparotomy. In most circumstances, however, the experienced vascular surgeon will return the patient to the operating room with the knowledge that a second anesthesia is better tolerated than is continued bleeding, with the possibility of a delayed operation after the patient's reserves have been exhausted. If there is serious doubt in the matter, it is usually better to explore the abdomen. More than once such secondary exploration has failed to reveal any large bleeding point, but removal of accumulated hematoma has benefited the patient by allowing the diaphragms to descend and also preventing the necessity of absorbing a large hematoma.

INTESTINAL ISCHEMIA

Although the small intestine is occasionally the site of intestinal ischemia following aortic reconstruction (if so, it is usually deadly) more often the colon is affected. The majority of these cases follow resection of aneurysms rather than grafting for aortoiliac occlusive disease because the latter is ordinarily associated with considerably more development of the collateral circulation.[1]

Illustrative Case

A 72-year-old male had a woven Dacron tube graft replacement of a 7-cm abdominal aortic aneurysm and a concomitant aorta–left renal 6-mm polytetrafluoroethylene (PTFE) graft for renovascular hypertension with associated elevation in creatinine. Postoperatively there was rapid return to normal of the blood pressure and of the creatinine level.

The first bowel movement occurred on the fourth postoperative day, but thereafter abdominal distention increased, and left abdominal tenderness developed by the seventh postoperative day, with a fever spike on the following day. Left colon ischemia was tentatively diagnosed.

A plain film of the abdomen (Figure 7-1) showed an area in the left colon suggestive of ischemic colitis. Colonoscopy confirmed this. A nonoperative program of clear fluids and antibiotics was chosen. Low fever spikes continued throughout the rest of the hospitalization, and a tender mass became palpable in the left flank. There was diarrhea but no blood.

The entire clinical course was improvement. Repeated sodium diatrizoate (Hypaque) colon studies (Figure 7-2) and colonoscopy also indicated improvement. He was discharged on the twenty-sixth postoperative day.

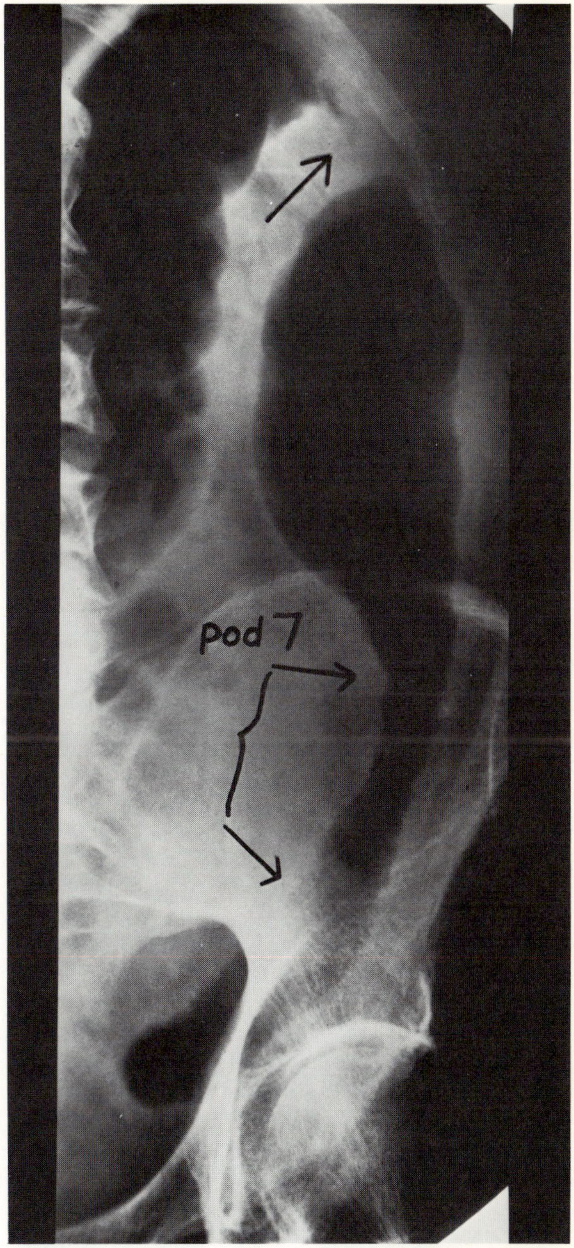

FIGURE 7-1 Ischemic colitis 7 days after resection of aortic aneurysm. The *upper arrow* shows area of tight spasm; the *lower, bracketed arrows* show another spastic region.

Comment During the operation the inferior mesenteric artery was suture-ligated within the aneurysmal sac without any particular consideration of its transposition. The insidious development of signs of colon ischemia was initially interpreted as continuing postoperative ileus, but the occurrence of left abdominal tenderness followed by a fever spike strongly suggested the correct diagnosis. It was feared that an immediate resection of the colon with colostomy would inevitably lead to contamination of the PTFE graft from the aorta to the left renal artery and an eventually fatal outcome, so a nonoperative course was chosen with considerable trepidation. Close observation over the next few days indicated stabilization and improvement.

Improvement continued at home (Figure 7-3), but after 7 months stenosis of the splenic flexure of the colon, with abcess, required temporary colostomy and later resection of the left colon.

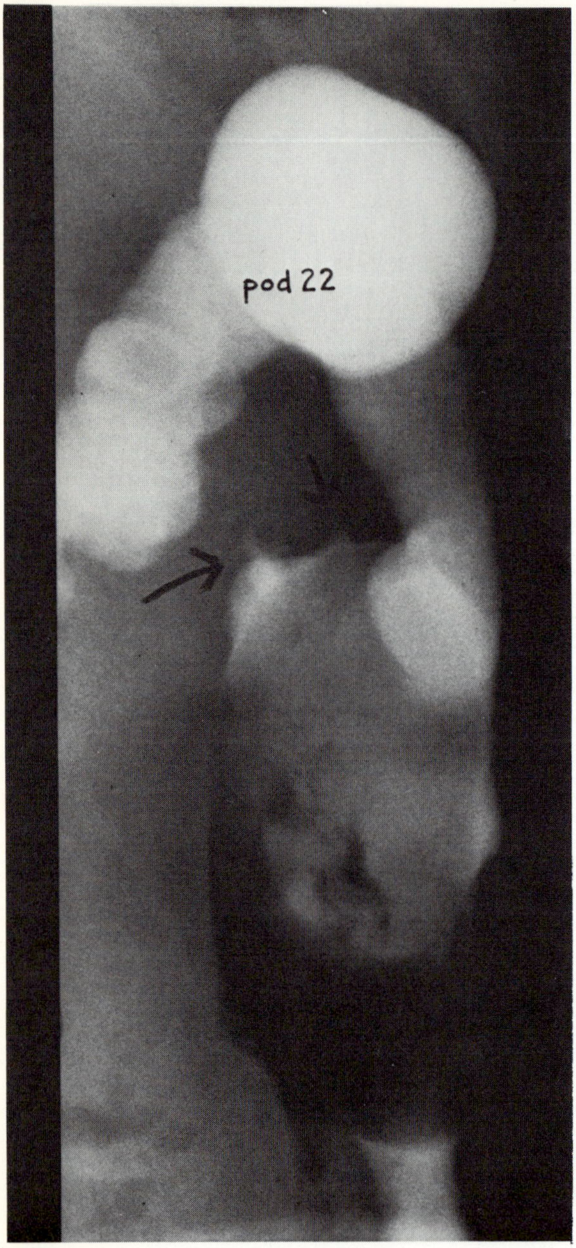

FIGURE 7-2 Twenty-two days after operation the spastic region of the upper left colon is apparent. *Arrows* show deep ulcers.

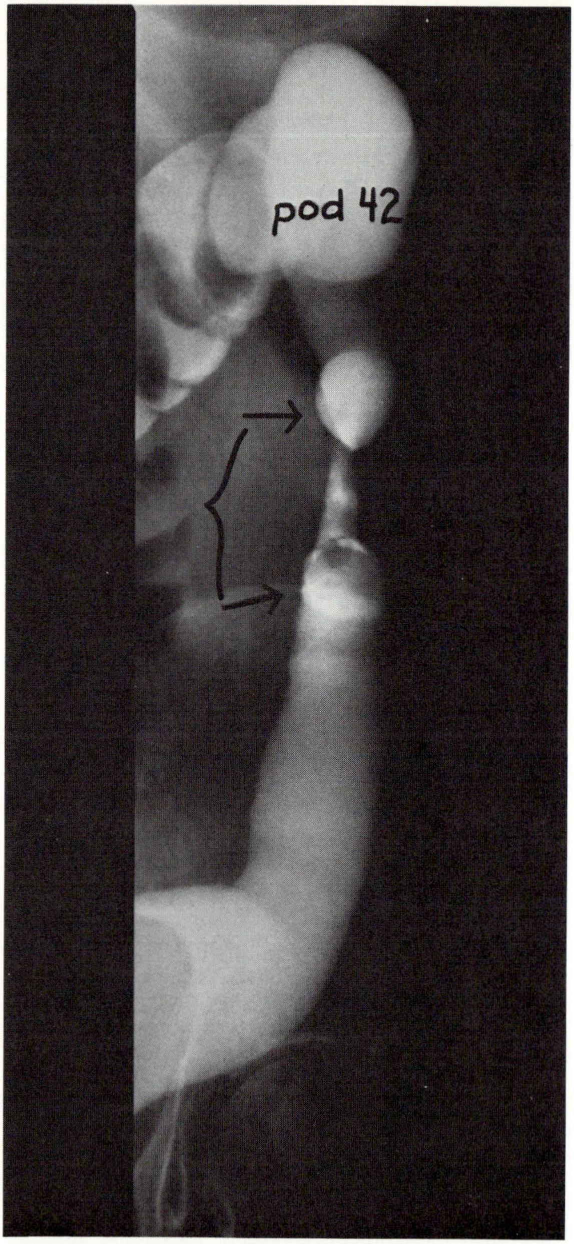

FIGURE 7-3 Forty-two days after operation the left colon is essentially normal except in the region denoted by the *bracketed arrows,* where spasm has progressed to stenosis.

Incidence

It has long been recognized that many patients develop temporary diarrhea following aortic grafts, presumably because of dissection around the root of the sigmoid colon but perhaps, in the light of increasing experience, as a result of some degree of colon ischemia. Ernst's group found evidence of ischemia in 6.7 percent of 163 patients whose colons were examined with the colonoscope after aortic reconstruction. The incidence was considerably higher following repair of a ruptured aneurysm in that series. The overall mortality rate approximated 50 percent.[2]

Intraoperative Diagnosis

The surgeon should be alert for the possibility of intestinal ischemia in every patient undergoing aortic reconstruction. Patients with the greatest risk include those with ruptured aneurysms, patients having long periods of hypotension, those with angiographic evidence of a large flow in the inferior mesenteric artery, and those with occlusion or stenosis of the celiac and superior mesenteric arteries.

Simple inspection of the left colon following aortic reconstruction is not a critical examination because the ischemic changes are slow to appear and difficult to detect and also because the ischemia may be caused not by the initial arterial occlusion but by later secondary thrombosis.

Hobson and associates have described intraoperative Doppler study of the flow within the inferior mesenteric artery (IMA) and in its branches following its interruption,[3] and Ernst has recommended measurement of the stump blood pressure to help in determination of whether to reimplant or to ligate the IMA. Ernst used 40 mm as the critical pressure in a 64-patient series.[4]

If the IMA is not to be preserved, its orifice should be sutured from within the opened wall of the aneurysm rather than by external ligation at a more distant point, which may excessively remove collateral circulation. If there is little back bleeding from the IMA orifice, or if its measured pressure is below 40 mm, the orifice probably should be preserved by removal of a button of surrounding aortic wall for later implantation into the side of the replacement graft to preserve blood flow into the IMA. The facts are not clear because most of us have never reimplanted the IMA and have had few severe problems due to colon ischemia. Further, no one knows the long-term fate of the transplanted patch button of tissue, which is a part of the original thin aneurysmal sac.

If occlusion or tight stenosis of the superior mesenteric and/or celiac artery is recognized on the preoperative aortogram, a simultaneous bypass to that artery should be considered.

Postoperative Diagnosis

The clinical manifestations of ischemia may be masked by other postoperative responses. Prolonged ileus or unusual left abdominal pain may be early symptoms, along with somewhat later diarrhea, which may become bloody. Evidence of sepsis or metabolic acidosis should also alert the clinician to this possibility.

Arteriography has a limited role in the diagnosis of intestinal ischemia. Fiberoptic colonoscopy may be easily performed at the bedside, and repeat examinations usually allow recognition of the changing pattern of hemorrhages, edema, erosions, and ulcers within the left colon. Radiographic studies of the left colon, using radiopaque contrast material other than barium, are also useful in following the progress of the lesion.

Treatment

Ischemia of the small intestine is rare, and when it occurs, it usually produces a fatality. If it is recognized, immediate laparotomy and intestinal resection are necessary.

The nonoperative management of lesser degrees of ischemic colitis requires careful observation of the clinical course as well as repetitive colonoscopy and colon x-rays. Persistent diarrhea, particularly with bleeding, or any systemic evidence of perforation or local walling off requires a shift in strategy to operation.

The operation is performed to prevent perforation and probable death. The entire area of ischemic colon must be removed, and a proximal end colostomy must be established. The surgeon must pay considerable attention to prevention of fecal contamination of the indwelling graft, by closing the posterior tissues and appropriate walling off, before cutting across the bowel.

Occasional patients tolerate the ischemic colon but later develop a stricture which requires resection. The risk for this should be lower than for an earlier resection and colostomy, although that should not be delayed in hopes of tolerance if it is needed.

INFECTION

The treatment of infected grafts is discussed in Chapter 24, so will not be repeated here beyond the brief recognition that contaminated synthetic grafts ordinarily require complete removal with concomitant extraanatomic bypass.

AORTOENTERIC FISTULA

A fistulous communication which develops between an aortic graft and the duodenum (or less commonly the jejunum) usually occurs at the suture line and rarely is due to breakdown of the graft, with direct communication into the gut. It has been commonly thought that there is erosion of the duodenum by the adjacent pulsating suture line, with infection and later breakdown of the anastomosis so that bleeding occurs. It is perhaps just as likely that the process is the result of a false aneurysm due to sutures cutting through the proximal aorta because they were placed too superficially, which is similar to what happens when a false aneurysm develops in the groin.

Clinical Presentation

A patient who presents with any form of gastrointestinal bleeding and who has had a previous aortic graft should be considered likely to have an aortoenteric fistula until absolutely proven otherwise. Gastrointestinal endoscopy should be performed immediately to determine a possible source of bleeding in the distal esophagus, stomach, or duodenum. If no bleeding lesion is found, the tentative diagnosis of aortoenteric fistula is considerably strengthened. Demonstration of gastritis or another lesion which is not causing massive bleeding may cause confusion and delay the necessary abdominal operation.

In any event minor "herald" bleeding begins to warn of an impending major hemorrhage. Presentation with severe bleeding without such previous minor episodes is unusual.

Diagnostic Studies

Angiography sometimes demonstrates a false aneurysm but usually is not particularly helpful. Colonic bleeding should be ruled out by colonoscopy whenever possible.

Perdue and associates in 1980 discussed the sensitivity of diagnostic examinations, finding that both computerized tomography (CT) scan (four of four) and citrate gallium 67 scan (five of five) were better than endoscopy (three of eight) in making a positive preoperative diagnosis.[5] This, of course, means not that endoscopy should not be used but that negative findings do not rule out a fistula.

Plan of Management

In 1979 Victor Bernhard and his associates summarized several reports of aortoenteric fistulas, finding 83 patients with a perioperative mortality rate of 73 percent. They discussed their own data on 20 patients, noting that the average onset of symptoms was 4 to 6 years after the original aortic graft operation and that all but one patient had a herald bleed prior to life-threatening hemorrhage. They described a rational plan of management, beginning with upper gastrointestinal endoscopy rather than barium study, and pointed out that angiography is not often diagnostic. Seventy-eight percent of their patients who underwent removal of the graft with an extraanatomic bypass survived.[6]

Exploratory laparotomy may be necessary for making a final determination of whether or not there is a fistula. In this event the proximal aorta should be controlled by one method or another so that if massive hemorrhage occurs during separation of the duodenum from the scar tissue, the bleeding can be controlled.

Optimum surgical management includes placing an extraanatomic axillobifemoral bypass prior to opening the abdomen if the diagnosis has been established. The abdomen may then be opened and the prosthesis completely removed, the proximal end of the aorta being suitably closed, without contamination of the extraanatomic bypass.

PARAPLEGIA DUE TO ANTERIOR SPINAL CORD SYNDROME

Neurologic complications rarely follow abdominal aneurysmectomy. Grace and Mattox in 1974 found only 28 recorded instances, of which there were 5 recoveries.[7] Elliott, Szilagyi, Hageman, and Smith in 1980 increased the collected number to 46, including their own 8.[8]

Incidence

Undoubtedly, there are many unreported cases of this unusual and unpredictable complication. A show of hands at the 1984 meeting of the Southern Association for Vascular Surgery indicated that half those present had seen such, though not necessarily as the operating surgeon. The Elliott series from Detroit had 8 among 861 (0.43 percent) abdominal aneurysmectomies, with the incidence tenfold higher among operations for rupture (1.9 percent) than for elective (0.19 percent) procedures. I am fortunate to have had no personal experience, although I have observed one such at a safe distance.

Etiology

While several factors have been suspected as contributory, including the extent of atherosclerosis, age, coagulation problems, level and length of aortic cross-clamping, and hypotension, none of these appear significant when patients with and without cord damage are compared. Variations of the blood supply to the cord are a more likely cause, although information on this is still evolving.

The blood supply of the lower spinal cord where the lesion occurs consists of extraspinal arteries derived from vessels in the neck, the intercostals, and the lumbar and sacral arteries. In the embryo their branches are paired to each segment, but the branches disappear later, leaving irregularly spaced vessels entering the spinal cord via intervertebral foramina. The largest of these, the great radicular artery (of Adamkiewicz), varies in its origin but in 75 percent of people arises from T9 to T12.[9] When the artery originates proximally, it is often supplemented by a more distal one. This distal artery is occasionally the dominant vessel and therefore indispensable.

Even though the blood supply to the spinal cord and the lumbar region is rather precarious, the collateral is ordinarily sufficient to maintain flow through the anterior spinal artery, which furnishes most of the blood supply.

If the radicular artery is blocked and the collateral flow is insufficient to maintain the nutrition of the cord, there may occur paraplegia with disassociated sensory loss (absence of pain and temperature sensation with intact proprioception and vibration awareness) and sphincter incontinence.

Prevention

There are at present no absolutely certain ways to prevent this rare complication, although prevention of hypotension and reimplantation of any large vessel which appears to be the artery of Adamkiewicz has been recommended,[7] as well as several other techniques of demonstration of the extraspinal arteries, which are impractical.

The interested reader will find a discussion by Elliott and colleagues superb and encyclopedic. Elliott's final conclusion is pessimistic but accurate: "spinal cord damage following intra-abdominal vascular reconstructive procedures is a totally unpredictable and therefore unpreventable postoperative complication."[8]

URETERAL OBSTRUCTION

Ureteral obstruction secondary to aortoiliac or aortofemoral grafting is unusual, perhaps because its true incidence is not recognized, and only seven cases have been reported. Batson, Frusha, and Parker performed intravenous pyelograms on 50 asymptomatic patients 6 to 46 months after aortofemoral grafting and found 14 percent to have some degree of unilateral hydronephrosis. None required operation for relief.[10]

Such occurrences without clinical symptoms are well-known to urologists. Roth noted that it is not really unusual for a urologist to find a functionless kidney with a totally occluded ureter with a history of prior pelvic surgery in a patient with no or few symptoms.[11]

My experience comprises three cases, one of which is shown in Figure 7-4, where the dilated, twisted right ureter was clearly visualized by retrograde catheterization. Despite the alternative of ureteral division and transposition, many of these problems will eventuate, as did this patient's, in nephrectomy.

The second personal patient likewise had nephrectomy, and the third did not require operation, since the hydroureter subsided after a few weeks.

Prevention

Several reported entrapments of the ureter between a graft limb and the underlying native iliac artery[12] reinforce the usual advice to tunnel the graft posterior to the ureter. However, placing the ureter anterior to the graft limb does not always prevent the problem, as attested by the three cases of Antkowiak and D'Altorio where a periuretal fibrosis of an anteriorly coursing ureter occurred. The importance of fibrosis, rather than mere position, was emphasized by their collection of 15 cases; in 6 the ureter was anterior, in 8 it was posterior to the graft, and in 1 the position was unknown.[13]

Clinical Diagnosis

Complaints of flank or abdominal pain or urinary symptoms should suggest the possibility of ureteral entrapment. Cases have occurred as early as 12 days and as late as 29 months postoperatively. Unilateral lesions are usual, but 4 of the 12 cases collected by Hagedorn and associates were bilateral.[14] The bilateral cases presented with more acute symptoms of oliguria or anuria and uremia.

Intravenous pyelography usually shows the problem, but retrograde study is sometimes necessary.

Treatment

Division of the ureter, with transposition anterior to the graft and anastomosis there,[12] is a procedure which saves the kidney and is obviously the choice when it is possible. The less desirable nephrectomy should be avoided.

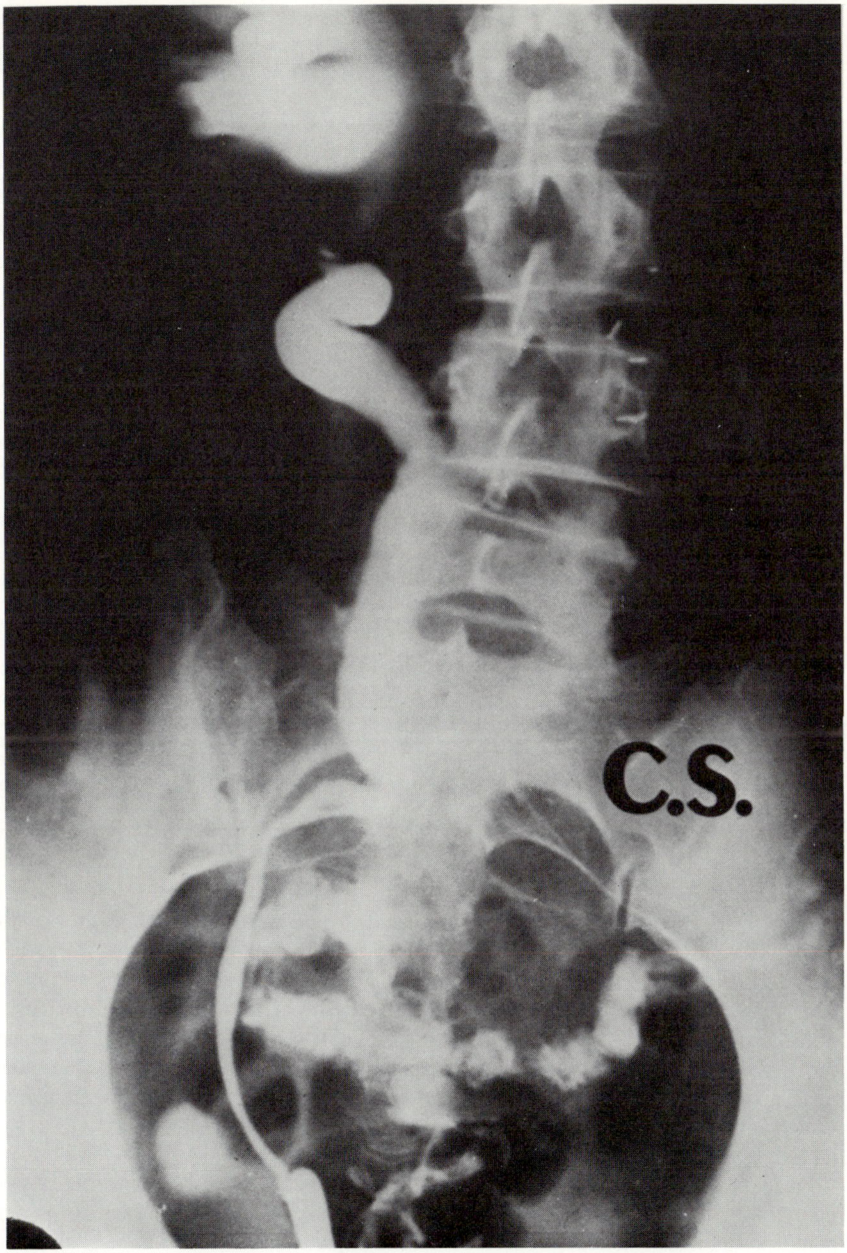

FIGURE 7-4 Hydroureter and hydronephrosis following aorto-bifemoral grafting eventuated in nephrectomy.

REFERENCES

1 Papadopoulos CD, Mancini HW, Marino AWM Jr: Ischemic necrosis of the colon following aortic aneurysmectomy. *J Cardiovasc Surg* (Torino) 1974, 15:494.

2 Hagihara PF, Ernst CB, Griffen WO Jr: Incidence of ischemic colitis following abdominal aortic reconstruction. *Surg Gynecol Obstet* 1979, 149:571.

3 Hobson RW III, Wright CB, O'Donnell JA, Zamil Z, Lamberth WC, Najem Z: Determination of intestinal viability by Doppler ultrasound. *Arch Surg* 1979, 114:165.
4 Ernst, CB: Aortoenteric Fistulas, in Haimovici H (ed.): *Vascular Emergencies*, Appleton-Century-Crofts, New York, 1982, pp 365–385.
5 Perdue GD, Smith RB, Ansley JD, Constantino MJ: Impending aortoenteric hemorrhage and the effect of early recognition on improved outcome. *Ann Surg* 1980, 192:273.
6 Kleinman LH, Towne JB, Bernhard VM: A diagnostic and therapeutic approach to aorto-enteric fistulas: Clinical experience with 20 patients. *Surgery* 1979, 86:868.
7 Grace RR, Mattox KL: Anterior spinal artery syndrome following abdominal aortic aneurysmectomy. *Arch Surg* 1977, 112:813.
8 Elliott JP, Szilagyi E, Hageman JH, Smith RF: Spinal cord damage secondary to surgery of the abdominal aorta, in Bernhard VM, Towne JB (eds): *Complication in Vascular Surgery.* Grune & Stratton, New York, 1980, p 407.
9 Djindjian R: *Angiography of the Spinal Cord.* University Park, Baltimore, 1970.
10 Batson RC. Frusha J, Porter JA: Hydronephrosis following aortofemoral bypass using Dacron venous grafts. *J Cardiovasc Surg* (Torino) 1981, 22:491.
11 Roth RB: *Surgical Injuries to the Ureter. Proceedings of the Sectional Meeting of the American College of Surgeons in Cooperation with Deutsche Gesellschaft fur Chirurgie in Munich, June 26–9, 1968.* Springer-Verlag, Berlin, 1969.
12 Petrone AF, Dudzinski PJ, Mantiatis W: Ureteral obstruction secondary to aortic femoral bypass. *Ann Surg* 1974, 179:192.
13 Antkowiak JH, D'Altorio RA: Ureteral obstruction secondary to bifurcated aortic graft. *Arch Surg* 1979, 114:8533.
14 Hagedorn CH, Tannenbaum MD, Stone WJ: Ureteral obstruction following aortofemoral or aortoiliac bypass graft. *J Tenn Med Assoc* May 1979, p 339.

Invited Commentary

Calvin B. Ernst, M.D.
Baltimore, Maryland

This succinct review of the major complications of abdominal aortic reconstruction focuses on the important aspects of diagnosis and treatment. These entities are not extensively detailed with supportive data, but there are ample references for the reader interested in further details.

Complications of abdominal aortic reconstruction may be classified as (1) those that occur early in the perioperative period, including acute renal failure, distal embolization (trash foot), impotence, spinal cord ischemia, and ischemic colitis and (2) those that are recognized late following reconstruction, including ureteral obstruction, graft infection, pseudoaneurysm development, and aortoenteric fistula. All present challenges in prevention and management, but clearly some, such as acute renal failure, bowel ischemia, and aortoenteric fistula, because of their potential lethality, are more important than others.

Patients undergoing aortic reconstruction may be at risk of developing postoperative acute renal failure because of decreased functional renal reserve secondary to associated diseases, including diabetes mellitus, hypertension causing renal arteriolosclerosis, and poor renal perfusion secondary to renal arterial occlusive disease or compromised myocardial function. Most instances of acute renal failure relate to renal ischemia secondary to impaired perfusion. Strict attention to maintenance of optimal cardiac function and extracellular fluid volume, by hydration and by monitoring of cardiac output and ventricular performance using Swan-Ganz catheter data, will minimize low-perfusion renal failure. Optimal volume replacement, indicated by pulmonary artery wedge pressures of 10 to 12 Torr and a cardiac index of 3.0 l/m^2, has been shown to be much more accurate than rapid urine flow and central venous pressure (CVP) measurements in preventing renal failure. In addition, renal complications of contrast media may be minimized by adequate hydration both before and after arteriography. This is particularly true for diabetics. It is suggested that elective aortic reconstruction be delayed for 24 hours following aortography, to allow time for adequate hydration and to minimize contrast media toxicity. Finally, administration of 12.5 g of mannitol before aortic clamping and another 12.5 g before declamping may minimize renal cortical ischemia. Mannitol has been shown to be an effective oxygen-free radical scavenger which diminishes tubular cell injury associated with ischemia and reperfusion.

Intestinal ischemia following aortic reconstruction almost always affects the colon. The overall mortality rate of ischemic colitis approximates 50 percent and approaches 90 percent for transmural involvement. Prevention of ischemic bowel complications requires identification of the patient at high risk and also depends on precise, gentle, meticulous operative technique, on knowledge of bowel blood supply, and on determination of when the inferior or superior mesenteric arteries must be reconstructed or when the inferior mesenteric artery (IMA) may be safely ligated. As indicated, once it has been determined that colonic collateral blood flow is adequate to prevent development of colon ischemia, the IMA must be oversewn from within the aneurysmal sac. If reconstruction is required, indicated by IMA stump blood pressure of less than 40 Torr or loss of left colon mesentery Doppler sounds, I prefer to reconstruct the IMA by suturing the orifice of the IMA, without removing a Carrell patch, to the aortic graft—the inclusion technique popularized by Stanley Crawford.

Progression or resolution of ischemic colitis can be determined only by repeated colonoscopy. Resolution of ischemic colitis requires about 10 to 14 days, during which time the bowel is put at rest by nasogastric suction. Optimal intravenous nutrition and fluid balance are maintained, and broad-spectrum antibiotic coverage is provided to prevent bacteremia from the involved bowel and potential hematogenous graft infection. Progression requires colectomy with construction of a colostomy and Hartmann's pouch. Care must be taken to avoid opening the pelvic retroperitoneum during colectomy, lest contamination of the prosthesis occur.

Massive gastrointestinal hemorrhage in a patient who has undergone prosthetic aortic reconstruction signals aortoenteric fistula until proved otherwise. Often the only way to make the diagnosis is by operation because, in spite of sophisticated diagnostic studies, preoperative confirmation of aortoenteric fistula is possible in only one-third of patients. A high index of suspicion and early operation are essential to making the diagnosis.

Two critical factors in the equation of successful management are control of hemorrhage and secure closure of the aortic stump. Temporary occlusion of the supraceliac aorta through the lesser space has proved successful for control of bleeding. An alternative is to open the fistula or graft distal to the fistula and thread a balloon-tipped catheter into the aorta. After inflation of the balloon, which often resides at or above the renal artery ostium, the graft–aortic anastomosis is dismantled and the fistula closed.

Secure, lasting closure of the aortic stump is mandatory, but up to one-third of patients die as a result of dehiscence of the closure. Two layers of nonabsorbable monofilament suture are required. In addition, a buttress of omentum transposed through the transverse mesocolon provides additional fresh tissue to reinforce the aortic stump and, probably more important, provides well-vascularized coverage, which facilitates resolution of periaortic infection.

Technical factors at the time of aortic reconstruction are paramount in preventing development of secondary aortoenteric fistula. Gentle dissection of the duodenum from the underlying aneurysm is required for prevention of duodenal injury or ischemia. Since contact between the duodenum and prosthesis predisposes to fistulization, interposition of viable tissue between the duodenum and graft during retroperitonealization is mandatory. Debrided aneurysmal sac sutured over the prosthesis effectively separates the graft and enteric tract. Where aneurysmal sac is not available and retroperitoneal tissue is lacking to adequately isolate the duodenum from the graft, a transposed pedicle of omentum sutured into the retroperitoneum over the graft has proved effective.

8 PERIPHERAL ANEURYSMS

Aneurysms of peripheral arteries were treated surgically long before aortic ones. Much of the early history of vascular reconstruction evolved through efforts to correct these lesions.

The earliest attempts to treat peripheral aneurysms aimed to produce thrombosis by continued obliterative pressure, by intraluminal injection or by surgical ligation. The Greek surgeon Antyllus in the second century A.D. performed proximal and distal ligations of popliteal aneurysms along with packing of the opened sac. Desault in France and John Hunter in England first ligated the superficial femoral artery proximally in the thigh in 1785, but it was the latter who recognized that collateral circulation allowed the limb to remain viable.*

Sir Astley Cooper first ligated the carotid artery for aneurysms in 1805. The patient died of infection. In 1808 another patient survived the procedure. Further experience indicated that 20 to 30 percent of such carotid ligations produced cerebral complications.

In an effort to avoid the dangers of sudden arterial occlusion, several devices were invented to reduce the lumen of the artery while collateral circulation developed. Selverstone and Crutchfield clamps[2] represent examples of these, along with the external band developed by William S. Halsted (Figure 8-1).[3]

The great innovator Rudolph Matas, from New Orleans, introduced endoaneurysmorrhaphy in 1888. By 1920 he had operated upon 154 popliteal aneurysms with 0.6 per cent mortality and 95 percent limb salvage. Bernheim used the Halsted technique of gradual occlusion of the proximal iliac artery, along with endoaneurysmorrhaphy, to correct 66 femoral aneurysms with 92 percent recovery and 6.3 percent amputation.[4]

These precursor operations were outmoded by Voorhees's introduction of the synthetic graft to replace a diseased vessel.[5] Reconstruction has now been a standard procedure for peripheral aneurysms for 30 years.

CLINICAL MANIFESTATIONS

The common multiplicity of peripheral arterial aneurysms, as well as the occurrence of hidden intracavitary aneurysms, necessitates a search for others when one is found. There were concomitant aneurysms (28 percent aortic) among 81 percent of Pappas's 89 patients,[6] and Cutler and Darling reported 75 percent.[7] A British series of 116 popliteal aneurysms had 86 percent multiplicity.[8] The entire vascular system should be searched for other vascular lesions, since most patients with a peripheral aneurysm will have other manifestations of atherosclerosis; hyperten-

*The historically inclined reader will enjoy W. R. Chitwood's interesting account of the Hunter brothers and their contributions to vascular surgery.[1]

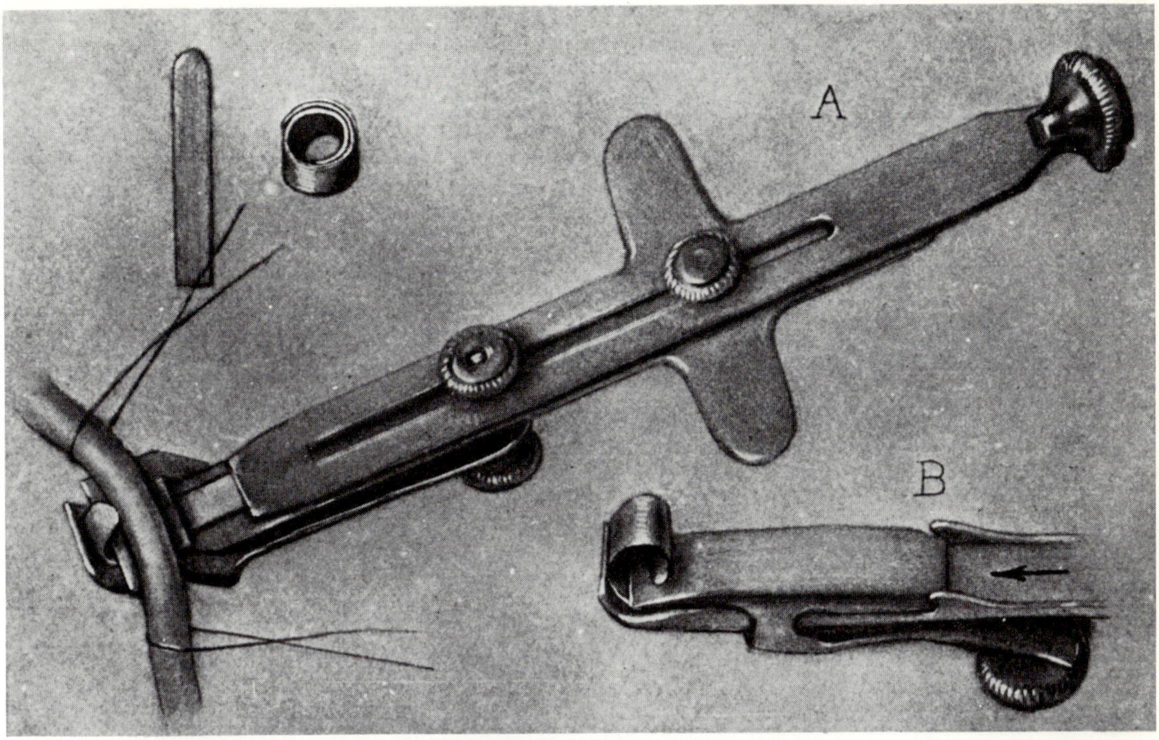

FIGURE 8-1 Halsted's original instrument to apply an aluminum band to constrict an artery proximally to produce thrombosis of a peripheral aneurysm. (Courtesy *Surg* 1974, 76:858.)

sion, angina and coronary artery disease, cerebrovascular disease, and limb ischemia are common.

Many peripheral aneurysms present initially as a pulsatile mass, but small ones may not be easily detected. Thus, a subclavian aneurysm due to pressure of a cervical rib may not be evident until a distal embolus causes toe symptoms. Thrombosis of a popliteal aneurysm often progresses to the extent that the original lesion is overlooked in the midst of a femoropopliteal graft to bypass the extensive thrombosis.

SPECIFIC LESIONS

Carotid Aneurysms

True aneurysms of the extracranial carotid arterial system are unusual, but once they are present, their progression is to be expected and their complication rate is high, so resection with arterial reconstruction is indicated.

A pulsatile mass in the neck makes an obvious presentation, but a high, deep mass in the nasopharynx may be mistaken for tumor or even for a peritonsillar abscess requiring drainage. Rupture occasionally occurs into the adjacent tissue.

Elongation of a carotid artery with twisting or coiling, as well as a carotid body tumor, may mimic an aneurysm. Arteriograms differentiate these.

Neurologic symptoms of amaurosis fugax, transient ischemic attacks and stroke occurred in 50 percent of the 21-patient series at the University of Michigan. These threats were confirmed by the 50 percent stroke rate among their patients who did not have operative correction, whereas none had later strokes after operation.[9]

Since simple excision and ligation of either the common or internal carotid artery is dangerous to the brain, the artery should be reconstructed with an autogenous vein or a synthetic tube. Certain patients with high carotid stump pressures may not require a shunt, but it seems prudent to consider this, although there may be considerable technical difficulty in placement if the distal stump is high. A Fogarty catheter may be useful in that event. Since the complete removal of a large carotid aneurysm may lead to damage to adjacent nerves, such aneurysms may be better treated by inlaying the graft and leaving the deep wall of the aneurysm intact in the neck.

Exposure of the cephalad portion of the internal carotid artery may be obtained by removing the mastoid process and the inferior portion of the auditory canal, as described by Purdue, Pellegrini and Arena.[10] Aneurysms which extend cephalad to or beyond the base of the skull may be inoperable.

Subclavian and Axillary Aneurysms

Atherosclerosis accounts for some of these. Others are secondary to the continued trauma of a crutch (Figure 8-2), thoracic outlet pressure,[11] or a poorly healed rib or clavicular fracture.

Local symptoms due to the mass often lead the patient to seek medical care. Acute or chronic

FIGURE 8-2 Axillary aneurysm due to the long-continued intermittent pressure of a crutch.

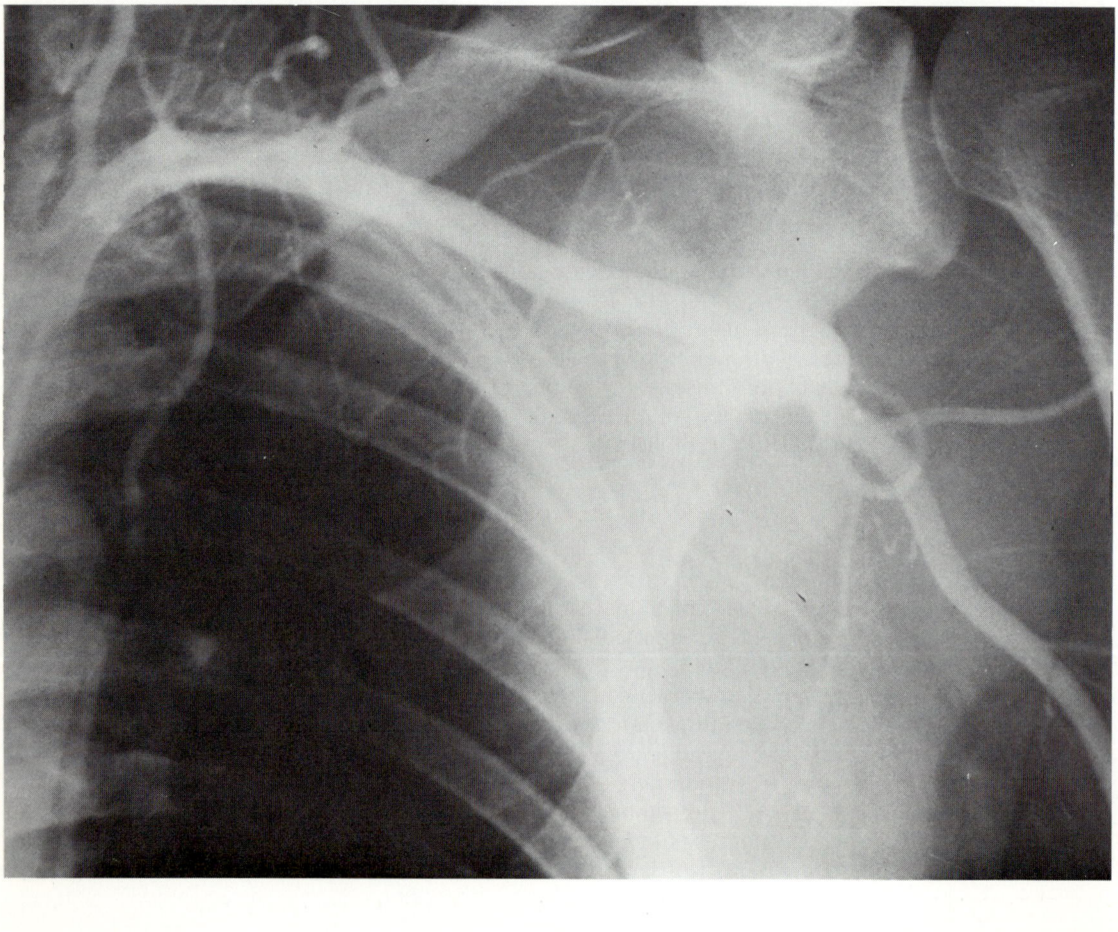

thrombosis with or without distal ischemia or embolism also occurs. Angiography is the key to diagnosis and surgical management.

The proximal control required for the resection and graft can often be achieved through a supraclavicular incision. Sometimes the entire procedure can be accomplished within the neck. If not, another incision, inferior to the clavicle, is carried through the pectoralis major muscle to expose the axillary artery there (Figure 8-3). The clavicle may often be left in place, but its resection is not functionally harmful to most people (excepting certain athletes).

The majority of the series (86 percent) of 14 aneurysms treated by DeBakey's group required one or another form of intrathoracic approach.[12] It is likely that these were severe problems in a group in whom smaller lesions were repaired elsewhere by less extensive procedures.

An autogenous vein from the thigh or, alternatively, a synthetic tube may be used for reconstruction of the artery.

Femoral Aneurysms

True femoral aneurysms are rare lesions, usually found in males with hypertension. They present as an asymptomatic pulsatile mass or as thrombosis with distal ischemia (Figures 8-4 to 8-7). Rupture occasionally forces an emergency operation. Distal embolization occasionally occurs.

As usual, arteriographic mapping is the key to proper treatment.

Since clinical progression is likely, femoral aneurysms should be repaired. Total excision with

FIGURE 8-3 The aneurysm-containing portion of the subclavian-axillary artery was resected and replaced by a knit Dacron graft, which was tunneled posterior to the clavicle.

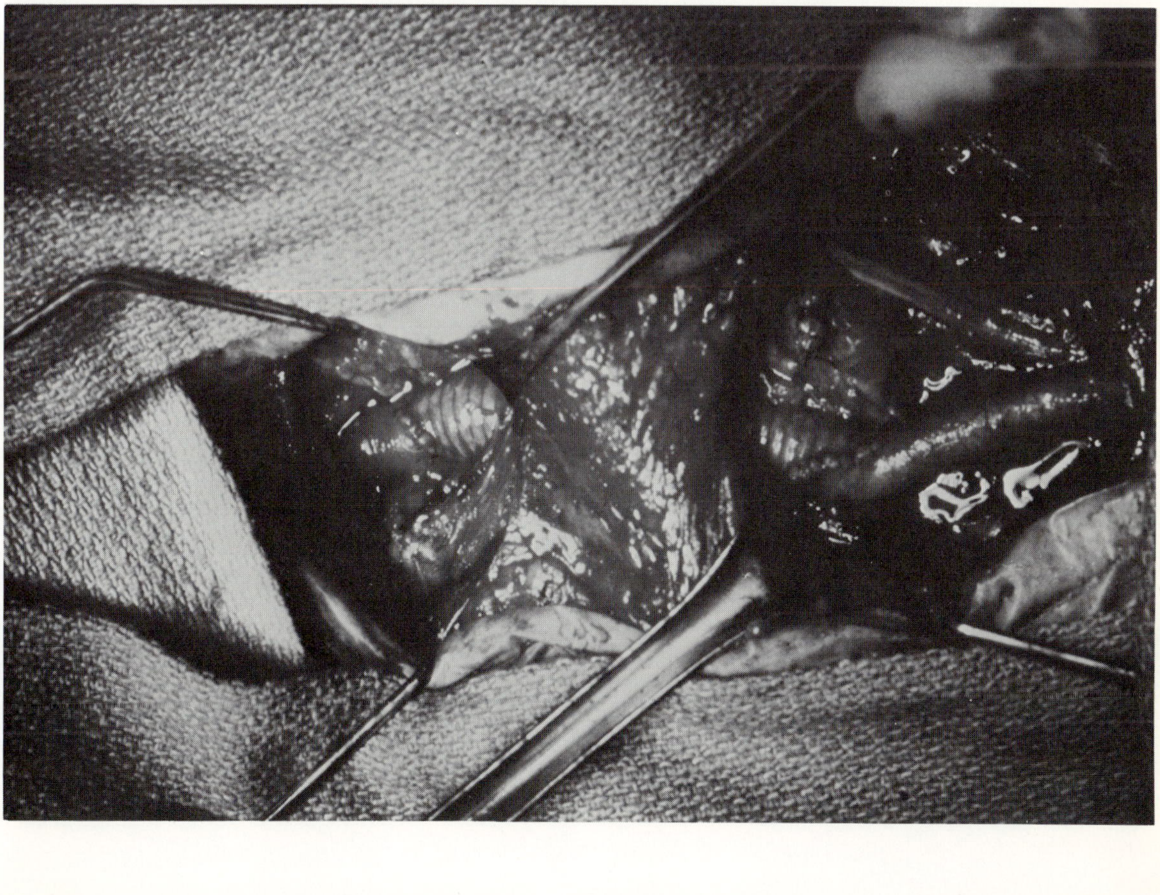

graft replacement usually requires a synthetic tube because a vein graft is too small. The revascularization should particularly provide flow into the profunda femoris artery.

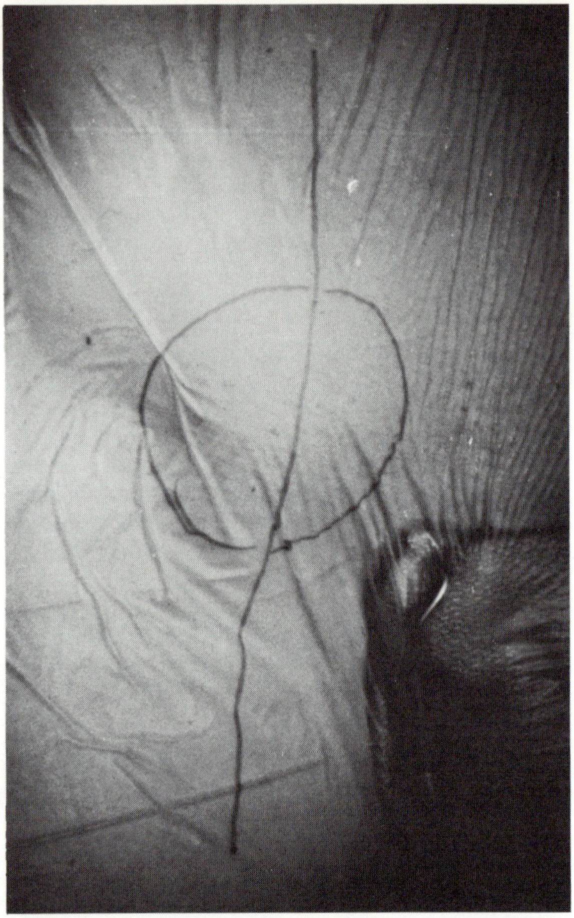

FIGURE 8-4 The aneurysmal mass in the right groin is *encircled.* The *line* indicates the skin incision over the femoral aneurysm.

Popliteal Aneurysms

Second only to aortic aneurysms in frequency, these aneurysms often lie hidden in the popliteal space, asymptomatic until their sudden thrombosis with distal ischemia or embolization. Less frequent presentations include pain due to pressure on adjacent nerves, venous thrombosis, and rupture. Nevertheless, among the 147 popliteal aneurysms in the Vermilion series, a third were asymptomatic, almost half had claudication, a third had rest pain, and 7 percent each had venous obstruction or ulceration. Rupture occurred in 3 percent.[13]

Thirty-odd years ago Robert Linton recognized the grave risk of limb-threatening complications with popliteal aneurysms—77 percent limb loss over an 18-year period.[14] The risk is now well-recognized.[15,13] The common occurrence of concomitant aneurysms elsewhere (60 percent in the University of Michigan series)[16] indicates the importance of searching for other lesions. Most are due to arteriosclerosis,[17] and almost half are bilateral.[18,16]

Arteriography will map blood supply and "run-off," but partial intraluminal thrombosis characteristically masks the true size of the lesion. Ultrasound is more accurate to delineate size.

Large and/or symptomatic popliteal aneurysms obviously require repair. There is also a clear-cut indication for repair of the acutely thrombosed lesion with ischemia secondary to occlusion of the blood supply to the leg and foot (Figure 8-8).

The asymptomatic popliteal aneurysm requires more thought. Observation without operation avoids costs, loss of work, pain, and the inevitable (even though small) risk of a surgical mishap. The decision for or against surgical repair must therefore rest upon the probable results of one or the other course of action. However, the risk of limb-threatening complication is so great that the advice of Vermilion, Kimmins, Pace, and Evans for surgical treatment, even for small lesions, is sound.[13] Repair of a lesion which has caused no problem demands a good result, or at least one which surpasses the prognosis for an untreated lesion. Published statistics usually reflect the results (33 percent bad) of nontreatment of all, rather than completely asymptomatic, popliteal aneurysms. Nevertheless, among the 21 unoperated noncomplicated popliteal aneurysms reported by Evans, 76 percent developed problems within 5 years.[19] Fifteen years ago a series of

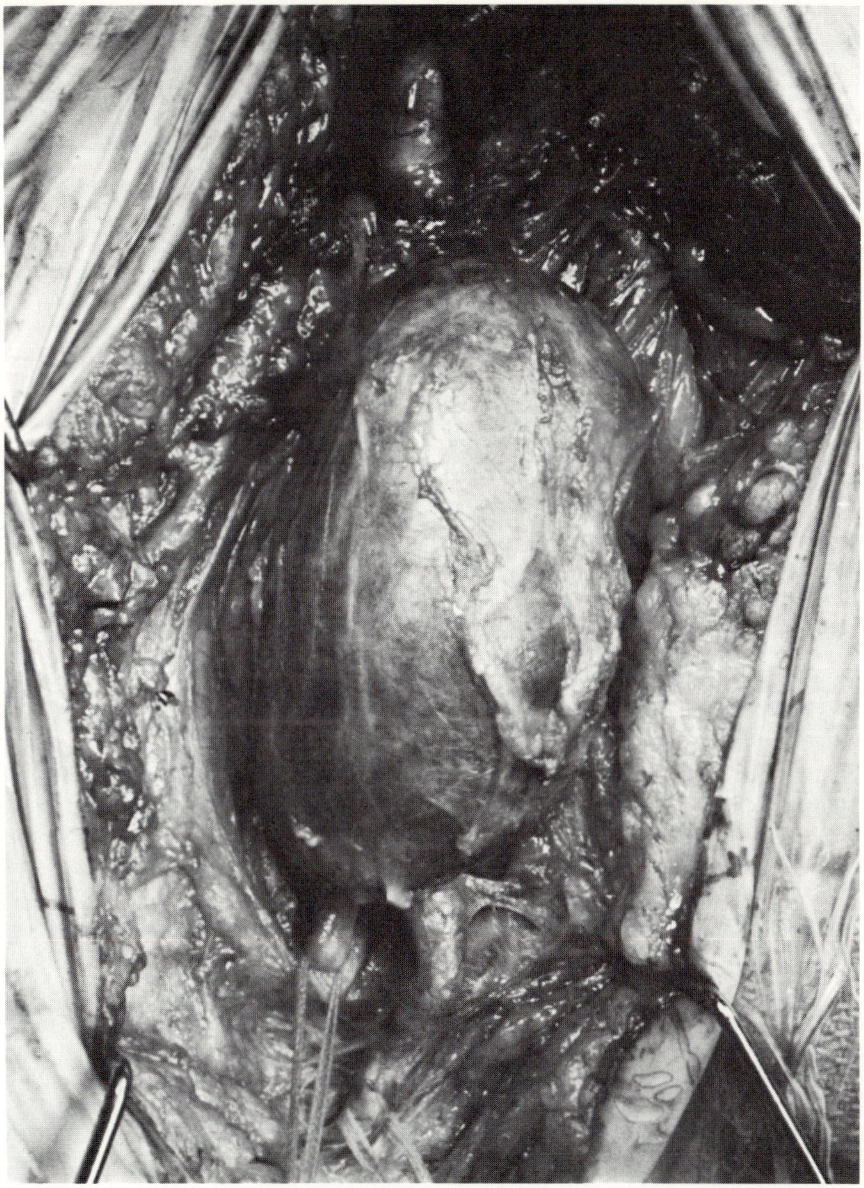

FIGURE 8-5 The arteriosclerotic femoral aneurysm has been dissected to allow its complete removal. *Above,* the external artery enters, and *below,* the superficial femoral and profunda femoris arteries exit the aneurysm.

87 asymptomatic popliteal aneurysms followed without operation showed that 31 percent developed complications, with loss of limb in 3.5 percent.[17]

After surveying 61 patients with popliteal aneurysms, the Michigan group recommended "earlier surgical treatment of asymptomatic aneurysms," but this multiple-author series over a 39-year period (1943–1982) does not necessarily represent the authoritative opinion.[16]

The old procedures of endoaneurysmorrhaphy and, later, resection and grafting have been superseded by the preferable operation of a bypass graft, remote to the aneurysm, with ligation of the vessels entering and exiting, so that thrombosis of the aneurysm is accompanied by provision of a blood supply to the distal tissues (Figure 8-9). Further, this obviates the need to remove the aneurysm, with risk to the adjacent vein and nerves (Figure 8-10). Autogenous saphenous vein is the conduit of choice (Figure 8-11),[20] although knit Dacron tubes had a 50 percent patency rate at 7 years in Towne's report of 42 operations.[18]

Rarely the aneurysm thereafter persists as a large mass with pressure symptoms after its successful bypass and thrombosis (Figure 8-12). This may require a posterior exposure to open the sac and empty its contents. Entering collateral vessels will require control from within the sac. A suction drainage tube should be placed to aid removal of fluid during the healing process.

In one elderly male a large thrombosed aneurysm was associated with an excellent collateral arterial circulation. It was evacuated via a posterior approach without the necessity for an accompanying graft.

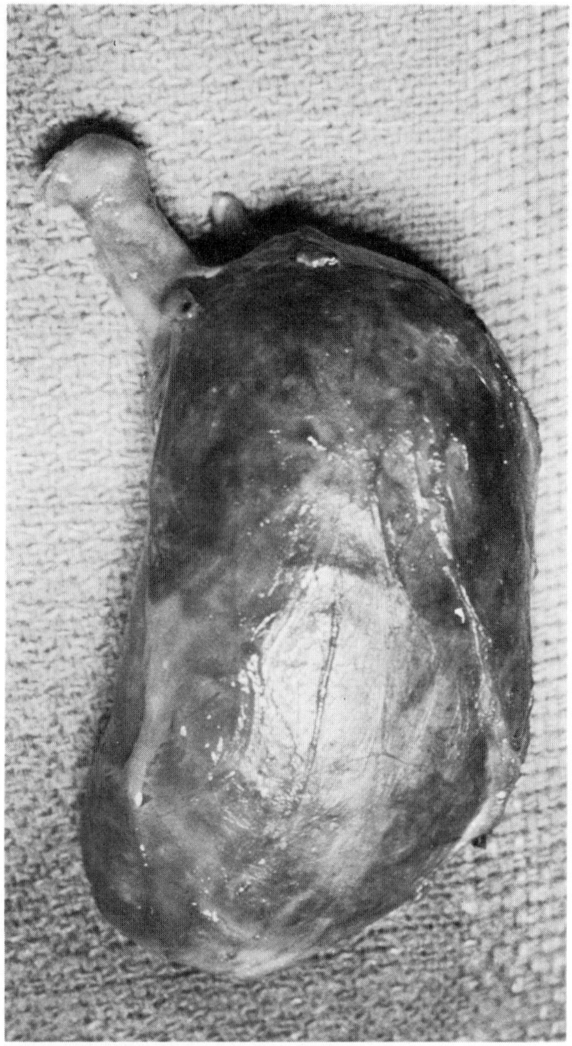

FIGURE 8-6 The femoral aneurysm, along with a portion of external iliac artery, has been excised.

FALSE ANEURYSMS

Aneurysms which do not include all layers of the arterial wall are *false* (atypical, curious). In some locations, such as femoral, they are more common than true ones (Figure 8-13). Femoral false aneurysms are the prototype, although any location subject to trauma (surgical or otherwise) may be the site of origin. More common than violent trauma today is the false aneurysm which occurs months after a prosthetic graft is anastomosed to an artery.*

The risk of development of anastomotic aneurysms of the femoral artery was 2.6 percent in the 43-limb experience of Nichols and associates[22] and 3 percent among Szilagyi's computer-collected 4303 cases.[23]

The older idea that dissolution of silk suture material led to false aneurysms is a good example of specious reasoning, since they still occur with new, stronger, permanent synthetic sutures.

*The 1981 collective review of Satiani is a concise, complete summary of information regarding false aneurysms.[21]

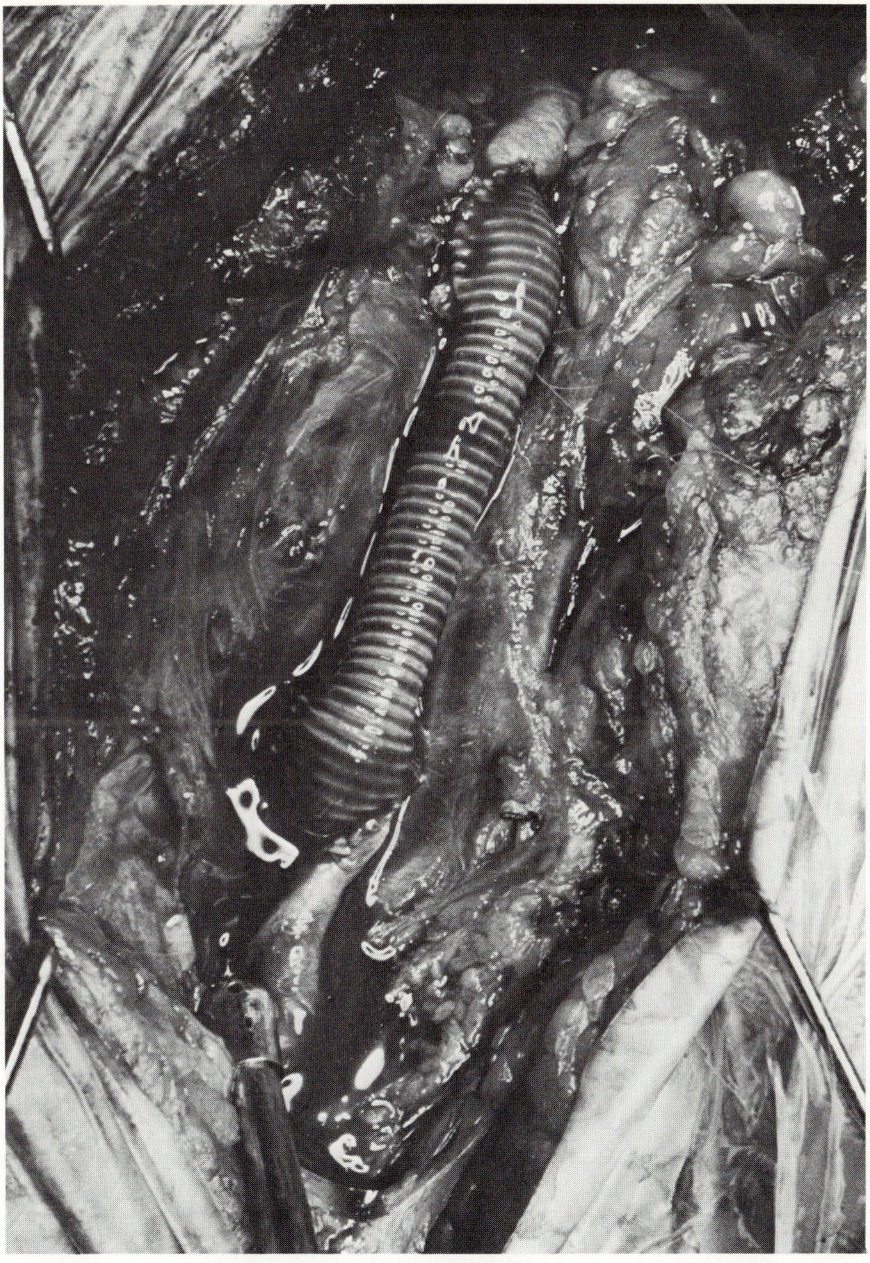

FIGURE 8-7 The femoral arterial system was reconstructed with a Dacron graft.

Nevertheless, false aneurysms continue to form, and sutures continue to receive the blame. A Houston group in 1979 recommended braided multifilament as superior to the monofilament polypropylene suture.[24] The latter, however, is preferred by most surgeons, with the proviso that it should not be crushed or handled by steel instruments during the procedure. This obvious precaution is widely ignored.

A few lesions may be due to dilatation of the graft[25] or to infection.

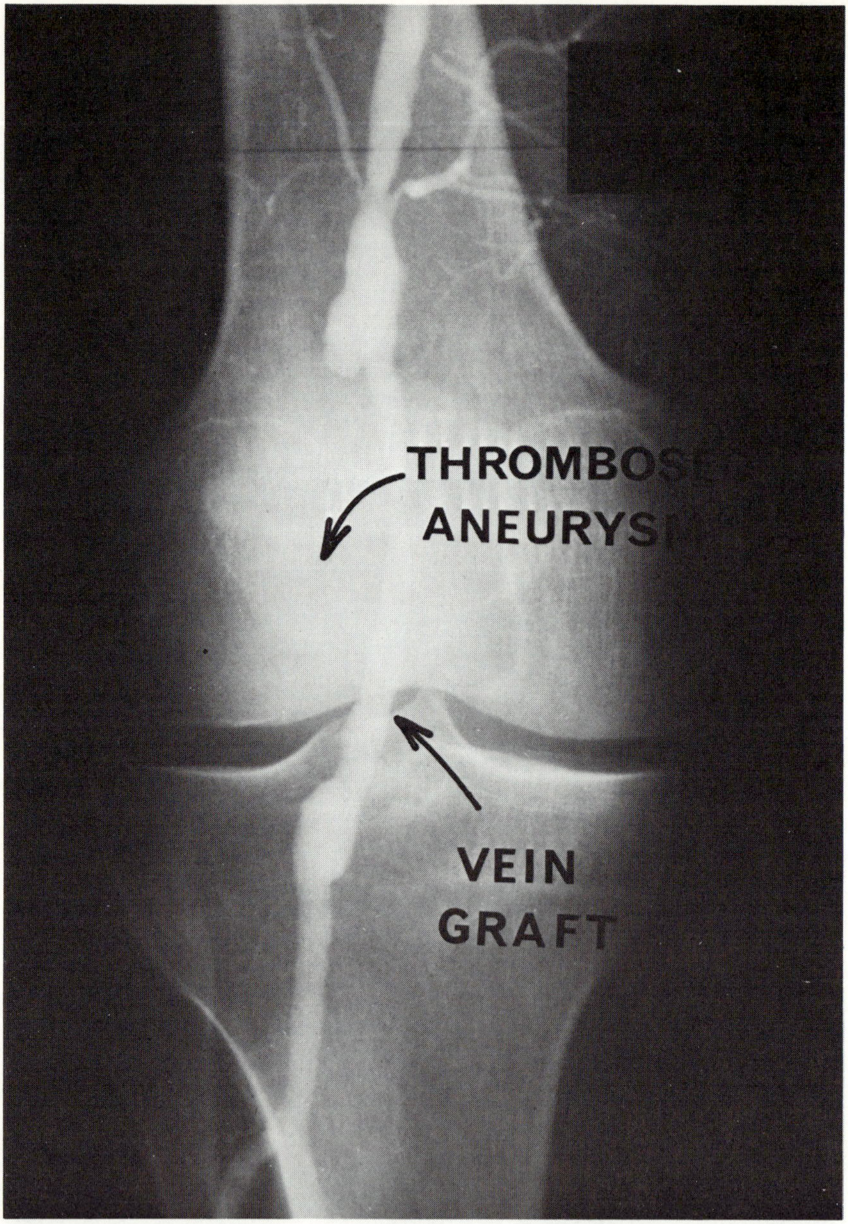

FIGURE 8-8 Acute thrombosis of a popliteal aneurysm with distal ischemia was repaired with a bypassing vein graft through the posterior approach used until 1968.

The most common cause of false aneurysms is disruption of the arterial wall. The suture line splits a portion away, and blood escapes into a hematoma, where it evokes a fibrous reaction and becomes encapsulated. The usual association of the problem with an aortofemoral graft rather than a femoropopliteal one (80 versus 2 in the Walter Reed Center group)[26] suggests a tightly stretched graft plus motion as an important causative factor. False aneurysms rarely occur

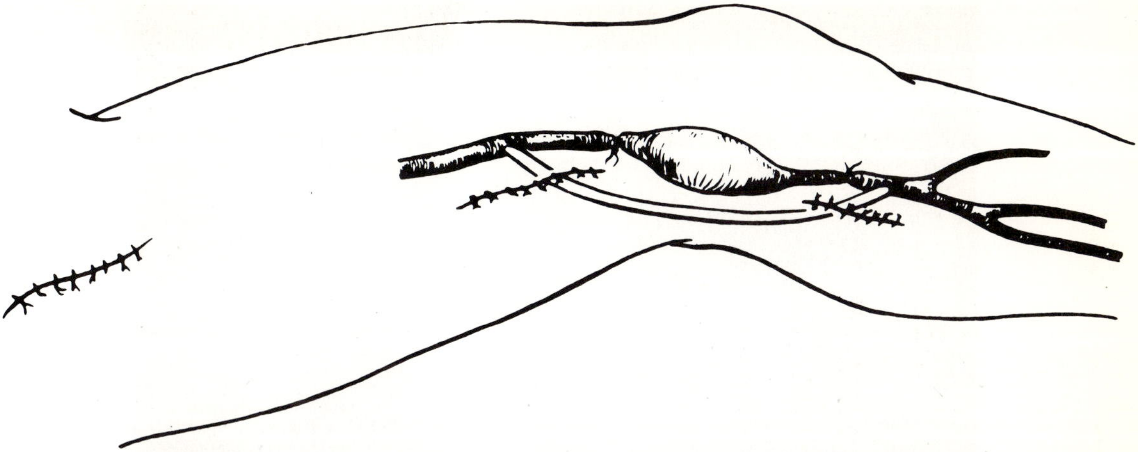

FIGURE 8-9 The modern operation for popliteal aneurysm bypasses the mass through a medial-thigh and upper-calf incision. The graft is autogenous saphenous vein removed from the groin. Proximal and distal ligatures cause thrombosis within the graft and also prevent distal embolism.

when the distal end of the graft is joined to the iliac artery within the pelvis—a worthwhile procedure which is hardly known today.

False aortic aneurysms are unusual. Their discovery is usually triggered by symptoms. Observation is dangerous because of the likelihood of extension with final free rupture without any external warning. Surgical repair of false aortic aneurysms should be done without delay. The broken aortic anastomosis must be replaced with a new segment or an entire graft. If there is infection, the graft must be removed and the distal circulation restored by an extraanatomic axillobifemoral graft.

It has been suggested that all intraabdominal grafts (which are hidden from clinical examination) should be inspected by ultrasound periodically.[27] The rare occurrence of false aneurysms in this position, along with the costs involved, leads to the conclusion that such is ultradefensive and not needed in the absence of symptoms.

The timing of repair of a femoral false aneurysm is less clear-cut. Small ones have often been observed for long periods, since the lesser ones rarely thrombose, embolize, or rupture. Each will progress, so as soon as the decision is accepted by the patient, the lesion should be corrected. Repairs of bilateral false aneurysms are staged to allow recovery without complications after the initial procedure (Figures 8-14, 8-15).

The technique of repair of a femoral aneurysm should stress simplicity (a worthy aim for any procedure). Spinal anesthesia is a good choice. Incision over the mass should be carried proximally in the groin to expose the inguinal ligament. This is incised to allow the graft, with its fibrous sheath coursing down from within the pelvis, to be exposed. A vascular clamp is used to control the inflow of blood.

Distally the superficial and profunda branches of the femoral artery may be dissected from the surrounding scar tissue. It is, however, easier to open the aneurysmal sac, scoop out the contained thrombus, and control back bleeding by indwelling Fogarty balloon catheters. A new segment of polytetrafluoroethylene (PTFE) or Dacron graft is then fashioned appropriately, anastomosing the new conduit proximally end-to-end to the old graft and distally to the anterior surface of the femoral arterial system.

The Nichols group has suggested a variation for this reconstruction to prevent recurrence: buttress the femoral segment by encircling it with a split synthetic tube, which is closed about

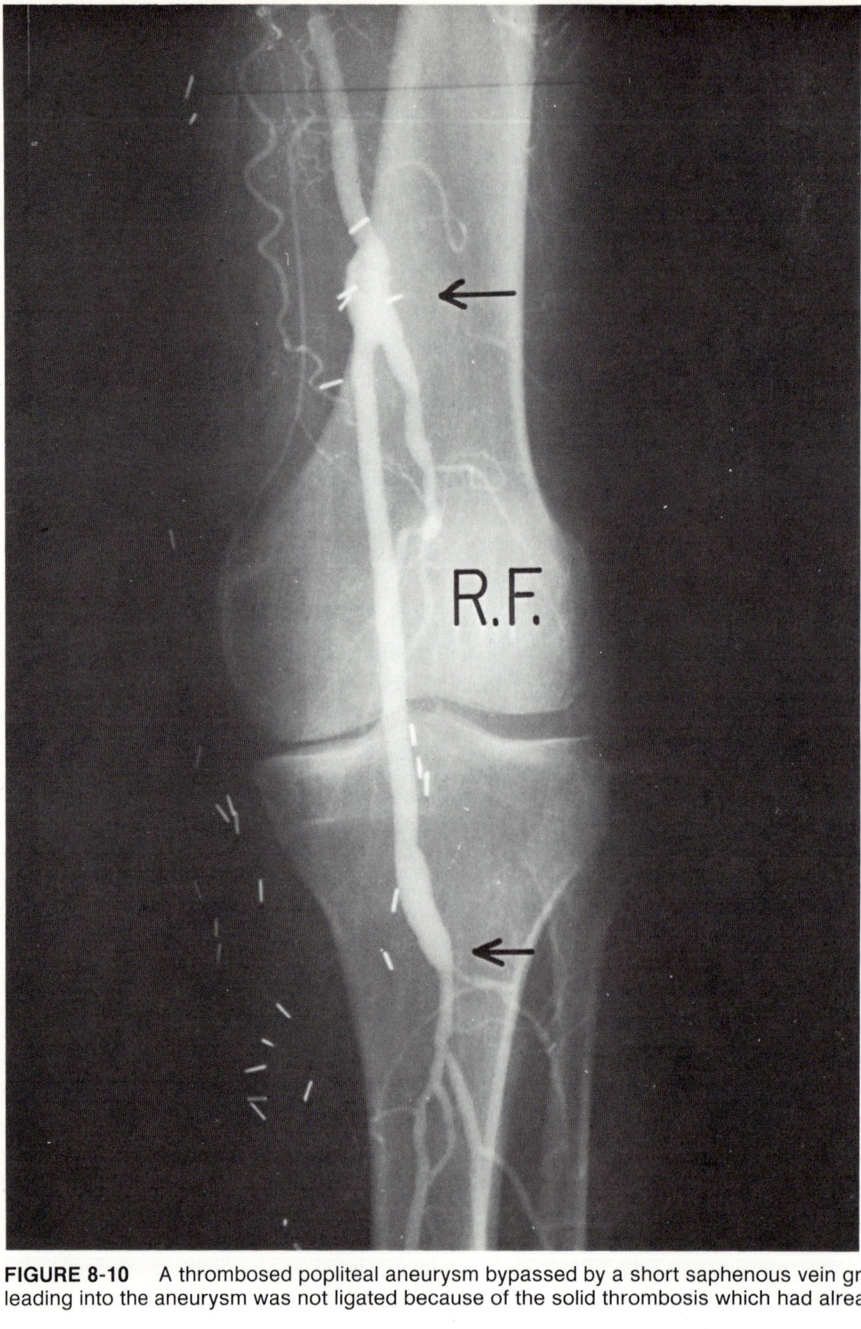

FIGURE 8-10 A thrombosed popliteal aneurysm bypassed by a short saphenous vein graft. The artery leading into the aneurysm was not ligated because of the solid thrombosis which had already occurred.

the host vessel and attached to the prosthetic as it enters.[22] It might be even better to resect the diseased femoral artery, replace it with a synthetic tube, and attach the end of the new graft to the side of this so that the suture line will not tend to pull off the side of the artery. There is no personal experience with such a complicated variation—simplicity is the rule.

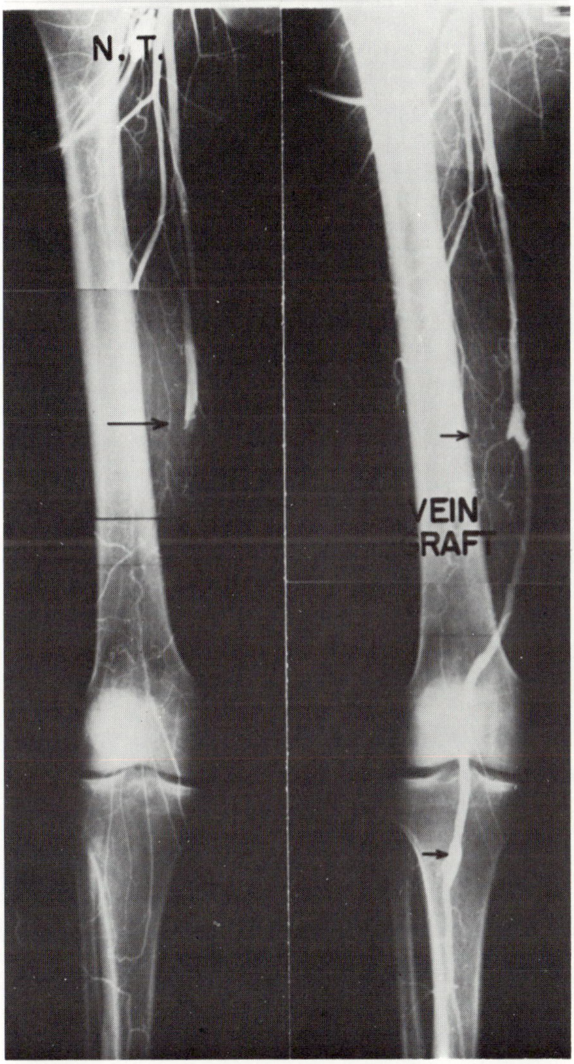

FIGURE 8-11 Acute thrombosis of a popliteal aneurysm with progression of the clot proximally. A long segment of saphenous vein was used for the reconstructive bypass.

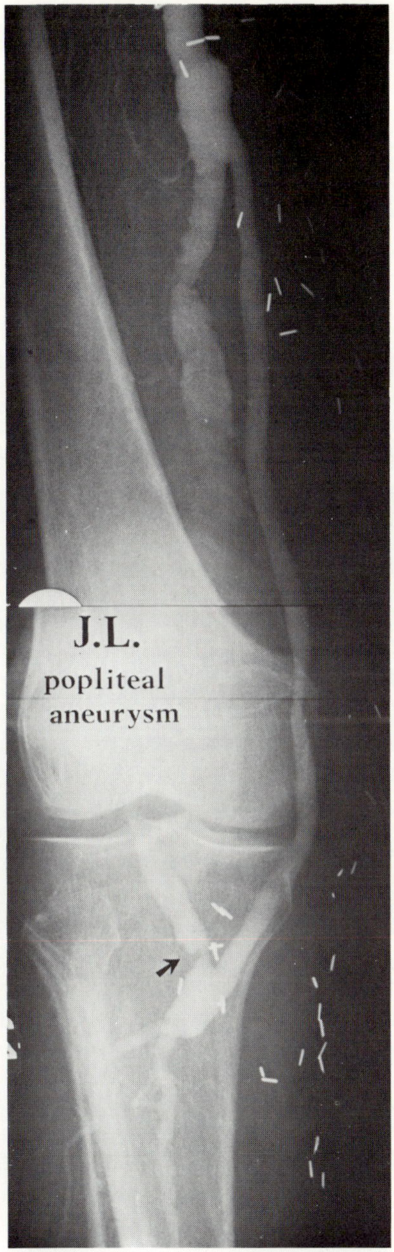

FIGURE 8-12 This popliteal aneurysm was bypassed with saphenous vein and a distal ligature *(arrow)* placed to prevent embolism. The lead-in proximal artery was not ligated. The aneurysm did not thrombose, continued to be pulsatile and painful, and required secondary proximal ligation. The double ligation should be performed at the original operation.

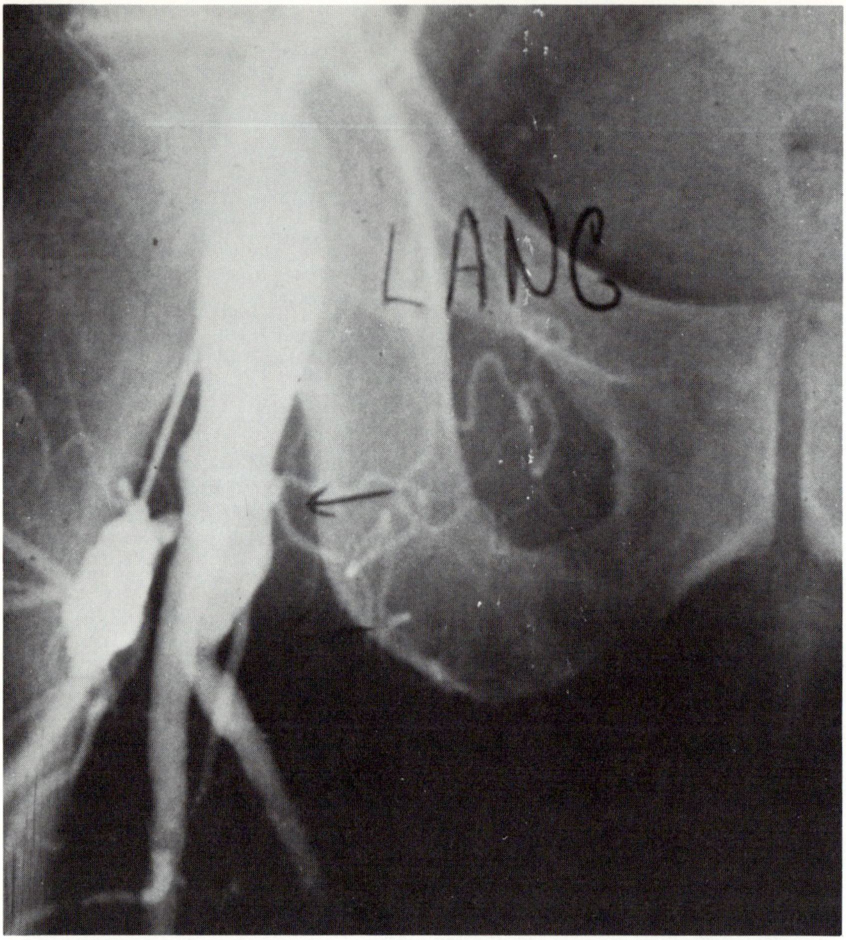

FIGURE 8-13 This true aneurysm of the common femoral artery occurred proximal to the origin of a femoropopliteal venous bypass. It was removed and replaced without disturbing that anastomosis.

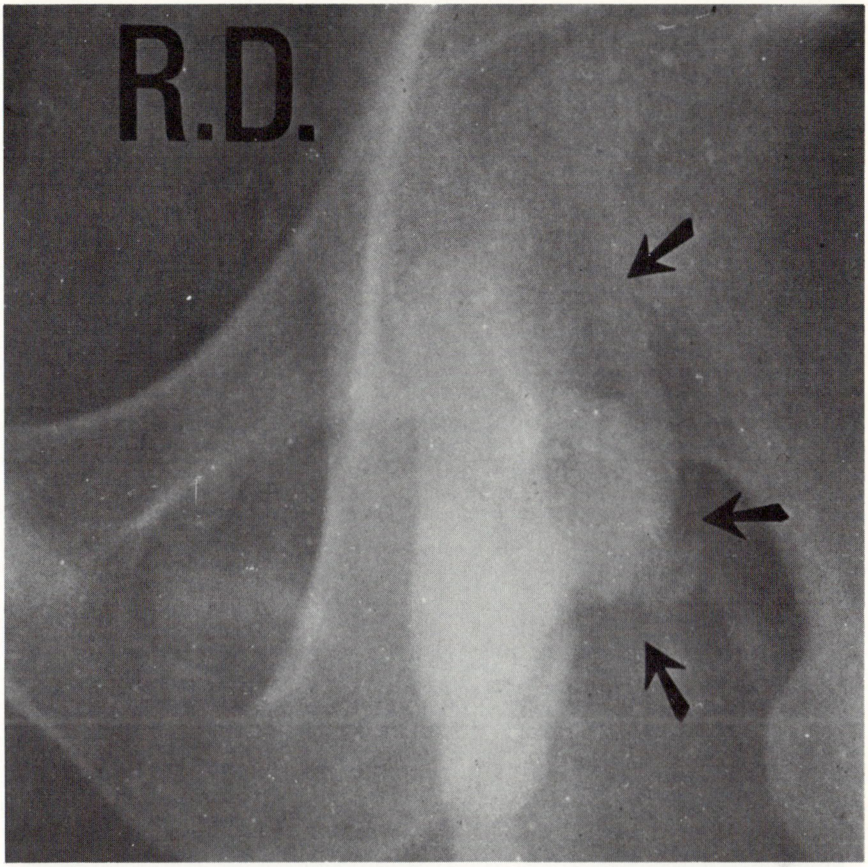

FIGURE 8-14 *Arrows* delineate contrast material in a false femoral aneurysm at the site of a Dacron tube anastomosis to the femoral artery.

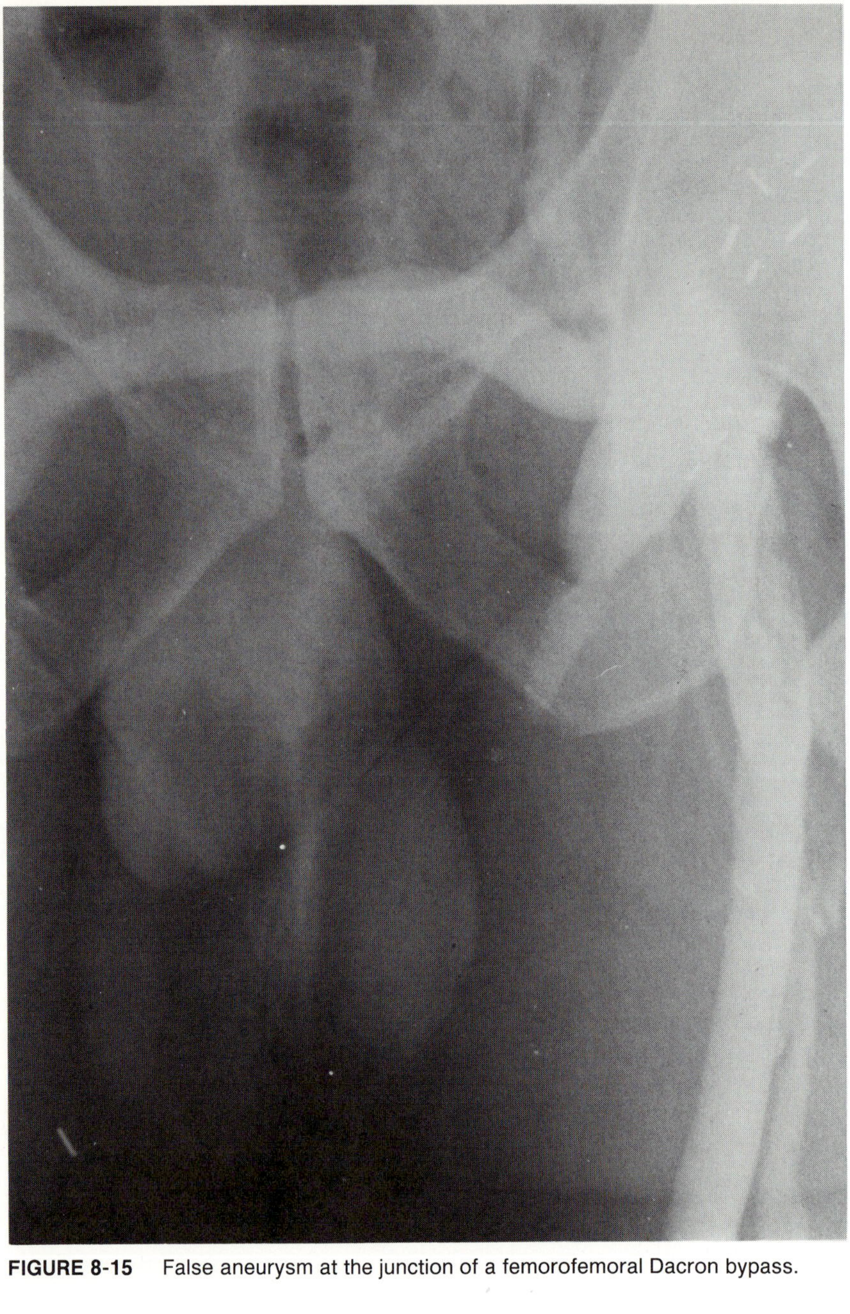

FIGURE 8-15 False aneurysm at the junction of a femorofemoral Dacron bypass.

REFERENCES

1 Chitwood WR: John and William Hunter on aneurysms. *Arch Surg* 1977, 112:829.
2 Crutchfield WG: Instruments for care in the treatment of certain intracranial vascular lesions. *J Neurosurg* 1959, 16:471.
3 Halsted WS: An experimental study of circumscribed dilatation of an artery immediately distal to a par-

tially occluding band, and its bearing on the dilatation of the subclavian artery observed in certain cases of cervical rib. *J Exp Med* 1916, 24:271.

4 Bernheim BM: *Surgery of the Vascular System.* JB Lippincott, Philadelphia, 1913.

5 Voorhees AB, Jaretski A, Blakemore AH: The use of tubes constructed from vinyon N cloth in bridging arterial defects. *Ann Surg* 1952, 135:332.

6 Pappas G, Janes JM, Bernatz PE, Shirger A: Femoral aneurysm. *JAMA* 1964, 190:489.

7 Cutler BS, Darling RC: Surgical management of arteriosclerotic femoral aneurysm. *Surgery* 1973, 74:764.

8 Bouhoutsos J, Martin P: Popliteal aneurysms: A review of 116 cases. *Brit J Surg* 1974, 61:469.

9 Zwolak RM, Whitehouse WM Jr, Knake JE, Bernfield BD, Zelenock GB, Cronenwett JL, Erlandson EE, Kazmers A, Graham LM, Lindenauer SM, Stanley JC: Atherosclerotic extracranial carotid artery aneurysms. *J Vasc Surg* 1984, 1:415.

10 Purdue GF, Pellegrini RV, Arena S: Aneurysms of the high internal carotid artery: A new approach. *Surgery* 1981, 89:268.

11 Lee BY, Thoden WR, Madden JL, McCann WJ: Subclavian artery aneurysm secondary to thoracic outlet syndrome. *Contemp Surg* 1984, 25:19.

12 McCollum CH, Da Gama AD, Noon GP, DeBakey ME: Aneurysm of the subclavian artery. *J Cardiovasc Surg* 1979, 20:159.

13 Vermilion BD, Kimmins SA, Pace WG, Evans WE: A review of 147 popliteal aneurysms with long-term follow-up. *Surgery* 1981, 90:1998.

14 Linton RR: The arteriosclerotic popliteal aneurysm. *Surgery* 1949, 26:41.

15 Gifford RW, Hines EA, Janes JM: An analysis of follow-up study of 100 popliteal aneurysms. *Surgery* 1953, 33:284.

16 Whitehouse WM Jr, Wakefield TW, Graham LM, Kazmers A, Celenock GB, Cronenwett JL, Dent TL, Lindenauer SM, Stanley JC: Limb-threatening potential of arteriosclerotic popliteal artery aneurysms. *Surgery* 1983, 93:694.

17 Wychulis AR, Spittell JA, Wallace RB: Popliteal aneurysms. *Surgery* 1970, 68:942.

18 Towne JB, Thompson JE, Patman DD, Persson AV: Progression of popliteal aneurysmal disease following popliteal aneurysm resection with graft: A 20 year experience. *Surgery* 1976, 80:426.

19 Evans WE, Steele O: Peripheral artery aneurysm (Chapter 78), in Rutherford RB (ed): *Vascular Surgery.* WB Saunders, Philadelphia, 1977.

20 Fry WJ: Popliteal artery aneurysm (Chapter 5-2), in Sabiston DC (ed): *Textbook of Surgery.* WB Saunders, Philadelphia, 1977.

21 Satiani B: False aneurysms following arterial reconstruction. *Surg Gynecol Obstet* 1981, 152:357.

22 Nichols WK, Stanton M, Silver D, Keitzer WF: Anastomotic aneurysms following lower extremity revascularization. *Surgery* 1980, 88:366.

23 Szilagyi DE, Smith RF, Elliott JP, Hageman JH, Dall'Olmo CA: Anastomotic aneurysms after vascular reconstruction: Problems of incidence, etiology and treatment. *Surgery* 1975, 78:800.

24 Starr DS, Weatherford SC, Lawrie GM, Morris GC Jr: Suture material as a factor in the occurrence of anastomotic false aneurysms. *Arch Surg* 1979, 114:412.

25 Clagett G, Salander J, Eddleman W, Cabellon S, Youkey J, Olson D, Hutton J, Rich N: Dilation of knitted Dacron aortic prostheses and anastomotic false aneurysms: Etiologic considerations. *Surgery* 1983, 93:9.

26 Youkey JR, Clagett GP, Rich NM, Brigham RA, Orecchia PM, Salander JM: Femoral anastomotic false aneurysms. *Ann Surg* 1984, 197:703.

27 Gaylis H: Pathogenesis of anastomotic aneurysms. *Surgery* 1981, 90:509.

Invited Commentary

W. Sterling Edwards, M.D.
Albuquerque, New Mexico

In the late 1950s and the early 1960s we were exposed to a large number of unruptured popliteal aneurysms. Some of these were asymptomatic, but some had thrombosed and presented with ischemic limbs. The standard posterior approach to the aneurysm was frustrating at times, since there was often a significant inflammatory reaction around the sac involving the popliteal vein. Thrombectomy was difficult, since this was before the invention of the Fogarty catheter. Some of these popliteal aneurysms were quite extensive, with ballooning of the artery for many centimeters up the superficial femoral, and removal of all this sac made an extensive procedure. This led us, in 1969, to bypass some of these aneurysms with the patient's own vein, and exclude the sac with its dangerous thrombotic material.* All this could be done through medial leg incisions with the patient in the usual supine position, and avoiding exposing the sac of the aneurysm at all. Its simplicity and safety has led us to recommend prophylactic surgery on asymptomatic patients, even those of advanced age, if the leg involved is still being actively used in walking.

I agree with Dr. Dale's thesis that too much graft tension is the major cause of false femoral aneurysms in the groin after aortofemoral grafting. An additional preventive measure I use is a cloth pledget as a buttress at the heel and toe of the graft to femoral anastomosis, to keep the sutures from pulling through the diseased artery at these two points of greatest stress.

Surgery of femoral false aneurysms has been greatly simplified by controlling back bleeding from profunda branches by Fogarty catheters, rather than trying to dissect these multiple small branches often encased in thick scar tissue. Sometimes, Hegar dilators or small metal coronary dilators work even better for this purpose and should always be available during these operations.

*Edwards, WS: Exclusion and saphenous vein bypass of popliteal aneurysms. *Surg Gynecol Obst* 1969, 128:829. This is, as far as I know, the first description of ligation and exclusion of popliteal aneurysms.

9 PERIPHERAL OCCLUSIVE DISEASE

The development of vascular surgery has centered around peripheral arterial reconstruction, whose benefits are increasingly needed by our ever-aging population to preserve function and save limbs. A recent survey in our hospital showed that 43 percent of the vascular procedures were directed toward such reconstructions (Table 9-1).

Broad indications for reconstructive procedures are twofold: to rehabilitate patients whose limb dysfunction is limiting their usual work or life habits, and to save limbs threatened with early loss due to ischemia. Long-term successful rehabilitation and salvage in many patients encourages continued efforts. Important clinical considerations will be discussed, particularly those which require a choice among alternatives.

ILLUSTRATIVE CASE

R.S., a 53-year-old man, was first examined in 1963 with a 6-year history of claudication in the buttocks and thighs. A bilateral aortoiliac thromboendarterectomy was performed for complete absence of the right common iliac artery and multiple stenoses of the left.

Fifteen years later, in 1978, a left femoropopliteal venous bypass was placed because of incapacitating claudication. Two months later the graft occluded (perhaps because the donor vein was only 4 mm in diameter). The limb was viable, so nothing further was done.

By 1979 there was night pain along with several unhealing necrotic areas on the third toe. A 6-mm polytetrafluoroethylene (PTFE) graft was placed from the left common iliac artery to the popliteal artery just above the knee (Figure 9-1). Five hours later postoperative thrombosis was corrected by thrombectomy.

Eighteen months afterward the graft occluded (Figure 9-2) and was replaced with a new 6-mm PTFE conduit from the left iliac to the popliteal artery, this time below the knee.

Two years later, in 1982, the patient returned with acute ischemia of 72-hour duration due to recurrent occlusion of the PTFE graft in the left thigh. The graft was opened in the groin and also at its entrance to the popliteal artery below the knee and cleaned of thrombosis with Fogarty catheters. The distal anastomosis was patched with a vein removed from the dorsum of the hand. A completion intraoperative arteriogram comparable to the intraoperative arteriogram made 2 years previously (Figure 9-3) showed runoff into two vessels.

Three hours later rethrombosis occurred. The distal anastomosis was opened, and Fogarty catheters were passed distally without encountering any clot. When a catheter was passed proximally, a 6-cm segment of neointima was removed. It apparently had rolled up and caused the acute thrombosis. Another intraoperative arteriogram showed restoration of flow into the two-vessel runoff. Patency continued for the 24 ensuing months.

Comment

After 21 years and eight operations this now 74-year-old man continues to walk on intact limbs.

TABLE 9-1 INCIDENCE OF VASCULAR PROCEDURES, ST. THOMAS HOSPITAL, AUGUST 1984

Procedure	No.	%
Aortofemoral graft	16	
Femoropopliteal or femorotibial graft	39	
Profundaplasty	2	
Graft thrombectomy	3	
Femoral false aneurysm	1	
Total peripheral arterial reconstruction	61	43
Renal artery graft	1	1
Aortic aneurysm repair	14	10
Arterial embolectomy	6	4
Carotid endarterectomy	60	42
Total	142	

MANAGEMENT OF INTERMITTENT CLAUDICATION

Claudication (from the Latin *claudicatio,* to limp)[1] refers to pain or discomfort in a limb being used or exercised beyond the functional capacity of its blood supply.

A Parisian veterinarian, Bouley, in 1831 first associated the disability with arterial occlusion in a horse.[2] The French neurologist Charcot in 1851 described the first human case.[3]

The clinical implication of claudication is occlusion of a main artery such as the superficial femoral proximal to the site of symptoms. Collateral circulation (in this instance the profunda femoris) maintains viability and nourishes the tissues at rest. The pain of claudication soon ceases when muscle activity ends but returns regularly with a resumption of exercise. It occurs even sooner with increased exertion such as walking uphill or running.

Warren delineated three criteria for true vascular claudication: it occurs as a muscle cramp after walking, it soon ceases during standing at rest, and it recurs when the patient walks again.[4] It does not persist during quiet standing, nor is it produced by certain positions during rest.

Intermittent claudication is usually easily differentiated from other causes of pains in the leg such as arthritis, sciatica, phlebitis, and tumor. It may, however, be confused with the pain resulting from intervertebral disc protrusion or from spinal stenosis, termed *spinal claudication* (Figures 9-4 and 9-5). This latter syndrome of nerve root pressure causes pain during standing (as well as walking), has a sciatic distribution, and is often associated with paresthesias or other neurologic signs; it does not affect normal distal pulses. The computerized tomography (CT) scan confirms the diagnosis of spinal stenosis. Goodreau and associates retrospectively reviewed 52 patients with spinal claudication, of whom 11 also had significant vascular disease. They recommended differentiation on the basis of (1) a careful history, (2) examination for pain or associated symptoms caused by nerve root compression, (3) noninvasive arterial studies, and (4) the delivery of relief by intrathecal injection of methylprednisone acetate (Depo-Medrol). They correctly predicted the value of the CT scan.[5]

Most patients with claudication exhibit slow progression as symptoms increase, although sudden ischemia due to acute arterial thrombosis occasionally occurs. Among the 5183 men and women studied at 6-month intervals in the Framingham Heart Disease Epidemiology Study, a subgroup of 162 claudicators developed major cardiovascular events within 8 years, which resulted in death in 20 percent of the males and 30 percent of the females. However, only a minority (2.5 percent) progressed to gangrene or infection with tissue loss or amputation.[6] Imparato and his group also noted that claudication is "relatively benign," since only 2.3 percent of their patients developed gangrene yearly.[7] Roberts's team surveyed five series and concluded that approximately 1.4 percent of claudicators come to amputation each year. Since there was no operative mortality in their own 100-patient operative series and at 5 years 69 percent of their grafts were patent and only three limbs had been lost, they suggested that reconstruction is safe and that it reduces the cumulative amputation rate.[8] Among 91 claudicators Cronenwett and his colleagues found a 9 percent yearly operation rate (along with a 5 percent mortality rate).[9]

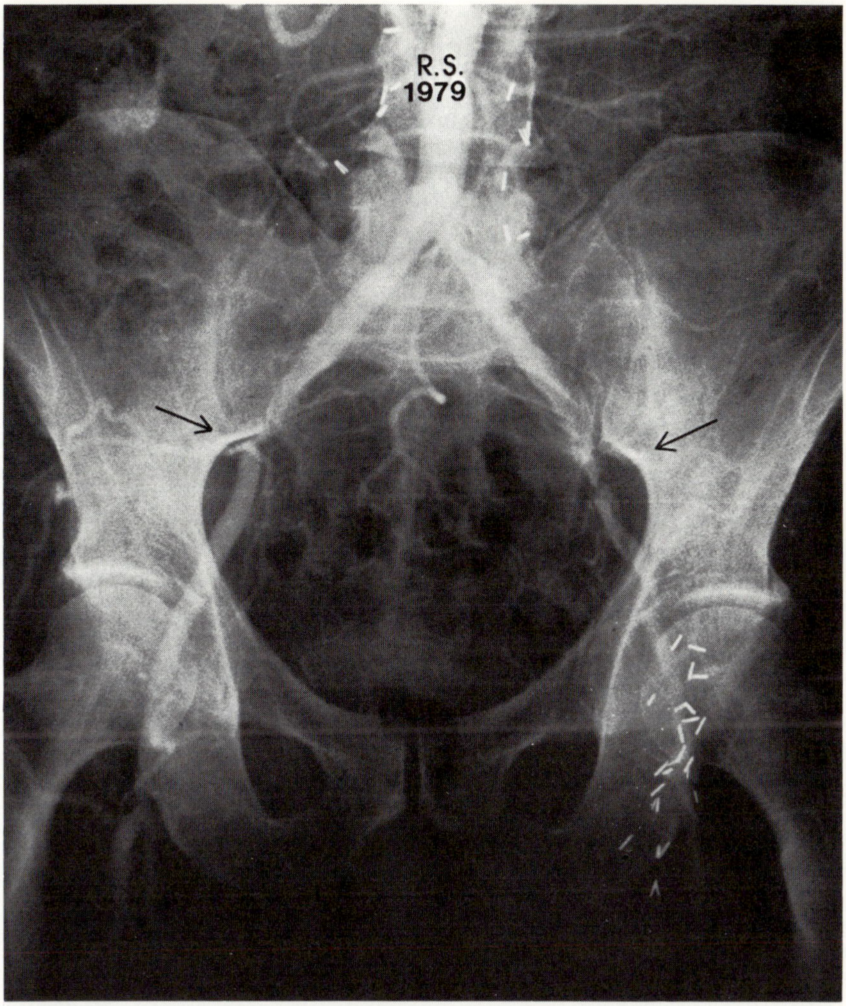

FIGURE 9-1 Occlusion of the left external iliac artery just beyond the iliac bifurcation at the *left arrow.* At the *right arrow* the film indicates apparent iliac stenosis, but other films indicated patency. The original aortoiliac repair was patent. Revascularization was achieved by placing a PTFE graft from the distal left common iliac artery to the popliteal artery just above the knee.

Such statistics suggest a generally conservative approach reserving surgical revascularization for those patients who are seriously discommoded at work or play and for the minority whose symptoms progress to rest pain or distal ischemia as other lesions occur.

Reconstructive procedures by experts produce good results with low risks for these patients. Limb loss rates approach zero. Operative mortality is similarly low, provided there is no disease in the cardiac or cerebrovascular circulation.

Salvage of Limbs

Pain at rest denotes a later stage of occlusive disease involving insufficient collateral circulation either because it has not developed or, more often, because multiple arterial occlusions exist.

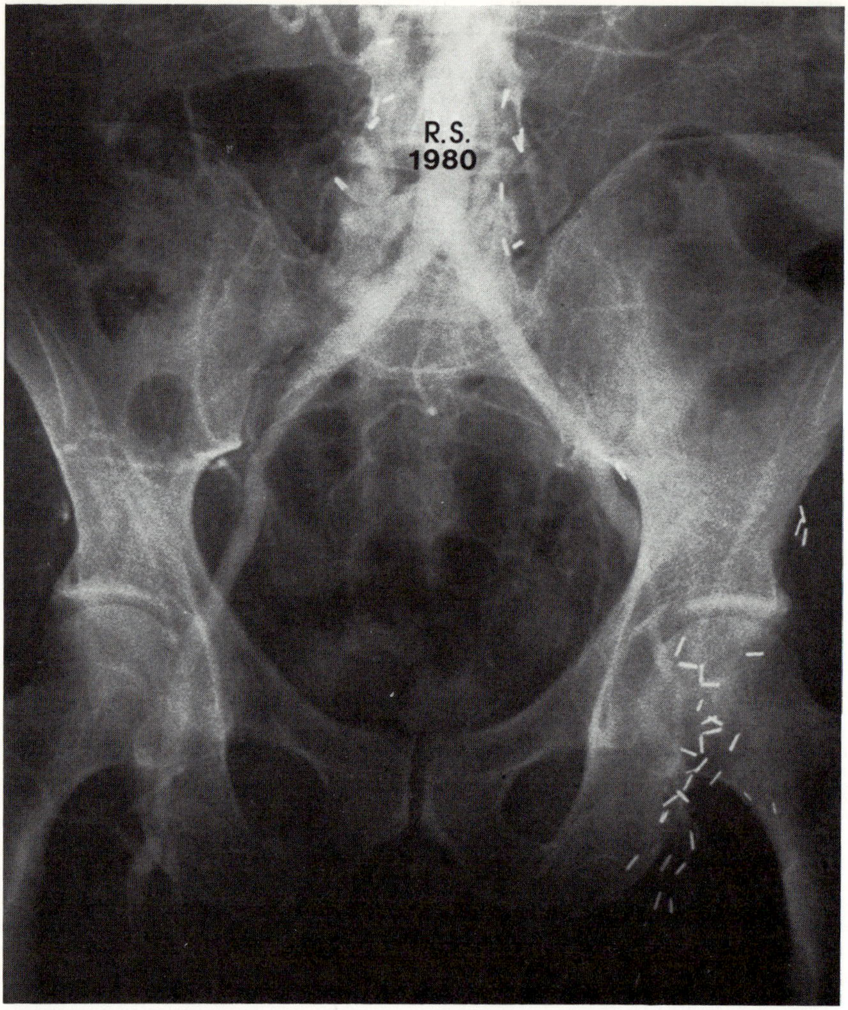

FIGURE 9-2 Eighteen months after the iliac-to-popliteal PTFE graft was placed, it thrombosed. It was replaced with a new PTFE graft, this time to the popliteal artery below the knee.

"Night pain" may simply be rest pain which occurs at night. Sometimes, however, it is due to diminished arterial flow when the cardiac output diminishes during sleep. Sometimes the patient relieves it by arising and walking. This interferes with sleep as well as points to the serious prognosis of the arterial occlusion. Claudication may be tolerated without operation with little risk to the extremity, but pain at rest and/or at night indicates the need for early revascularization.

Twenty-odd years ago it became apparent that most ischemic extremities facing early amputation because of tissue necrosis or rest pain could be saved for a reasonable time. In 1967 I reported a 64 percent salvage rate among 100 consecutive such limbs.[10] The surgical procedures were varied but were all directed at revascularization. Other similar reports soon confirmed this *aggressive approach to limb salvage.*

Veith's group in 1981 reported limb salvage among 551 patients to be 73 percent at 1 month

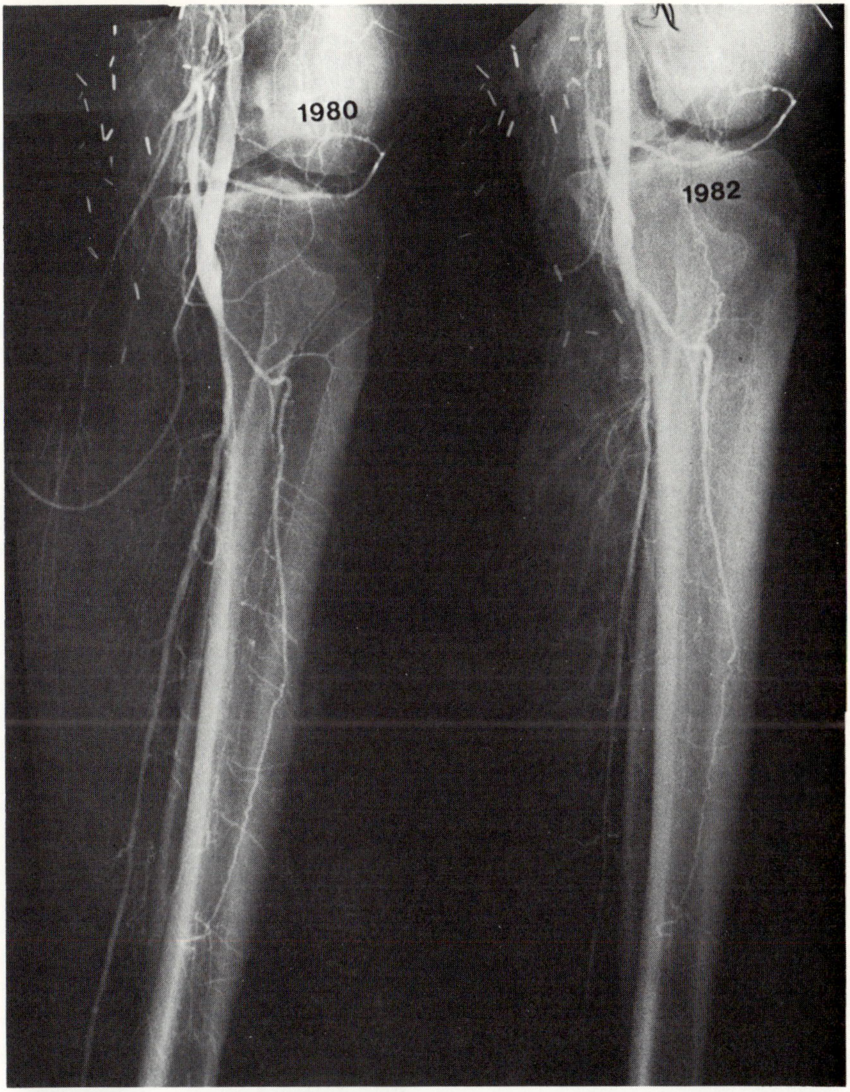

FIGURE 9-3 Two years later the old PTFE graft was thrombectomized and the distal anastomosis patched with a vein. *Right,* a completion arteriogram demonstrated a technically correct anastomosis with run-off into two vessels. *Left,* the appearance was similar to the completion arteriogram made 2 years previously.

and 66 percent at 5 years.[11] Today such limbs should at once be studied angiographically to determine the proper procedure for revascularization (Figures 9-6 and 9-7). Primary amputation is rarely needed (with a few exceptions of life-threatening infection or progression of necrosis so that the heel cannot be saved). The matter is discussed more fully in Chapter 25.

*The comprehensive discussion of rationale, methods, and results by Veith and associates will interest some readers.[12]

Angiography

Angiography is a preoperative planning tool. It is not usually needed to establish the clinical diagnosis or to determine whether an operation is needed.

Complete visualization, including that of the distal arteries of the ankles and feet and of the larger abdominal and leg vessels, allows selection of the procedure that is most likely to produce long-term revascularization that has a reasonable risk factor. Concomitant views of the renal and other visceral arteries are often indicated, since these can be obtained with little additional risk, as noted in Chapter 15.

Modern expertise with transfemoral catheter techniques has generally outmoded direct needle injections into the aorta or femoral arteries, although in the latter they are still useful in some situations. Thus, occlusion of both iliac arteries forces a choice between passing a needle or catheter by the left translumbar route or passing it via an axillary artery. The danger of nerve damage associated with the transaxillary route explains my preference for translumbar injection and for entering the aorta proximal to the visceral arteries (to avoid direct injection into them as well as to visualize them). Although accidents and complications have been reported, I have not personally observed life, limb, or organ loss by translumbar aortography during a thirty-odd-year experience.

Another indication for needle injection is the need to place the contrast material directly into a femoral artery to produce clearer distal opacification, which may be dim if the material is injected proximal to an iliac occlusion.

Finally, it may be safer to inject a synthetic graft residual in the groin than to place a catheter within it, although the latter procedure can usually be done without a complication.[13]

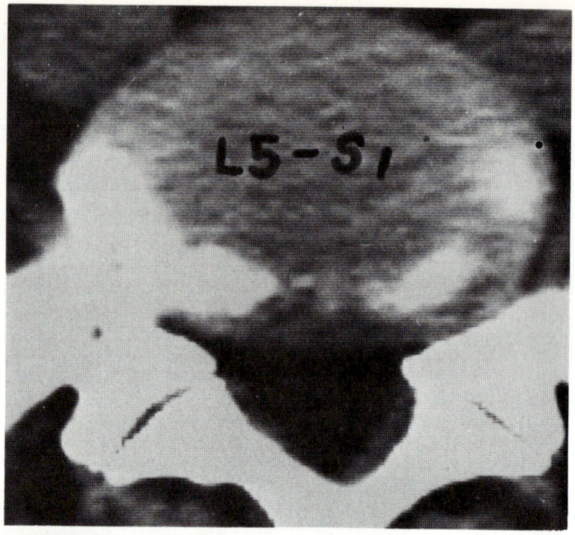

FIGURE 9-4 A CT scan at the L5-S1 level shows a wide-open spinal canal.

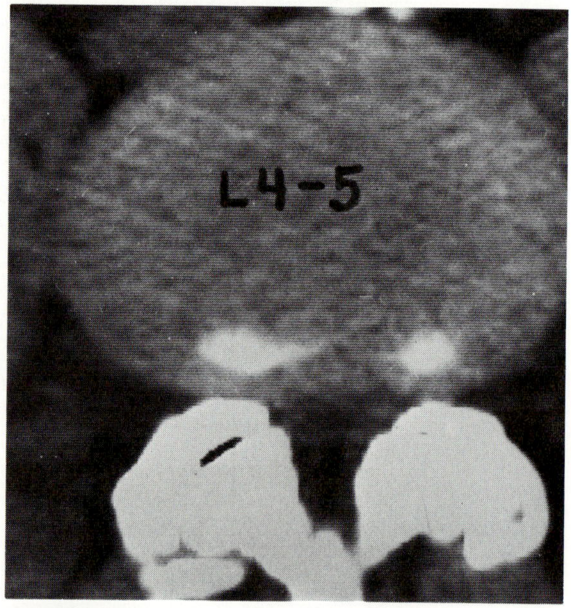

FIGURE 9-5 A CT scan at the L4-L5 level shows spinal stenosis resulting in spinal claudication.

Occasionally the severe extent of arterial occlusion prevents distal opacification by any technique preoperatively. Intraoperative arteriography at the beginning of the operative procedure then becomes mandatory, to allow the optimal procedure to be selected.[14,15] A needle or catheter

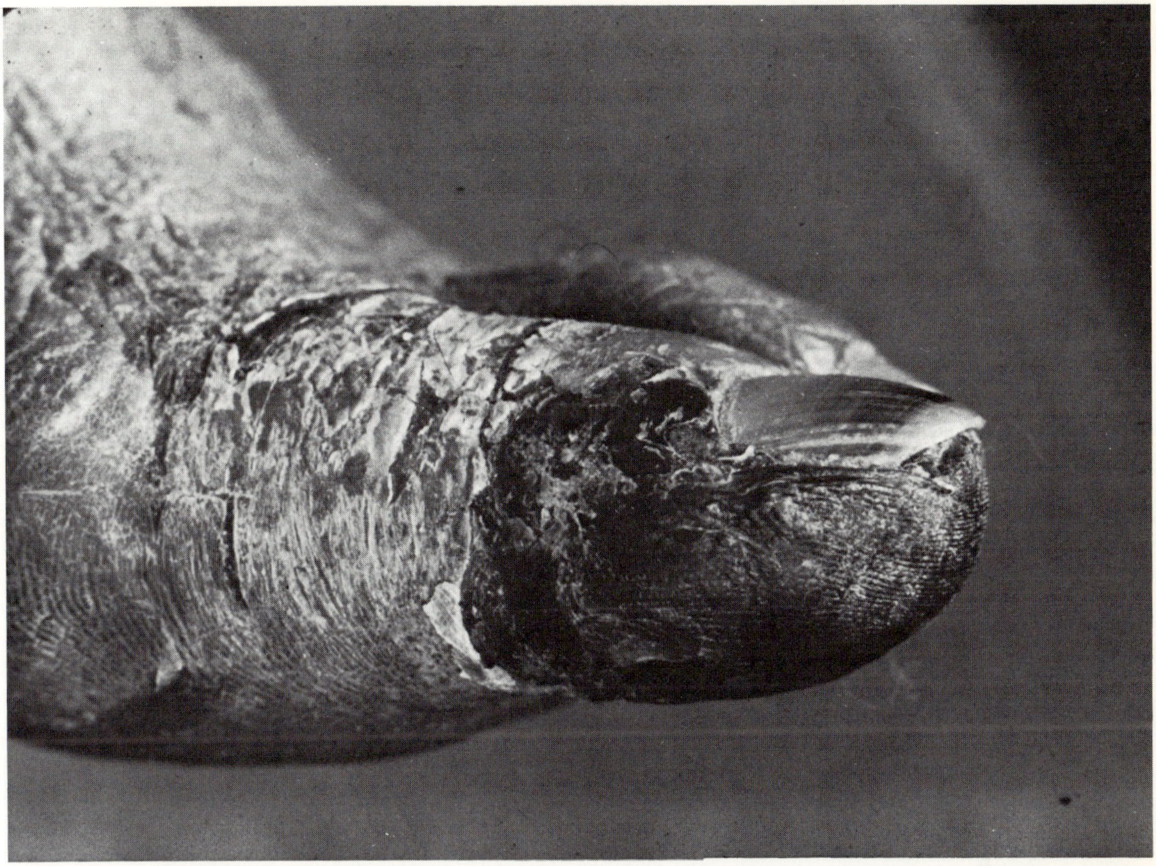

FIGURE 9-6 Ischemic gangrene of the left great toe due to femoropopliteal occlusive disease.

injection into the exposed common femoral artery, profunda branch, or popliteal artery will provide the needed information. Such arteriograms are more accurate in determining the intraluminal situation than is palpation, which also is useless in finding stenoses and occlusions distal to the site of injection.

The importance of complete, well-defined angiography should discourage angiographic study in an outlying hospital where the actual reconstructive procedure will not be done. Too often those arteriograms must be repeated because of incompleteness or poor visualization.

Selecting the Best Procedure

Optimal revascularization procedures lie somewhere between doing too little, with early failure or recurrence of disease, and doing too much, thereby incurring unneeded risks to limb, organ, or life. Knowledge of one's own results and those of others is required in selecting the operation most likely to achieve long-term success with a reasonable risk.

Twenty years ago lengthy procedures to completely replace the distal aorta and the iliac, femoral, and popliteal arteries bilaterally at one time[16] produced excessively high morbidity and mortality rates. These risks were thereafter reduced by the aorta-to-femoral (or -to-profunda) artery bypass without a primary attempt to include a bypass of the occluded femoral vessels. Only a minority of patients require secondary procedures for the popliteal arteries.

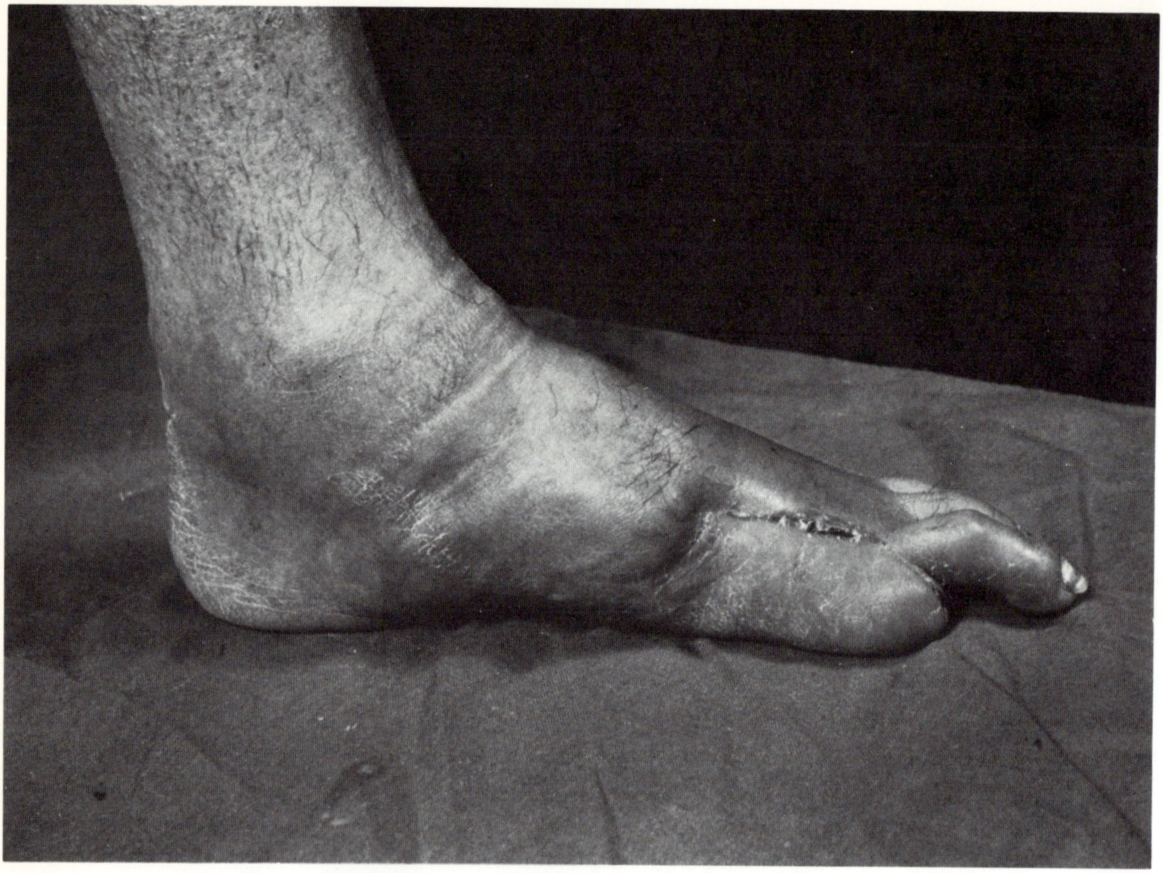

FIGURE 9-7 Following femoropopliteal revascularization, the nonviable toe and adjacent metatarsal head were amputated. Healing was immediate and the ability to walk was maintained.

During the same era the "too little" procedure of local and aortic and/or iliac endarterectomy often led to early postoperative occlusion because the external iliac-femoral arteries were diseased. The general adoption of aortobifemoral bypass grafting (Figure 9-8) improved results without increasing risks.

Aortic Endarterectomy versus Grafting Most patients have extensive iliac disease if the aorta is stenotic or occluded. Indeed, the atherosclerotic process usually involves the common femoral artery as well, especially posteriorly. A limited endarterectomy is not often feasible; immediate or early postoperative occlusion is common if that is done. A bypass graft to the femoral artery provides a wide anastomosis there, since the anterior portion of the graft functions as a patch and enlarges the lumen. Brewster and associates noted that endarterectomies were indicated in only 10 percent of their recent aortoiliac reconstructions, specifically for patients in whom the disease ended at the iliac bifurcation, thus allowing a satisfactory end point for the internal dissection.[17] Most vascular surgeons agree that proximal aortic disease and external iliac and femoral thickening are better treated by aortobifemoral grafts and that thromboendarterectomies are not often suitable procedures.[18,19]

The early patency rate of aortobifemoral grafts now approaches 100 percent and the 5-year rate is over 80 percent in a number of series. Mannick's group documented a 5-year cumulative

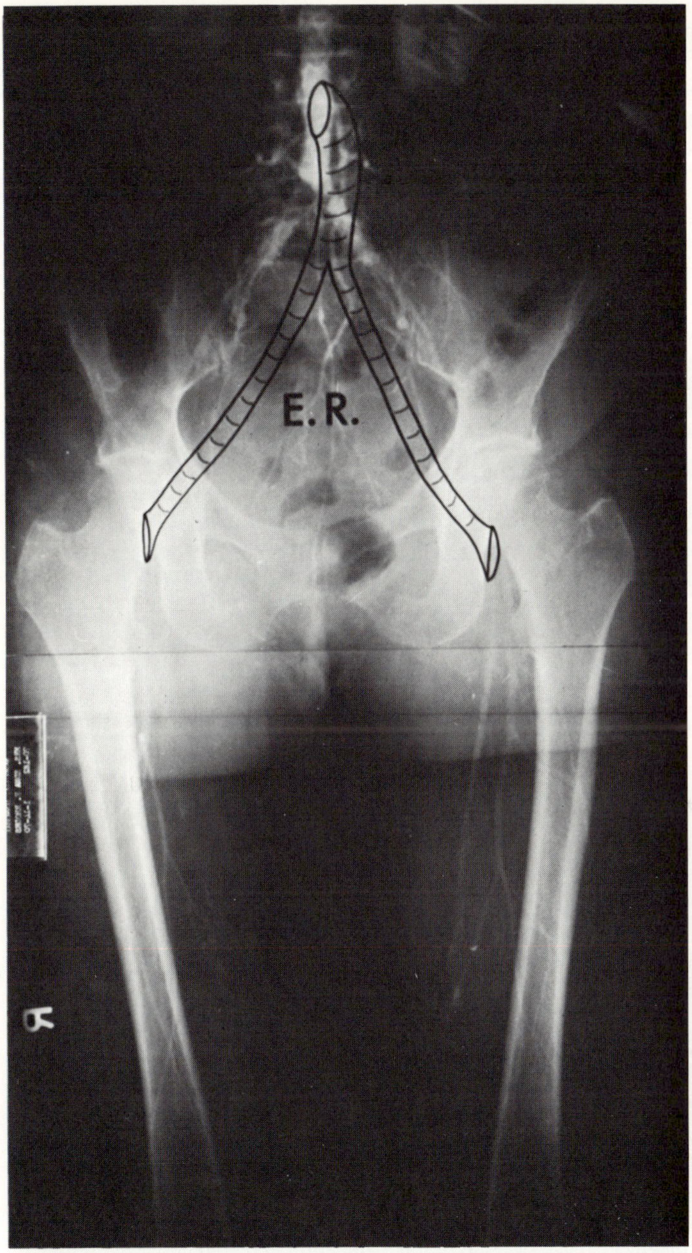

FIGURE 9-8 A standard aortobifemoral Dacron bypass graft revascularized these extremities. These iliac arteries were bilaterally occluded.

patency rate of 86 percent among 168 aortobifemoral grafts.[20] Edwards and associates followed for a short period 330 aortic reconstructions for occlusive disease and reported only 0.4 percent early failure and 0.8 percent later failure of graft limbs.[21]

Occasionally there occurs a limited distribution of the atherosclerotic process, making endarterectomy (Figure 9-9) or transluminal angioplasty proper. For such it must be possible to

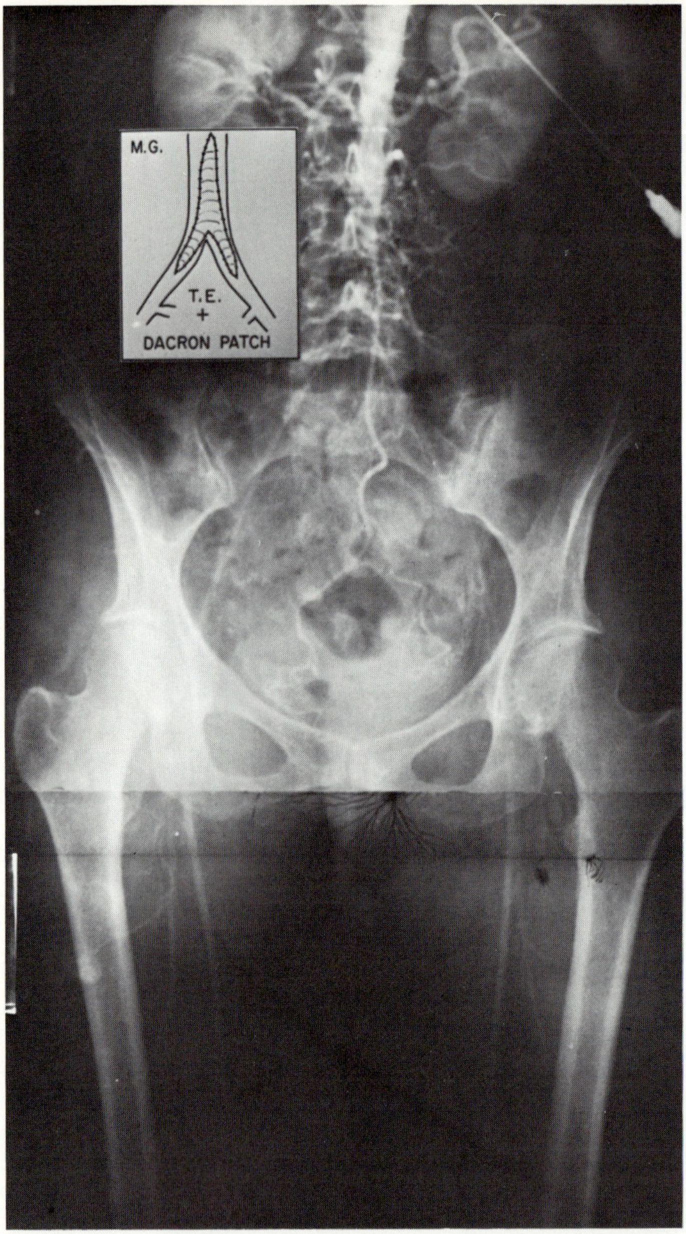

FIGURE 9-9 Limited occlusive disease of the distal aorta and common iliac arteries may be treated by direct open endarterectomy with a Dacron patch closure.

remove completely the thickened area through a longitudinal arteriotomy. Closure with a Dacron patch is usually advisable (Figure 9-10). So-called blind endarterectomies through short incisions are dangerous, since tags and shreds are often left to attract thrombosis.

An endarterectomy deep within the pelvis (Figure 9-11) is considerably more difficult to con-

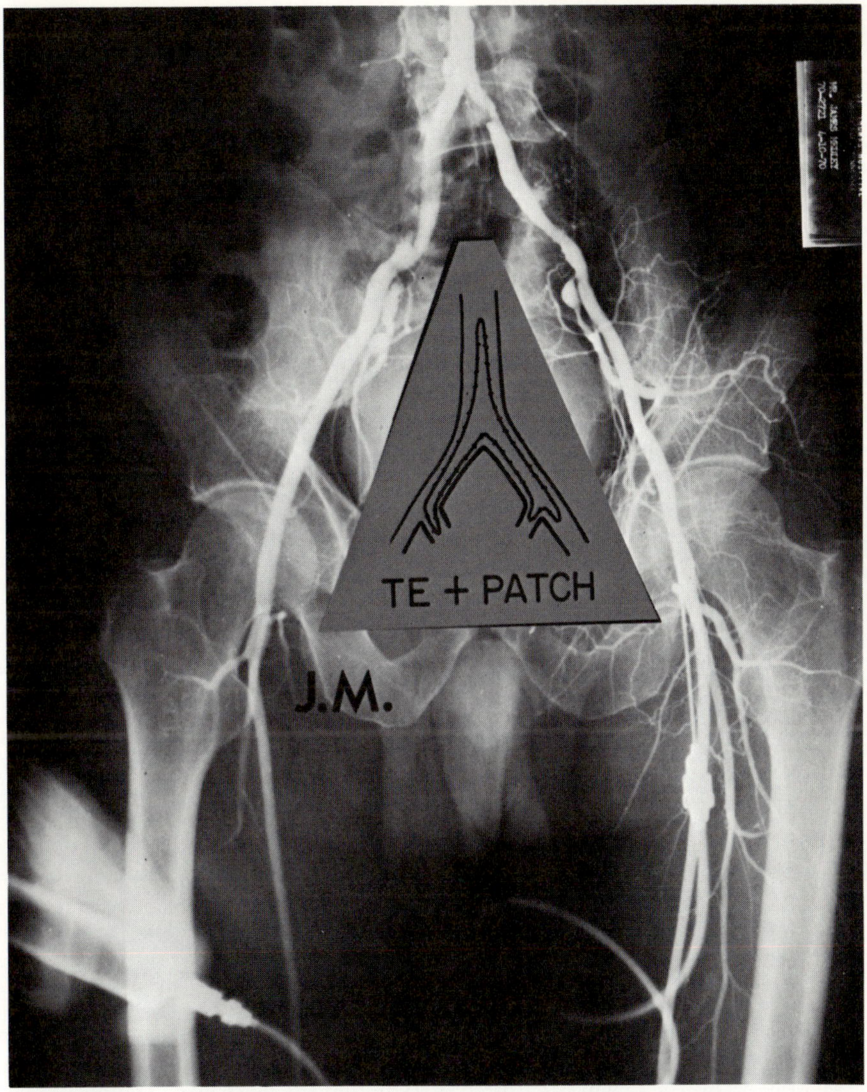

FIGURE 9-10 Limited stenotic areas of both common iliac arteries may be managed by direct open thromboendarterectomy with Dacron patch closure, in this instance extending over the origins of the hypogastric arteries bilaterally.

duct properly than is an aortobifemoral graft. The procedure is optimal for an experienced surgeon for a few patients.

The Choice of Synthetic Graft

Over the years there has continued the search for a synthetic material to replace arteries without causing a foreign-body reaction, rejection due to infection, or thrombosis as time passes and the disease progresses. Despite the fusing, braiding, weaving, and knitting of a variety of fibers, the

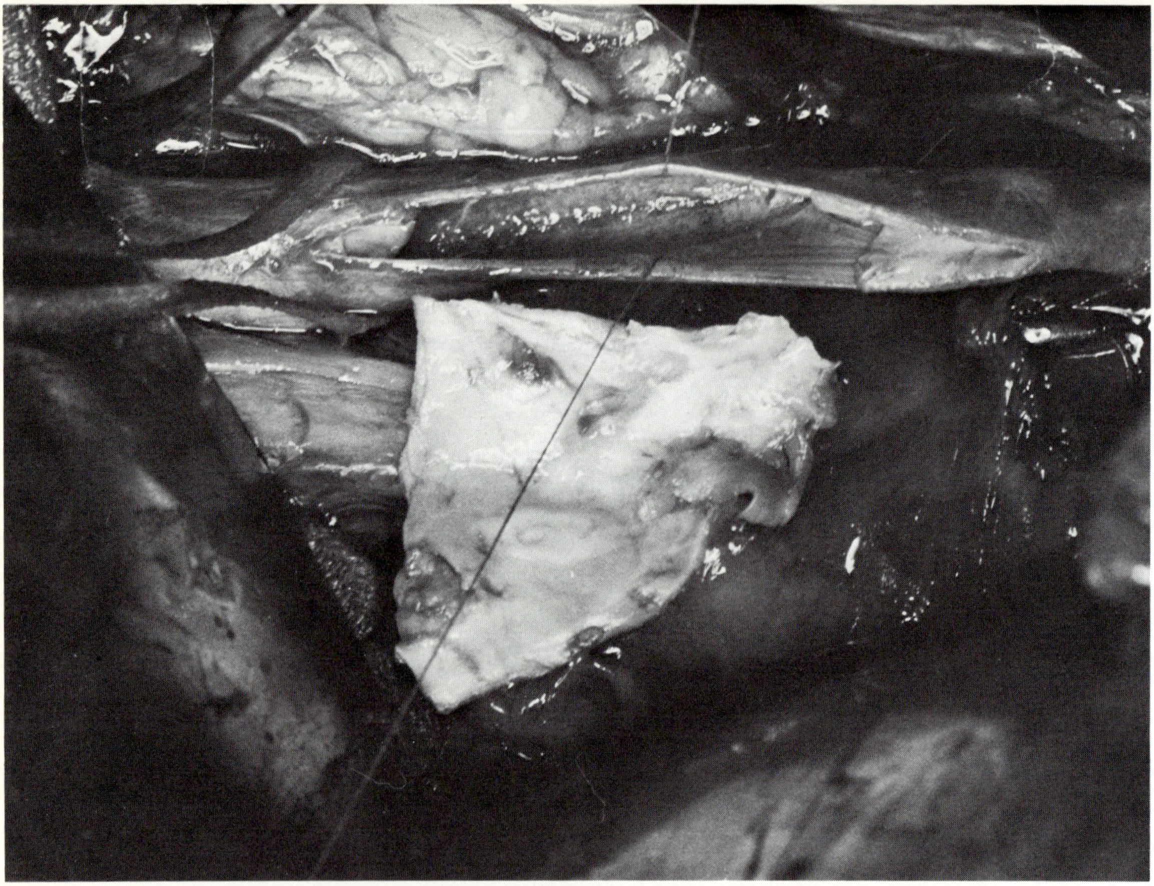

FIGURE 9-11 Common iliac endarterectomy has been partially accomplished and the specimen laid alongside as a demonstration. The distal dissection is ended so that the patch graft extends well beyond it. Proximally the endarterectomy has not yet been completed.

synthetic graft remains imperfect. Indeed, when one is recovered some years later, its interior irregularities, plagues, and uncovered areas evoke wonder that any of these remain patent.*

After Voorhees's team discovered in 1951 that the dog's aorta could be replaced with a vinyon-N tube,[23] it was learned that a variety of synthetic materials could be successfully used. The parade of successively favored grafts is a lengthy one: vinyon-N, Ivalon, nylon, Teflon, Dacron, and PTFE, not to mention lesser-knowns which are hardly remembered. Indeed, in the decade of the fifties there was hardly a young surgeon without a special graft or method of production.

Despite the advertisements of manufacturers today there is little difference in long-term results between the several synthetic grafts which are available to replace the aortoiliac arterial system. Some, however, are easier to use, require less preliminary preparation, and are consequently preferred by one or another surgeon. One such is the crimped woven double-velour graft,

*The widespread opinion that the interior of a synthetic graft becomes smoothly covered reflects the fact that surgeons place thousands of these conduits but rarely examine one which has been recovered later. After reviewing the various available graft materials in 1983, Stanley's group stated that "complete healing and endothelialization of the inner surface of a prosthesis has never been achieved in a human implanted fabric graft recovered to date."[22]

which provides a relatively soft material that accepts a needle and suture easily, adapts to contours well, and requires no preclotting.

Close attention to the continuous over-and-over posterior aortic suture line should avoid leaks with this material. It is, however, advisable to open the graft to blood, cross-clamping it distally, in order to examine the posterior anastomosis for leaks prior to placing the distal anastomoses. After a few minutes of opening and closing the proximal aortic clamp, there should be no further seepage of blood through the interstices, and the distal portions of the procedure may be done.

End-to-End versus Onlay Aortic Grafts

The common use of end-to-side, onlay anastomoses in the femoropopliteal system as well as elsewhere for small vessels was early extended to aortic anastomoses. It must be remembered that internal lesions and various stages of clot formation require interior cleaning prior to the anastomosis. Onlay grafts are easy to accomplish, and if there remains any flow into or through the iliac arteries, that is not disturbed.

The concept of interruption of the proximal aorta with end-to-end graft anastomosis to a less-diseased vessel occurred later. Direct linear flow rather than diversion into a tangential stream, often with a bulging anastomosis, is also theoretically attractive, provided the graft remains patent and the pelvis is perfused by retrograde flow.

It has been proposed that the incidence of long-term patency of the graft is related to the type of proximal anastomosis. Whether the statistics represent a real difference or occur as a result of more experience, better grafts, and sutures is not clear, because the reports are of uncontrolled experiences. For example, after $3\frac{1}{2}$ years of follow-up Pierce and associates report a "significantly higher" graft limb patency rate of 100 percent for 41 end-to-end anastomoses compared with 91 percent for 38 end-to-side procedures. At the same time, the rates of sexual dysfunction were worse for the end-to-end anostomoses—27 percent compared with 13 percent for the end-to-side procedures.[24] Not only are the numbers small, but the two series were performed at different times; also the statistical differences are not great. When the sexual problems are recognized, the report argues more for the end-to-side technique.

The incidence of aortoenteric fistula formation has been supposed to be less when there is not a bulging anterior aortic end-to-side anastomosis. While frequently stated, this is an undocumented clinical opinion, as noted by Mannick.[20]

In the absence of absolute knowledge I continue to use the onlay, end-to-side graft (with internal endarterectomy as needed) for patients in whom one iliac artery is receiving blood or in whom the inferior mesenteric artery is patent, in order not to chance their retrograde perfusion. Perfusion of an anomalous renal artery may also be ensured (Figures 9-12 and 9-13). If, on the other hand, the aorta is completely occluded without flow into the iliac arteries, it is simpler to perform an end-to-end anastomosis just distal to the renal arteries and oversew the distal aortic end. Flow into the inferior mesenteric artery may be preserved by transposing the artery to the side of an end-to-end graft.[21]

Both methods of proximal anastomoses are useful; it is dogmatic to *always* use one or the other. Individualization is a more rational policy. Rutherford's comments are apropos: "There is no exclusively right way," and "If one limb of a bifurcated graft fails, can the proximal anastomosis be to blame?"[25]

The graft size is chosen to correspond to the femoral vessels; limbs which are too large (as were often used in the past) should be avoided. The limbs are passed posterior to the ureters to emerge in the groin, where accurate length is established to prevent the tightness and proximal pull that may lead to a false aneurysm later.

Provision of a widely patent outflow encourages patency of the proximal graft. Particular attention to the orifice of the profunda femoris is therefore necessary, including profundaplasty

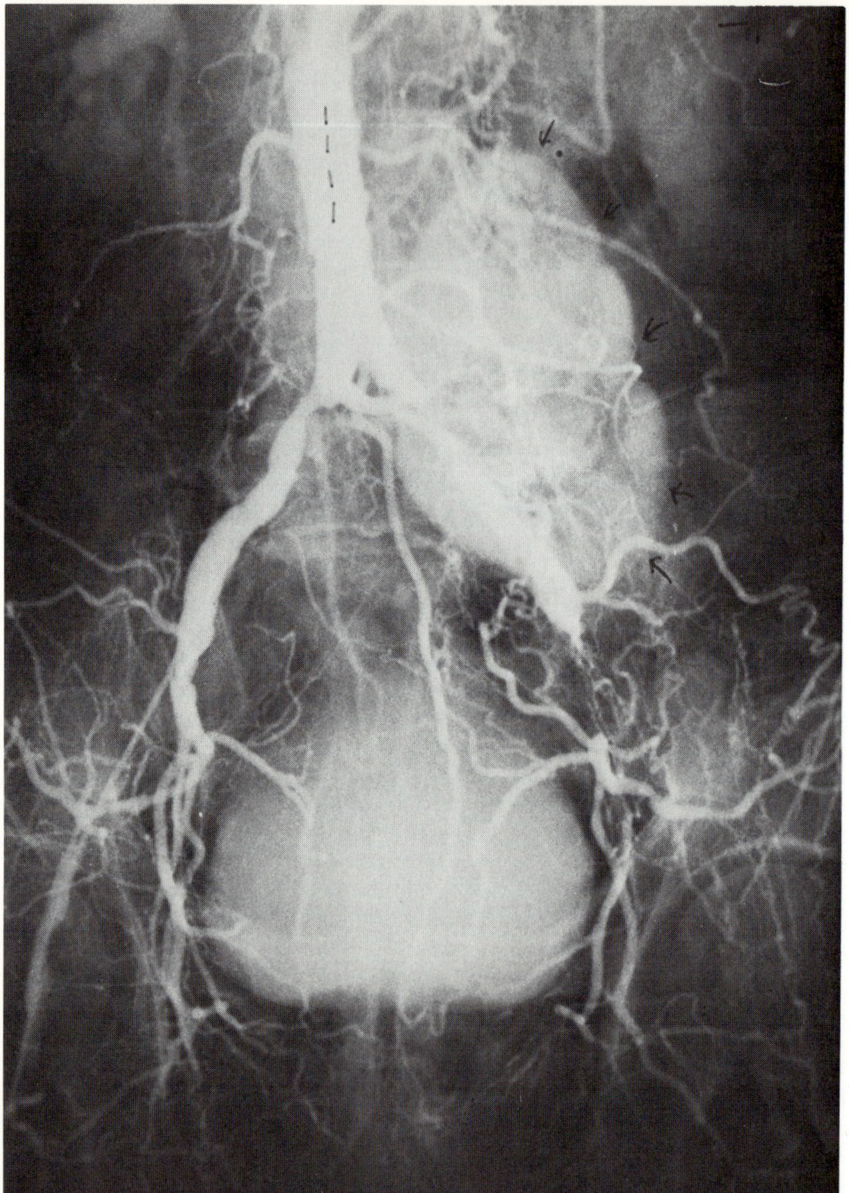

FIGURE 9-12 A preoperative aortogram demonstrated a distally placed left kidney (as outlined by *arrows*) with multiple supplying arteries. An onlay graft was placed at the *broken line.*

when needed. In such a case an elongated toe of the graft is useful to provide patch closure of the profunda to the point of complete distal patency. If, on the other hand, the proximal portion of the profunda is soft and patent, it is usually preferable to place the toe of the graft to the superficial femoral artery, thus "covering" the orifice of the profunda without disturbing it in any way.

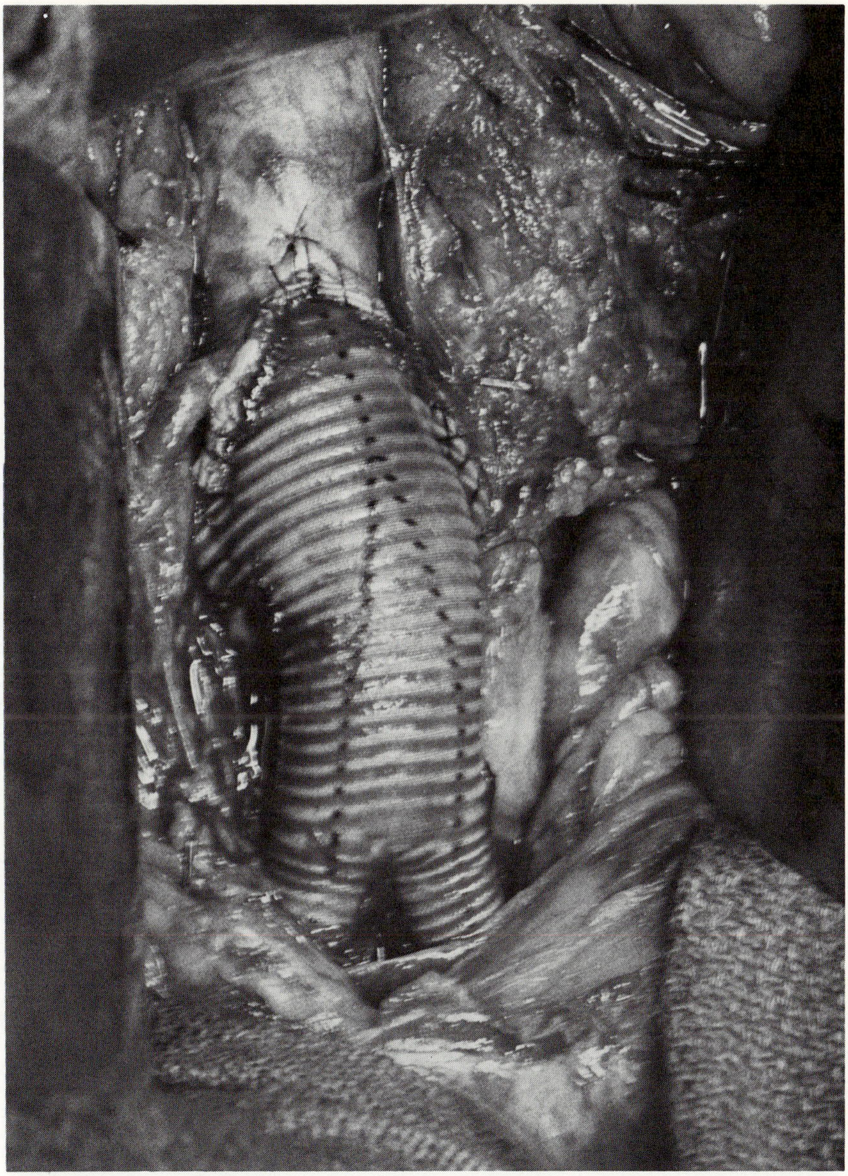

FIGURE 9-13 A double-velour woven Dacron aortobifemoral graft was placed end-to-side because of a distally placed left kidney with multiple vessels.

High Proximal Aortic Occlusion

Occasionally the infrarenal aorta is completely blocked and the total outflow occurs into the visceral arteries, of which the renal arteries are most distal (Figure 9-14). Placement of the proximal anatomosis of a graft above the visceral arteries is needlessly complex and therefore dangerous. A better plan is to clean out an inch of aorta just below the renal vessels by endarterectomy, then attach the graft to that segment. This safer procedure involves opening the aorta well below the contemplated line of suture, performing the endarterectomy so as to leave a long area

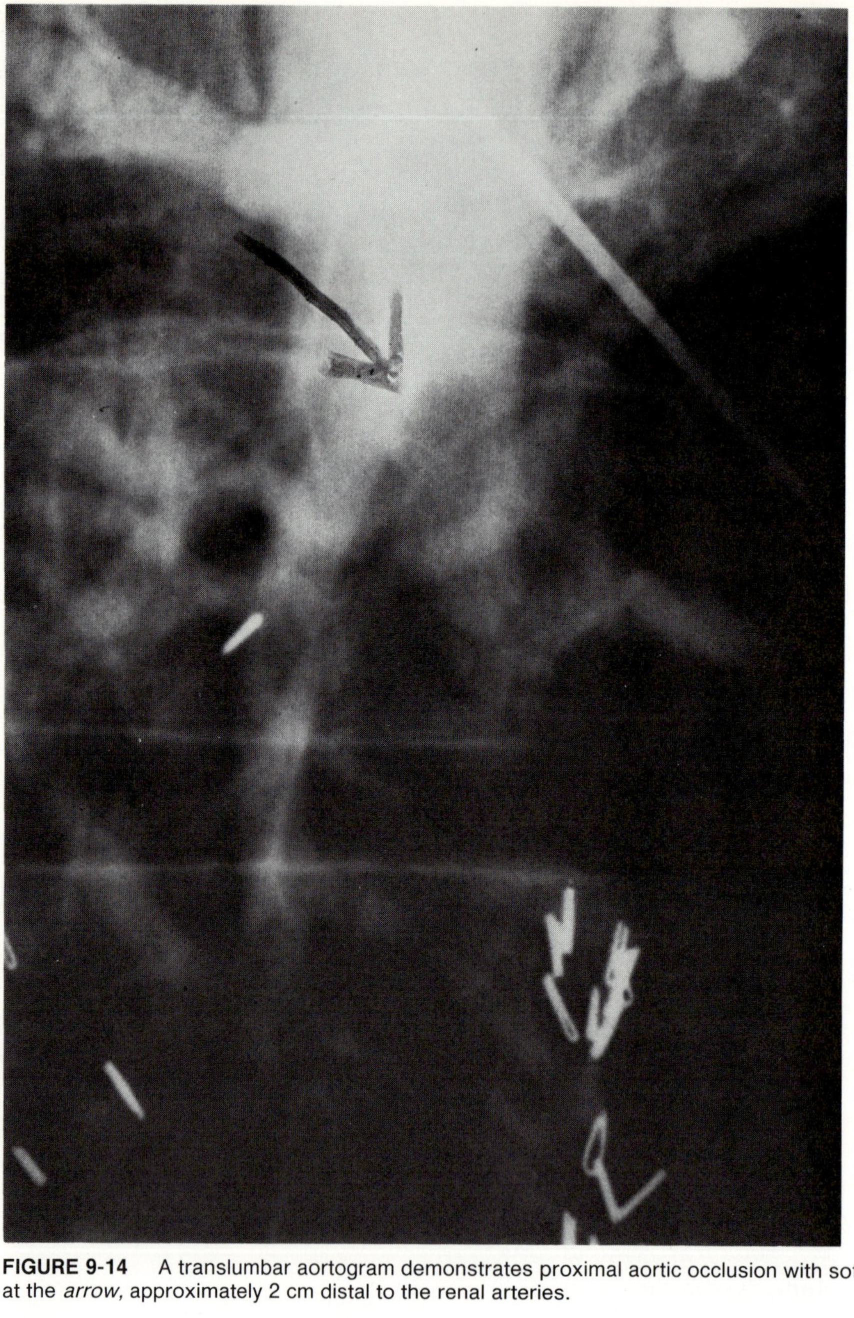

FIGURE 9-14 A translumbar aortogram demonstrates proximal aortic occlusion with soft thrombosis at the *arrow,* approximately 2 cm distal to the renal arteries.

of wall posteriorly, and performing an oblique anastomosis, rather than cutting across the dangerously thin endarterectomized aorta posteriorly.

Since the endarterectomy must be carried up to the renal arterial orifices, there is the possibility of embolism to the kidneys. It has been suggested that both renal arteries must be dissected and clamped to prevent this. There is a simpler method, which I have used in approximately 20 such cases without evidence of renal dysfunction. After the aorta is opened longitudinally well below the renal vessels, the endarterectomy is performed carefully to within 1 to 2 cm of the renal orifices. The aorta is then transected distally, and its proximal ends are held open with a stay suture on each side.

The posterior half of the oblique anastomosis is completed. The suprarenal aorta is then pressed firmly against the vertebrae (by the fingers or the occluder, Figure 6-7) to occlude the aortic flow proximally. The proximal portion of the endarterectomy is completed, with direct vision up into the aorta and the renal orifices. Some bleeding from the latter is picked up by the autotransfusion suction unit. The proximal aorta is cleaned, irrigated with saline, and well flushed. The anastomosis is then completed and opened and the graft is cross-clamped. No doubt, the flushing and retrograde renal bleeding explain the lack of embolism to the kidneys.

The University of California at Los Angeles group similarly had no renal difficulties using this technique of brief manual occlusion to allow proximal aortic clean-out and flushing. There was only one instance of transient postoperative creatinemia among their 20 cases. Survey of three other series indicated a similarly low risk of renal complications.[26]

Proximal extension of the dissection to allow renal artery clamping along with further opening of the aorta will allow direct open endarterectomy of one or both renal arteries, should that be required.

Concomitant Shunts to Visceral Arteries

The widespread segmental occurrence of atherosclerotic lesions may involve important visceral arteries at the same time that the aortoiliac system is compromised. Preoperative recognition of this, suggested by the clinical pattern, confirmed by angiography, and further delineated by appropriate functional tests, allows simultaneous correction for many patients.

The extended procedure with a concomitant shunt to one or more visceral arteries is clearly indicated to correct malfunction of organs. Whether renal stenoses and occlusions of mesenteric vessels should be prophylactically bypassed is not clear. Edwards's group has reported renal bypasses in 15 percent of 584 aortic grafts for occlusive and/or aneurysmal disease. Another 8 patients had mesenteric bypasses. An unstated number of these were performed prophylactically.[27] The overall 2.3 percent mortality of the entire group is favorable. Smith commented briefly upon 47 patients undergoing concomitant aortic and visceral grafting who had 4.3 percent mortality, along with loss of a kidney in 1 patient. Seventeen percent of those visceral bypasses were prophylactic.[28]

There are not yet facts to judge whether prophylactic concomitant visceral grafts are justified in terms of low risk and prevention of later problems. To say the least, prophylactic operations are controversial and their need is unproven. Neither low risk nor an abnormal x-ray is a primary surgical indication; the "Everest syndrome" was discussed in Chapter 3.

Correct preoperative assessment allows an optimal plan for the entire reconstruction, which involves not only appropriate incisions but also orderly dissection of multiple sites and a correct sequence of the necessary grafts and anastomoses.

First, in order to expose the viscera as briefly as possible and to prevent hypothermia, the incisions and dissection should be conducted so that the abdominal (and/or thoracic) cavity is opened only after completion of the necessary peripheral dissections.

Second, the internal dissection of branch vessels such as the renal arteries should usually be accomplished prior to systemic heparinization. An exception is dissection of the right renal artery, whose exposure may at times be delayed until the time for grafting, to avoid tumbling of the intestine back and forth, in and out of the abdomen.

Third, the main or most important graft should usually be completed before a side shunt is undertaken. This not only restores peripheral flow as quickly as possible but also allows retreat from an extensive procedure should time or blood loss be excessive or the patient's condition deteriorate. Thus, an aortobifemoral graft should be completed and opened prior to construction of a side shunt to a renal artery.

Fourth, while secondary bypasses can be added to an aortic graft which is partially occluded or side-clamped, it is usually better to temporarily occlude the main graft above and below the proposed site of anastomosis. This allows more accurate and efficient placement of the sutures as well as preventing an orificial malposition of the side shunt.

Finally, the extended operation should not be forced in the event that time, blood loss, or deterioration of the patient's condition indicates termination of the procedure before a contemplated secondary shunt is added.

Most patients do tolerate necessary concomitant procedures and thereby escape the additive risks of two different anesthesias, operations, and postoperative complications, along with the hazards of a secondary dissection through scar tissue. Two different procedures for the renal arteries are no longer acceptable for an experienced team.

Unilateral Repair

Often one limb is asymptomatic, its pulses are present, and the angiogram shows no significant lesion, thereby suggesting reconstruction of only one side of the arterial supply to the lower extremity. Such a procedure would also be followed for a patient who has already lost one limb (Figure 9-15).

If a unilateral lesion exists in the arteries of the thigh or leg, there is of course no consideration of a contralateral prophylactic procedure for mere stenosis, even though some will later progress and require revascularization. If, however, the unilateral lesion be iliac, there are advocates of a bilateral (aorto-bi-iliac or bifemoral) repair even though the contralateral vessel is minimally affected or moderately affected without complete occlusion (Figure 9-16). The recommendation is based upon (1) the probable progression of the contralateral disease,[18] (2) the technical ease of performing the second side at the same time, (3) the problems associated with a later operation upon the other side, and (4) the little added morbidity and mortality asssociated with a bilateral rather than a unilateral repair.

Reasons not to perform bilateral grafting when one side is minimally involved are several. First is the need for an intraabdominal procedure rather than a safer unilateral extraperitoneal operation (either aortofemoral graft, iliac-femoral graft, iliac endarterectomy, or femorofemoral graft). Second, an extraperitoneal iliac-femoral repair or a femoral crossover graft is not likely to produce the sexual dysfunction which may accompany an aortic graft in a male. Third is the 2 to 5 percent incidence of false aneurysms which follow graft anastomoses to the femoral arteries. Finally, there is the risk of infection of the groin wound, which, even if minimal in some hands, is a devastating complication for any patient, since it at once threatens the limb, or even life.

This is another matter which is still controversial. Prophylactic operations require further documentation before the principle is established.

Sexual Dysfunction after Aortic Surgery

Rene Leriche long ago recognized the association of sexual dysfunction with aortoiliac disease in males.[29] May, DeWeese, and Rob in 1969 alerted surgeons to the considerable risk of such after aortic surgery. Some degree of preoperative sexual dysfunction was recognized among their 70 patients; 8 percent of the 26 with aneurysms and 49 percent of the 44 with occlusive disease had preoperative failure of erection. Aortic operations produced further impairment in 21 percent of aneurysm patients and 34 percent of those with occlusive disease. Ejaculatory impairment of one or another sort was produced in 63 percent of those with aneurysms and 44 percent of those with occlusive disease.[30] DePalma has recently described methods of study and surgical techniques designed to avoid such problems.[31-33]

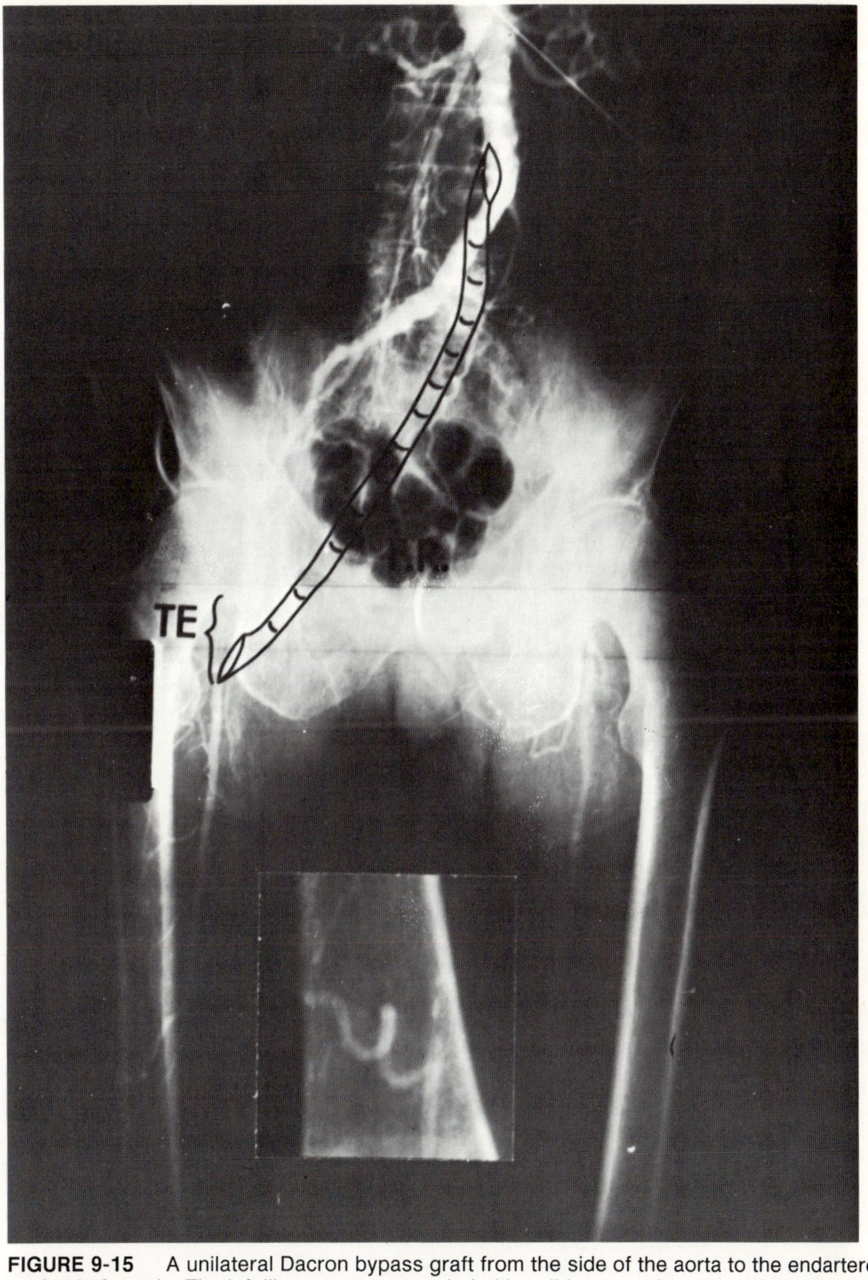

FIGURE 9-15 A unilateral Dacron bypass graft from the side of the aorta to the endarterectomized profunda femoris. The left iliac artery was occluded but did not require revascularization because an above-knee amputation on that side was well-vascularized by collateral circulation.

Several techniques are useful to diminish the chance of postoperative sexual dysfunction: (1) nerve damage around the aortic bifurcation is avoided by limiting the dissection and placing an end-to-side anastomosis on the right side of the aorta to avoid the nerves accompanying the inferior mesenteric artery, (2) internal iliac perfusion is maintained or increased by correct choice

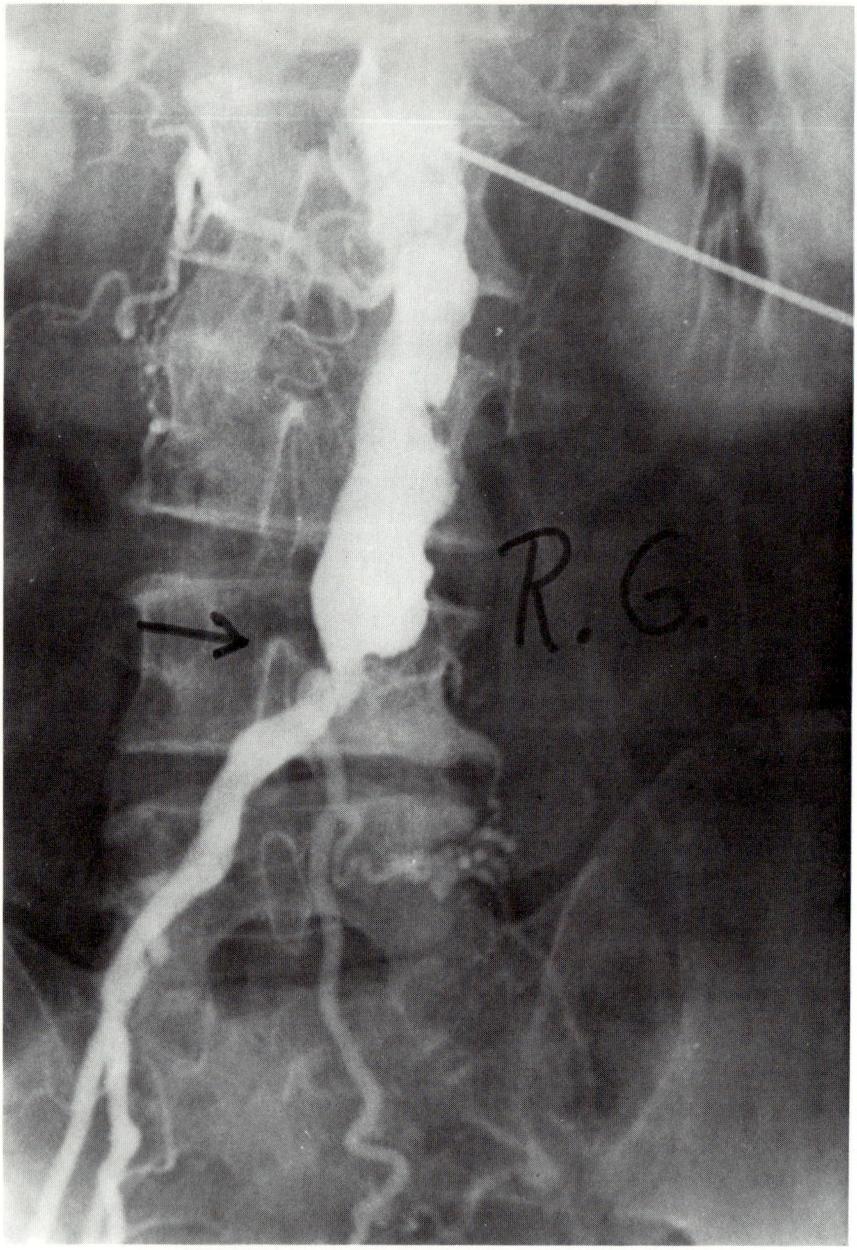

FIGURE 9-16 Aortic irregularities, right common iliac stenosis, and an occluded left iliac artery indicated a standard aortobifemoral graft.

of the reconstruction along with suitable endarterectomy where needed, (3) flushing into the internal iliac system is avoided to prevent embolization there, and (4) femorofemoral bypasses (rather than aortobifemoral grafts) avoid these problems and sometimes improve sexual function. DePalma noted this benefit in 9 of 13 men who had femorofemoral grafts for unilateral iliac occlusion.[33]

Despite these studies and others[34,35] the actual risk of any particular procedure is not known, particularly since psychogenic problems as well as organic changes influence the matter. These risks are now well-recognized by surgeons and are becoming increasingly so by patients. The situation requires preoperative consideration of the risks along with alternative methods to avoid them. These include femorofemoral shunts and transluminal angioplasty for unilateral iliac disease in males.

Extraanatomic versus Aortofemoral Grafts

The discussion of results in Chapter 13 leads to the belief that femoral-to-femoral bypasses provide a 5-year patency rate about 10 percent below that of the standard aortobifemoral graft. Axillary bifemoral grafts have not become widely used but are reported to have patency rates another 10 to 15 percent below the femoral crossover graft (and therefore 20 to 25 percent less than aortobifemoral grafts). These extraanatomic shunts, especially the short femoral-to-femoral ones, should be considered for patients in whom there is an elevated risk from an intraabdominal "Y" graft. However, as Rutherford notes, the extraanatomic bypasses are still "second-best procedures, to be performed only with clear-cut indications and should not be considered a substitute for lack of technical skill or intensive care facilities."[36]

Femorofemoral bypasses should also be considered for the male (any in general, and the younger in particular) because of the risk of sexual dysfunction after an aortic procedure.

Concomitant Sympathectomy

Lumbar sympathectomy is at best an indirect method to increase blood flow to the distal tissues. Its worth clearly does not approach that of direct revascularization,[37] yet there continue to occur instances of limb salvage apparently due to it.

The matter is discussed in Chapter 20. In brief, there are two indications for sympathectomy. The first is aortic revascularization. During the exposure for revascularization both ganglionated chains are removed over a distance of an inch. The added operational time is 5 to 10 minutes. There is no evidence that long-term graft patency is improved, but warm feet in the recovery room attest to diminution of peripheral arterial resistance during the early postoperative period.[38] The procedure adds no risk if it is abandoned at the first hint of technical difficulty (in about 5 percent).

The other indication for lumbar sympathectomy for atherosclerosis arises when the distal vessels are diseased without possibility of reconstruction, particularly if there is skin involvement without severe pain at rest. Sometimes there is the possibility of a distal repair to a poor vessel with diminished likelihood of success. In this circumstance a lumbar sympathectomy may be performed while another team exposes the distal leg artery. The wound is packed during heparinization and thereafter closed along with the leg wounds.

Femoropopliteal Grafts

The standard saphenous bypass between the common femoral and popliteal arteries requires little discussion, since it is generally agreed that its early and long-term results are superior to other grafts (Figure 9-17).[39] Successive alternative conduits have been introduced, but follow-up studies still indicate them to be second best. Even ardent exponents of PTFE, such as Veith's group, say "we still believe ipsilateral autologous saphenous vein to be the graft material of choice for femoral-popliteal bypass."[40]

The various alternatives to (Chapter 10) and complications of (Chapter 12) femoropopliteal bypass are discussed elsewhere. Other matters of interest are noted below.

Placing the vein graft in the subcutaneous tissue rather than beneath the muscle allows easy examination and simple access if it is needed later. Passing the graft through the popliteal space

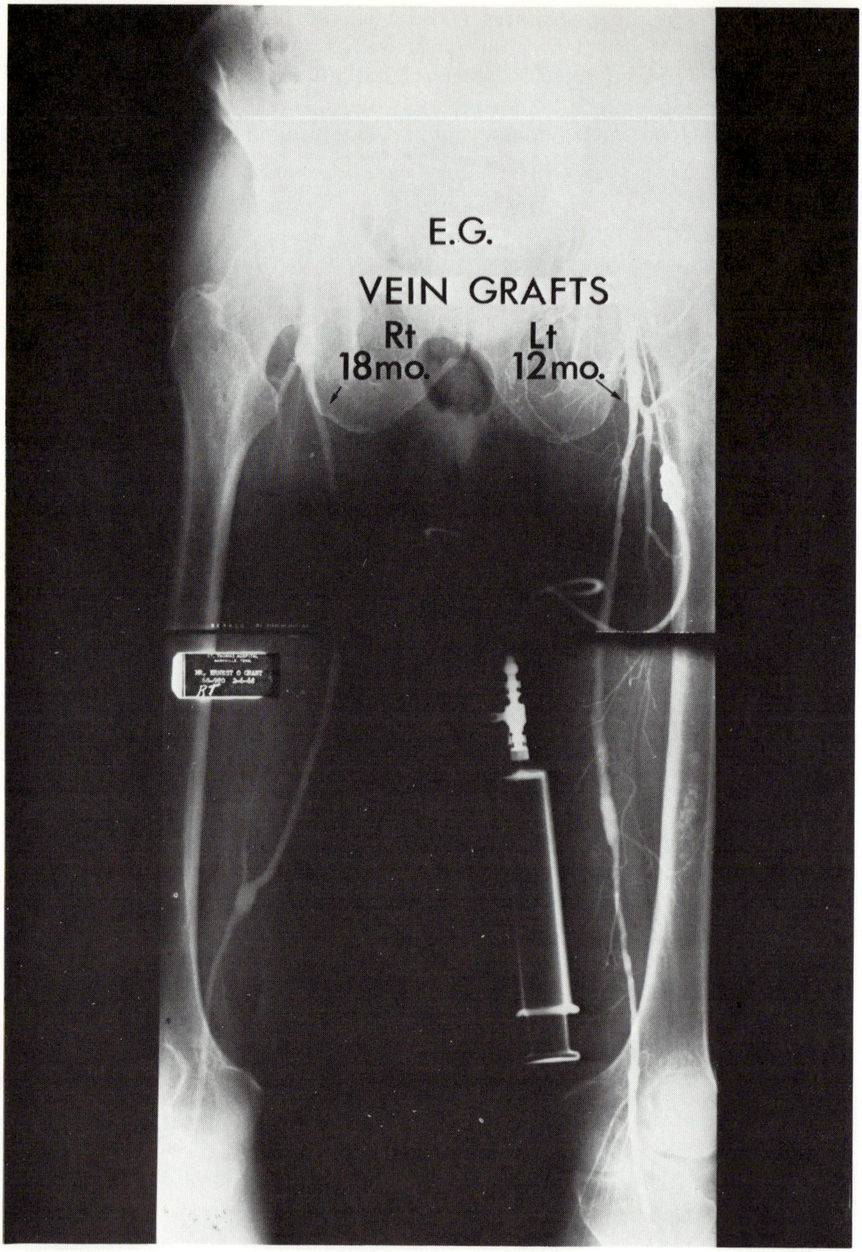

FIGURE 9-17 Bilateral autogenous saphenous vein grafts to above-knee anastomoses are demonstrated to be patent 12 and 18 months postoperatively.

alongside the host artery affords it protection at the knee and allows a parallel course at its entry into the popliteal artery below the knee.

The vein is removed without tying its tributaries, which are then ligated at a side table while the arteries are dissected from their beds by another team. A vein holder (Figure 12-2) allows a single person to tie off the vein's tributaries, distend it, and mark it to prevent twisting. Contrary to some cardiac surgeons I prepare the vein personally and delegate the arterial dissections to other members of the team.

Despite reports of microscopic changes dependent upon the solution used to clear and distend the vein graft, there are no documented differences in long-term patency rates. Heparinized Ringer's solution is suitable, but other irrigants are comparable.

The vein graft can hardly be too long—it will curve and remain patent—but too short means too tight and the possibility of occlusion due to that. Similarly, the anastomoses can hardly be made too long. A 3:1 ratio of the length of the anastomosis to arterial diameter is a good one (Figure 9-18). This allows room for technical error as well as for the constriction which occurs during healing. The most likely place for constriction of the anastomosis is at the toe of the distal anastomosis; next is the heel of the femoral junction (Figure 9-19). Avoidance is the best measure; a Linton vein patch is occasionally needed.

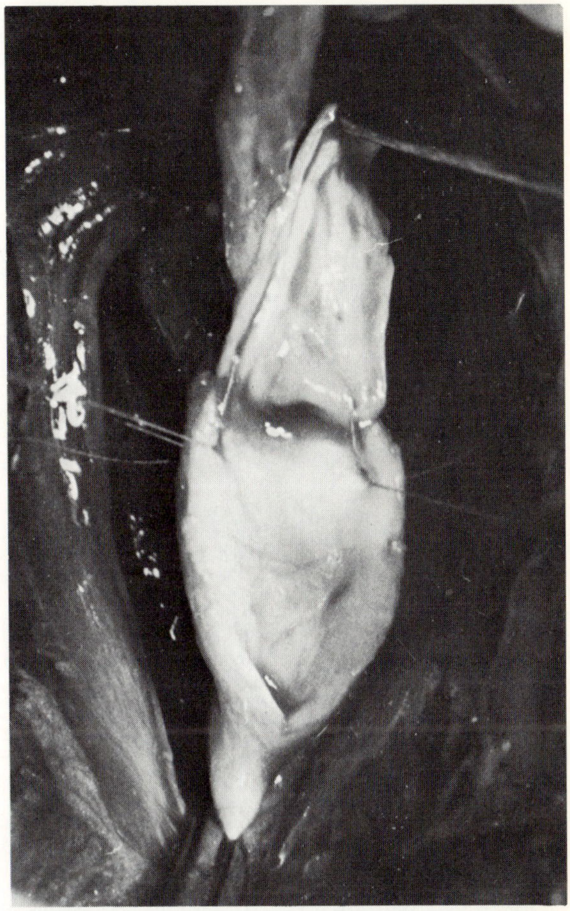

FIGURE 9-18 The length of the anastomosis between the autogenous vein and the femoral artery is emphasized.

Routine completion angiography (Chapter 14) will increase the patency rate of these and other peripheral reconstructions (Figures 9-20 to 9-23). Patency rates at the time of hospital discharge at 7 to 9 days should be 90 to 95 percent and the 5-year rate should be 60 to 70 percent.

The reversed autogenous saphenous vein graft remains the standard against which other femoral popliteal revascularizations are measured.

Profundaplasty

Compromise or loss of the collateral circulation provided by the profunda branch of the femoral artery often threatens loss of and always reduces the function of a limb whose superficial femoral or popliteal artery is occluded.* Its patency is thereby always a consideration when revascularization is performed. Profundaplasty should accompany femoropopliteal grafting, to provide an additional blood flow via its branches. In the case of aortofemoral grafting an additional purpose is to maximize blood flow through the graft.

Whether profundaplasty alone (Figure 9-24) will improve distal tissue perfusion enough to salvage a threatened extremity is less certain (Table 9-2). David and Drezner reported a high

*Bernhard's excellent discussion of profundaplasty is recommended[41]

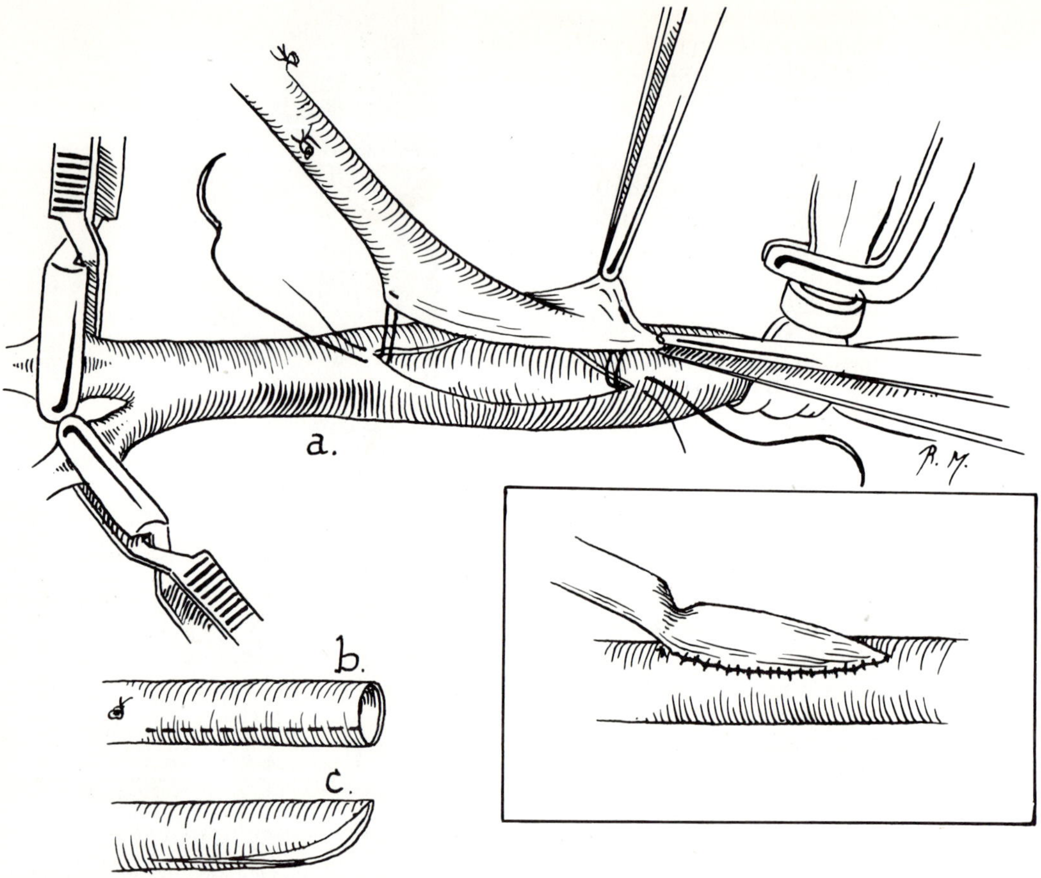

FIGURE 9-19 This old drawing (made 25 years ago, when modern vascular occlusive devices were not available) demonstrates the beginning of the anastomosis of the vein to the femoral artery. In the insert diagram there is stenosis at the heel of the anastomosis because the sutures were placed too deeply.

success rate—86 percent salvage of 50 limbs, 95 percent relief of rest pain in 39, and 55 percent salvage of tissue necrosis in 11.[42] Bernhard's success rate was 50 percent of 10.[41] Leather, Shah, and Karmody had 100 percent relief of rest pain among 34 patients and 78 percent salvage among 28 with tissue necrosis.[43] On the other hand, Mitchell's group had a high complication rate, and less than half their 27 profundaplasties were successful.[44]

Cotton and Roberts's experiences with 74 profundaplasties, largely for claudication, led them in 1975 to suggest that it could replace femoral popliteal grafting.[45] This latter proposal has not been generally accepted. If there is any reasonable chance of carrying blood distally via a graft, that should obviously be done. Otherwise, lumbar sympathectomy plus profundaplasty may be acceptable in an effort to avoid an amputation.

Profundaplasty should be carried distally beyond all plaques and thickening, far enough to provide a real increase in blood flow.[42] Closure of the arteriotomy may be done using a patch of vein, or a patch of endarterectomized superficial femoral artery, or by creating a common wall between the profunda and the superficial femoral artery.

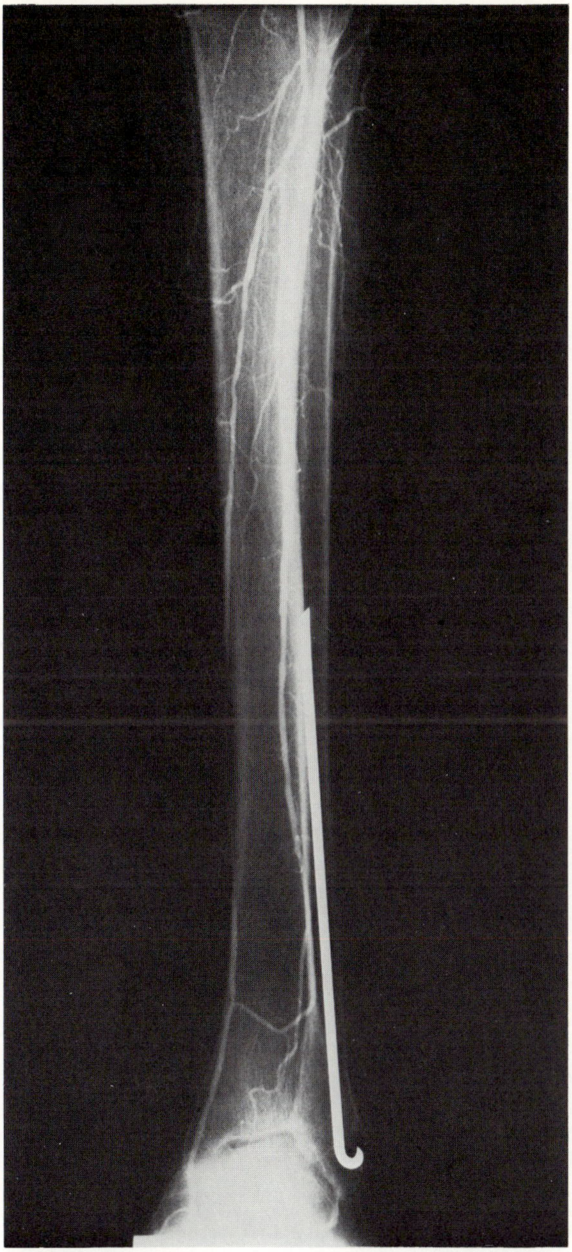

FIGURE 9-20 A preoperative arteriogram demonstrated a patent popliteal artery with poor run-off.

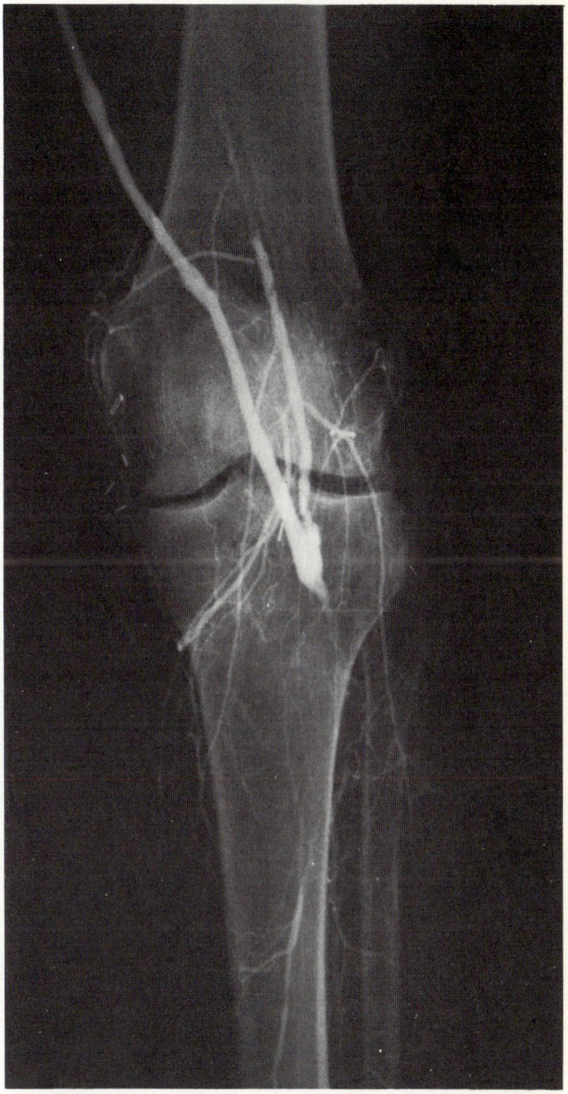

FIGURE 9-21 Completion angiography demonstrated a technically correct anastomosis but failure of flow a centimeter distal to that.

Occasionally, when the length of available vein is short, a large profunda may be used as the origin of a graft extending distally.

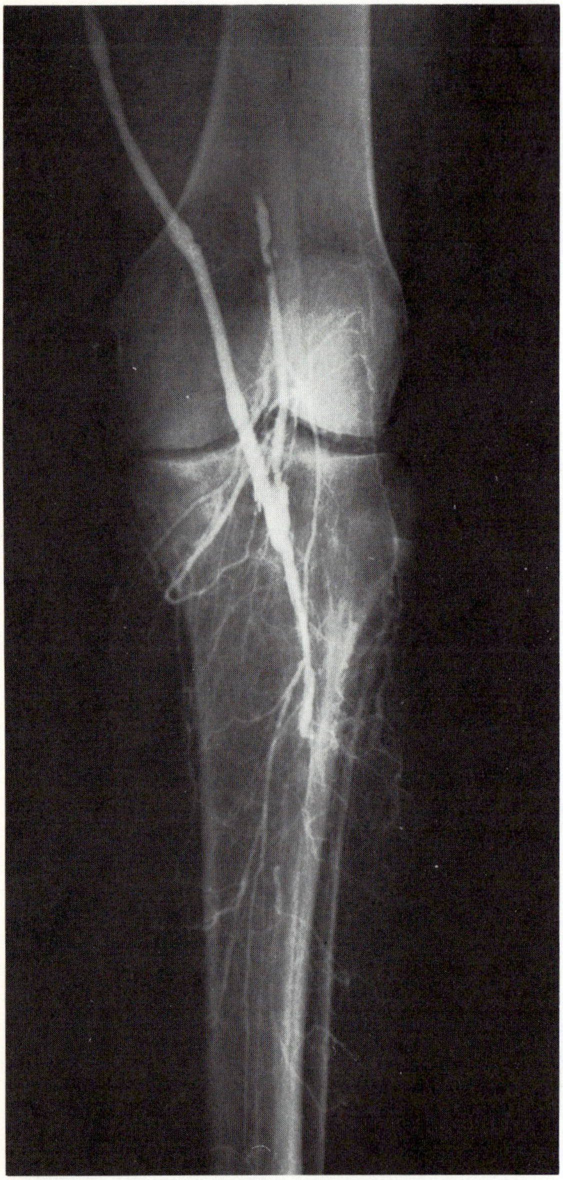

FIGURE 9-22 Following Fogarty thrombectomy, a second intraoperative arteriogram demonstrated improvement but continued failure of penetration of the material distally.

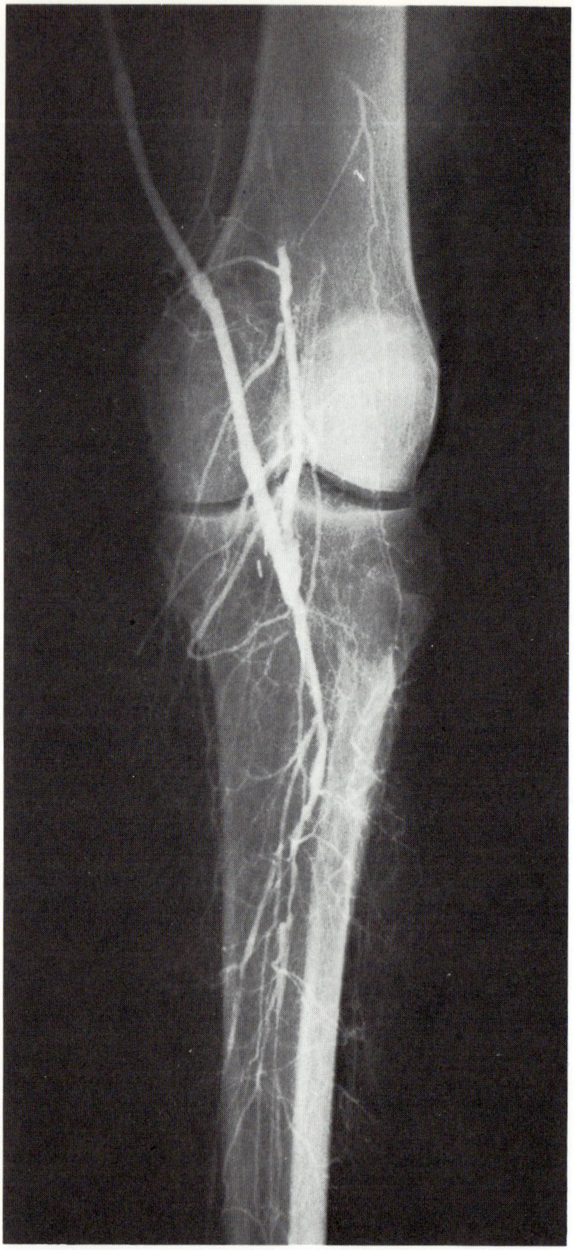

FIGURE 9-23 Following further Fogarty catheter thrombectomy, the distal circulation was open although limited, as indicated by preoperative evaluation.

Concomitant Proximal and Distal Reconstruction

The excellent revascularization achieved through the profunda branch, even if the superficial femoral artery is occluded, makes distal reconstruction unnecessary after proximal arterial recon-

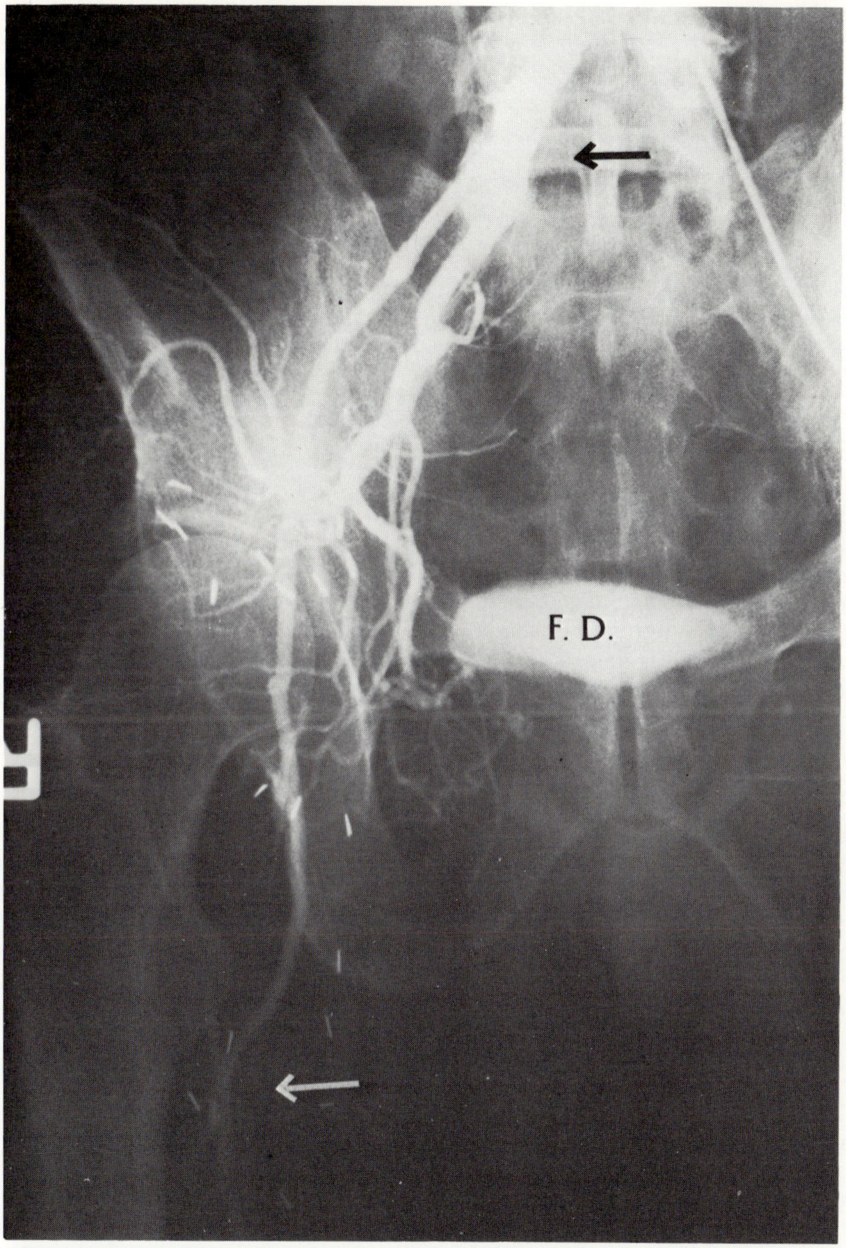

FIGURE 9-24 Revascularization of the profunda femoris was achieved by a reversed autogenous saphenous vein from the common iliac artery *(black arrow)* to the profunda *(white arrow)* via an extraperitoneal approach.

struction for most patients. Aortobifemoral grafts alone solve the problems of 80 to 90 percent of patients.

Royster's group reported combined segment occlusive disease in 58 percent of 140 patients. Only 1 of those having aortobifemoral grafting for threatened limb loss required a distal recon-

TABLE 9-2 RESULTS OF PROFUNDAPLASTY ALONE FOR LIMB SALVAGE

First author	Ref no.	Year	No.	Salvage results	Time
Cotton	45	1975	74	59% success	NA*
Hill	80	1977	7	2 successes	NA*
David	42	1978	50	86% success (55% for gangrene)	4 mo to 3 yr
Hull	69	1978	19	Benefit to 3 claudicators	
				Benefit to 7 of 16 salvage patients	
Leather	43	1978	62	100% relief for 34 rest pain patients	NA*
				78% success with 28 necrosis patients	
Mitchell	44	1979	27	40% success with 5 claudicators	
				45% success with 22 salvage patients	9 to 29 mo
Bernhard	41	1982	10	50% success	NA*

*Not available.

struction in the immediate postoperative period, along with 6 others done for continued claudication. Thus 13 percent of the 53 required additional distal revascularization.[46] Other reports of similar statistics indicate that about half of patients with aortic disease will have concomitant femoral occlusion and that 10 to 20 percent will require distal revascularization.[42,47–49]

Occasionally, the distal ischemia is so severe that it is at once clear that a femoropopliteal (or more distal) graft is needed at the same time as an aortobifemoral graft. Edwards's group performed such concomitantly in 6 percent of 330 aortic reconstructions,[47] while Brewster's group performed synchronous distal grafting for 2 percent of 368 patients.[17] Usually it is better to complete the proximal revascularization and reevaluate the possible need for a more distal procedure after a few days or weeks.

There has been continued difficulty in selection of the appropriate procedure when there are associated aortoiliac and femoropopliteal lesions, particularly when the proximal one is stenosis rather than complete occlusion. A variety of noninvasive tests, as well as pressure studies and radiographic techniques, have not completely solved the problem.[50] The best practical method presently is to explore the femoral artery first, with the planned procedure in mind but with wide preparation to allow a shift either proximally or distally after examining the artery and its pulse. Sometimes it must be opened before the final decision can be made to bring a graft from above or to restrict the procedure to a femoropopliteal revascularization.

Position of the Femoral Anastomosis

Sometimes the available autogenous vein is not long enough to span the distance from the common femoral artery to the popliteal artery, especially below the knee. If the superficial femoral artery is patent, the vein may be attached to it in the mid or distal thigh to form a shorter bypass to the distal artery. Another solution is endarterectomy of enough length of the superficial femoral artery to allow it to supply the vein with blood (Figure 9-25). In rare instances the origin of the vein graft is the lower end of a well-developed profunda femoris artery. There are usually better alternatives than this latter one.

Above-Knee or Below-Knee Anastomoses

For many years it was the conventional wisdom that grafts which crossed joints and thereby moved frequently performed poorly, with the exception of autogenous veins. The placement of the distal vein anastomosis to the above-knee segment of the popliteal artery was done because it was simpler and required a shorter segment of vein.

Later, as the medial-calf approach to the popliteal artery became well-known, it was recognized that some above-knee anastomoses lay proximal to stenotic lesions in the popliteal artery which would be bypassed if the graft were carried further down to the artery below the knee. This led on to the concept that perhaps all vein grafts should be anastomosed below the knee, in order to bypass lesions which might later develop just at the knee level. The prophylactic result of this idea has not been documented, although the procedure is widely practiced.

It is, however, clear that an above-knee anastomosis should be used only if the artery distal to it is relatively normal. Otherwise, it is safer to carry the graft distally to bypass all the disease.

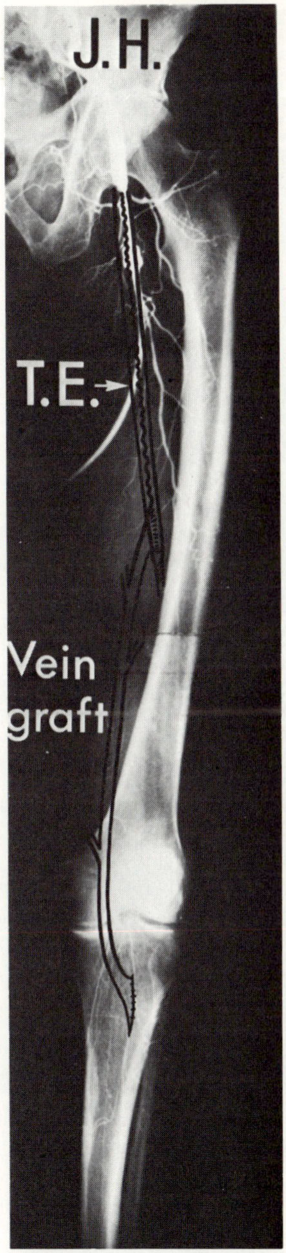

FIGURE 9-25 The vein graft was not long enough to reach from the common femoral artery to the popliteal artery below the knee. Endarterectomy of the superficial artery provided sufficient extra length to allow a completely autogenous reconstruction to be achieved.

Grafts to Isolated Popliteal Segments and to Distal Arteries

It has been thought that the quality of the distal run-off arteries directly influenced the patency of a femoropopliteal graft. DeWeese and Rob documented lower 10-year patency rates in vein grafts to popliteal arteries with no run-off or one-vessel run-off than in grafts to arteries with two- or three-vessel run-off (29 percent versus 41 percent respectively).[51] Such data suggest that delivering blood to an "isolated" popliteal artery will not produce good results, since there will be no large arteries to carry the blood on down the leg (or in a retrograde direction either). Correct determination of the matter is important, since about 20 percent of patients needing femoropopliteal reconstruction have such an isolated popliteal segment.[52,53]

Further investigation of the long-term patency of grafts to such isolated popliteal segments (Figure 9-26) refutes this pessimism, as shown in Table 9-3. These several series report 61 to 84 percent patency rates 4 to 5 years after operation. They clearly suggest that salvage, rather than primary amputation, should be attempted.

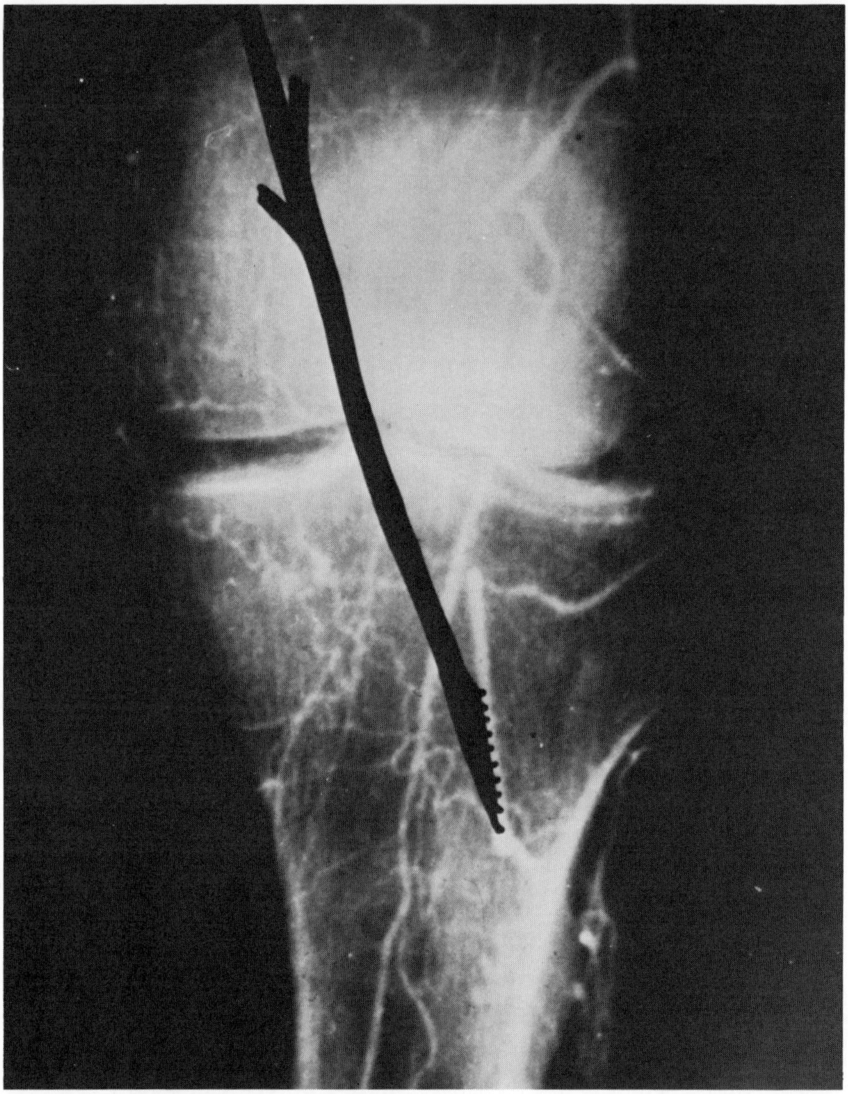

FIGURE 9-26 This isolated popliteal arterial segment was revascularized by an autogenous saphenous vein graft.

TABLE 9-3 GRAFTS TO ISOLATED POPLITEAL ARTERIAL SEGMENTS

First author	Ref no.	Year	No.	Type graft	% patent	Time
Mannick	52	1967	31	Vein	65	9 mo to $4\frac{1}{2}$ yr
Darling	81	1975	51	Vein	61	5 yr
Davis	70	1975	17	Vein	70	4 yr
Corson	54	1982	51	Vein	65	5 yr
			14	Prosthetic	17	5 yr
Veith	40	1982	48	PTFE	84	47 mo

Whether others can produce as good results with PTFE as Veith[40] is unknown. Corson's group reported only a 17 percent 5-year patency rate for PTFE versus 65 percent for vein grafts to isolated popliteal segments. Further, their 5-year rate to infrapopliteal arteries was 66 percent, suggesting the simpler procedure of using the isolated popliteal segment.[54] However, when there is extensive distal necrosis, the graft probably needs to be placed (either sequentially or directly) to a patent distal artery.[55]

If the thesis of aggressive efforts to salvage extremities rather than to amputate be accepted, there remains the question of whether to (1) end the graft at the isolated segment, (2) add a distal extension to a patent tibial vessel (to form a sequential graft) or (3) skip the isolated segment and go directly to a patent distal tibial or peroneal artery.

DeLaurentis and Friedman in 1971 described three successful sequential Dacron and vein bypasses[56] and by 1981 had produced 80 percent patency among 33 such grafts.[57] Sterling Edward's group in 1976 reported six sequential femoral-popliteal-tibial vein grafts, but two failed within 3 months.[58] Bliss and Fonseka had 11 successes among 16 "hitch-hike" grafts in 1976.[59] Flinn and associates in 1980 noted that the length of vein available in many patients was insufficient for a long sequential graft. In fact, only 3 of their 40 reconstructions used veins alone; others used PTFE. They also reported that failure of the more distal segment in 12 limbs was not critical, since loss of the limb did not follow.[60] Jarrett reported a 4-year 62 percent success rate among 23 sequential grafts to the tibial arteries,[61] and Clayson had a 63 percent 3-year patency rate among 17 grafts.[62]

The vein sequential graft needs no defense. Its several techniques show imaginative variations. It probably offers something more than grafting to an isolated popliteal segment, but at the expense of a considerable increase in dissection and time. There are no available statistics to contrast the complication rates of the two procedures. Further, there at once occurs the idea of omitting the anastomosis at the popliteal level and carrying the pressurized blood flow directly to a patent distal artery.

Vein grafts to the distal calf and ankle vessels (Figures 9-27 and 9-28) have been quite successful (Table 9-4). The large series of Reichle and associates is notable because there are follow-ups as long as 7 years. Their cumulative patency rate for femorotibial vein grafts at 7 years was 43 percent and for femoroperoneal grafts was 38 percent. They salvaged over half the limbs which had infrapopliteal revascularizations.[74]

Recently the Albany group's successful experiences with in situ vein grafts to small distal arteries (80 percent of 242 patent at 2 years) has suggested to them that few grafts need be ter-

TABLE 9-4 GRAFTS TO TIBIAL OR PERONEAL ARTERIES

First author	Ref no.	Year	Number and type	% patent	Time
Davis	70	1975	38 vein	63	4 yr
Edwards	47	1976	97 vein	81	1 to 2 yr
Dardik	71	1979	61 umbilical cord vein (peroneal)	38	30 mo
Karmody	72	1979	59 in situ vein	90	30 mo
Sumner	73	1979	31 vein (tibial)	59	30 mo
Reichle	74	1980	137 vein and Dacron (femorotibial)	43	7 yr
			27 (femoroperoneal)	38	7 yr
Auer	75	1981	124 vein	59	5 yr
Graham	76	1981	58 vein (femoroperoneal)	51	3 yr
Imparato	77	1981	7 vein	51	10 yr
Kacoyanis	78	1981	105 vein	60	5 yr
Welsh	79	1981	105 vein	50	2 yr

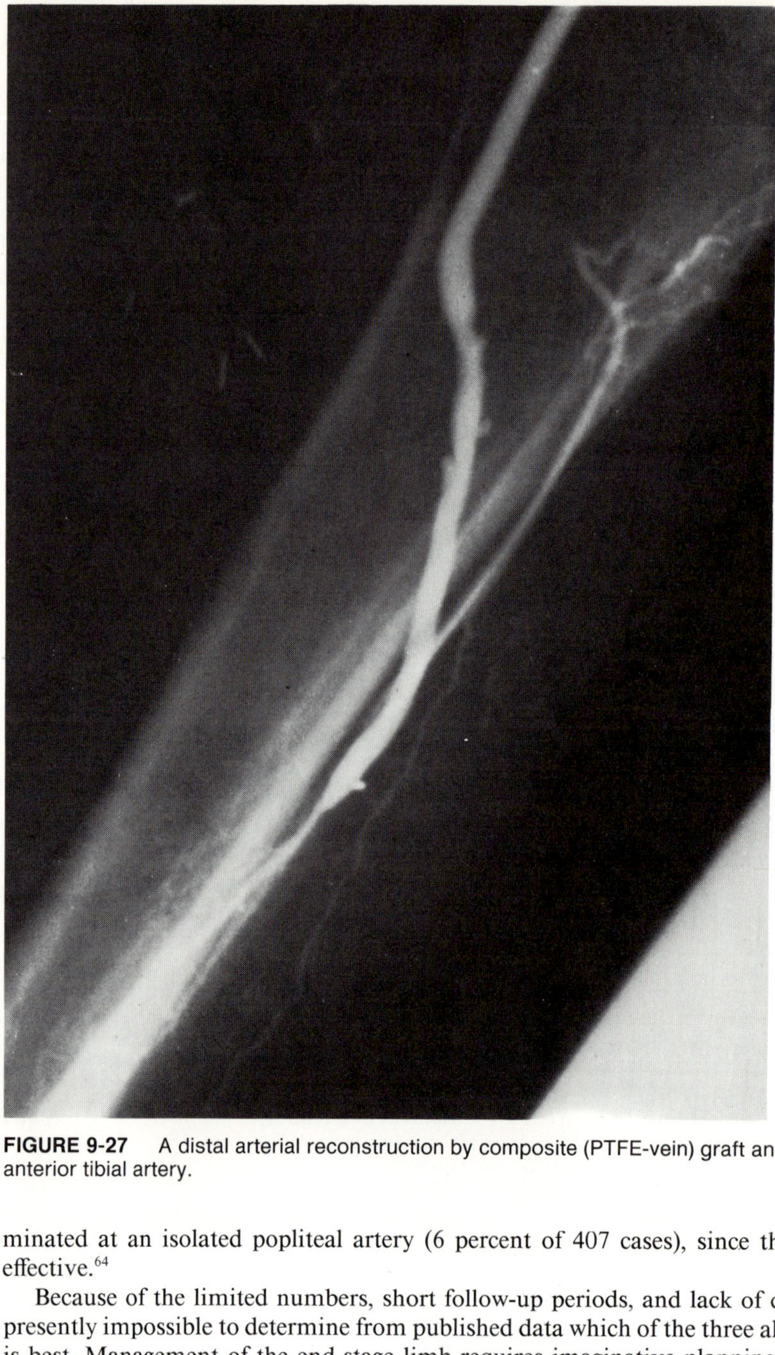

FIGURE 9-27 A distal arterial reconstruction by composite (PTFE-vein) graft anastomosed to the anterior tibial artery.

minated at an isolated popliteal artery (6 percent of 407 cases), since the distal site is more effective.[64]

Because of the limited numbers, short follow-up periods, and lack of controlled series, it is presently impossible to determine from published data which of the three alternatives for salvage is best. Management of the end-stage limb requires imaginative planning, which often reflects the art more than the science, the skill of the individual rather than a standard approach, and pragmatism over theory. A choice must be made based upon the surgeon's experience and judgment of the individual problem.

A sound recommendation has been made by Gupta and Veith, who have studied the matter

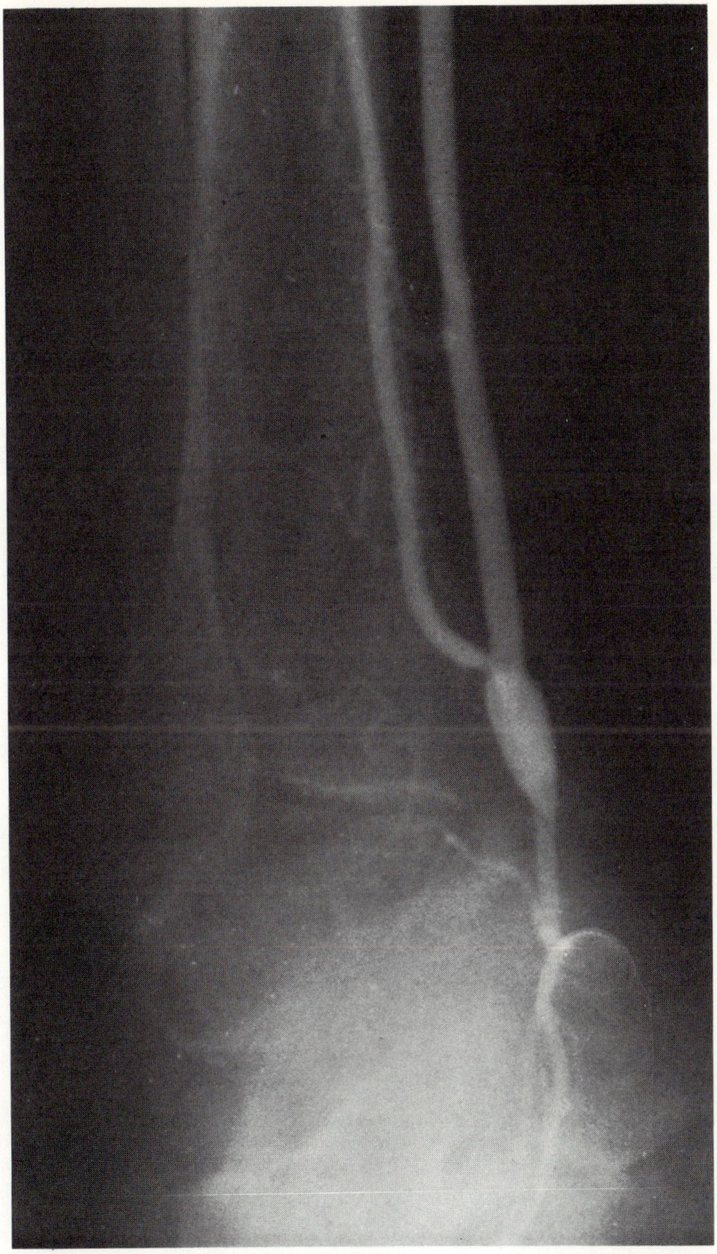

FIGURE 9-28 A distal arterial revascularization by autogenous vein graft anastomosed to the posterior tibial artery.

extensively.[53] They recommend using the isolated segment alone for patients with rest pain and minimal or no distal tissue necrosis. If there is extensive tissue necrosis, a sequential or direct bypass to a tibial or peroneal artery will carry blood under pressure further distally with a better chance of salvage of the foot (Figures 9-29 and 9-30).

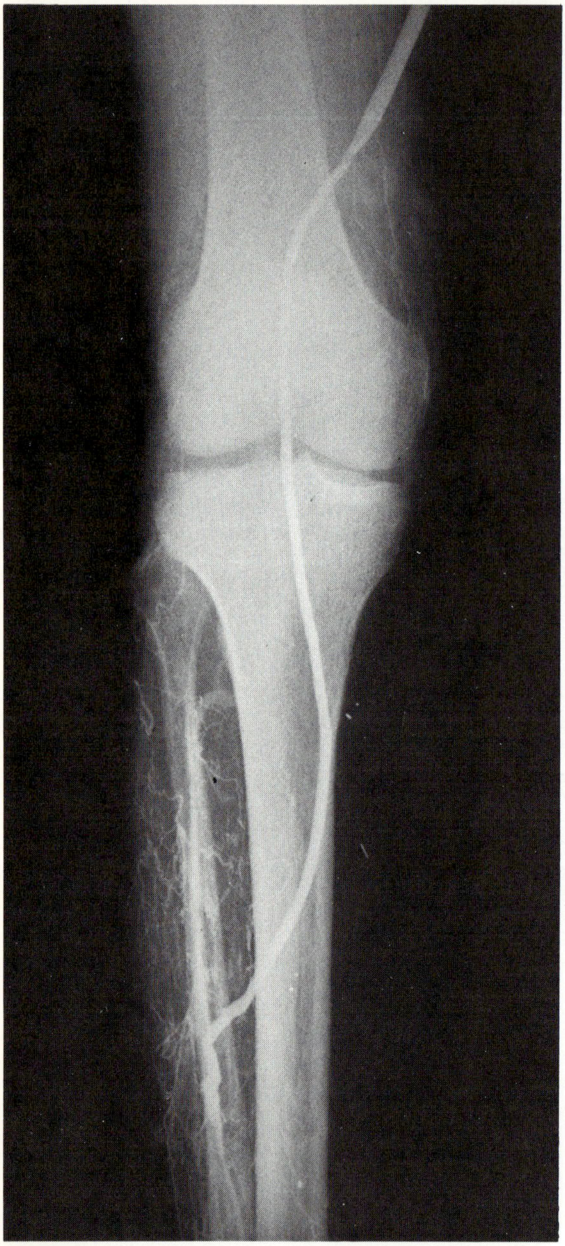

FIGURE 9-29 A composite PTFE-vein graft was passed through the popliteal space alongside the occluded popliteal artery, thence crossed through an opening in the interosseous membrane, and then anastomosed to the still-patent anterior tibial artery. The anastomosis between the PTFE and vein graft is hardly visible above the condyles of the femur because the diameters were well matched.

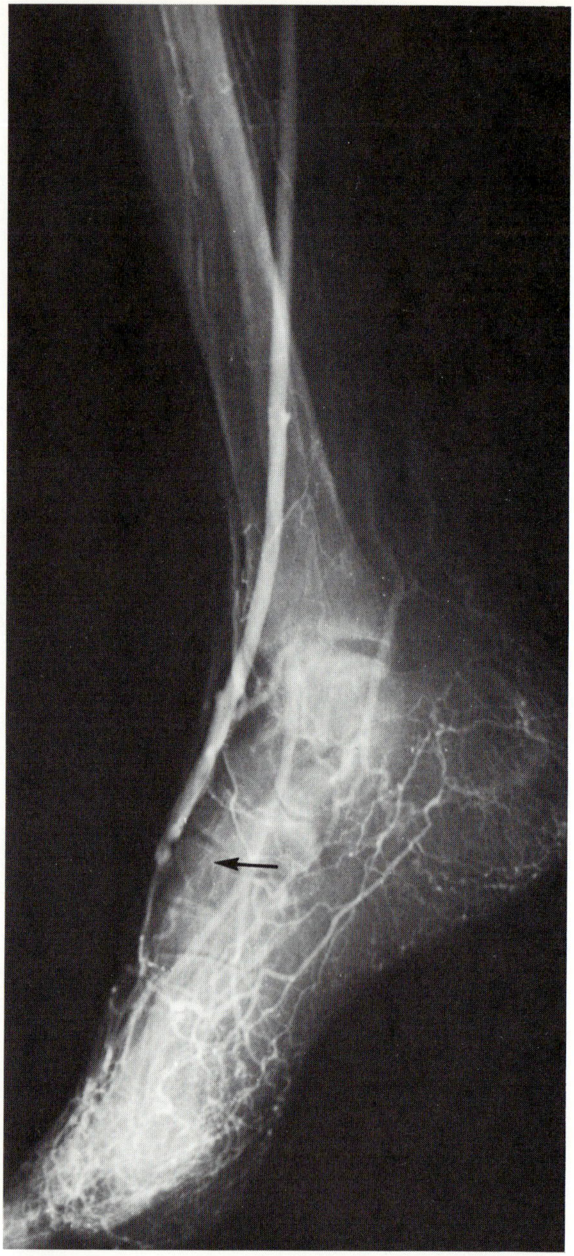

FIGURE 9-30 A vein graft anastomosed to the dorsalis pedis artery in the foot.

Distal Femoropopliteal Endarterectomy

Endarterectomies of the arteries of the lower extremities fell into disrepute for several reasons. First, they were attempted for long segments of diseased vessel, where there was the likelihood of technical error as well as of leaving areas of disease untreated. Second, lateral patches were used, which often produced aneurysmal segments of the vessels, which attracted thrombosis.[65] Third, the procedure was applied to distal vessels whose diameters, even when restored, were unlikely to be large enough for continued patency. Finally, the technique required for endarterectomies is more demanding than for a bypass graft. Their high failure rate led to general abandonment in favor of the femoropopliteal bypass graft.

Nonetheless, there are some situations for which a femoropopliteal endarterectomy is a good choice (Figures 9-31 to 9-34).[66] First is a short segment of tight stenosis or occlusion. Next, there is the same lesion where transluminal dilation has failed. Such endarterectomies should be approached through an incision well away from the saphenous vein, which may be needed later. Either incise the tissues 3 to 4 cm anterior to the course of that vein, or operate through the posterior approach to the popliteal artery. This latter approach, not well known today, allows easy exposure of the artery without severing any muscle or nerve. It also exposes the popliteal

FIGURE 9-31 Multiple ischemic lesions of the great toe due to a short popliteal arterial occlusion.

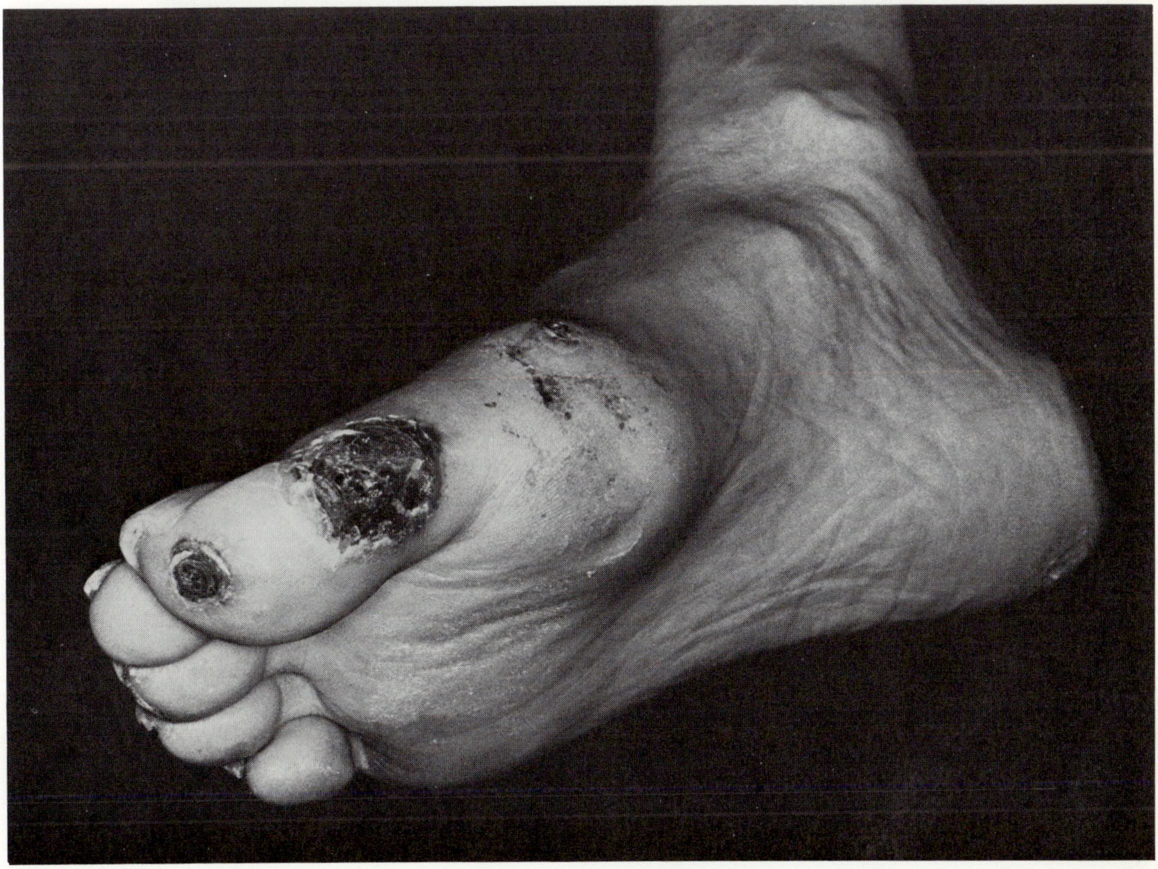

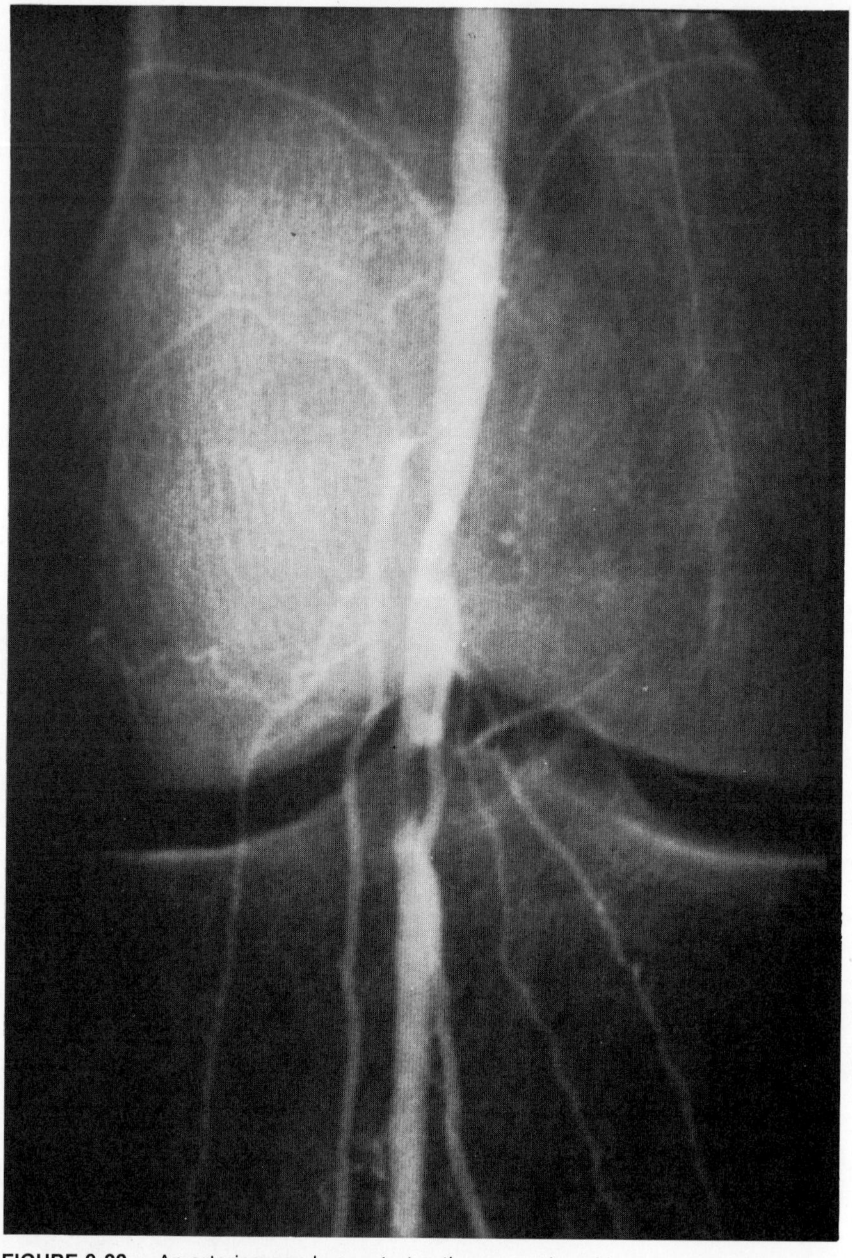

FIGURE 9-32 An arteriogram demonstrates the unusual position of a short popliteal arterial occlusion with a prominent collateral bypassing it.

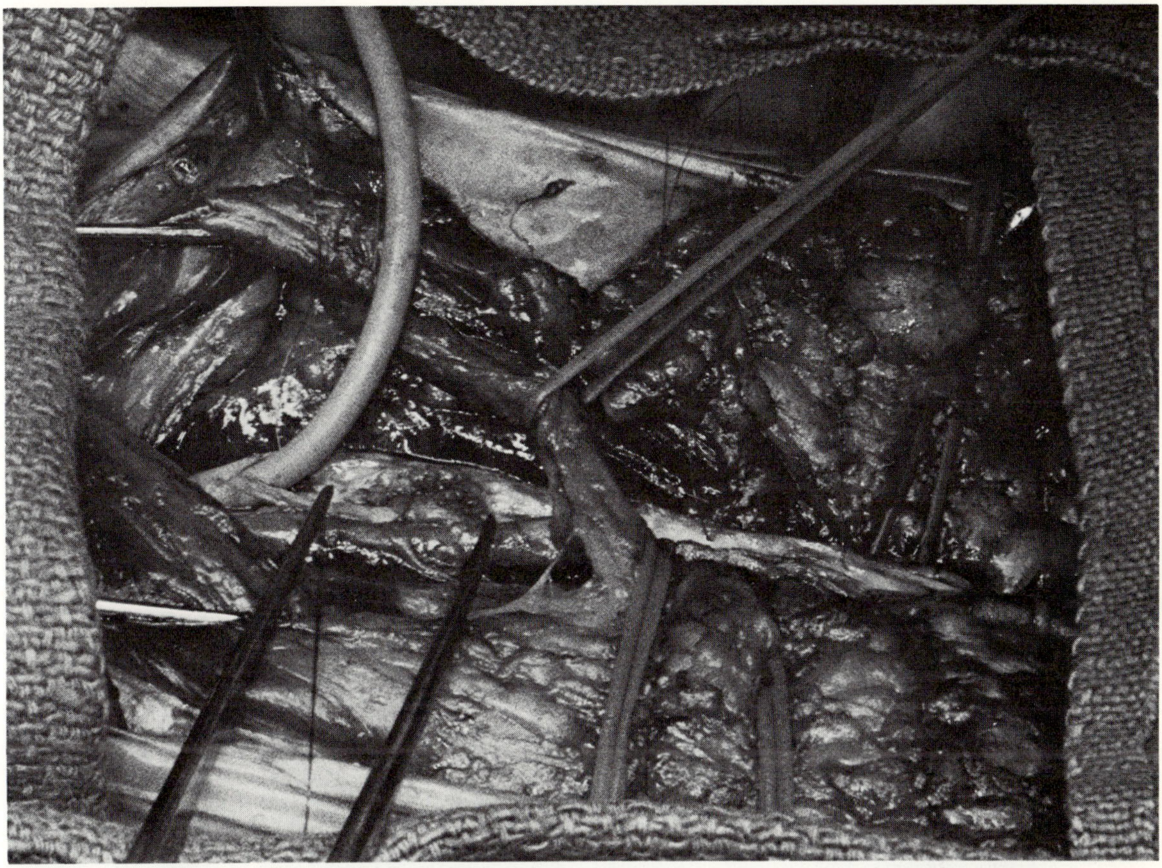

FIGURE 9-33 Endarterectomy is underway with a no. 8 urethral catheter indwelling during the reconstruction, to allow distal heparinization and also to aid correct tailoring closure.

end of the lesser saphenous vein, which may be useful as a short tailoring patch to cover the distal end of the endarterectomy (Figures 9-35 and 9-36).

Personal experience with these repairs for properly selected cases has been favorable (Figure 9-37). Inahara and Scott's excellent results among 104 limbs of 100 patients paralleled those of vein grafts. There were no failures of short-segment superficial femoral endarterectomy while the patients were in the hospital, and the 5-year patency rate of 70 percent and 10-year rate of 50 percent confirm the appropriate patient selection as well as the excellent surgical technique.[67]

Distal Thrombosis and Embolism

Clotting of the femoral and/or more distal arteries must be risked whenever the blood flow to them is reduced. It may occur during sleep, during anesthesia for a remote lesion, or during a vascular procedure. However, the cross-clamping which accompanies revascularization does not usually much reduce flow, so occlusion is more likely due to clot "washing down" from above or from the graft itself. Systemic heparinization prior to clamping, along with placing heparin-saline directly into the distal vessels, usually prevents thrombosis.

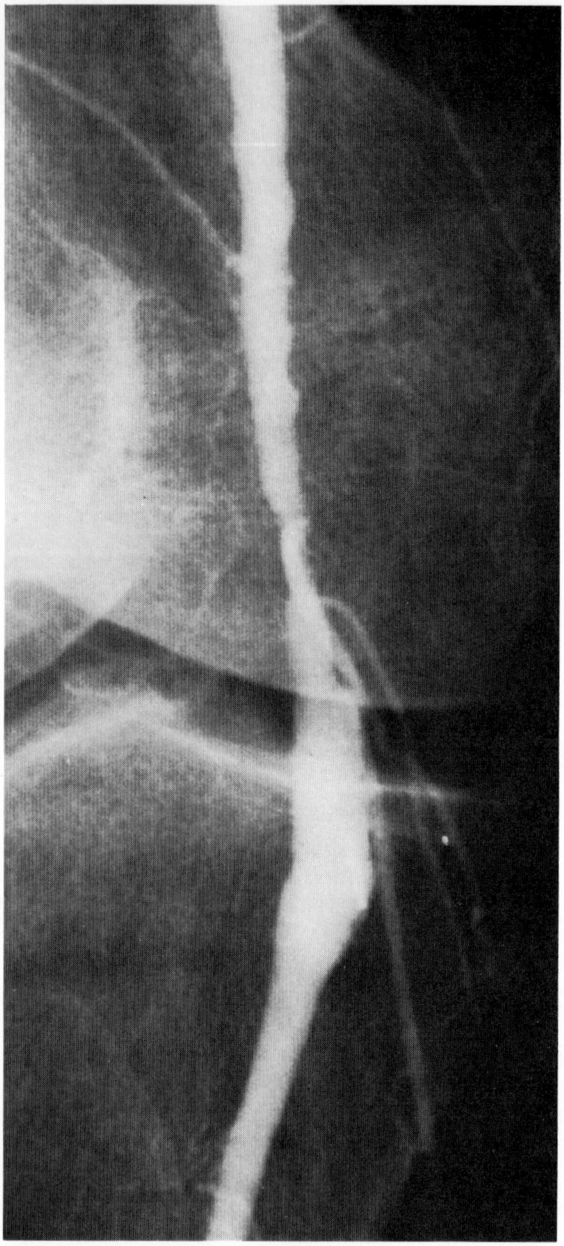

FIGURE 9-34 The completion arteriogram demonstrated that despite efforts to prevent placing the venous patch graft too loosely, the accomplishment was imperfect.

Clotting due to embolism ("trash foot") and other more proximal problems can usually be prevented by properly cleaning the graft of debris prior to opening the flow of blood into it, as well as by flushing the proximal vessel to rid it of clot accumulated above a chronically occluded area or even during the time of cross-clamping. Since the autotransfusion unit has encouraged more vigorous flushing, distal embolism has become uncommon. The trade-off between blood loss (recovered via the unit) and embolism problems favors flushing.

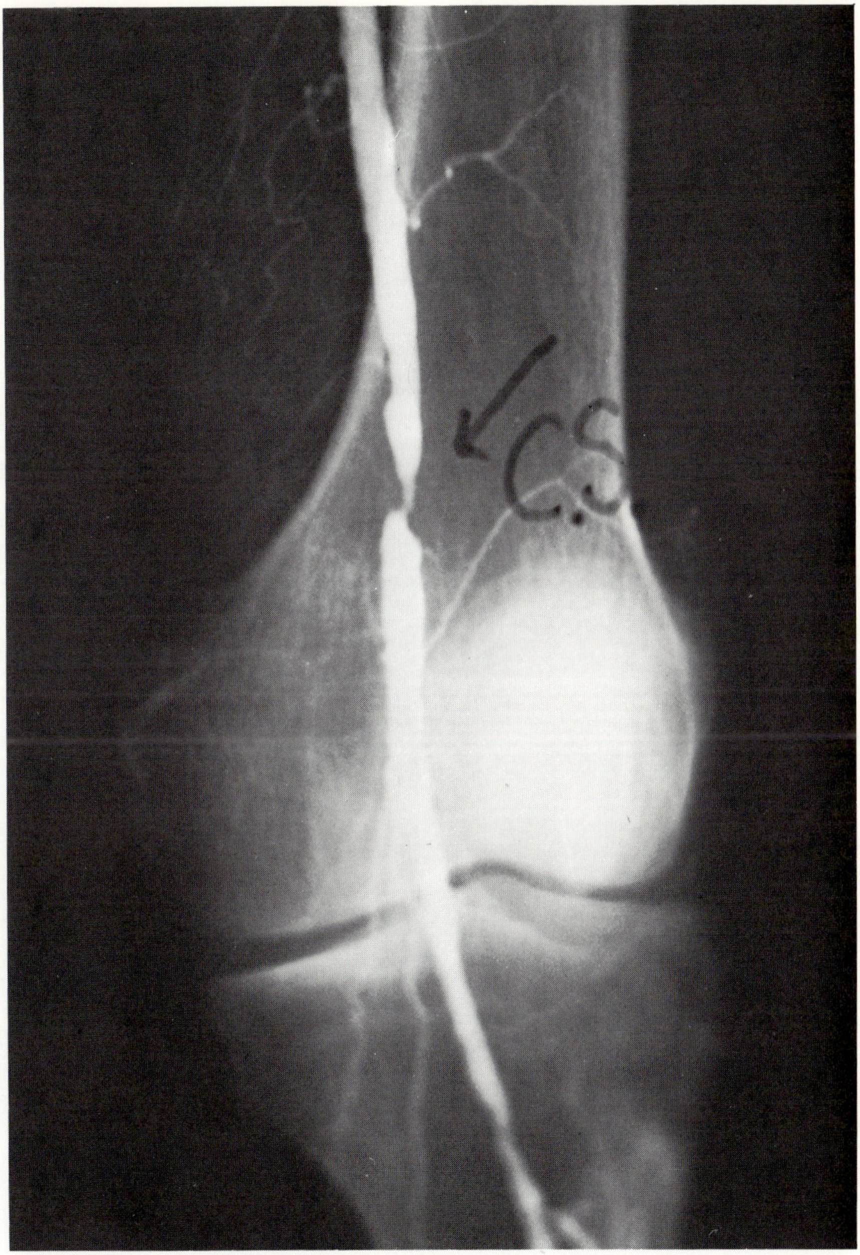

FIGURE 9-35 Limited arteriosclerotic occlusion of the popliteal artery.

Early Reoperation for Acute Thrombosis

Thirty years ago the failure of a vascular repair in the immediate postoperative period usually was managed by an overnight period of observation and then reoperation the following day if ischemia persisted or became devitalizing. The poor results of this plan were soon recognized,

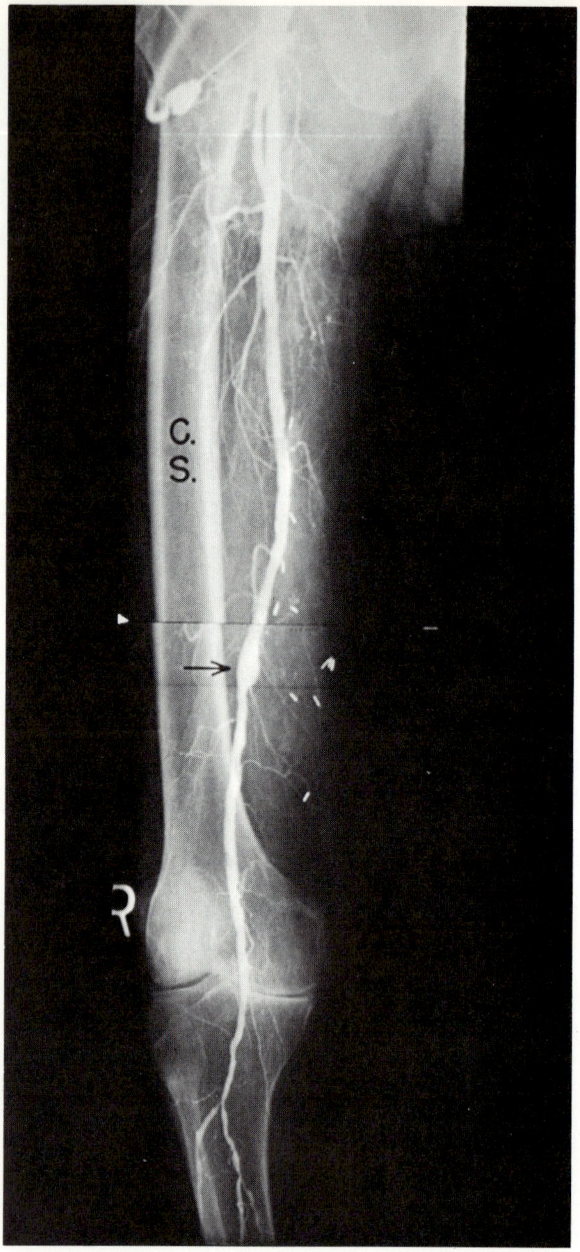

FIGURE 9-36 Direct-vision endarterectomy and patch graft closure at the *arrow*.

and middle-of-the-night secondary explorations became more commonplace. There is an even more aggressive approach today.

Our plan begins with the recognition that vascular surgery allows little or no room for error and that a technical defect must be corrected at once. Completion angiography provides a visible check while the patient and surgery team are still in the operating room (and is discussed more fully in Chapter 14).

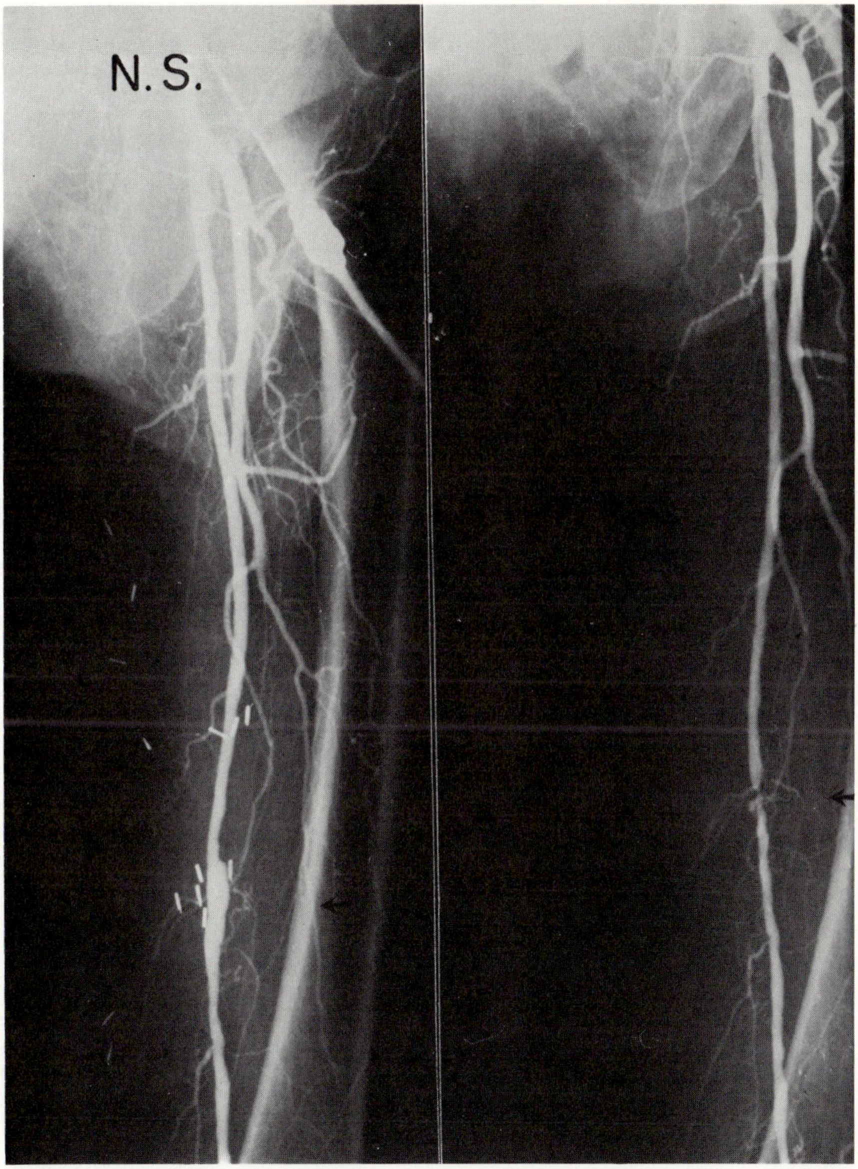

FIGURE 9-37 *Right,* limited occlusion of the superficial femoral artery in the midthigh was treated, *left,* by direct open endarterectomy and a patch graft which is a bit large.

An experienced member of the team evaluates the situation of each newly-operated-on patient in the Recovery Room in the late afternoon or a few hours after termination of the procedure, to be certain that warmth of the extremity and the expected pulses are present. Delegation of this responsibility to an inexperienced attendant invariably delays early recognition of vascular thrombosis. Immediate return to the operating room for thrombectomy, embolectomy, or extension of the original procedure if needed is a sine qua non for good results. We reported our results with early reoperation of 81 patients for either acute thrombosis or hemorrhage (4.7 percent of the 1703 total). Sixty percent of the 58 limbs which had acute thrombosis were salvaged. The success rate for the 30 femoropopliteal grafts that needed reoperation was 63 percent.[68]

The surgeon who undertakes peripheral arterial revascularization accepts the necessity to recognize early failures and correct them at once. Limbs and lives are risked not by early reoperation but by delay. Hopeful observation leads to tragedy.

REFERENCES

1 *Dorland's Medical Dictionary,* 24th ed. W. B. Saunders, Philadelphia, 1965, p 313.
2 Bouley: Observations of intermittent claudication. *Recuiel de Medecine Veterinaire et Comparee* 1831, 8:517.
3 Charcot JM: On intermittent claudication, observed in a case of complete obliteration of the iliac artery. *Comptes Rendus des Seances et Memoires de la Societe de Biologie,* 1858.
4 Warren R: Two kinds of intermittent claudication. *Arch Surg,* 1976, 111:739.
5 Goodreau JJ, Creasy JK, Flanigan P, Burnham SJ, Kudrna JC, Schafer MF, Bergan JJ, Yao JST: Rational approach to the differentiation of vascular and neurogenic claudication. *Surgery* 1978, 84:749.
6 Peabody CN, Kannel WB, McNamara PM: Intermittent claudication: surgical significance. *Arch Surg.* 1974, 109:693.
7 Imparato AM, Kim GE, Davidson T, Crowley GJ: Intermittent claudication: its natural course. *Surgery* 1975, 78:795.
8 Naji A, Barker CF, Berkowitz HO, Chu J, Roberts B: Femoropopliteal vein grafts for claudication: analysis of 100 consecutive cases. *Ann Surg,* 1978, 188:79.
9 Cronenwett JL, Warner KG, Zelenock GB, Whitehouse WM Jr, Graham LM, Lindenauer SM, Stanley JC: Intermittent claudication: current results of nonoperative management. *Arch Surg,* 1984, 119:430.
10 Dale WA: Salvage of arteriosclerotic legs by vascular repair. *Ann Surg,* 1967, 165:844.
11 Veith FJ, Gupta SK, Samson RH, Scher LA, Fell SC, Weiss P, Janko G, Flores SW, Rifkin H, Bernstein G. Haimovici H, Gliedman ML, Sprayregen S: Progress in limb salvage by reconstructive arterial surgery combined with new or improved adjunctive procedures. *Ann Surg,* 1981, 194:386.
12 Veith FJ, Gupta SK, Samson RH, Scher LA, Ascer E, Sprayregen S: Femoral-popliteal-tibial occlusive disease, in Moore WS (ed): *Vascular Surgery.* Grune & Stratton, New York, 1983, Chap 14.
13 Eisenberg RL, Mani RL, McDonald EJ Jr: The complication rate of catheter angiography by direct puncture through aorto-femoral bypass grafts. *Am J Roent,* 1976, 126:814.
14 Flanigan DP, Williams LR, Keifer T, Schuler JJ, Behrend AJ: Prebypass operative arteriography. *Surgery* 1982, 92:627.
15 Scarpato R, Gembarowiez R, Farber S, O'Donnell TF, Kelly JJ, Callow AD, Deterling RA: Intraoperative prereconstruction arteriography. *Arch Surg,* 1981, 116:1053.
16 Dale WA: Extensive aortic-iliac-femoral grafting: report of three cases. *Arch Surg,* 1959, 78:133.
17 Brewster D, Perler B, Robison J, Darling R: Aortofemoral graft for multilevel occlusive disease: predictors of success and need for distal bypass. *Arch Surg,* 1982, 117:1593.
18 Wylie EJ, Olcott C, String ST: Endarterectomy versus bypass operation for aorto-iliac occlusive disease, in Varco RL, Delaney IP (eds): *Controversy in Surgery.* W. B. Saunders, Philadelphia, 1976, p 437.
19 Humphries AW, Corrigan TP: Aorto-iliac Occlusive Disease: advantages of bypass grafting, in Varco RL, Delaney IP (eds): *Controversy in Surgery.* W. B. Saunders, Philadelphia, 1976, p 451.
20 Mannick JA, Whittemore AD, Couch NP: Aortoiliac occlusive disease, in Moore WS (ed): *Vascular Surgery.* Grune & Stratton, New York, 1983, Chap 13.
21 Davidson J, Benkart D, Edwards WH, Mulherin J: The role of graft material in aortic reconstructive surgery. *Ann Surg,* 1983, 197:714.
22 Stanley JC, Lindenauer SM, Graham LM, Whitehouse WM, Cronenwett JL, Zelenock GB: Vascular grafts, in Moore WS (ed): *Vascular Surgery.* Grune & Stratton, New York, 1983, Chap 9.
23 Voorhees AB, Jaretski A, Blakemore AH: The use of tubes constructed from vinyon N cloth in bridging arterial defects. *Ann Surg,* 1952, 135:332.
24 Pierce G, Turrentine M, Stringfield S, Iliopoulos J, Hardin C, Hermreck A, Thomas J: Evaluation of end to side vs. end to end proximal anastomosis in aortobifemoral bypass. *Arch Surg,* 1982, 117:1580.
25 Rutherford RB: In discussion of Ref. 24.
26 Traverso LW, Baker JD, Dainko EA, Machleder HI: Infrarenal aortic occlusion. *Ann Surg,* 187:397, 1978.

27 Davidson JT: Discussion of Davidson J, Benkart D, Edwards WH, Mulherin J: The role of graft material in aortic reconstructive surgery. *Ann Surg,* 1983, 197:714.
28 Smith RB: Discussion of Davidson J, Benkart D, Edwards WH, Mulherin J: The role of graft material in aortic reconstructive surgery. *Ann Surg,* 1983, 197:714.
29 Leriche R: Des obliterationsarterielle hautes (obliteration la terminasion de l'aorte) comme causes des insuffisances culatoires des membres inferieurs. *Bull Mem Soc Chir,* 1923, 49:14.
30 May AG, DeWeese JA, Rob CG: Changes in sexual function following operation on the abdominal aorta. *Surgery* 1969, 65:41.
31 DePalma RG: Impotence in vascular disease: relationship to vascular surgery. *Br J Surg,* 1982, 69:514.
32 Merchant RF Jr, DePalma RG: The effects of femorofemoral grafts on postoperative sexual function: correlation with penile pulse volume recordings. *Surgery* 1981, 90:962.
33 DePalma RG: Etiology and management of sexual problems related to aorto-iliac disease and surgery, in Veith FJ (ed): *Critical Problems in Vascular Surgery.* Appleton-Century Croft, New York, 1982, Chap 29.
34 Schwartz SI: Sexual dysfunction. *Contemp Surg,* 1980, 17:31.
35 Kempczinski RF: Role of the vascular laboratory in the evaluation of male impotence. *Am J Surg,* 1979, 138:278.
36 Rutherford RB: Results of extra-anatomic bypass: reasons for variance and relationship to indications, in Greenhalgh RM (ed): *Extraanatomic and Secondary Arterial Reconstructions.* Pitman, London, 1981, Chap 13.
37 Barnes RW, Baker WH, Shanik G, Maixner W, Hayes AC, Lin R, Clark W: Value of concomitant sympathectomy in aortoiliac reconstruction. *Arch Surg,* 1977, 112:1325.
38 Callow AD, Simeone FA: The Grimonster symposium on the occasion of the 50th anniversary of the first lumbar sympathectomy. *Arch Surg,* 1978, 113:295.
39 Cranley JJ, Hafner CD: Newer prosthetic material compared with autogenous saphenous vein for occlusive arterial disease of the lower extremity. *Surgery* 1981, 89:8.
40 Veith FJ, Gupta SK, Samson RH, Scher LA, Ascer E, Sprayregen S: Femoral-popliteal-occlusive disease, in Moore WS (ed): *Vascular Surgery.* Grune & Stratton, New York, 1983, Chap 14.
41 Bernard VM: Limitations of profunda femoris revascularization, in Veith FJ (ed): *Critical Problems in Vascular Surgery.* Appleton-Century Croft, New York, 1982, Chap 17.
42 David TE, Drezner AD: Extended profundaplasty for limb salvage. *Surgery* 1978, 84:758.
43 Leather RP, Shah DM, Karmody AM: The use of extended profundaplasty in limb salvage. *Am J Surg,* 1978, 136:359.
44 Mitchell RA, Bone, GE, Bridges R, Pomajzl MJ, Fry WJ: Patient selection for isolated profundaplasty: arteriographic correlates of operative results. *Am J Surg,* 1979, 138:912.
45 Cotton LT, Roberts VC: Extended deep femoral angioplasty: an alternative to femoropopliteal bypass. *Br J Surg,* 1975, 62:340.
46 Royster TS, Lynn R, Mulcare RJ: Combined aortoiliac and femoropopliteal occlusive disease. *Surg Gynecol Obstet,* 1976, 143:949.
47 Edwards WH, Wright R: Tibial and peroneal bypass in severe occlusive disease of the lower extremities. *Ann Surg,* 1976, 183:710.
48 Perdue GD, Long WD, Smith RB: Perspective concerning aortofemoral arterial reconstruction. *Ann Surg,* 1971, 173:940.
49 Crawford ES, Bomberger RA, Glaeser DH, Saleh SA, Russell WL: Aortoiliac occlusive disease: factors influencing survival and function following reconstructive operation over a 25 year period. *Surgery* 1981, 90:1055.
50 Flanigan DP, Williams LR, Schwartz JA, Schuer JJ, Gray B: Hemodynamic evaluation of the aortoiliac system based on pharmocologic vasodilatation. *Surgery* 1983, 93:709.
51 DeWeese JA, Rob CG: Autogenous venous grafts ten years later. *Surgery* 1975, 82:775.
52 Mannick JA, Jackson BT, Coffman JD, Hume DM: Sources of bypass vein grafts in patients with isolated popliteal artery segments. *Surgery* 1967, 61:171.
53 Gupta SK, Veith FJ: Fate of patients with a blind popliteal segment: limb loss with a patent femoralpopliteal graft, in Veith FJ (ed): *Critical Problems in Vascular Surgery.* Appleton-Century Croft, New York, 1982, Chap 16.
54 Corson JD, Brewster DC, LaSalle J, Darling RC: Comparative analysis of vein and prosthetic bypass grafts to the isolated popliteal artery. *Surgery* 1982, 91:448.

55 Watelet J, Philippe JM, Chamoun S, Testart J: When can revascularization by limited to the isolated popliteal artery?, letter. *Surgery* 1983, 93:725.
56 DeLaurentis DA, Friedman P: Arterial reconstruction about and below the knee: another look. *Am J Surg,* 1971, 121:392.
57 Rosenfeld JC, Savarese RP, Friedmann P, DeLaurentis DA: Sequential femoral popliteal and femoral tibial bypasses, *Arch Surg,* 1981, 116:1538.
58 Edwards WS, Gerety E, Larkin J, Hoyt TW: Multiple sequential femoral tibial grafting for severe ischemia. *Surgery* 1976, 80:711.
59 Bliss BP, Fonseka N: "Hitch-hike" grafts for limb salvage in peripheral arterial disease. *Br J Surg,* 1976, 63:562.
60 Flinn WR, Flanigan DP, Verta MJ, Bergan JJ, Yao JST: Sequential femoral-tibial bypass for severe limb ischemia. *Surgery* 1980, 88:357.
61 Jarrett F, Berkoff HA, Crummy AB, Bezer FO: Femorotibial bypass grafts with sequential technique: clinical results. *Arch Surg,* 1981, 116:709.
62 Clayson KR: Discussion of Rosenfeld JC, Savarese RP, Friedmann P, DeLaurentis DA: Sequential femoral popliteal and femoral tibial bypasses, *Arch Surg,* 1981, 116:1538.
63 Reichle FA, Rankin KD, Tysa RR, Finestone AJ, Shuman C: Long-term results of 474 arterial reconstructions for severely ischemic limbs: a 14 year follow-up study. *Surgery* 1979, 85:93.
64 Corson J, Karmody A, Shah D, Naraynsingh V, Leather R: When can revascularization be limited to the isolated popliteal artery? *Surgery* 1984, 95:127.
65 Dale WA, Lewis MR: Lateral vascular patch grafts. *Surgery* 1965, 57:36.
66 Wittenstein GJ: To ream or to graft? Time for a reappraisal. *Surgery* 1977, 82:774.
67 Inahara T, Scott CM: Endarterectomy for segmental occlusion of the superficial femoral artery. *Arch Surg,* 1981, 116:1547.
68 Mulherin JL, Allen TR, Edwards WH, Dale WA: Management of early post-operative complications of arterial repairs. *Arch Surg,* 1971, 112:1371.
69 Hull DA, Babcock GK, Hyde GL, Stoeckinger JM, McGee EM: Femoral artery profundaplasty. *Am J Surg,* 1978, 136:356.
70 Davis RC, Davies WT, Mannick JA: Bypass vein grafts in patients with distal popliteal artery occlusion. *Am J Surg,* 1975, 129:421.
71 Dardik H, Ibrahim IM, Dardik II: The role of the peroneal artery for limb salvage. *Ann Surg,* 1979, 189:189.
72 Karmody AM: Discussion of Sumner DS, Strandness DE: Hemodynamic studies before and after extended bypass grafts to the tibial and peroneal arteries. *Surgery* 1979, 86:442.
73 Sumner DS, Strandness DE: Hemodynamic studies before and after extended bypass grafts to the tibial and peroneal arteries. *Surgery* 1979, 86:442.
74 Reichle FA, Martinson MW, Rankin KP: Infrapopliteal arterial reconstruction in the severely ischemic lower extremity: a comparison of long-term results of peroneal and tibial bypasses. *Ann Surg,* 1980, 191:59.
75 Auer AI: Discussion of Kacoyanis GP, Whittemore AD, Couch NP, Mannick JA: Femorotibial and femoroperoneal bypass vein grafts: a 15 year experience. *Arch Surg,* 1981, 116:1529.
76 Graham JW, Hanel KC: Vein grafts to the peroneal artery. *Surgery* 1981, 89:264.
77 Imparato AM: Discussion of Kacoyanis GP, Whittemore AD, Couch NP, Mannick JA: Femorotibial and femoroperoneal bypass vein grafts: a 15 year experience. *Arch Surg,* 1981, 116:1529.
78 Kacoyanis GP, Whittemore AD, Couch NP, Mannick JA: Femorotibial and femoroperoneal bypass vein grafts: a 15 year experience. *Arch Surg,* 1981, 116:1529.
79 Welsh P: Discussion of Kacoyanis GP, Whittemore AD, Couch NP, Mannick JA: Femorotibial and femoroperoneal bypass vein grafts: a 15 year experience. *Arch Surg,* 1981, 116:1529.
80 Hill DA, Jamieson CW: The results of arterial reconstruction utilizing the profunda femoris artery in the treatment of rest pain and pregangrene. *Br J Surg,* 1977, 64:359.
81 Darling RC: Discussion of Davis RC, Davies WT, Mannick JA: Bypass vein grafts in patients with distal popliteal artery occlusion. *Am J Surg,* 1975, 129:421.

Invited Commentary

William H. Edwards, M.D.
Nashville, Tennessee

Dr. Dale has covered the important area of peripheral arterial occlusive disease with his usual thorough, clear, and concise review. He has the unique advantage of having been on the forefront of many of the advances that have occurred in vascular surgery since that Vinyon-N tube graft was first implanted over 30 years ago.

A positive, firm approach to the patient with symptomatic peripheral arterial disease by a surgeon familiar with the proper evaluation of and need for direct arterial reconstruction will yield good results and satisfied, active patients.

Vascular surgeons, either by choice or political necessity, have, for the most part, abdicated their role in the angiographic evaluation of the patient with peripheral arterial disease. The surgeon who is called upon to attempt restoration of flow has the best understanding of the pathophysiology that has produced the patient's symptoms, and the best understanding of what he or she, as a surgeon, needs to visualize in order to ensure the best chance for success of an operation. The technique of angiography is secondary to the necessity for high-quality films.

The type of synthetic graft material to be chosen for aortic reconstructive surgery is secondary to the need for adequate inflow and outflow. This is best accomplished with an end-to-end aortic anastomosis and particular care to be certain that the femoral outflow is the best possible. As stated, we found that distal bypass, in conjunction with the aortofemoral graft, was necessary in only 6 percent of aortic reconstructions.

I feel that bypass to a patent distal tibial vessel offers better long-term patency than an isolated popliteal segment. The unavailability of sufficient autogenous tissue will at times alter this approach.

I prefer the greater saphenous vein for all arterial reconstructions below the groin. If the diameter of the vein seems inadequate or if the greater vein is unavailable, I will perform an above-knee Dacron or polytetrafluoroethylene (PTFE) anastomosis if that segment of popliteal artery is patent without extensive disease.

If good tibial arteries are present and the greater saphenous vein cannot be used, I will harvest the lesser saphenous vein from both legs and fashion a long vein graft with an end-to-end anastomosis. My experience has been limited, but I have been pleased with the results.

In a previous report, we reported on the use of arm veins. While recognizing their fragile characteristics, we still feel that they offer satisfactory autogenous tissue.

If inadequate autogenous tissue is not available for a bypass, a composite graft of autogenous vein and PTFE has frequently been constructed. The vein is used for the distal anastomosis, and a 6-mm PTFE is used for the upper anastomosis. The composite graft is made by joining the two in an end-to-end fashion with a long, tapering suture line to reduce turbulence at the point of anastomosis. All patients with PTFE grafts are maintained on antiplatelet drugs.

A continued effort to maintain arterial flow into an extremity usually provides relief of symptoms and prevents amputation. The ideal graft material has yet to be developed. Advances in techniques along with better graft material will allow even better long-term results for those extremities whose viability can be maintained.

10 ALTERNATIVES FOR FEMOROPOPLITEAL RECONSTRUCTION

Autogenous tissues are preferable to synthetic grafts, which, however well-advertised, do remain foreign bodies. While occasionally someone preaches the virtues of one or another substitute for particular indications,[1,2] most opinion still interprets the reported results as favorable to autogenous vein grafts. The patient's own saphenous vein remains the standard for a femoropopliteal graft, against which other materials must be measured.

Fortunately most patients have saphenous veins with sufficient diameter, length, and strength to be used as arterial conduits. The supply has decreased with their use as aortocoronary bypasses, but many of these patients still retain a useful segment of vein. Fortunately there is a negative correlation between varicose veins and clinically significant atherosclerotic arterial disease, so patients with the latter rarely have veins which cannot be used.

The percentage of patients with a suitable saphenous vein varies with the individual surgeon's criteria. At one time I thought 90 percent of veins were suitable.[3] Presently a vein which is bifid, has any evidence of previous phlebitis, or is borderline in size will not be used, leading to a current availability rate of about 80 percent. This includes some short vein grafts based proximally on the mid or distal superficial femoral artery, since that seems preferable to a synthetic tube.

Nevertheless, there are patients who require a different technique or material, either because (1) they fall into the minority who do not have a suitable vein or (2) the vein has already been placed in the femoropopliteal position and has failed. Let us examine the alternatives (Table 10-1).

AUTOGENOUS TISSUE

Autogenous Veins

Unsuitability or absence of the main saphenous vein does not absolutely prevent an autogenous vein repair using a source other than the ipsilateral saphenous vein. Not infrequently there is a proximal or distal remnant of the saphenous vein which is long enough to span the distance between an anastomosis placed in the distal portion of the superficial femoral artery and a patent vessel below the knee.

Recent information has reversed the old opinion that the proximal anastomosis should invariably be based on the common femoral artery. Veith in 1981 reported 81 percent patency at 6 years for 60 grafts originating from the distal femoral or popliteal artery, compared with 66 percent patency for 290 grafts based on the common femoral artery.[4] Schuler and associates confirmed this in 23 patients having similar short vein grafts with 84 percent patency 31 months later.[5] My experience is similar. Given a choice of placing a short segment of saphenous vein from a distal femoral anastomosis of an artery which has a normal angiographic appearance and which at operation is not extensively diseased versus the alternative of placing a long synthetic tube, I would choose the autogenous repair (Figure 10-1). It should also be recalled that a segment of the proximal portion of the superficial femoral artery can be cleaned out by eversion thromboendarterectomy to allow its use as an autogenous tube leading onto a short segment of autogenous vein graft (Figure 10-2).

TABLE 10-1 ALTERNATIVES FOR FEMOROPOPLITEAL REPAIRS

1	Autogenous vessels
	Veins
	Ipsilateral standard femoropopliteal
	Contralateral saphenous
	Arm
	Lesser saphenous
	In situ saphenous
	Endarterectomy
	Alone
	With distal vein graft
	Profundaplasty
	Dilation
	Collagenous tubes (on mandrels)
2	*Homologous* vessels
	Arteries
	Veins
	Umbilical cord veins
3	Heterologous arteries
4	Synthetic grafts
	Dacron
	PTFE
5	Composite grafts

Arm Veins Arm veins furnish suitable substitutes for some patients. It may be necessary to anastomose two of these to obtain sufficient length. I have not hestiated to use these when needed, although recent condemnation of arm veins does require another look at them.

The basilic, cephalic, and combinations of these veins have been occasionally used by many surgeons since Kakkar's report in 1969.[6] Our early experience with 32 cases confirmed their usefulness in 1976.[7] Since then others have similarly approved arm veins, particularly when the distal anastomosis must be made to a small vessel in the calf or at the ankle.

Campbell and associates reported their results with arm vein grafts in 33 patients. Four grafts failed and two patients died. This 82 percent patency rate for 1 to 41 months is probably a maximum, since the time was short and some of the good results were determined by the lack of symptoms rather than by arteriograms.[8] Whittemore in 1982 updated his earlier report[9] with a continued recommendation for arm veins in secondary reconstructions.[10]

The discussion of Schulman and Badhey of arm veins is worthwhile and unique in providing long-term follow-up of 68 long arm vein grafts in 62 patients for a minimum of 2 years. Their cumulative life table patency rates for both femoropopliteal (31 percent at 5 years) and femorotibial (6 percent at 5 years) arm vein grafts were lower than reported with autogenous saphenous veins in other series. Their documentation is weak because they cite the statistics of others rather than their own rates using saphenous vein grafts.[11] The Australian surgeons Graham and Lusby found a cumulative 5-year patency of 49 percent of 37 arm vein–arm vein grafts, concluding that arm veins should be the first alternative if the saphenous is not available.[12] Andros supported this position, discussing 70 arm vein bypasses with 80 percent 5-year patency for grafts to the tibial level.[13]

The recent report of 56 late arteriograms of arm veins used for coronary artery bypasses in our hospital indicates that 43 percent failed and that 22 percent of the patent ones had local areas of stenosis. This has led these cardiac surgeons to prefer the internal mammary artery as an alternative to the saphenous vein.[14] This series indeed paints a dismal outlook for arm vein grafts. There are no details of the method of removal of these veins, or of how they were handled, but the authors suggest that "the thin wall of the . . . graft is more likely to be traumatized" as it is removed and that "the injured vein may subsequently develop stenosis." These statements

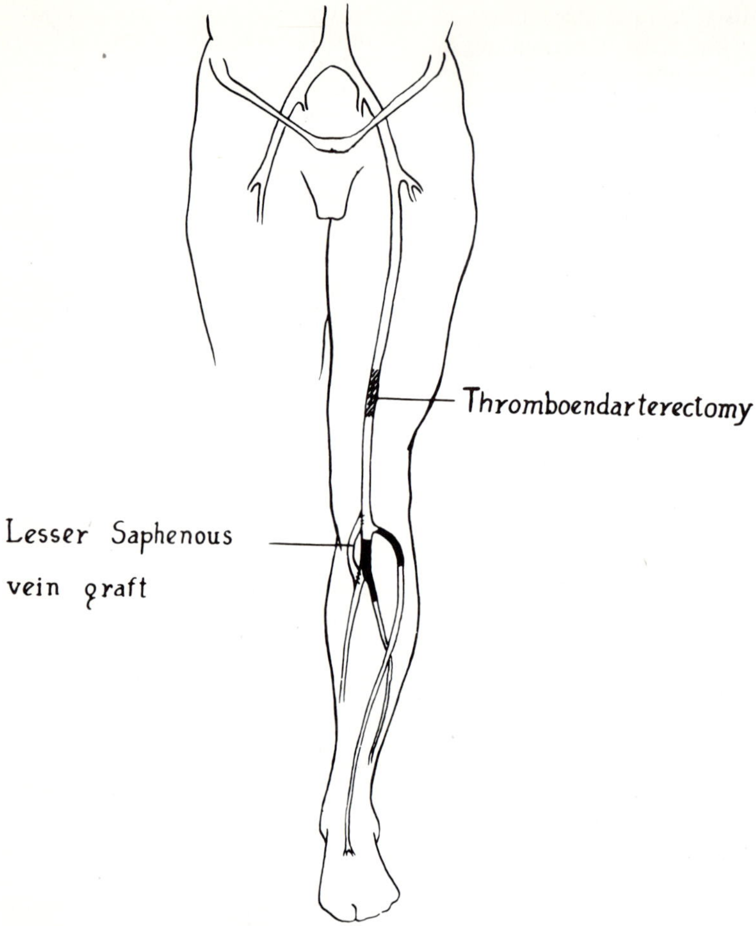

FIGURE 10-1 The saphenous vein was too small to be used as a long bypass from the common femoral to the tibial artery below the knee. Alternatively, a limited thromboendarterectomy of the distal superficial femoral artery was performed along with a short lesser saphenous vein bypass just below the knee.

are correct. They confirm the opinion of vascular surgeons that dissection of the vein graft is an important part of the operation which should not be lightly assigned to a technician.

Thus, arm veins have detractors as well as advocates. Further experience is needed to allow correct judgment. In difficult situations involving small below-knee arteries, I still use arm veins preferentially to synthetics and note that knowledgeable colleagues also follow that plan.

Lesser Saphenous Vein The lesser saphenous is suitable (Figure 10-3), although its position may make it difficult to obtain.

Contralateral Saphenous Vein The contralateral saphenous is a good source of autogenous tissue. Because of the high incidence of the eventual occurrence of bilateral arterial disease, however, the contralateral extremity should not be lightly robbed of its saphenous vein. If there is any other method with a reasonably good chance of success, that should be preferred to the use of the contralateral saphenous vein in most circumstances. However, if the limb will be lost otherwise and the distal anastomosis must be to a small calf or ankle vessel, it is justifiable to use the contralateral saphenous vein.

In Situ Saphenous Vein Bypass Twenty-odd years have elapsed since the nonreversed saphenous vein, its valves cut or avulsed by one or another technique, but still lying in its original position in the subcutaneous tissue of the lower limb, was first used as a femoropopliteal arterial bypass graft. The early experiences of May, DeWeese, and Rob[15] and of Hall[16] produced poor results, perhaps because of the methods used to remove the valves, and the technique never became well-known or accepted.

Two groups, led by Connolly and Kwaan in California[17] and Leather and Karmody in Albany,[18] persisted, improved the procedure, and recently reported patency results paralleling those of the presently standard reversed saphenous vein graft for femoropopliteal bypasses. Thus, the 10-year patency rates for the reversed (43 percent) and in situ (41 percent) grafts were the same in the Connolly and Kwaan series of 300 each, while the Albany team found a 69 percent cumulative patency rate at 3 years.[18]

This alternative technique allows use of a saphenous vein as small as 2 mm distally, which would be unsuitable for the usual reversed vein graft.

Critics have cited its more complicated technique (which becomes less difficult with experience), the possibility of leaving arteriovenous connections (which are not a real problem if few and small), and the possibility of later stenoses at the sites of valve destruction. Finally, the best method of valve destruction is still debatable. Despite these problems the technique now is established and may offer a good alternative for some patients.

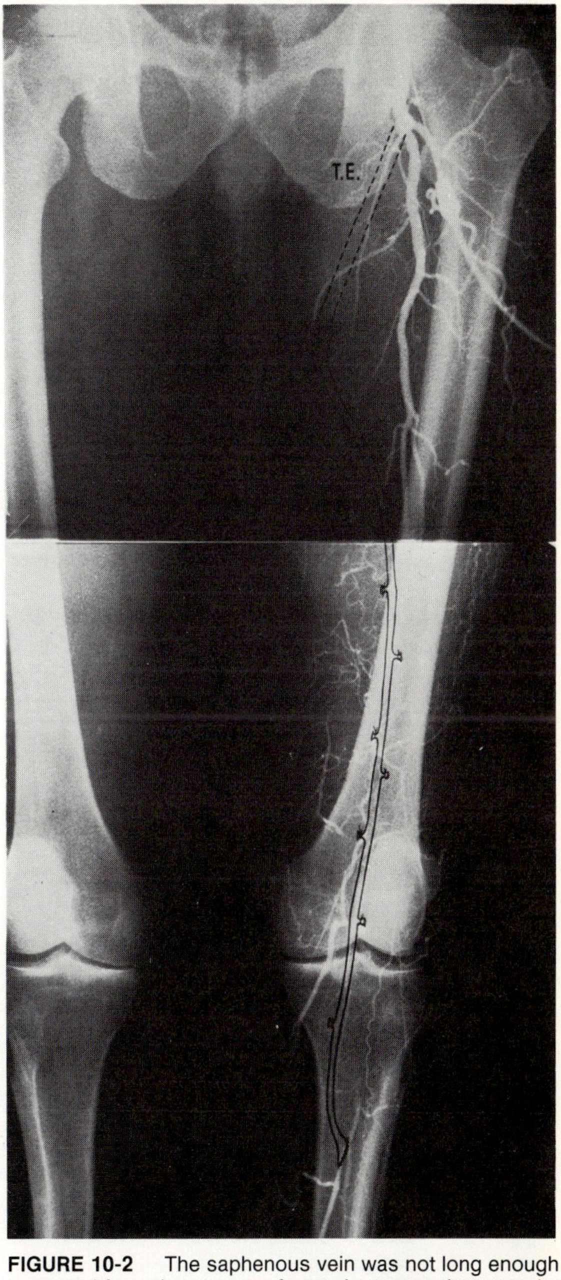

FIGURE 10-2 The saphenous vein was not long enough to extend from the common femoral artery to the posterior tibial artery. The alternative consisted of proximal eversion thromboendarterectomy with the available saphenous vein anastomosed from this to the posterior tibial artery.

Proximal Femoral Endarterectomy and Distal Vein Graft An autogenous artery may also be obtained for a conduit by an eversion endarterectomy and use of the residual medial-adventitial shell. The superficial femoral artery may thus become the proximal portion of the reconstruction, and a short segment of autogenous vein may be anastomosed to its distal end. This is a good alternative when there is an insufficient length of vein available (Figure 10-2).

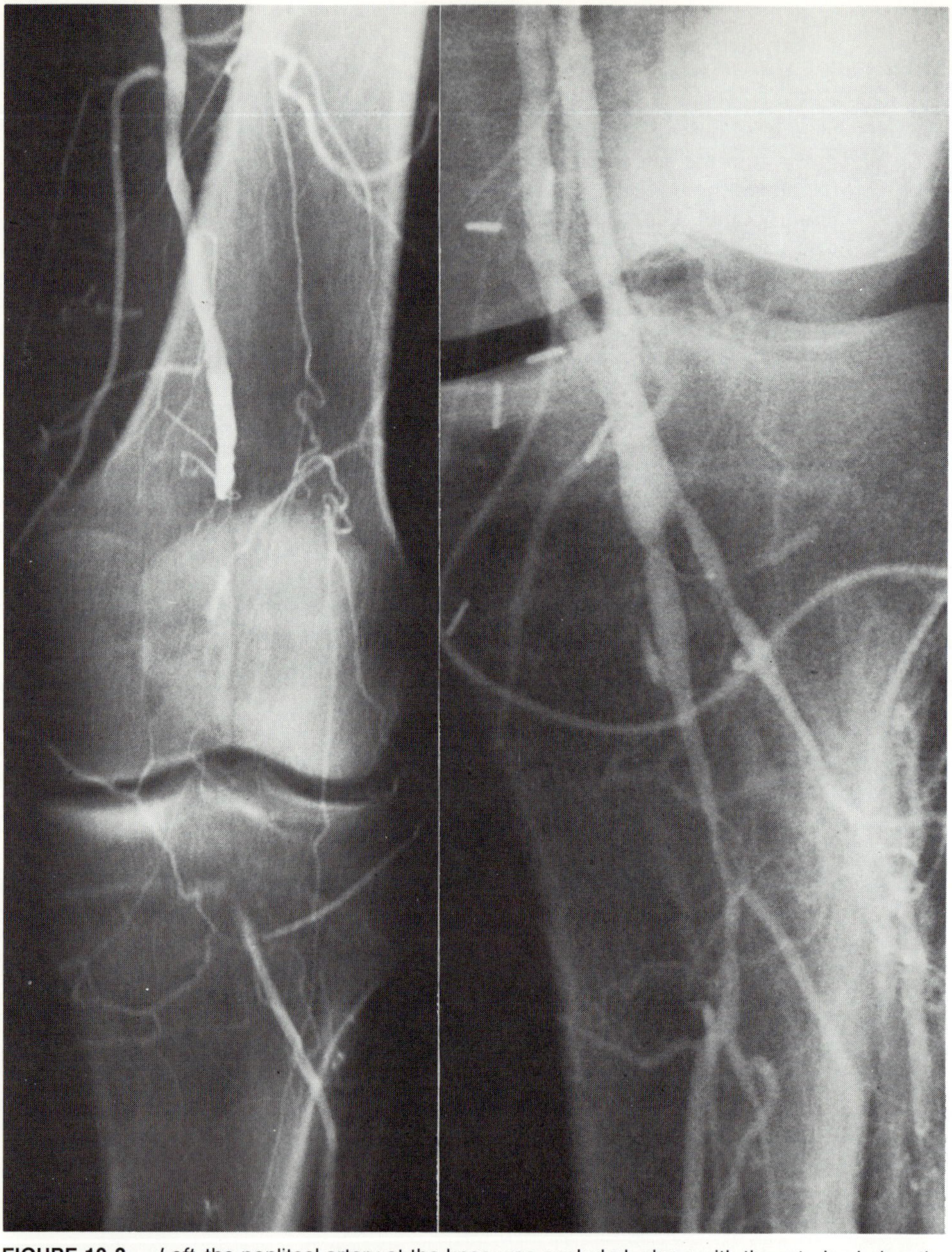

FIGURE 10-3 *Left,* the popliteal artery at the knee was occluded, along with the arteries below the joint except for a patent anterior tibial artery. *Right,* through a posterior approach the lesser saphenous vein was used for a reconstructive bypass graft.

Autogenous Artery

Ehrenfeld, Stoney, and Wylie have particularly advocated the use of short lengths of the hypogastric artery or the iliac artery (replaced by a synthetic tube) to bypass renal arterial lesions in children and to replace infected grafts in adults.[19] These vessels are not long enough to form a femoropopliteal bypass.

Endarterectomy The clean-out procedure in the femoral arterial system has fallen into general disfavor because of poor results, the additional time which is necessary to perform it, and recent general unfamiliarity. In times past, endarterectomies were attempted in long segments by crude techniques with high failure rates. The lateral patch grafting technique for a time seemed to offer promise of improved patency results. These did not follow, probably because of difficulty in properly tailoring the venous patch graft, resulting in aneurysmal dilatation created by the revascularization operation, a situation which is known to result in thromboses both experimentally and clinically (Figures 10-4 and 10-5).[20] If careful closure is performed, a patch is not often needed (Figures 10-6 and 10-7). It is often wise to place a short venous patch at the distal end of a femoral thromboendarterectomy, to prevent sudden stenosis there.

Blind techniques of thromboendarterectomy are not recommended; the clean-out should be performed under direct vision, either by suitable incisions or by the eversion technique.

Inahara and Scott's results with popliteal endarterectomy and patch grafting are comparable to those for vein grafting at that level. Among 100 procedures the cumulative patency rate at 5 years was 70 percent and at 10 years was 50 percent. Six (8 percent) early acute thromboses required immediate secondary operations, of which five were corrective and one led to below-knee amputation.[21]

The results of 123 long superficial femoral thromboendarterectomies done by a semiclosed technique with venous patch grafts at the arteriotomy sites were comparable to results for autogenous vein grafting in the hands of Imparato's group. Their cumulative patency rates of 76 percent at 1 year, 46 percent at 5 years, and 26 percent at 10 years indicate that even long segments may be disobliterated by experts with the expectation of success. They stress the importance of at least one distal vessel run-off.[22]

Patching an endarterectomy does not require the use of the greater saphenous vein, since a dorsal hand vein or the lesser saphenous vein may be used for the patch.

Transluminal Dilation Accumulating experience with percutaneous transluminal dilation indicates considerably better results with large vessels such as the iliac artery than with smaller ones such as the distal portion of the superficial femoral or popliteal artery. Early popliteal recurrences suggest that the more distal ones will require surgical revascularization of one sort or another. It does seem worthwhile, however, to perform intraoperative dilation of a short area of the superficial femoral or popliteal artery at the time that a common femoral procedure or a profundaplasty is performed. Proper instruments and radiologic facilities, along with technical expertise, should be readily available in the vascular surgical operating room.

Profundaplasty If the origin of the profunda femoris is found (by either angiogram or operative exposure) to be stenotic, this should be corrected along with whatever other procedure is indicated. If the main procedure is a bypass from the aorta, the profundaplasty offers an additional arterial bed, thereby increasing blood flow through the graft. When a femoropopliteal repair is the order of the day, the profundaplasty provides a secondary source of blood to the distal tissues in the event that the graft fails.

Profundaplasty alone is less likely to be of success (Figure 10-8). It offers too little and should be accompanied by a bypass graft to a distal vessel.

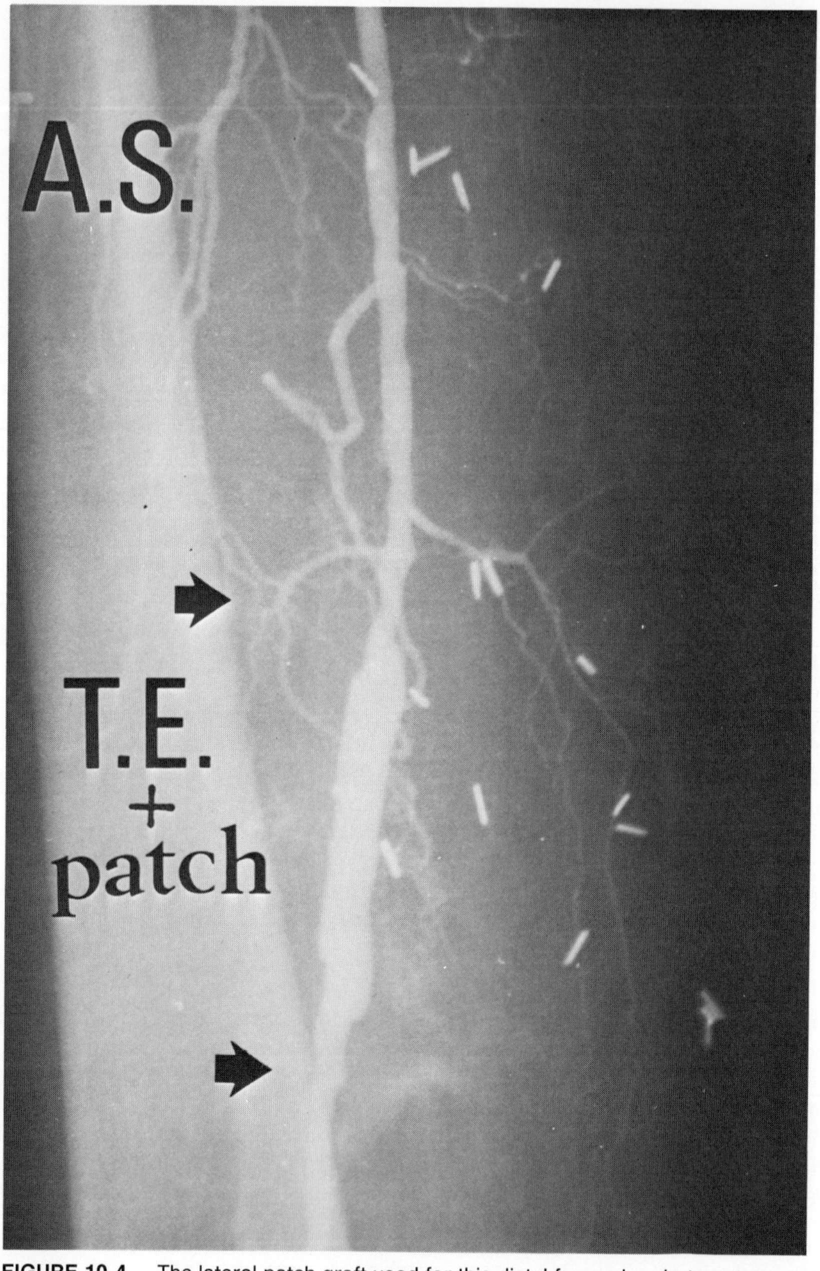

FIGURE 10-4 The lateral patch graft used for this distal femoral endarterectomy was placed too loosely and resulted in dilatation *(arrows)*.

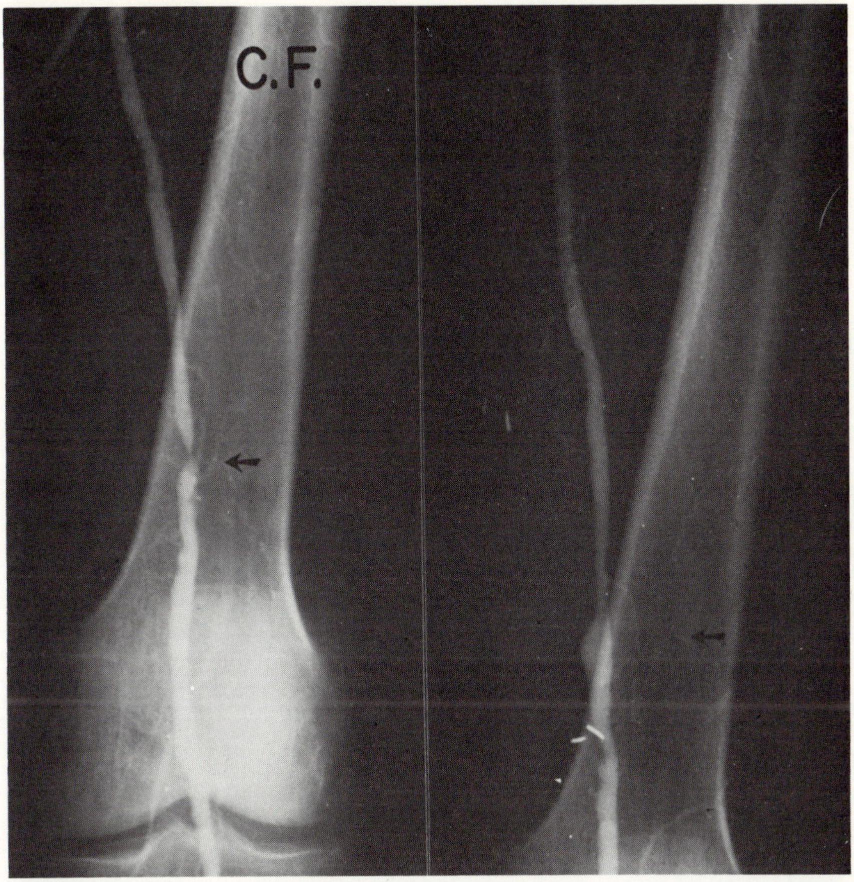

FIGURE 10-5 A short arteriosclerotic occlusion at the junction of the femoral and popliteal arteries *(left arrow)* was corrected by endarterectomy with a lateral patch graft, which was placed too loosely, resulting in an aneurysmal dilatation *(right arrow).*

Mandrel-Developed Collagenous Tubes For 20 years there have been sporadic efforts to produce an autogenous tube from the patient's own collagen for arterial replacement. Pierce in 1953[23] and Eiken in 1960 implanted plastic rods in dogs and used the tissue which developed around them to replace canine arteries.[24] Schilling made somewhat similar wire-screen tubes,[25] and Hufnagel studied the matter further.[26] In the early 1960s I implanted similar rods with a Dacron mesh cover, thereby forming a synthetic-supported collagen tube which performed well in the dog's aorta.

C. H. Sparks of Portland developed the idea further and eventually performed 17 revascularizations of the human femoropopliteal system by this technique.[27] Results were poor generally,[28] including two personal attempts, because the details were never completely worked out: incomplete collagenization was frequent. Currently the matter lies in limbo, essentially abandoned, awaiting further laboratory study to determine whether or not the method has a potential for clinical use.

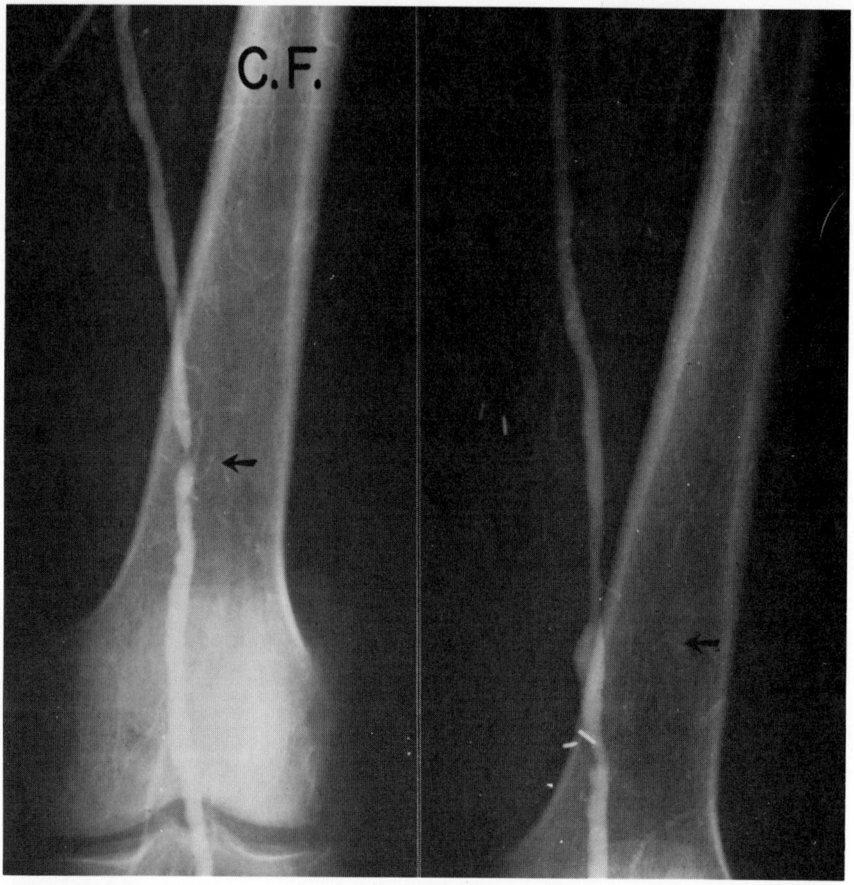

FIGURE 10-6 *Left,* the short occlusion *(arrow)* of the superficial femoral artery suggested local endarterectomy. *Right,* the endarterectomy was closed without a patch graft, resulting in normal restoration of the lumen *(arrow).*

HOMOLOGOUS TISSUES

Homologous Arteries

The arterial banks maintained by medical centers 25 years ago are of historical interest now, yet all results were not bad and many patients maintained viable, functioning limbs for years following peripheral placement of these arteries. There is no known experience with the use of homologous arterial grafts to carry blood to the distal calf and ankle vessels, but the dismal results of synthetics anastomosed to these small arteries suggest that we are perhaps overlooking the possibility that, if not perfect, might be better than polytetrafluoroethylene (PTFE) or Dacron for occasional patients.

Difficulties with procurement and storage of homologous arterial grafts, along with their complications of aneurysm, rupture, and thrombosis, led to their general abandonment 25 years ago. My experience with 90 was similar to the reports of others, and none have been used personally since 1959.[29]

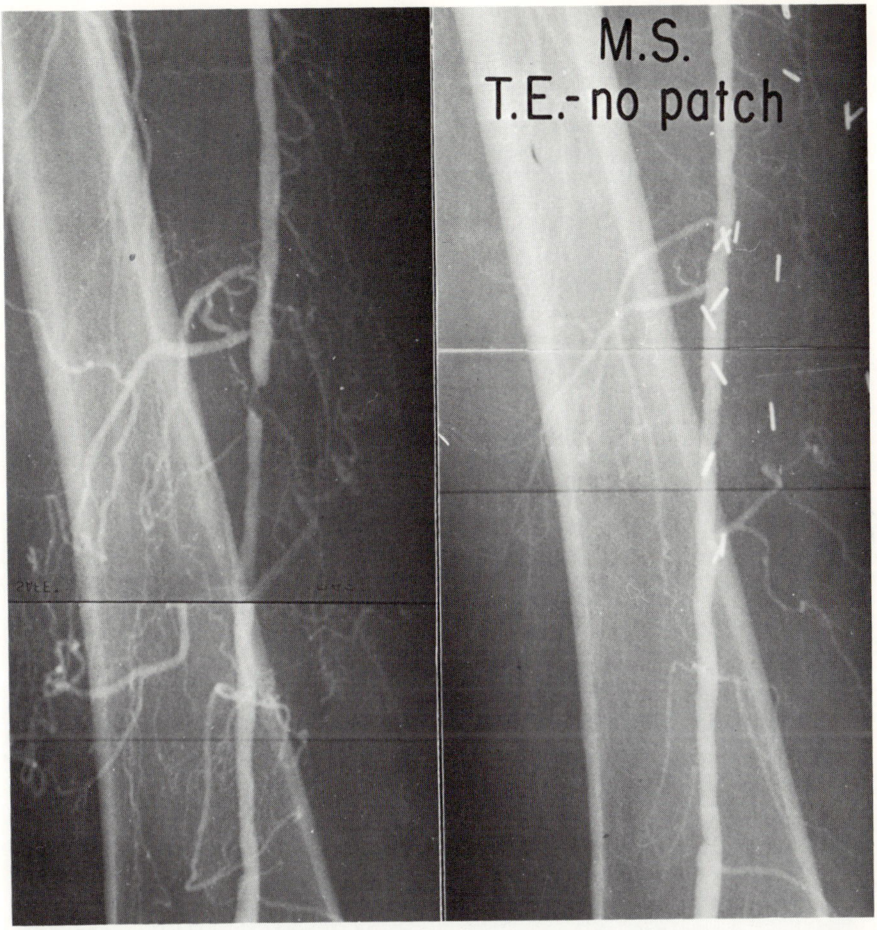

FIGURE 10-7 *Left,* short arteriosclerotic occlusion of the superficial femoral artery in the midthigh. *Right,* correction was accomplished by endarterectomy without a patch graft.

Homologous Veins

Homologous veins were long ago found deficient by laboratory experience and have thereafter been used only occasionally in patients.

Recent hope that the antigenic response of homologous vein grafts could be reduced by dimethyl sulfoxide[30] or cryopreservation[31] was chilled by the experiments of Axthelm and associates using rat models: there was no diminution of antigenicity. They concluded in 1979 that "there is no known way to reduce the antigenicity of viable venous allografts."[32] This probably explains the high failure rate of homologous veins, such as the 10 of 11 reported by Stephens's team.[33]

These recognized antigenic properties of homologous vein[34] do cause pessimism. Ochsner's original 1971 report[35] was later modified to indicate that occlusion was common even when blood groups were matched and that it might be expected that all would "eventually have problems."[36] His 1984 account of 129 homologous veins placed in various positions in 91 patients

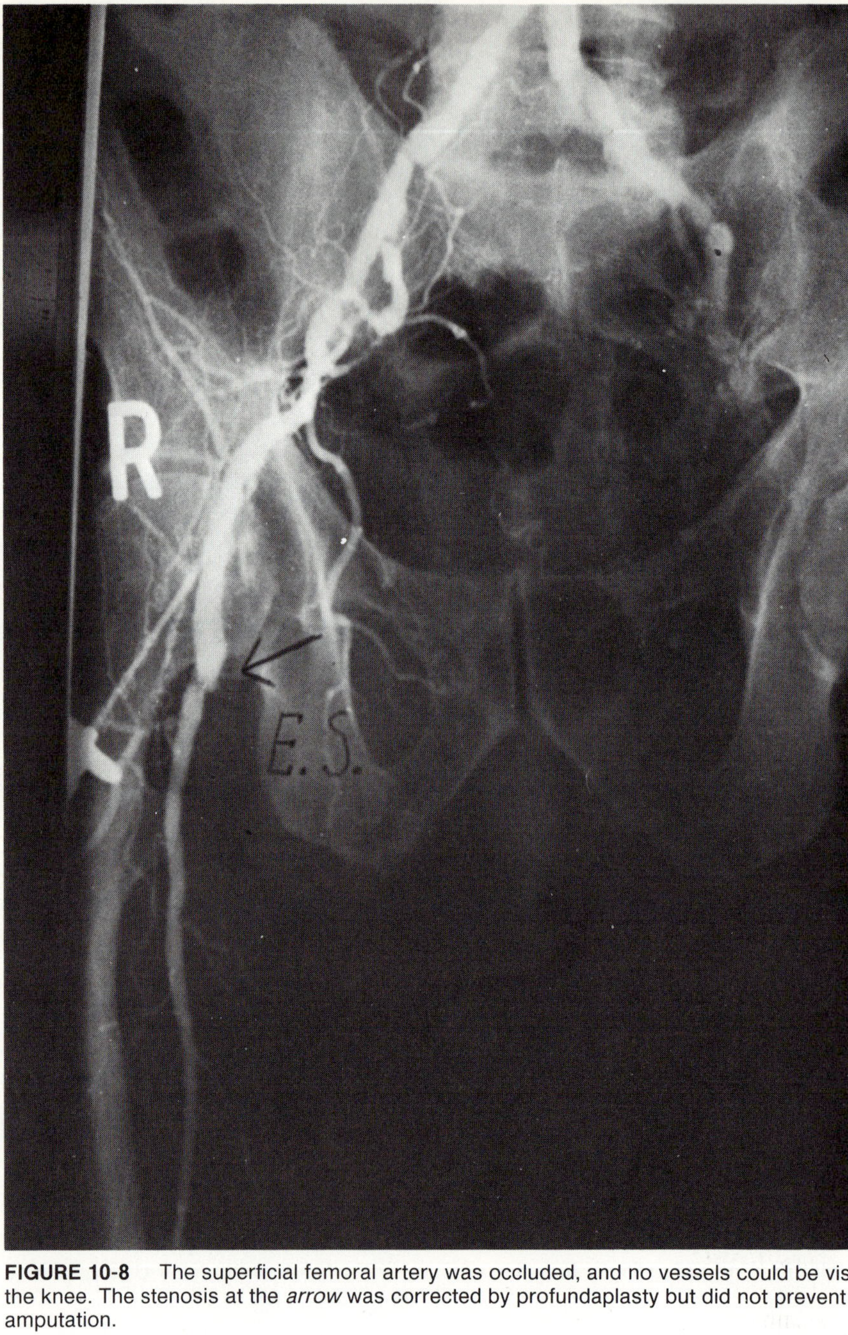

FIGURE 10-8 The superficial femoral artery was occluded, and no vessels could be visualized below the knee. The stenosis at the *arrow* was corrected by profundaplasty but did not prevent subsequent amputation.

showed that while half occluded within a year, 37 percent of the remainder did remain patent for 5 years.[37]

These experiences rule against the use as arterial bypasses of homologous veins in their present state.

SYNTHETIC TUBES

Dacron Tubes

For 30 years vascular surgeons have hoped that one or another synthetic tube graft would be highly successful as an arterial conduit. This goal has not been achieved: the autogenous vein remains the standard against which other materials must be measured. Frank Veith, an advocate of the PTFE graft, in 1982 found "autologous saphenous vein to be the graft material of choice for femoro-popliteal bypass." He recommends the PTFE graft if an autogenous vein is not available.[38]

Nevertheless, one or another form of synthetic graft has been widely used for arterial replacement for a quarter century. Indeed, it was widely believed to be superior to the autogenous vein graft for a few years in the late 1950s and early 1960s, but subsequent evidence invalidated that concept.

Woven, knit, velour, and double-velour variations have been advocated, to the extent that uncertainty exists regarding which version is best. Though none produces patency rates to rival a good vein graft placed between the femoral and below-knee popliteal or tibial arteries, the outlook for a Dacron graft whose distal end lies above the knee joint is relatively favorable. It is therefore a suitable method if there is no way to use autogenous tissue.

Whether Dacron or PTFE is preferable is not known, although various surgeons have expressed strong opinions. I prefer PTFE because it does not require preclotting, is easy to use, and may be easily reopened if thrombosis occurs.

Polytetrafluoroethylene

Expanded Teflon (PTFE) is a nontextile polymer of carbon and fluorine whose pore size is in the range of 12 to 30 μm. It is electronegative, which suggests an antithrombotic effect. Aneurysmal dilatation occurred in some of the early grafts.[39] This was stopped by covering the PTFE tubes with a thin Teflon coating.

In preparing this chapter, an attempt to provide tabular information of results proved to be worthless, since most reports compared results against the series of others or against assumed patency rates. None were controlled prospective studies, so it is not certain that patients in the comparative groups were similar. The Cranley and Hafner experience showed little difference between autogenous vein and umbilical cord grafts when used for claudication or for salvage procedures at the popliteal level (both were better than PTFE), but they showed slightly better results for tibial salvage procedures with autogenous vein than with either of the other materials (47 percent patency versus 27 percent and 35 percent at 4 years).[40] Bergentyz of Sweden agreed that PTFE was poorer.[41] Hobson's team found that autogenous vein grafts were better than PTFE (65 percent versus 53 percent), (55 percent versus 7 percent distally).[42] Hallett's group concurred.[43] The best statistics to be found are those of O'Donnell and associates, who in 1983 reported a 3-year patency rate of 63 percent for PTFE versus 72 percent for veins.[44] Similarly, Christenson noted 6-year patencies of 70 percent above-knee, 65 percent below-knee, and 63 percent for tibial arterial repairs with PTFE.[45] The encouraging results of McAuley, Steed, and Webster should be noted: a cumulative patency rate of 40 percent at 5 years and of 35 percent at 7 years.[46] The poor results of PTFE below the knee in our hospital from Edwards and Mulherin (24 percent 1-year PTFE patency versus 82 percent 1-year patency for autogenous vein) have led us away from the PTFE graft for below-knee procedures (Figure 10-9).[47]

Veith has recently stated that a multicenter randomized comparison of graft materials shows no significant difference at 3 years between PTFE and autogenous veins, both placed above the knee. When the distal anastomosis was made to a tibial artery, the vein grafts were somewhat better than PTFE (58 percent patency versus 45 percent at 3 years).[48]

Early enthusiasm for PTFE, such as "the results . . . are comparable with the autogenous vein graft,"[49] has been considerably modified as experience has increased. It is now especially thought that PTFE is far inferior to autogenous vein graft when anastomosed to distal calf or ankle vessels.

Umbilical Cord Vein Grafts

In the early 1960s umbilical cord vein grafts were briefly evaluated and abandoned.[50] Ten-odd years later the umbilical cord vein graft was reintroduced in an improved form, and it has now been reported in many patients as the best available material for femoropopliteal bypass grafting.[51]

Newborn umbilical cords are collected in delivery rooms, cleaned, and refrigerated during transport to the manufacturer. There they are placed on mandrels and tanned with 1 percent glutaraldehyde solution, which produces a relatively nonantigenic conduit. A loose-meshed Dacron tube is placed about the graft to prevent aneurysmal dilatation after its implantation.

Specific operative techniques are necessary to ensure proper placement. The graft may not be clamped or handled roughly, for fear of intimal fracture with mural dissection. The variable thickness of the wall may present difficulties. The graft may not be pulled through a tissue tunnel but must be placed through a hollow tube so that the mesh is not dragged away from the umbilical cord vein graft by the friction incurred.

The externally reinforced umbilical vein graft remains a controversial material. Dardik's 1982 report of 600 grafts (1975–1980) showed cumulative 4-year patency rates of 61 percent for femoropopliteal grafts, 38 percent for femorotibial and 25 percent femoroperoneal (Table 10-2). He continues to use the umbilical cord vein graft as his number-one choice, even above the saphenous vein.[52]

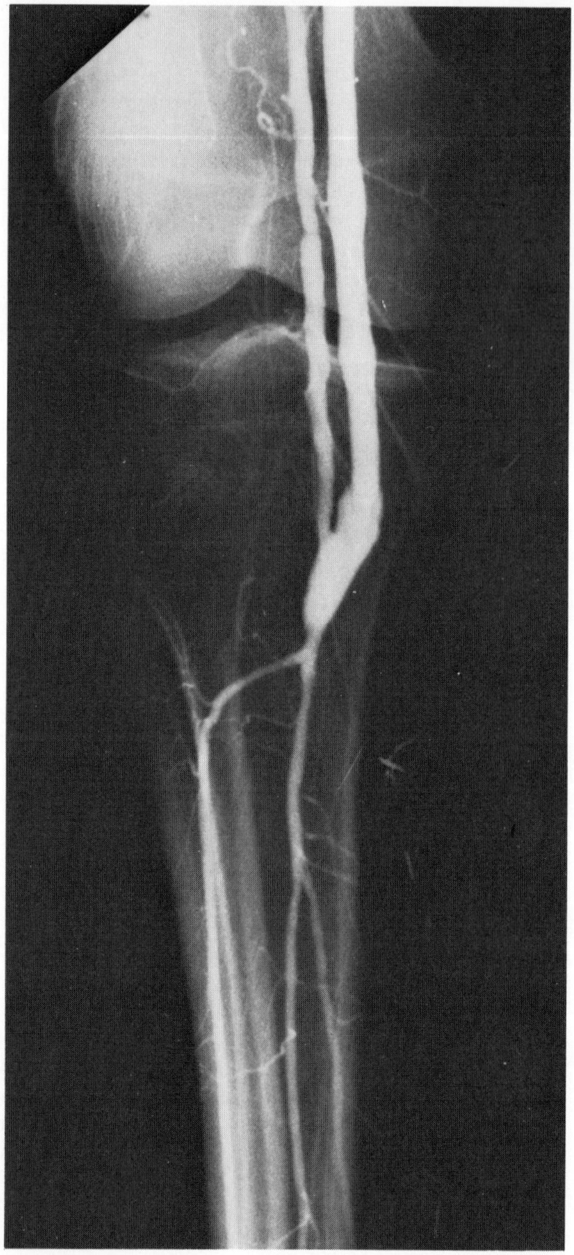

FIGURE 10-9 PTFE grafts ordinarily function better when the distal end is anastomosed proximal to the knee joint. This one, placed to the popliteal artery just above its bifurcation below the knee, has functioned well for 2 years.

The results of the Massachusetts General Hospital group in 1983 were less impressive when compared to those for vein grafts, but the umbilical vein performed better than PTFE below the knee (43 percent patency versus 32 percent).[53] Three European groups combined 104 patients to compare PTFE and umbilical vein grafts, finding the umbilical vein 2-year patency rate to be 57 percent while the PTFE rate was 30 percent. Another European team also reported better results with umbilical vein versus PTFE.[54] Weisel's group in Toronto in 1981 reported the 3-year cumulative patency rates of umbilical vein grafts as follows: above-knee 50 percent for 16, below-knee 30 percent for 36, and tibial 25 percent for 12.[55] Edwards and Mulherin's dismal experience with 15 umbilical cord grafts to tibial arteries (10 percent patent at 1 year) has discouraged its use in our hospital.[47]

TABLE 10-2 UMBILICAL VEIN CUMULATIVE 4-YEAR GRAFT PATENCY RATES, %

	Years				
Graft type	**1**	**2**	**3**	**4**	**5**
Femoropopliteal	82	73	65	61	61
Femorotibial	57	52	48	38	NA*
Femoroperoneal	58	57	28	25	NA*

*Not available.

Source: Dardik H, Baier RE, Meenaghan M, et al: Morphologic and biophysical assessment of long-term human umbilical cord vein implants used as vascular conduits. *Surg Gynecol Obstet* 1982, 154:17.

Aneurysms may develop at any point in the native arterial system. They also may develop in replacement grafts, including the autogenous saphenous vein.[56] Their increasing incidence over the course of time was an important factor in the demise of the replacement of peripheral arteries with homologous arteries in the early 1960s and of the heterologous bovine artery replacement in the 1970s. The earliest PTFE grafts were also subject to the development of aneurysms, but this was largely corrected by placement of an external Teflon sleeve. True aneurysms have not occurred frequently in umbilical cord grafts, but as Figure 10-10 indicates, occasional ones do occur. This is further documented by the three cases reported by Giordano and Keshishian.[57] Dardik's series, the largest in the world, had 7 (1 percent) aneurysms among 756 grafts. Whether the number will increase with time and eventually preclude its use has not yet been determined. Dardik recommends periodic follow-up to detect these, as well as their removal if present.[51]

The Choice between Dacron, PTFE, and Umbilical Cord Veins

Most vascular surgeons currently interpret the facts as favoring vein grafts over all others. The question of PTFE versus Dacron tubes and umbilical cord vein grafts is not yet decided.

If PTFE versus Dacron versus umbilical cord vein grafts be declared a standoff at present, one must choose between them on the bases of ease of use and secondary clean-outs. I think PTFE is easier to use; some experienced and skillful colleagues disagree. It can certainly be salvaged after late thrombosis in many instances; others interpret this adversely and prefer Dacron, which may have fewer late thromboses. Thus, at present the preference is not clear, leading to the recommendation that the individual surgeon use his or her personal experience as a guide—a pragmatic answer.

HETEROLOGOUS BOVINE ARTERIAL GRAFTS

There was considerable interest during the 20-year period after 1956 in the ficin-digested carotid artery of the cow, which was tanned into a nonantigenic tube. Bovine heterografts were easy to use and performed well for short periods in both the femoropopliteal position and the femorofemoral position. As time passed, however, aneurysms began to develop and thromboses occurred, indicating their unsuitability for general use. Our report of bovine arterial grafts in 1976 not only discussed personal experience with 96 such grafts but included a national survey of their results in the hands of others, which amounted to a requiem for the heterograft.[58] They are still useful in arterial access procedures.

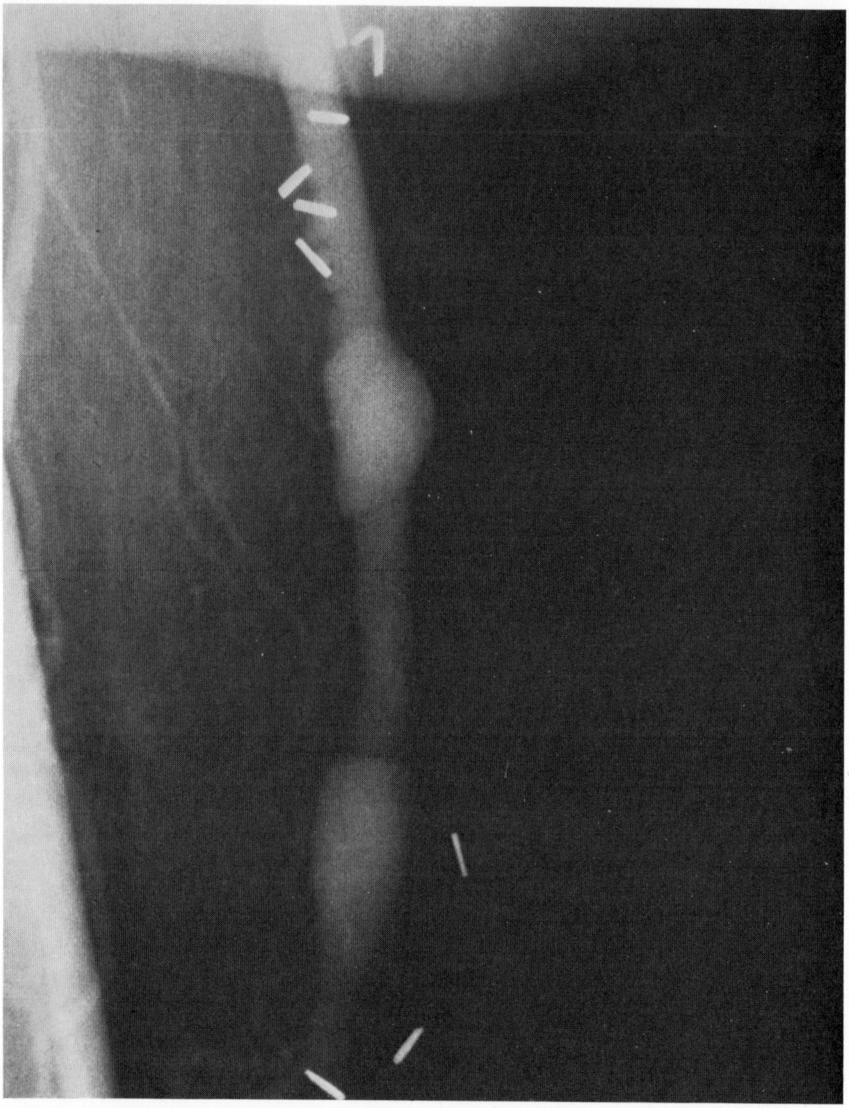

FIGURE 10-10 Two small aneurysms have developed in this umbilical cord vein graft 2 years following its placement. The lesions were originally detected by routine ultrasonography.

Composite Grafts

Composites fashioned from different veins, or proximal thromboendarterectomy and a short vein, are quite useful. They will not be discussed further. Ordinarily the term *composite graft* implies a proximal length of Dacron or PTFE attached to a segment of autogenous vein to cross the knee joint and allow distal anastomosis to a small artery (Figure 10-11).

Insufficient length of the saphenous vein long ago led to construction of composite grafts, whereby one or another synthetic tube was joined to the available segment of vein. We reported the early promise of these in dogs, using an end-to-end Teflon-vein graft.[59] The promise did not materialize when the same technique was applied to atherosclerotic human arteries. Of 16 such

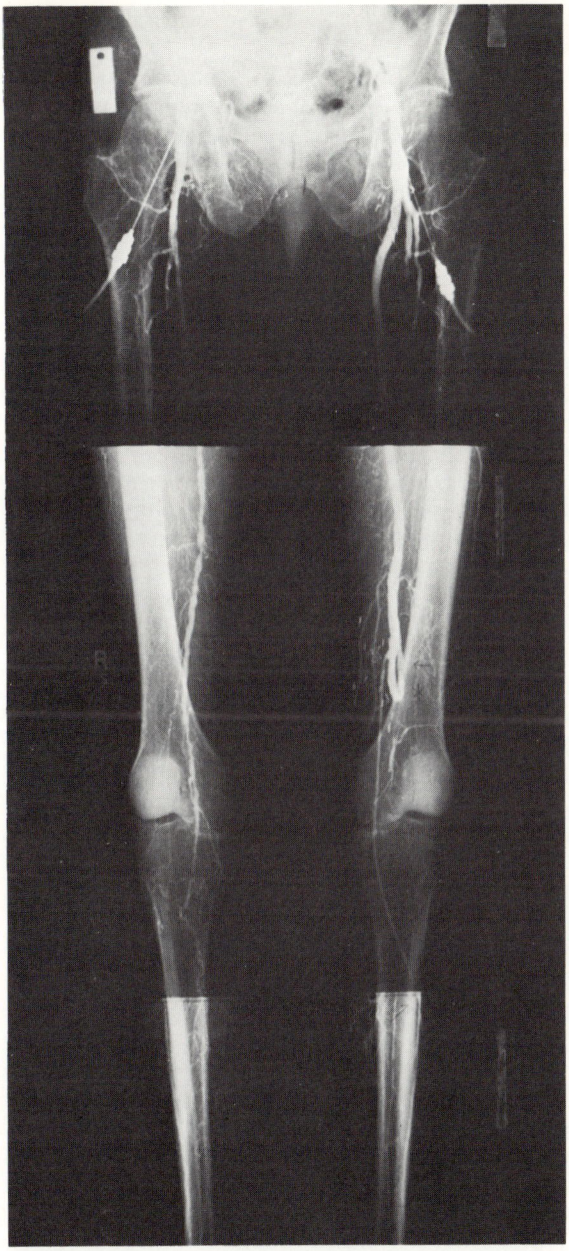

FIGURE 10-11 The saphenous vein was too short to allow a long bypass to the below-knee tibial vessel. The alternative solution consisted of a PTFE graft to the popliteal artery above the knee and a sequential attachment of the available saphenous vein to carry blood down to the tibial artery.

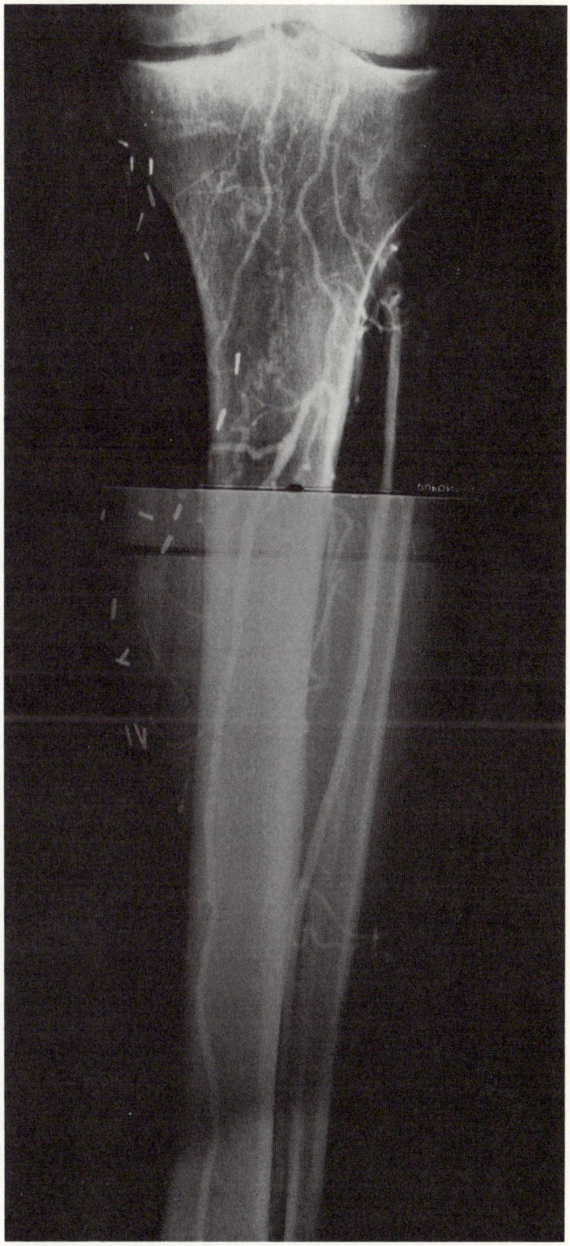

FIGURE 10-12 Extensive occlusion left only tibial arteries available below the knee.

there were 15 failures within a year, and the other 1 failed soon after.[60] No further patients were personally managed by this method for many years.

In 1973 Linton described 40 successful composite (Dacron-vein) femoropopliteal grafts, whose 5-year patency rate was 53 percent, compared with 345 saphenous vein grafts with 72 percent patency. The difference was significant, but the composite seemed useful as a "second-string" procedure.[61] There followed a number of other reports concerning composite grafts of Dacron, and later of PTFE, with veins. Despite two pessimistic accounts, each with less than 10 cases,[62,63] the others indicate rather good success, with 5-year composite patency rates (CPRs) of 40 to 63 percent. Verta's high 4-year CPR of 72 percent may be partly explained by the sequential nature of his procedures (rather than simple one-vessel distal anastomosis).[64] Snyder's group in Norfolk has the largest number, 68 with a 58 percent CPR at 4 years, distinctly better than their results with plain PTFE.[65] On the contrary, the Massachusetts General Hospital report of LaSalle found no real difference between composite and plain prosthetic grafts and suggested that the less-complicated synthetic tube be used.[66] The causes of these differences is unclear but is typical of this field of surgery. A prospective randomized study of the matter is not available.

There are three real differences between these recent, encouraging reports and our poor results in 1962. First is the use of PTFE rather than woven Dacron, the latter usually associated with a relatively thick neointima as opposed to the thin layer deposited upon the luminal surface of PTFE. Second is the current recognition that the synthetic tube and vein size should be fairly similar. In our 1962 series larger Dacron tubes were used (to allow room for the neointima to form). Third, our anastomoses were fluted end-to-end, rather than the quite long, ovoid anastomoses constructed presently. Thus, the modern composite graft is considerably different from the 1962 model. It is a useful alternative (Figures 10-12 to 10-15).

Sequential Grafts

The establishment of two or more distal anastomoses provides more blood flow through the portion of the graft proximal to the first anastomosis, as well as a double run-off at different levels. This technique was established in coronary arterial bypasses[67] and has proved similarly useful in distal limb reconstructions.[68–70]

The graft may consist of a long venous segment, anastomosed side-to-side to the popliteal artery and end-to-side to a tibial vessel. Alternatively, a segment of vein may be placed piggyback near the end of a proximal synthetic or vein graft to carry blood distally. There is as yet no clear-cut long-term difference between the two methods, but the placement of a side anastomosis in the center of a long graft demands good tailoring to prevent stenosis there.

The advantages of a sequential graft include augmentation of blood flow with the double anastomosis open. Berkoff noted this to be in the order of 40 to 75 percent. Another positive feature is maintenance of proximal patency even though the distal portion of the graft fails.[71]

A disadvantage is the additional dissection and operative time which are required. Further, if only a short segment of vein is available, there is uncertainty as to whether it is better used as a bypass to an "isolated" popliteal artery or as the distal portion of a sequential graft using a synthetic proximally. I favor use of the vein to the isolated segment in most cases, to avoid the occlusion problems seen more commonly with synthetics placed to arteries with poor run-off vessels.

An Alternative for an Elderly Bad-Risk Patient

Not uncommonly, severe ischemia of the foot occurs in an elderly patient, whose overall risk is greater because of one or a combination of lesions, including coronary heart disease, chronic obstructive pulmonary disease, renal failure, and other chronic degenerative lesions. It thus becomes important to reduce the extent of dissection, blood loss, and total operating time by

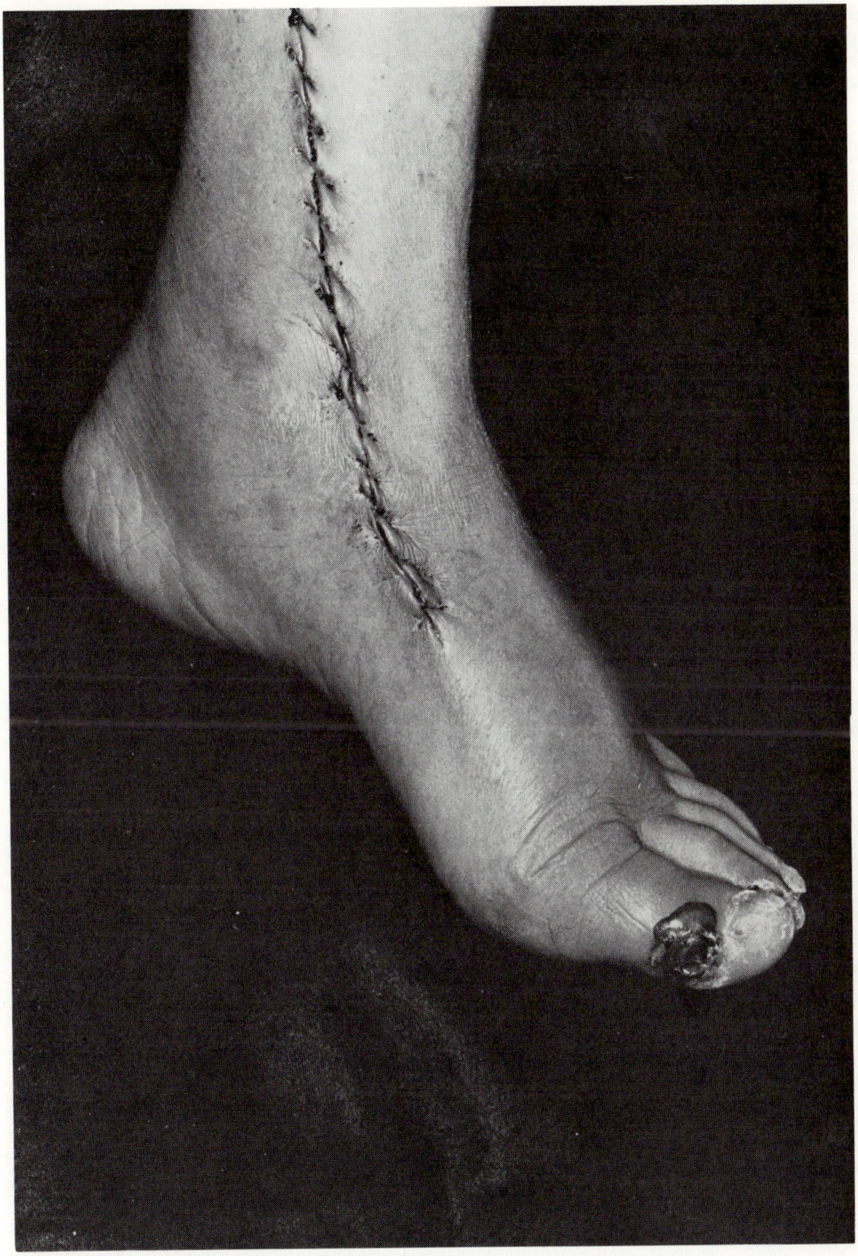

FIGURE 10-13 A remnant of the greater saphenous vein was removed from the lower leg and ankle through this incision. The gangrenous toe ulcer is visible.

providing the simplest vascular reconstruction. Femoropopliteal bypass with PTFE instead of autogenous vein may be the best procedure.

Illustrative Case T.A., an 80-year-old diabetic female with angina pectoris and severe obesity, developed continuous foot pain due to occlusion of the superficial femoral artery. An 8-mm

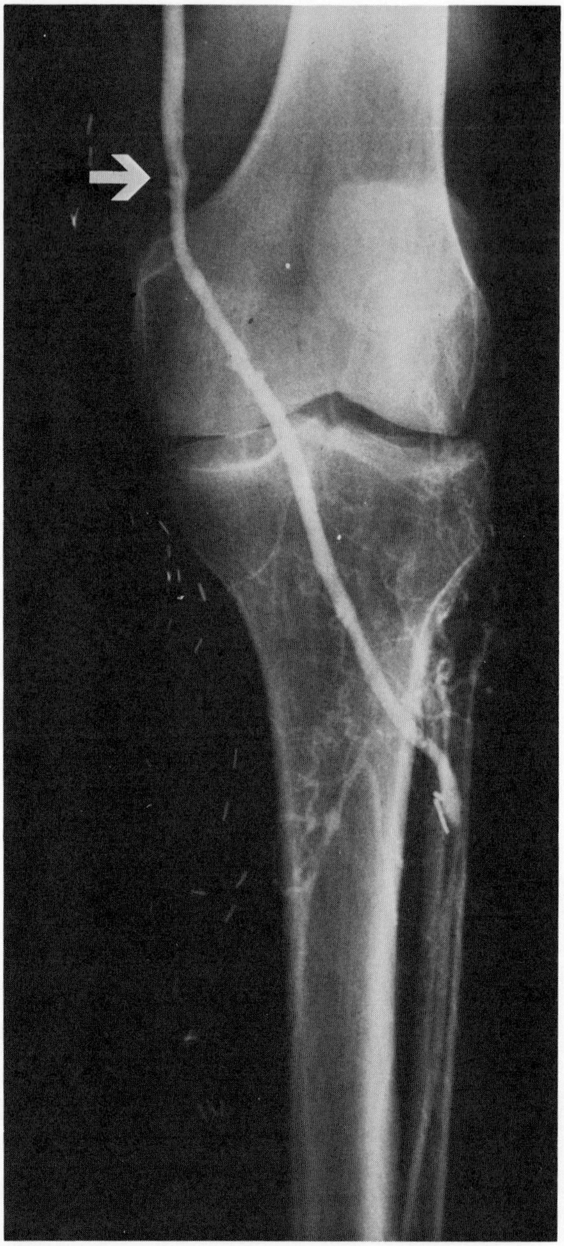

FIGURE 10-14 A composite was constructed of 6-mm PTFE and the available remnant vein graft, and the vein end was used to revascularize the anterior tibial artery from an origin on the common femoral artery in the groin. The *arrow* indicates the hardly visible anastomosis between the synthetic and the vein.

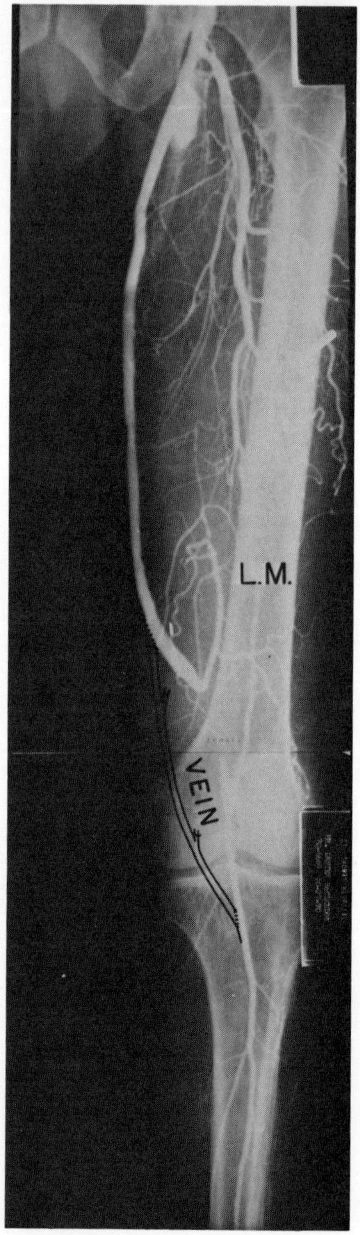

FIGURE 10-15 Another method for a composite graft whereby the PTFE was anastomosed to the popliteal artery above the knee and a short segment of vein was placed as a sequential graft to the distal popliteal artery.

PTFE graft placed in the femoropopliteal (above-knee) position relieved symptoms and produced a warm foot.

Comment There was no effort to use the vein, so the procedure was greatly simplified.

If the saphenous vein is not to be dissected, it is easy to perform both the groin and distal dissections simultaneously, attach the graft proximally, pass it behind the muscles, and anastomose the other end distally. Actually, both anastomoses may be done at the same time, but an accurate fit is less certain.

It is desirable to place the distal anastomosis to the popliteal artery as near as possible to the knee joint in order to bypass lesions in the proximal portion of the popliteal artery. The best approach is the little-known middle route.

Three different exposures of the popliteal artery may be described. The original above-knee dissection anterior to the sartorius muscle leads to the artery just as it emerges from Hunter's adductor canal. It may be traced distally to some extent.

The second approach to the popliteal artery, this time below the knee, just posterior to the tibia, is well known to all vascular surgeons. The third (middle) approach exposes the popliteal artery medially just above the knee joint (Figure 10-16). The skin incision lies two-thirds proximal and one-third distal to the joint. Dissection proceeds through the fat and fascia to the pes anserina tibial attachment of the semimembranosus and semitendinosus muscles. This is

FIGURE 10-16 The middle approach to the popliteal artery just posterior to the knee joint. The indicated muscles have been severed to allow exposure. This allows anastomosis of a synthetic graft just at the level of the joint but without actually crossing it.

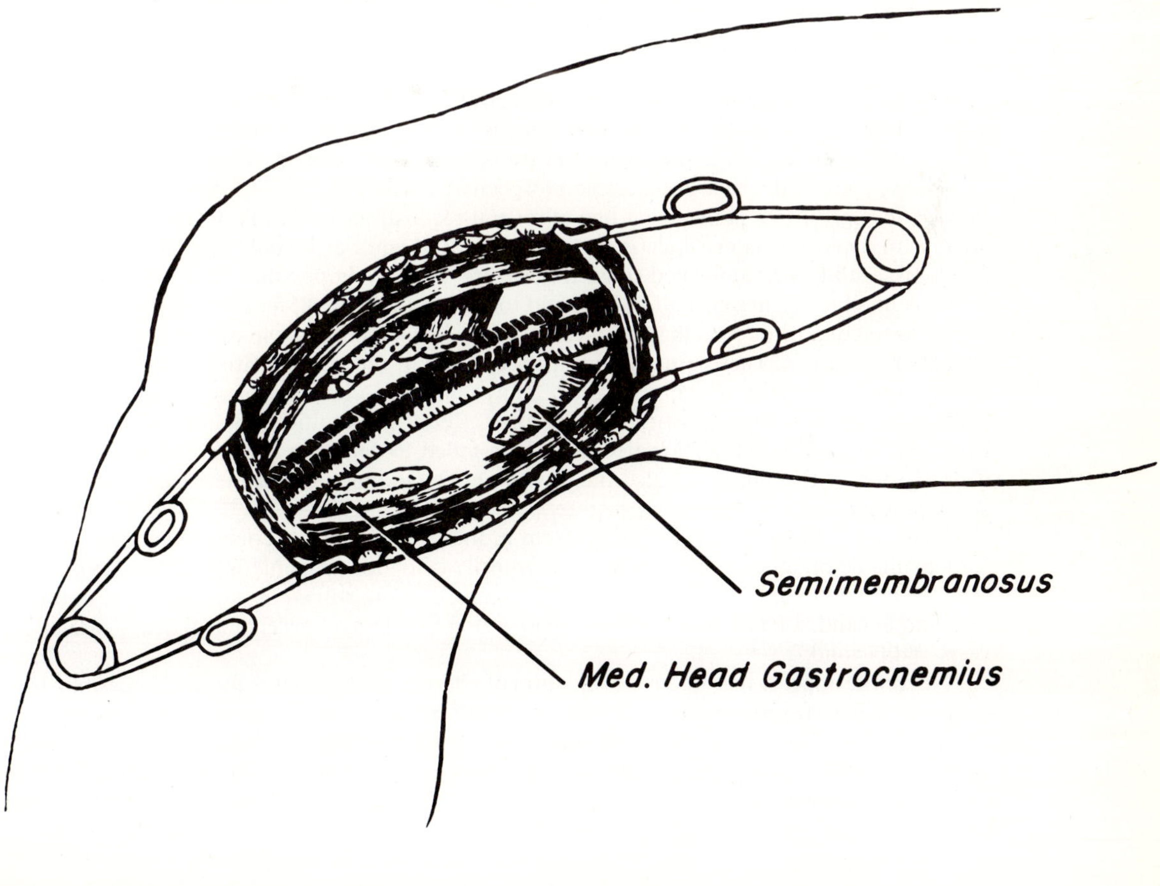

divided, with marking sutures placed to aid its later reconstitution. Deeper dissection discloses the popliteal artery as it passes distally under cover of the medial head of the gastrocnemius muscle. This may be retracted to allow the anastomosis. Occasionally it must be divided, in which case its later closure by sutures is difficult and not necessary in an elderly patient. The middle route is the best for a distal, but still above-knee, anastomosis.

A few surgeons recently have advocated preference for a synthetic tube graft if the distal anastomosis can be placed above the knee, not only to save the vein for future use, but also with the idea that at that level the prostheses rival the autogenous vein in patency rates. Brewster, LaSalle, and Darling, however, citing experience with 347 vein grafts and 208 prosthetics in 1981, concluded that "the superior results of autogenous vein grafts in femoral-popliteal reconstruction do not confirm recent reports that suggest equally satisfactory results with alternate grafts."[72] The thesis of equality of above-knee saphenous and synthetic tube grafting is attractive but unproven.

CHOICE OF TECHINQUES

There is presently no absolute way to determine the best alternative if an autogenous saphenous vein is not available or suitable for a femoral bypass.

The problem is at least threefold. First is the difficulty in assessing the reports of experience. Not only are there variations in the extent of disease, but the criteria of results are not the same. Few authors indicate whether patency of grafts is determined by angiography, by presence of pulses, or by letter or telephone reports. We must recognize the natural optimism of the surgeon, that nurses and residents are reluctant to report failures to their chief, and that most chiefs are far too busy to concern themselves personally with postoperative examination of patients. Further, long-term patients are reluctant to return, the majority having long since accepted their improved status or their limb loss.

Second, the reported results are variable in terms of statistics. Construction of tables to summarize these reports is, to say the least, frustrating and at worst is indeterminate. The tables which were made for this chapter were so confusing that they were omitted.

Finally, there is the lack of objective prospective studies. It is difficult or impossible for the surgeon to suggest to a patient that one of several reconstructive techniques may be used in an attempt to determine later which is preferable. Neither you nor I would submit to that. Such a prospective study with informed consent therefore becomes impossible, and without such consent it is unethical, since each of us is bound to perform the "best" for the individual.

The worst of all worlds is the "multicenter study" which proposes to obtain large numbers of patients for analysis. These usually end in uncertainty, if not chaos. Witness the English multicenter study of heparin, which resulted in many papers and later acrimony among the participants regarding how the statistics were handled. Recall the multicenter study of renovascular hypertension, in which I participated but which failed to delineate the problem until the Vanderbilt group, with John Foster, led the way to understanding. I doubt the results of any multicenter study.

Allen Callow recently viewed the problem in the light of long experience: "none of the presently available prostheses performs as satisfactorily below the inguinal ligament as above." He concluded that "there is no graft, whether Teflon or Dacron, woven or knitted, or . . . umbilical vein and expanded PTFE graft that can be expected to retain an acceptable patency rate at five years and beyond."[73]

It therefore appears that no final evaluation of alternative methods is presently possible. Individual vascular surgeons must select the procedure which in their hands is most likely to be successful. The situation is similar to that of the English surgeon, a panel member discussing several operations for duodenal ulcer, who was asked which procedure he had requested for his own recent personal operation. He replied, "I chose a surgeon in whom I had confidence and asked him to do what he thought was best for me."

REFERENCES

1 Rosenthal D, Levine K, Stanton PS, Lamis PA: Femoropopliteal bypass: The preferred site for distal anastomosis. *Surgery* 1983, 93:1.

2 Dardik H: *Graft Materials in Vascular Surgery.* Symposia Specialists, Miami, 1978.

3 Dale WA: *Autogenous Vein Grafts.* Charles C Thomas, Springfield, Illinois, 1959.

4 Veith FJ, Gupta SK, Samson RH, Flores SW, Janko G, Scher LA: Superficial femoral and popliteal arteries as inflow sites for distal bypasses. *Surgery* 1981, 90:980.

5 Schuler JJ, Flanigan DP, Williams LR, Ryan JJ, Castronuovo JJ: Early experience with popliteal to infrapopliteal bypass for limb salvage. *Arch Surg* 1983, 118:472.

6 Kakkar VV: The cephalic vein as a peripheral vascular graft. *Surg Gynecol Obstet* 1969, 128:551.

7 Clayson K, Edwards WH, Allen TR, Dale WA: Arm veins for peripheral arterial reconstructions. *Arch Surg* 1976, 111:1276.

8 Campbell DR, Hoar CS Jr, Gibbons GW: The use of arm veins in femoral-popliteal bypass grafts. *Ann Surg* 1979, 190:740.

9 Whittemore AD, Clowes AW, Couch NP, Mannick JA: Secondary femoropopliteal reconstruction. *Ann Surg* 1981, 193:35.

10 Whittemore AD: Discussion of Schulman ML, Bradhey MR: Late results and angiographic evaluation of arm veins as long by-pass grafts. *Surgery* 1982, 92:1040.

11 Schulman ML, Badhey MR: Late results and angiographic evaluation of arm veins as long by-pass grafts. *Surgery* 1982, 92:1032.

12 Graham JW, Lusby RJ: Infrapopliteal bypass grafting: Use of upper limb vein alone and in autogenous composite grafts. *Surgery* 1982, 91:646.

13 Andros G: Discussion of Ochsner JL, Lawson JD, Eskind SJ, Nills NL, DeCamp PT: Homologous veins as an arterial substitute: Long-term results. *J Vasc Surg* 1984, 1:312.

14 Stoney WS, Alford WC Jr, Burrus GR, Glassford DM Jr, Petracek MR, Thomas CS Jr: The fate of arm veins used for aortocoronary bypass grafts. *J Thorac Cardiovasc Surg* 1984, 88:522.

15 May AG, DeWeese JA, Rob CG: Arterialized in situ saphenous vein. *Surgery* 1965, 91:743.

16 Hall KV: The great saphenous vein used in situ as an arterial shunt after extirpation of the vein valves. *Surgery* 1962, 51:492.

17 Connolly J, Kwaan J: In situ saphenous vein bypass. *Arch Surg* 1982, 117:1551.

18 Leather R, Shah D, Corson J, Karmody A: Instrumental evolution of the valve incision method of in situ saphenous vein bypass. *J Vasc Surg* 1984, 1:113.

19 Ehrenfeld WK, Stoney RJ, Wylie EJ: Autogenous arterial grafts (Chapter 17), in Stanley JC (ed): *Biologic and Synthetic Vascular Prostheses.* Grune & Stratton, New York, 1982, p. 291.

20 Dale WA, Lewis MR: Lateral vascular patch grafts. *Surgery* 1965, 57:36.

21 Inahara T, Scott CM: Endarterectomy for segmental occlusive disease of the superficial femoral artery. *Arch Surg* 1981, 116:1547.

22 Walker PM, Imparato AM, Riles TS, Mintzer R, Kopelman I: Long-term results in superficial femoral artery endarterectomy. *Surgery* 1981, 89:23.

23 Pierce EC: Autologous tissue tubes for aortic grafts in dogs. *Surgery* 1953, 33:648.

24 Eiken O: Autogenous connective tissue tubes for replacement of small artery defects: A preliminary report of an experimental study in dogs. *Acta Chir Scand* 1960, 120:47.

25 Schilling JA, Shurley HM, Joel W, Richter KM, White BN: Fibrocollagenous tubes structured in vivo. *Arch Path* 1961, 71:548.

26 Hufnagel CA: Discussion of Schilling JA, Shurley HM, Joel W, White BN, Bradford RH: Abdominal aortic grafts: Use of in vivo structured autologous and homologous fibrocollagenous tubes. *Ann Surg* 1964, 159:828.

27 Sparks CH: Silicone mandril method for growing reinforced autogenous femoro-popliteal artery grafts in situ. *Ann Surg* 1973, 177:293.

28 Hallin RW, Swetman WR: The Sparks mandril graft. *Am J Surg* 1976, 132:221.

29 DeWeese JA, Woods WD, Dale WA: Failure of homografts as arterial replacements. *Surgery* 1959, 46:565.

30 Weber TR, Lindenauer SM, Dent LL, Allen E, Salles CA, Weatherbee L: Long-term patency of vein grafts preserved in liquid nitrogen in dimethyl sulfoxide. *Ann Surg* 1976, 184:709.

31 Perloff LJ, Reckard CR, Rowlands DR Jr, Barker CF: The venous homograft: An immunological question. *Surgery* 1972, 72:961.

32 Axthelm SC, Porter JM, Strickland S, Baur BA: Antigenicity of venous allografts. *Ann Surg* 1979, 189:290.

33 Stephens M, Sheil AGR, Wong J: Allograft vein arterial bypass. *Arch Surg* 1978, 113:591.

34 Williams GM, Hoar AT, Krajewski C, Parks LC, Roth J: Rejection and repair of endothelium in major vessel transplants. *Surgery* 1975, 78:694.

35 Ochsner JL, DeCamp PT, Leonard GL: Experience with fresh venous allografts as an arterial substitute. *Ann Surg* 1971, 173:933.

36 Ochsner JL: Discussion of Williams GM, Hoar AT, Krajewski C, Parks LC, Roth J: Rejection and repair of endothelium in major vessel transplants. *Surgery* 1975, 78:694.

37 Ochsner JL, Lawson JD, Eskind SJ, Mills NL, DeCamp PT: Homologous veins as an arterial substitute: Long-term results. *J Vasc Surg* 1984, 1:307.

38 Veith FJ, Gupta SK, Samson RH, Scher LA, Ascer E, Spraygen S: Femoral-popliteal-tibial occlusive disease (Chapter 14), in Moore WS (ed): *Vascular Surgery: A Comprehensive Review.* Grune & Stratton, New York, 1983.

39 Campbell CD, Brooks DH, Webster MW, Bondi RP, Lloyd JC, Haynes MF, Bahnson HT: Aneurysm formation in expanded polytetrafluoroethylene prosthesis. *Surgery* 1976, 79:491.

40 Cranley JJ, Hafner CD: Revascularization of the femoropopliteal arteries using saphenous vein, polytetrafluoroethylene and umbilical vein grafts: Five and six year results. *Arch Surg* 1982, 117:1543.

41 Bergentyz SE: Discussion of Cranley JJ, Hafner CD: Revascularization of the femoropopliteal arteries using saphenous vein, polytetrafluoroethylene and umbilical vein grafts: Five and six year results. *Arch Surg* 1982, 117:1543.

42 Hobson RW II, Yeager RA, Glynch TG, Jamil Z, Padberg FT, Lee BC: Failure of polytetrafluoroethylene (PTFE) in femoro-tibial bypass for limb salvage. *J Cardiovasc Surg* (Torino) 1983, 24:361.

43 Hallett JW Jr, Brewster DC, Darling RC: The limitations of polytetrafluoroethylene in the reconstruction of femoropopliteal and tibial arteries. *Surg Gynecol Obstet* 1982, 152:819.

44 O'Donnell T, Farber S, Richmand D, Deterling R, Callow A: Above-knee polytetrafluoroethylene femoropopliteal bypass graft: Is it a reasonable alternative to the below-knee reversed autogenous vein graft? *Surgery* 1983, 94:26.

45 Christenson JT, Broome A, Norgren L, Eklof B: PTFE grafts for lower limb reconstructions: Results of 281 Goretex graft implantations, a six year follow-up. *J Cardiovasc Surg* (Torino) 1983, 24:360.

46 McAuley C, Steed D, Webster M: Seven year follow-up of expanded polytetrafluoroethylene (PTFE) femoropopliteal bypass grafts. *Ann Surg* 1984, 199:57.

47 Edwards WH, Mulherin JL: The role of graft material in femoropopliteal bypass grafts. *Ann Surg* 1980, 191:721.

48 Veith FJ: Letter, May 1984.

49 Haimov H, Giron F, Jacobson JH: The expanded polytetrafluoroethylene graft. *Arch Surg* 1979, 114:673.

50 Nabseth DC, Wilson JT, Tan B, McDonough EF, Weiner J, Child CG: Fetal arterial heterografts. *Arch Surg* 1960, 81:929.

51 Dardik H, Ibrahim I, Sussman B, Kahn M, Sanchez M, Klausner S, Baier R, Meyer A, Dardik I: Biodegradation and aneurysm formation in umbilical vein grafts: Observations and a realistic strategy. *Ann Surg* 1984, 199:61.

52 Dardik H, Baier RE, Meenaghan M, Natiella J, Weinberg S, Turner R, Sussman B, Ibrahim IM, Dardik I: Morphologic and biophysical assessment of long-term human umbilical cord vein implants used as vascular conduits. *Surg Gynecol Obstet* 1982, 154:17.

53 Robison J, Brewster D, Abbott W, Darling C: Femoropopliteal and tibioperoneal artery reconstruction using human umbilical vein. *Arch Surg* 1983, 118:1039.

54 Raithel D, Schweiger J: The Dardik biograft in reconstructive arterial surgery: Report on a five year experience in 94 cases. *World J Surg* 1984, 8:113.

55 Weisel RD, Johnson KW, Baird RJ, Drezner AD, Oates TK, Lipton IH: Comparison of conduits for leg revascularization. *Surgery* 1981, 89:8.

56 Szilagyi DE, Elliot JP, Hageman JJ, Smith RF, Dall'Olmo CA: Biologic fate of autogenous vein implants as arterial substitutes: Clinical and histopathologic observations in femoral-popliteal operations for arteriosclerosis. *Ann Surg* 1973, 178:232.

57 Giordano J, Keshishian J: Aneurysm formation in human umbilical vein grafts. *Surgery* 1982, 91:343.

58 Dale WA, Lewis MR: Further experience with bovine arterial grafts. *Surgery* 1976, 80:711.

59 Pridgen W, Dale WA: Composite (Teflon and autogenous vein) grafts in small canine arteries. *Ann Surg* 1962, 28:7.
60 Dale WA, Pridgen W: Failure of composite (Teflon-vein) grafts in human arteries. *Surgery* 1962, 51:258.
61 Linton RR, Wirthlin LS: Femoropopliteal composite Dacron and autogenous vein bypass grafts. *Arch Surg* 1973, 107:748.
62 Burnham SJ, Flanigan P, Goodreau JJ, Yao JST, Bergan JJ: Nonvein bypass in below knee reoperation for lower limb ischemia. *Surgery* 1978, 84:417.
63 Hobson RW II, O'Donnell JA, Jamil Z, Mehta K: Below knee bypass for limb salvage. Comparison of autogenous saphenous vein, polytetrafluoroethylene, and composite Dacron-autogenous vein grafts. *Arch Surg* 1980, 115:833.
64 Verta MJ: Composite sequential bypasses to the ankle and beyond for limb salvage. *J Vasc Surg* 1984, 1:381.
65 Snyder S, Gregory RT, Wheeler JR, Gaygle RG: Femoropopliteal composite bypass grafts (letter). *Surgery* 1983, 93:729.
66 LaSalle AJ, Brewster DC, Corson JD, Darling RC: Femoropopliteal composite bypass grafts: Current status. *Surgery* 1982, 92:36.
67 Bartley TD, Bigelow JC, Page US: Aortocoronary bypass grafting with multiple sequential anastomoses to a single vein. *Arch Surg* 1972, 105:915.
68 Edwards WS, Gerety E, Larkin J, Hoyt TW: Multiple sequential femoral tibial grafting for severe ischemia. *Surgery* 1976, 80:722.
69 Edwards WH, Wright RS: Tibial and peroneal bypass in severe occlusive disease of the lower extremities. *Ann Surg* 1976, 183:710.
70 Jarrett F, Berkoff HA, Crummy AB: Sequential femoral-tibial bypass grafting for limb salvage. *Ann Surg* 1978, 188:685.
71 Berkoff HA, Flinn WR, Flanigan P, Verta MJ, Bergan JJ, Yao JST: Sequential femoral-tibial bypass for severe limb ischemia. *Surgery* 1980, 88:357.
72 Brewster DC, LaSalle AJ, Darling RC: Comparison of above knee and below knee anastomosis in femoropopliteal bypass grafts. *Arch Surg* 1981, 116:1013.
73 Callow AD: Historical overview of experimental and clinical development of vascular grafts (Chapter 2), in Stanley JC (ed): *Biologic and Synthetic Vascular Prostheses.* Grune & Stratton, New York, 1982.

Invited Commentary

Frank J. Veith, M.D.
New York, New York

This is a lucid review of one of the controversial topics in vascular surgery. I am in general agreement with many of the author's conclusions.

It must be emphasized that a major reason for much of the controversy in this area is the fact that the choice of graft material and the operation performed are only two factors in determining the short- and long-term success of femoropopliteal arterial reconstructions. Several other factors play roles which I believe are of equal or greater importance in determining the outcome. These include the quality of preoperative arteriography, the indications for operation and, most importantly, the care and commitment which the vascular surgeon and radiologist devote to operative and nonoperative aspects of patient care. Variability in these crucial factors probably accounts for the differences in results. These differing results from various centers are bound to give rise to controversy. Rarely do surgeons who cannot make a particular graft or operation work take the time or trouble to visit another center reporting better results to see why they cannot obtain similarly good results. It is easier to assume that the more optimistic report is somehow inaccurate.

Because of the importance in determining outcome of factors other than the choice of graft, valid comparisons between different grafts can be based on the results of only adequately performed randomized prospective studies in which large numbers of patients are entered and then followed for long periods of time. Although such studies are difficult, they are not impossible. Our group, together with Drs. Bergan, Yao, Flinn, Bernhard, and Towne, have performed such a study over the past 6 years.[1] More than 800 limb salvage patients have been entered into the study. Informed consent has been obtained, and substantial numbers of patients have been followed over 3 years.

To date, with meaningful numbers of patients followed $3\frac{1}{2}$ years, *no statistically significant differences ($p > 0.5$) in primary ($3\frac{1}{2}$ year) patency have been observed between randomized PTFE femoropopliteal bypass grafts (59 percent) and randomized saphenous vein femoropopliteal bypass grafts (68 percent).* This is true whether the graft crosses the knee joint or not. Secondary patency rates and limb salvage rates are better for both groups, underscoring the importance of the vascular surgeon's commitment to repeated angiography and appropriately performed reintervention (angioplasty or reoperation) in this group of patients.[2,3] Reintervention is particularly easy and fruitful if failing arterial reconstructions are detected before graft thrombosis has occurred.[4]

Because there are as yet no conclusive long-term results that allow accurate comparison of vein and PTFE grafts, we still believe that ipsilateral autogenous saphenous vein is the material of choice for femoropopliteal bypass if the patient's life expectancy is over 3 years. A PTFE graft is the preferred alternative in poor-risk patients and in those whose veins are missing or of poor quality (about 40 percent of our patients). Other prosthetics or the umbilical vein graft probably perform equally well, but this should be proved by a properly conducted randomized prospective study.

Our ongoing randomized prospective study has also shown that *vein grafts are superior to PTFE grafts if the distal anastomosis is carried to an infrapopliteal artery (58 percent versus 37 percent 3-year patency, $p < 0.5$).* However, with secondary operations, 3-year limb salvage rates with PTFE grafts to small arteries exceed 50 percent, and such operations should be performed in preference to amputation if no saphenous vein is available. When bypasses to distal small vessels are required, we are particularly enthusiastic about the results of short vein grafts from the popliteal artery to arteries at the ankle or in the foot.[5] Particularly in this setting, the value of in situ vein bypass remains to be shown; use of reversed vein grafts may be superior and facilitate the operations, since many patients may have a usable segment of thigh saphenous vein with a diseased saphenous segment in the leg.

Finally, a percutaneous transluminal angioplasty should be attempted in preference to a bypass operation when a short hemodynamically significant stenosis of the superficial femoral or popliteal artery is associated with a threatened limb. If an appropriately skilled and committed interventional radiologist is available, good results (50 percent at 2 years) can be obtained in this setting. Failures and serious complications can be easily managed by the vascular surgeon, resulting in low morbidity and mortality.[6]

COMMENTARY REFERENCES

1 Bergan JJ, Veith FJ, Bernhard VM, et al: Randomization of autogenous vein and polytetrafluoroethylene grafts in femoral-distal reconstruction. *Surgery* 1982, 92:921.

2 Veith FJ, Gupta SK, Daly V: Management of early and late thrombosis of expanded polytetrafluoroethylene (PTFE) femoropopliteal bypass grafts: Favorable prognosis with appropriate reoperation. *Surgery* 1980, 87:581.

3 Veith FJ, Gupta SK, Samson RH, et al: Progress in limb salvage by reconstructive arterial surgery combined with new or improved adjunctive procedures. *Ann Surg* 1981, 194:386.

4 Veith FJ, Weiser RK, Gupta SK, et al: Diagnosis and management of failing lower extremity arterial reconstructions prior to graft occlusion. *J Cardiovasc Surg* (Torino) (in press).

5 Veith FJ, Gupta SK, Weiser RK, et al: Short vein grafts in limb salvate arterial reconstructions, in Bergan JJ, Yao JST (eds): *Evaluation and Treatment of Upper and Lower Extremity Circulatory Disorders.* Grune & Stratton, New York, 1984, p. 309.

6 Samson RH, Sprayregen S, Veith FJ, et al: Management of angioplasty complications, unsuccessful procedures and early and late failures. *Ann Surg* 1984, 189:234.

11 SECONDARY ARTERIAL OPERATIONS

The patient presenting with symptoms after failure of a revascularization procedure may at once be categorized as a difficult problem in terms of judgment, as well as of technique, and as less likely to receive long-term benefit despite the best management. The best chance is the first: "occasional" operators who choose the wrong alternative or perform less skillfully for the initial procedure violate the axiom of no harm to the patient. The veteran also may perceive in retrospect that the initial strategy was not the best and may place the error in a storehouse of experience for future reference. Hence the importance of long-term follow-up of results.

CHOOSING A SECONDARY PROCEDURE

Several questions at once occur in the evaluation of a patient for a secondary procedure.

Why Did the Initial Procedure Fail or a Complication Occur? The common causes of late failure of revascularization include (1) progression of the degenerative atherosclerotic process, (2) degenerative changes in the wall of the graft, (3) overgrowth of the neointima, so-called intimal hyperplasia, (4) disproportion of graft and host vessel size, and (5) changes in the clotting mechanism, such as those caused by smoking.[1,2]

The inexorable progression of degenerative processes such as arteriosclerosis undoubtedly explains some failures: the tibial arteries thicken and occlude, so the proximal graft has no runoff and clots, or a stroke occurs due to intracranial arterial thrombosis despite continuing patency of a previous carotid endarterectomy.

The vascular surgeon, however, must choose a procedure with foreknowledge of the likely course of the disease process. The popliteal anastomosis must be placed distal to a popliteal stenosis so that its later complete occlusion will be tolerable. The diseased gallbladder must be removed prior to final closure after aneurysmectomy, to prevent early postoperative inflammation. Catheter thrombectomy of acute arterial thrombosis is so prone to recurrence that a more certain form of revascularization is indicated from the start. The initial management strategy therefore must consider the probable future course or complications as well as provide a technically correct procedure.

Neointimal hyperplasia typically occurs near the anastomosis of polytetrafluoroethylene (PTFE) to an artery. Its cause is unknown, although eddy currents are an obvious suspect. Whether antiplatelet medication will prevent this, as is suggested by canine experiments,[3] is unknown. Currently there is no general agreement regarding either the drugs [aspirin, dipyridamole, or ibuprofen (Motrin)] or their optimal dose. In the absence of facts I use the cheapest and least dangerous, a "baby aspirin" with breakfast daily.

It is generally agreed that graft-host artery disproportion produces abnormal flow patterns and an increased chance of thrombus deposition, which goes on in uncontrolled fashion until thrombosis results. Animal tests of patch grafts placed snugly versus those placed loosely to form an aneurysmal dilatation clearly showed that the latter had a much higher rate of clotting.[4] This has led to using even smaller aortobifemoral grafts to approximate more closely the size of the femoral arteries.

Finally, there is the matter of smoking tobacco, long suspected of causing arterial thrombosis. There are at least two series which show this association. The series of Wray, DePalma, and Hubay speaks for itself. They followed 100 patients having aortic surgery, 50 each for aneurysms and for occlusive disease. None of the aneurysm replacement grafts failed. Among the 29 smokers with occlusive disease there was a 31 percent rate of thrombosis of some part of the graft over a 3- to 6-year period. None of the 17 nonsmokers thrombosed a graft. Four patients were lost to follow-up.[1]

What Are the Alternatives for Secondary Repair? Imagination, as well as mere recollection of the available techniques, is important in determining the best strategy after an initial failure. Three things are of primary importance. First, the run-off must be assured: often it requires enlargement or a more distal bypass. Second, clot must be completely removed from whatever graft or vessel remains in place. Third, graft and artery damaged during the procedure must be bypassed or replaced.[5]

Graft stenoses may be patched as well as replaced (Figure 11-1). Taking an extraanatomic pathway may be easier and safer than ploughing through a field of cicatrix or of infection, and a peripheral aneurysm persistent after a successful bypass may be better treated by endoaneurysmorrhaphy than by further polar ligations.

It is worthwhile to discuss all the options with all interested team members. More than once an inexperienced person has given a suggestion which has proved better than the conventional wisdom. Younger people "may not be educated but they are not stupid."*

The entire list of alternatives must be known and available to allow an optimal selection. These are discussed in Chapter 10 and will not be repeated here.

What Are the Probable Results? The worst as well as the best outcome must be visualized. If the expected patency rate for a PTFE graft to a tibial artery is only 10 to 25 percent, a below-knee amputation may be in order. When a carotid artery has occluded without symptoms, it is rash to advise an operation for improvement.

Informed consent by the patient and family is more than a legalistic protection (if it is that!). The surgeon's knowledge and statement of personal results allow a discussion of alternatives prior to the final choice. It is surely moral that the recipient understand the odds of various alternative methods, to allow participation in the decision. Indeed, it is sometimes difficult to dissuade a patient or family who wishes "one more chance" at a low-percentage reoperation rather than an ablative procedure.

TECHNICAL PRINCIPLES OF SECONDARY OPERATIONS

Avoid Dissecting Scar Tissue A completely new and different incision, such as one below the knee when the original was proximal to it, allows an efficient and bloodless approach to an artery. Place the proximal anastomosis to the external iliac artery beneath the severed inguinal ligament and the distal anastomosis to a tibial artery beyond the previous one. If the first graft lies in the subcutaneous tissue, place the second behind the muscle, and vice versa. Similarly, consider a crossover femorofemoral graft rather than complete replacement of an old aortic graft.

*I recall the advice of physiologist Hermann Rahn, who preferred the inexperienced person to use imagination in the laboratory rather than first to read everything published, which he thought tended to lead to mere repetition.

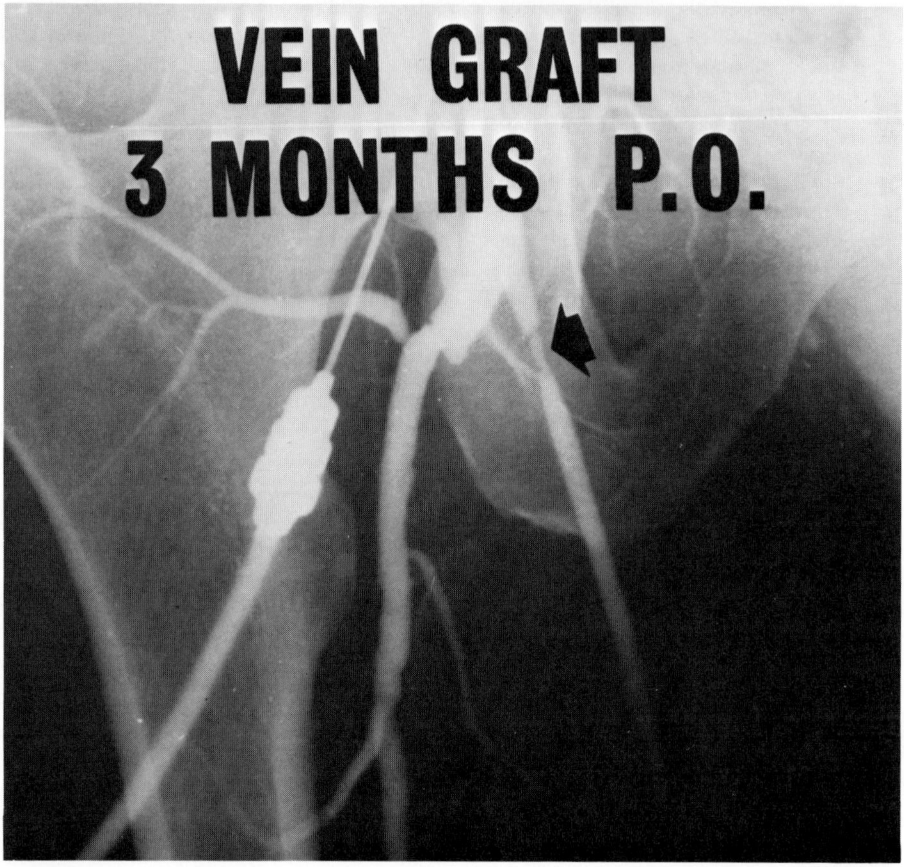

FIGURE 11-1 This short stenosis of a vein graft occurred just distal to the femoral anastomosis in the groin 3 months postoperatively. The saphenous vein graft was patched with a small segment of vein taken from the dorsum of the hand.

Obtain Early Arterial Control Obtain early proximal and distal arterial control by dissecting these vessels first. Established control allows later bold dissection with the assurance that bleeding can be controlled

Consider Quick Procedures Consider quick procedures for a direct arterial repair. A false aneurysm of a femoral anastomosis is easily handled by placement of a proximal clamp and the immediate opening of the sac and control of its arterial branches by balloon catheters. Such a "finesse" procedure allows an experienced team to complete a needed repair with minimal dissection, brief time, and little blood loss. It is an authoritative procedure, as opposed to a tentative and groping one.

Replace Rather Than Repair An old graft or anastomosis is usually better replaced than repaired. Thrombectomy is useful, especially to ensure that remaining portions of graft or artery harbor no clot, but new material is easier to suture and usually provides a better channel. The main body of the graft, if unclotted, is often usable if a new graft is added distally.

Achieve Hemostasis Achieve hemostasis by whatever method is needed. Although multiple ligatures, sutures, clips, and cauterizations may be done, the reopened wound usually oozes so much serum and blood that suction-drainage is needed. An accumulation of fluid is far better in a bottle than in the wound.

SPECIFIC REOPERATIONS

Carotid

Often the proximal portion of the common carotid artery lies outside the scar tissue, allowing an easier approach to its control there.

Adherence of nerves increases the likelihood of their injury. When the vagus lies anterior to the artery, its variation should be underlined in the original operative note. Inquiry of that original note or operation may be informative. The hypoglossal crossing requires a cautious approach, usually from the lateral aspect. Dissecting close to the internal artery is also protective (but of course has more danger to the vessel itself).

Dissection and elevation of the external carotid artery first allows a safer approach to the internal, which is more deeply embedded in scar tissue.

Sometimes it suffices and is safer to enlarge the carotid lumen by patching, making no attempt to remodel its interior.

While a patch graft should be immediately available for all carotid operations, the secondary ones particularly need these. Small ellipses of Dacron or PTFE are useful and easier to place than are vein grafts, which if used, should be obtained prior to the opening of the carotid artery.

Aorta

Knowledge of the original procedure and well-studied angiograms and scans often allow prediction of the optimal method of the proximal control which is requisite to aortic repair. If there remains a centimeter or more of the original infrarenal aorta, that may be dissected below all the visceral vessels and used for the proximal anastomosis (or closure, if an extraanatomic revascularization is needed). Sometimes a short segment of the original graft, well cleaned of thrombus, is useful. Otherwise, the aorta may be occluded above the renal arteries to allow the anastomosis, followed by clamping of the attached graft below the vessels during the remainder of the procedure. The "T"-shaped aortic occluder (Figure 6-7) may be used for such temporary proximal control.

An original end-to-side (piggyback) aortic graft may be completely removed and the new graft may be placed end-to-end, or alternatively, the original anastomosis may be preserved and a new lower end added. In the latter event all interior clot, in both the graft and the host aorta, must be cleaned and flushed to prevent early embolization or later stenosis.

The distal ends of a clotted limb or limbs of an aortic graft may be left indwelling in their retroperitoneal scar tissue bed or pulled out by inversion, using a clamp passed within the aortic lumen inferiorly.

Previous aortic and/or iliac endarterectomy failures are managed by aortobifemoral grafting without any attempt to reopen the previously cleaned segments.

Femorofemoral Graft

Occlusion of these crossovers usually occurs because of progression of the host arterial disease and not because of primary graft failure, so attention is directed toward the main disease problem rather than a local thrombectomy. An aortobifemoral graft is usually needed. Sometimes the new distal graft ends can be joined to the original ends of the crossover graft, but this hope is rarely achieved. Usually the distal anastomoses must be redone, in which case the central portion of the crossover graft may be left or removed, whichever seems easier.

Stenosis of one end of a femoral cross-over graft sometimes requires patching or, preferably, replacement of the end to a new femoral anastomosis.

Deterioration of the femoral arterial supply of one leg may require an extension from one or the other end of a femorofemoral bypass. The secondary femoropopliteal graft may be attached to the old femoral crossover or, preferably, to the femoral artery distal to that anastomosis so that the original is not disturbed. A useful technique to allow this is a short eversion endarterectomy of the superficial femoral artery, to which may be attached the secondary femoropopliteal graft (Figure 10-2).

Anastomoses in the Groin

False aneurysms at the site of femoral anastomoses may require repair while still patent or after their thrombosis. Early proximal control may be achieved by the opening of the tissues high in the groin. Immediate location of the inguinal ligament allows it to be severed and a retractor placed so that the fibrotic sheath can be opened and the graft encircled. With this protection one of two courses are available. The superficial and profunda femoral arteries may be exposed distal to the anastomosis and encircled for control and the false aneurysm or thrombosed anastomosis dissected last. Alternatively, the iliac limb of the graft may be opened distal to an occluding clamp, to allow multiple balloon catheters to be placed internally to control back bleeding from the orifices of the profunda and superficial femoral arteries. It should be recalled also that the proximal end of the common femoral artery may still be patent and require control. Thus three balloon catheters may be needed.

The internal balloon occlusion technique is awkward if an extended profundaplasty is required, in which event a long segment of profunda should be free to allow access to its branches as well as to its main lumen. The balloon technique and an internal dilator may, however, be useful in quickly locating the profunda and avoiding an extensive search from the outside.

In any event, the femoral anastomosis should be redone, using a new segment of graft which is attached to the retained proximal graft by a long ovoid anastomosis. The balloon occluders are withdrawn just before the final sutures are pulled up.

Preliminary, intraoperative, or completion angiography is done as indicated. Certainly, the status of the femoral, popliteal, and below-knee arteries must be clearly demonstrated now in the event that a more distal bypass is needed sooner or later.

Femoropopliteal Repairs

Late failure of a femoral or popliteal endarterectomy is easily managed by a femoropopliteal bypass performed at a distance as if no previous procedure had occurred (Figure 11-2). The same is true for failure of an angioplasty in the thigh.

An isolated stenosis of an autogenous venous bypass may be easily corrected by a longitudinal opening with autogenous venous patch closure (Figures 11-3 and 11-4). Access to the old graft is easy if it lies in the subcutaneous tissue of the thigh, where it is palpable.

If the original vein graft was placed deep to the muscles, more dissection is needed. In the distal thigh near the knee, where the vein graft often is tunneled through the popliteal space and between the gastrocnemius muscle heads to reach the popliteal artery below the knee, it may be simpler to approach the vein posteriorly through unscarred tissues. The posterior popliteal route is not well known today but offers good exposure without severed muscles. A lazy-"S" incision across the popliteal crease is followed by the opening of the fascia longitudinally, just beside the lesser saphenous vein (which may be used as a patch or as a shunt extension graft). The thigh

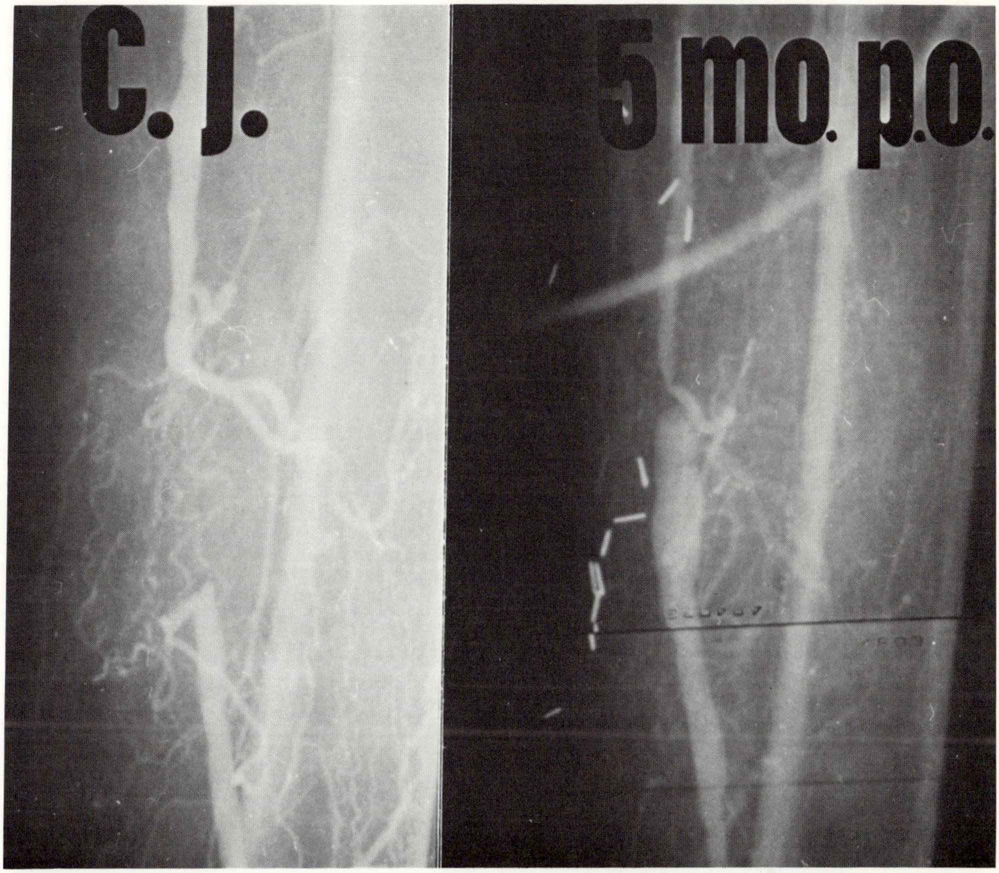

FIGURE 11-2 *Left,* direct open endarterectomy was performed originally to revascularize the short occlusion of this superficial femoral artery. *Right,* 5 months later there was proximal complete occlusion, which was due to progression of disease rather than thrombosis of the endarterectomized segment. Secondary repair consisted of femoropopliteal saphenous vein grafting.

muscles are spread apart, and the gastrocnemius heads are split to allow exposure of the popliteal vessels and the old graft.

The more commonly used medial approach to the previous graft, its anastomosis, and the popliteal artery is the alternative. It requires dissection of scar tissue but is a more familiar route for many surgeons.

If a new graft is used to replace the previous one, its route requires careful consideration. Many long-term successful grafts have been placed entirely in the subcutaneous tissues, but a pathway via the usual anatomic route is more attractive. Tunneling through scar tissue alongside the old graft in a cavalier fashion may cause severe venous injury in an unexposed location. Caution is the order of the day if that route is chosen.

Sometimes the original vein graft remains patent for a time after the run-off vessels thrombose. Early repair is indicated to save the graft from ultimate thrombosis. A new segment of vein may be added, its lower anastomosis being made to whatever distal artery remains patent (Figure 11-5).

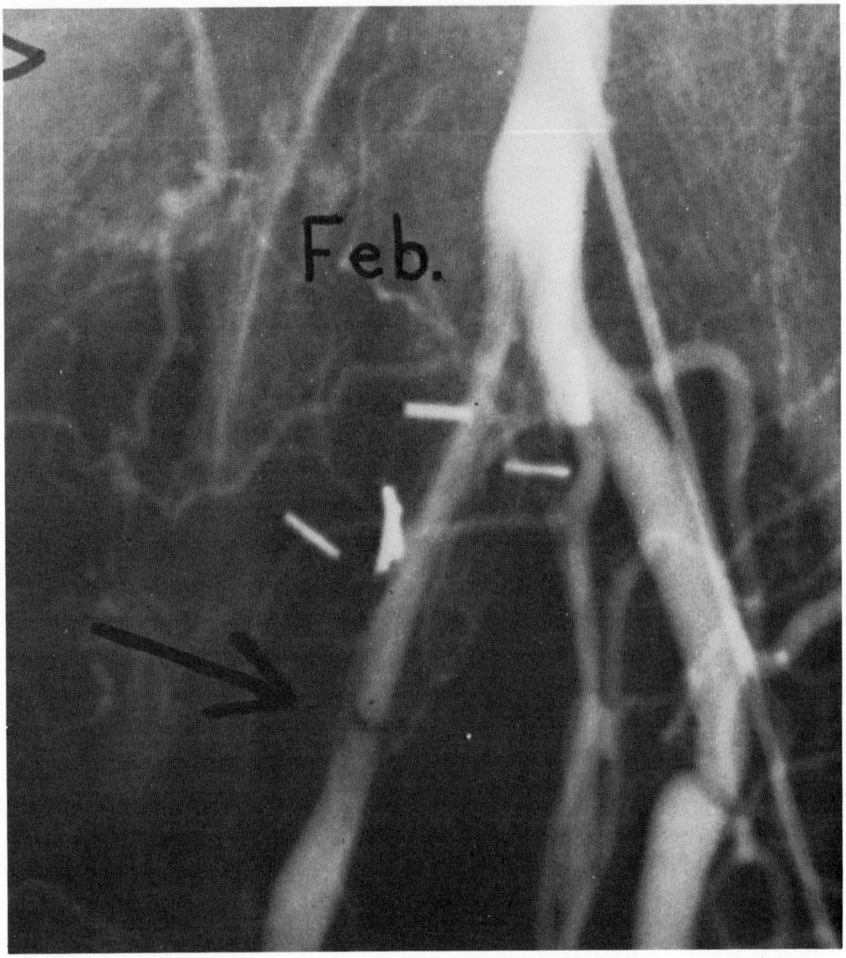

FIGURE 11-3 The proximal end of this autogenous saphenous vein graft was small originally and soon developed a quite tight stenosis *(arrow)* in February. The remainder of the graft remained patent, and the patient refused a secondary repair.

Late occlusion of a PTFE graft requires special consideration. The advocates of these grafts cite the good possibility of successful late thrombectomy as an advantage, since it can be done several times. Personal experience confirms these opinions and suggests thrombectomy with patch grafting of the anastomosis (especially distally) as the correct secondary procedure.

Even after many hours or several days have elapsed, the PTFE graft may often be salvaged. Both proximal and distal ends of the graft require exposure, to allow complete thrombectomy and correction of the anastomotic stenoses, which are usually causative. This commonly requires that a longitudinal arteriotomy be made in the distal artery so that a vein patch may be placed to enlarge the anastomosis after the hyperplastic intimal thickening is removed (Figure 11-6). It has even been suggested that the original anastomosis should be constructed with a vein patch as a part of it. Whether that modification will prevent later intimal hyperplastic occlusion of PTFE anastomoses is not yet determined.

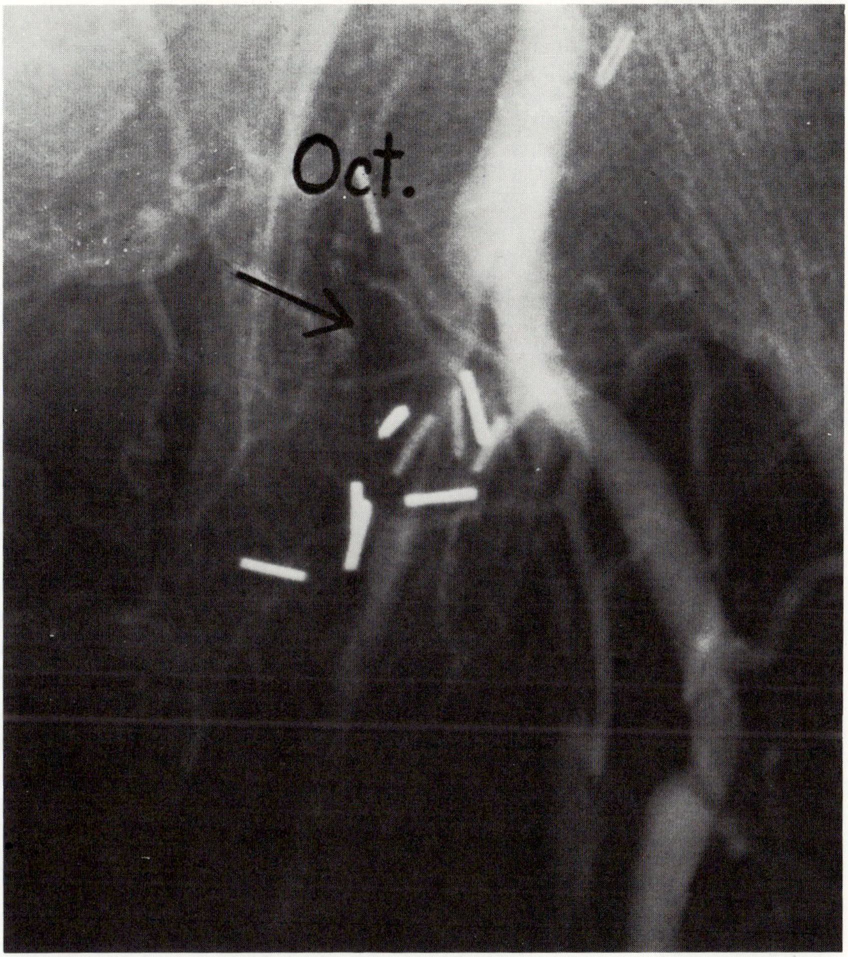

FIGURE 11-4 Nine months later, in October, the proximal portion of the graft had become completely occluded *(arrow)* and was repaired by placement of a completely new segment of vein.

An alternative secondary reconstruction of a PTFE graft after late thrombectomy is to extend it distally by new PTFE tubing or, preferably, by a short segment of autogenous vein, thus converting it to a composite graft.

Experience with PTFE grafts suggests that a series of occlusions, thrombectomies, and revisions are common prices for salvage of the limb by that technique. One such patient over a 10-year period had 18 vascular procedures of one or another sort, many of the latter ones using PTFE, prior to eventual bilateral amputation and later death.

Tibial Procedures

A failed tibial or peroneal revascularization cannot ordinarily be repaired. Occasionally another distal calf or ankle vessel may be used. The patient may be managed temporarily with pain medication in the hope that collateral circulation will develop. Most require amputation to relieve pain or control infection.

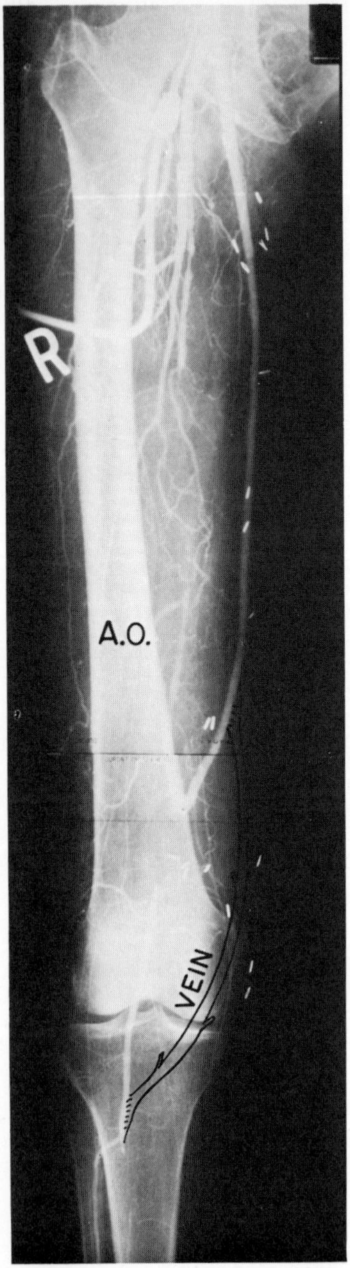

FIGURE 11-5 Originally the femoropopliteal vein graft was placed to the popliteal artery above the knee. Recurrence of symptoms led to an immediate investigation by arteriography, which demonstrated progression of the disease with continued patency of the vein graft. The new lesion was repaired by placement of a new segment of vein to carry blood to the popliteal artery below the knee.

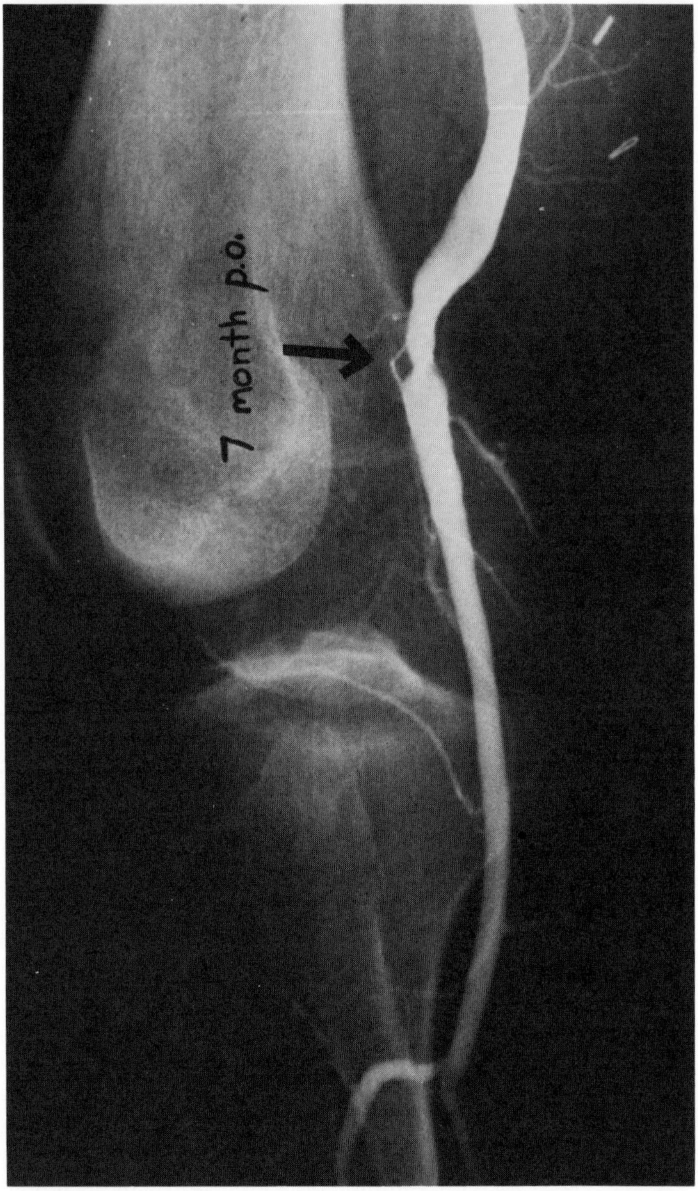

FIGURE 11-6 This PTFE graft after 7 months appeared to be patent, although calf symptoms had recurred. The arteriogram showed this irregularity *(arrow)* at the site of anastomosis just above the knee joint. It was repaired through a posterior approach by removal of the intimal wall hyperplasia and placement of a venous patch graft.

Renal Artery

Secondary dissection of this small vessel is difficult and often ends with nephrectomy. Three other courses are possible. First, percutaneous transluminal angioplasty may be performed. Second, hypertensive control by medication is often effective and usually is better over the long run than is renal ablation. Finally, nephrectomy may be performed but will result in loss of function and other recognized disadvantages.

REFERENCES

1 Myers VA: Smoking. *Br J Surg* 1978, 65:1267.
2 Wray R, DePalma RG, Hubay CH: Late occlusion of aortofemoral bypass grafts: Influence of cigarette smoking. *Surgery* 1971, 70:969.
3 Oblath RW, Buckley FO Jr, Green RM, Schwartz SI, DeWeese JA: Prevention of platelet aggregation and adherence to prosthetic vascular grafts by aspirin and dipyridamole. *Surgery* 1978, 84:37.
4 Dale WA, Lewis MR: Experimental arterial patch grafts. *J Cardiovasc Surg* (Torino) 1965, 6:24.
5 Macpherson DS, Bell PR: The unblocking of occluded Dacron grafts (Chapter 35), in Greenhalgh RM (ed): *Extra-Anatomic and Secondary Arterial Reconstruction.* Pitman, Bath, 1982, p 334.

Invited Commentary

Charles G. Rob, M.D.
Bethesda, Maryland

A secondary operation frequently is necessary because of a problem with the first procedure. It is essential that the first operation be done correctly.

Previously, surgeons (including myself) relied on clinical studies and the Doppler probe to judge the situation; even in expert hands some technical defects were not detected. The only way to be certain of the vascular procedure is by performing a completion angiogram. This should be done before the patient leaves the operating room. Exceptions may include the reconstruction of large arteries such as the aorta.

A diseased gallbladder should be removed before the incision is closed after an abdominal aortic graft has been inserted. But how does one manage associated lesions such as an inguinal hernia, carcinoma of the colon, or a stenotic renal artery? All may lead to a second operation. The bowel should be prepared before an elective operation on the abdominal aorta. It is then possible to resect a carcinoma at the time an aortic graft is inserted. An obvious exception is the presence of acute diverticulitis with an abscess, or the discovery of one of these lesions at the time of an emergency operation upon the aorta. Then the surgeon must use judgment, remembering at all times that the worst complication to be faced is an infected aortic prosthesis.

The author raises the question of informed consent in relation to secondary operations. The real objective should be to inform the patient and the family; the legal side is secondary. Informed consent can pave the way to full acceptance of a secondary operation such as an amputation. In this connection, I believe that we do not consult with our colleagues enough. A preoperative consultation with a trusted and respected colleague is usually welcomed by the patient and family and can be of great value if a predicted second operation becomes necessary.

Observing surgeons, one soon becomes aware that some perform more secondary operations than others. Often these surgeons are equally skillful. It is important to stress that an alternative to reoperation is conservative care. It is not necessary in many patients for all arteries to be open and pulsatile. With the advent of good noninvasive testing it has become apparent that the thrombosis and recurrent stenosis rate after carotid thromboendarterectomy is between 5 and 10 percent 1 year after the operation. Most of these patients are asymptomatic and would have been thought to have open carotids before the introduction of noninvasive laboratory techniques. Clearly these patients do not need more surgery. In the lower limbs many femoropopliteal or more distal bypasses occlude, but the limb survives as a useful part for the patient. The collateral circulation may have improved; an infected and ischemic lesion may have healed, reducing the demand on the circulation; or an associated procedure may have improved the inflow through the profunda femoris artery. Whatever the explanation, these patients do not need another operation.

It is sound practice to insist on a regular follow-up examination of all patients who have an arterial reconstruction operation for arterial disease. This may allow a small operation to prevent a complication. For example, the author describes a patient who had a femoropopliteal graft; mild claudication returned and the peripheral pulses disappeared with exercise, but moderate stenosis in the graft was easily corrected before the whole graft occluded. The surgeon's responsibility does not end when such patients leave the hospital; it ends when they die. The surgeon should either follow these patients personally or arrange to receive regular follow-up reports from the patients' own doctors.

Last, there is a tendency to blame progression of the patient's disease for problems which develop after an operation. It is true that this occurs, but the surgeon may be partially at fault. The surgeon must insist that hypertension be treated, that diabetes be controlled, and above all, that the patient with atherosclerosis be clearly and repeatedly told of the dangers of an improper or excessive diet and of continuing to use tobacco in any form.

12 ERRORS IN FEMOROPOPLITEAL OPERATIONS: PREVENTION AND CORRECTION

A voluminous literature describes the technique and results of femoropopliteal arterial reconstructive procedures, but the errors which cause failures are hardly mentioned or are omitted completely. The following discussion is directed toward avoidance of these hazards by knowledge of their possibility (Figure 12-1), by early recognition, and by prompt correction when required.

TOO LIMITED RECONSTRUCTION

Many vascular operations require a choice between doing too little, so unrelieved obstructions or stenoses compromise the repair, and doing too much, whereby the operative time, blood loss, and tissue trauma increase the risk of complications and even death.

Careful preoperative consideration of the clinical situation and complete angiography should allow a complete plan, with alternatives as needed, to be developed prior to the actual operation. The procedure itself then becomes a straightforward succession of steps without the necessity to stop for discussion of tactics unless some unusual and unforeseen circumstance occurs. Unconsidered problems should decrease as experience accumulates. They may also be diminished by full discussion of the procedure and possible variations prior to every operation. Vascular surgery is an unforgiving field. Its complexities penalize surgeons who free-lance as they go along.

There are situations where the plan can be completed only as the procedure progresses. It may be necessary to perform additional arteriograms after exposure of the distal vessels in the operating room to be certain that the anastomosis is not being placed proximal to a stenosis or obstruction which could not be seen preoperatively. Similarly, a femoropopliteal graft should not be placed without certainty that the aortoiliac system is providing sufficient inflow to maintain it. The recent addition of angioplasty to the armamentarium has provided a good answer to some of these combined problems. Thus, an iliac dilation may be performed concomitantly with a femoropopoliteal repair, or a few days prior to it.

Sometimes the preoperative plan must be revised, but the alternative should be well-recognized so that there is no confusion or delay in changing to it. If the vein graft is too small, or if it bifurcates early, that plan should be immediately abandoned in favor of an alternative. Similarly, if a contemplated femoral thromboendarterectomy is found to be too extensive, it is usually wise to change to a bypass graft without any attempt to clean out the vessel.

An indicated change of plan must be done promptly.

BLIND PROCEDURES ARE DANGEROUS

"Blind" thromboendarterectomy through small openings violates the axiom of good exposure, which allows ease and safety in surgical procedures. When the surgeon looks directly into a

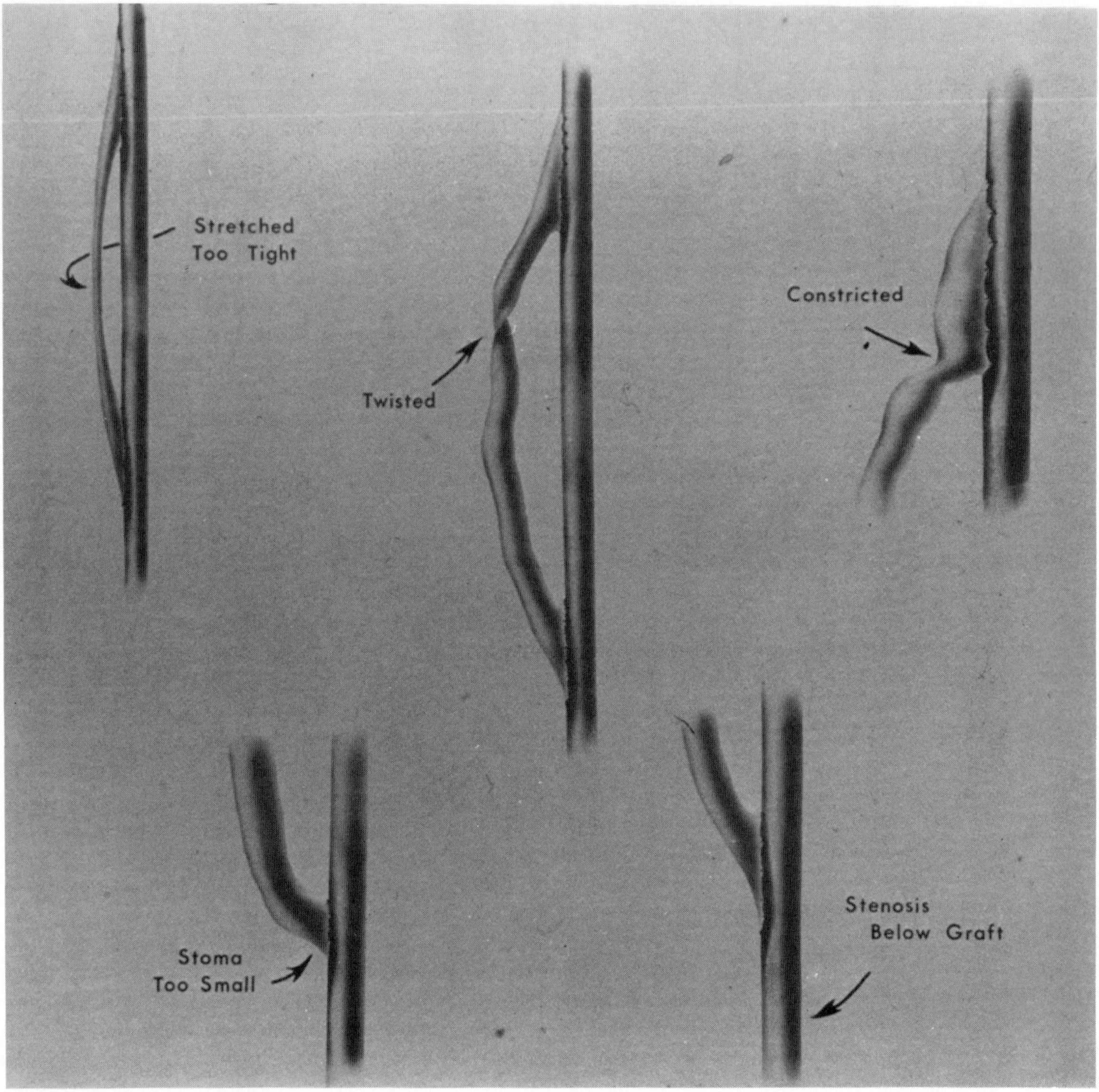

FIGURE 12-1 These common errors in femoropopliteal reconstructions are discussed in the text.

thromboendarterectomized segment while the operation is being performed in a completely open fashion, the tags and shreds of tissue show why a blind procedure may lead to thrombosis. The vessel should be opened to the full extent of the procedure and closed appropriately, with a patch if needed.

IS THE VEIN SUITABLE?

An autogenous vein continues to be the material of choice for peripheral arterial reconstructions. Approximately 80 percent of patients have a saphenous vein which is suitable for use.

The vein must be long enough. If not, there are a number of alternatives, including a vein from the arm or the other leg, a composite graft, a proximal thromboendarterectomy, or a synthetic tube bypass. These are discussed in Chapter 10.

The vein graft must have a diameter which is uniformly large enough. Whether this is 4 or 5 mm or more depends upon the experience of the individual surgeon. Perhaps the best advice is that any serious question about the size or length of the vein graft should at once trigger a shift to some other repair. Occasionally an isolated segmental stenosis may be excised and the vein anastomosed to allow its use.

If the vein has an area of thickening or other indication of previous phlebitis, it should be abandoned. Most of these ultimately thrombose.

DAMAGE TO THE GRAFT

Care in procuring an autogenous vein graft prevents later scarring or aneurysm formation. The graft should be handled delicately with the fingers or with rubber or Silastic tapes and should not be pinched with clamps or steel instruments. Such trauma leads to the sharply defined stenoses and occlusions which have been reported after a period of months or years.

Damage to the endothelium of the vein graft may be caused by the fluid used for irrigation of the graft. There are a number of reports indicating that one or another irrigating solution is better or worse.[1-4] Other studies suggest that the intimal endothelium may be damaged by distention of the graft during preparation.[5] These conclusions are largely based on electron microscopic findings which show endothelial damage. Whether or not this is reflected in a difference in the patency rate of grafts in humans has never been determined. I irrigate the interior of the vein graft with heparinized Ringer's solution and distend it with a hand-held syringe in order to detect leaking areas and to allow all communicating veins to be properly ligated, as well as to determine that the luminal size is sufficient.

FAILURE TO USE HEPARIN

It is recognized that a few competent vascular surgeons do not provide systemic heparinization during periods of vascular occlusion by clamping. There is no quarrel with such experienced surgeons, who rely upon speed and skillful technique to produce satisfactory results. Most of us produce better results by instilling heparin prior to the placement of any vascular clamp. My own results certainly improved markedly after heeding Robert Linton's advice in 1962 to use systemic heparin. Exceptions include ruptured aneurysms and certain intrathoracic grafts.

Omission of heparinization has occasionally occurred during either a portion of the procedure or the entire procedure and in some instances has been well tolerated. Recognition of this omission indicates immediate corrective heparinization, along with investigation and distal irrigation of the previously clamped vessels.

TWISTING THE GRAFT

There are several marking methods to prevent twisting. Some synthetic tubes are premarked; otherwise a line may be painted along one surface with a sterile pen such as the Codman surgical marker. The same marking may be placed as a line along one side of a vein graft. If the graft is held in the Codman vein holder (Figure 12-2), the marking is easily done.[6]

A synthetic graft should first be anastomosed proximally, then pulled through the tunnel in the tissues, clamped distally, and allowed to fill with blood. In this way the surgeon can be certain of its orientation and fit prior to cutting and tailoring it at the site of the distal anastomosis.

A vein graft is even more likely to become twisted. Care in orienting the vein graft before and after it is drawn through the tissue tunnel should prevent twisting. After the graft is pulled

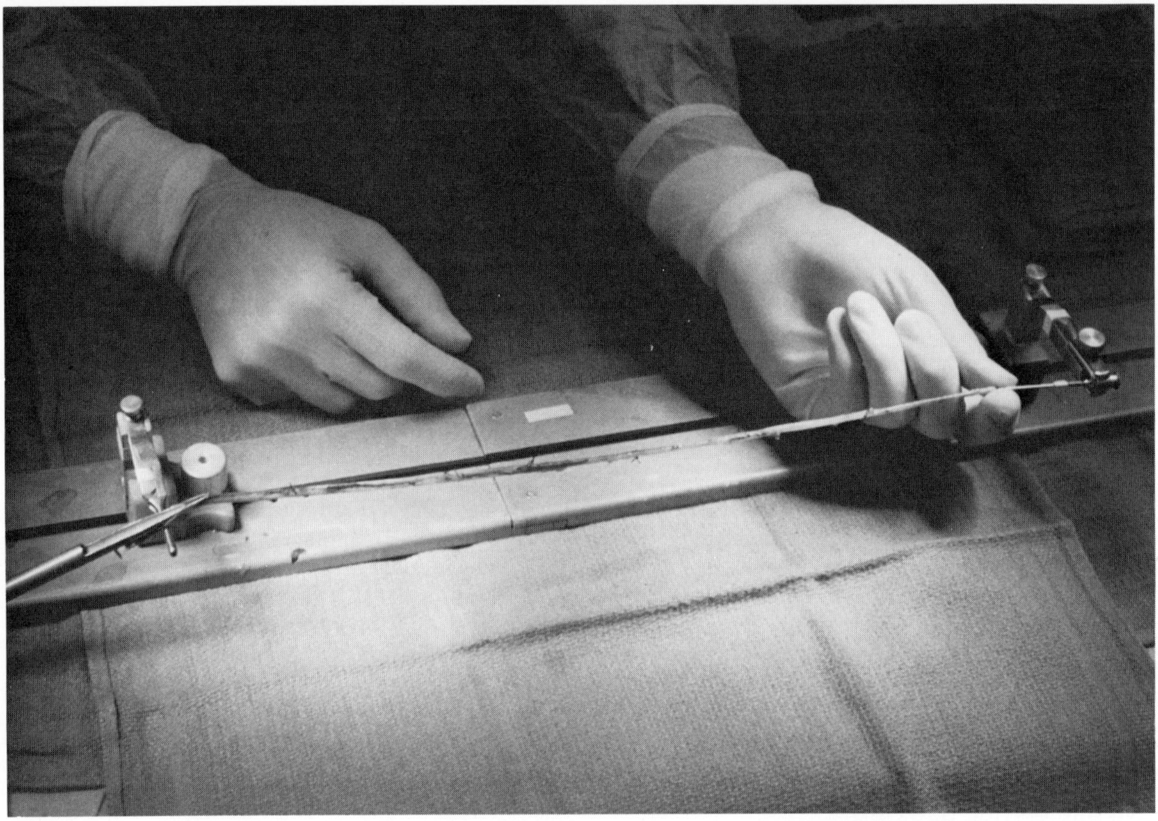

FIGURE 12-2 The vein holder[6] allows the saphenous vein to be handled by a single operator alone. *Right,* the autogenous saphenous vein is tied over the bulbous end of a small cannula held in the adjustable jaws of the apparatus. *Left,* the distal downstream end of the graft is held by the serrefine clamp shown near the operator's right hand. At this stage the tributaries have been tied, the graft has been marked, and the distal end has been removed from the clamp and mounted on the end of the Huang vein holder and is ready for the distal anastomosis.

through, the end should be clamped and fixed to prevent rotation until it is time for the anastomosis to be done.

Twisting should be suspected if the pulsation in the distal part of the vein graft is less than in its proximal portion. Immediate search for the twist is indicated. Since a part of the graft is tunneled, the twist may be difficult to locate. It may be necessary to assume a twist, divide the graft, open both divided ends completely to assure untwisting, and then rejoin the cut ends. The division and anastomosis should be diagonal, rather than an end-to-end butt anastomosis.

Illustrative Case

A 56-year-old diabetic male required femoropopliteal vein grafting for atherosclerotic occlusion of the superficial femoral artery. When the clamps were released at conclusion of the anastomoses, there was an excellent pulse in the proximal portion of the graft but only a feeble pulse in the hood of the distal anastomosis to the popliteal artery below the knee. Since the usual precautions to prevent twisting, including marking and careful passage of the graft through the tunnel, had been taken, it appeared that the problem lay within the lumen of the vein. Continued examination, however, indicated that there must be a twist within the tunnel. The graft was cut across tangentially in its midportion, and both ends were brought out for inspection with the clamps removed. It was apparent that there had been a 270° rotation. The cut ends were rejoined by an oblique anastomosis with 6-0 polypropylene. The distal pulse was strong. A completion arteriogram showed an excellent anastomosis and run-off vessels, and the posterior tibial pulse could be palpated.

Comment Despite the precautions of the entire team this technical error occurred in 1983. Even with a twist present, there was some distal pulse, but eventually the problem was recognized and corrected. It was an error, but its recognition led to correction and continued patency of the graft.

ANASTOMOTIC STENOSIS

A common technical error in vein grafting is improper suture placement at the heel of the proximal anastomosis or at the toe of the distal one. Bites placed too deeply cause stenosis and narrow the anastomosis.

Inspection at once reveals some of these. Completion arteriography demonstrates others. The ability to pass a dilator through the opening may provide a false signal, since the instrument expands the opening temporarily but leaves continued stenosis after its removal.

Anastomotic tightness may be relieved by resuturing. A surer method is to enlarge the anastomosis with a vein patch. Robert Linton, of Boston, publicized this patch graft, which bears his name. The proximal anastomosis is enlarged by the opening of the vein graft longitudinally just at the area of stenosis. It is closed with an oval portion of autogenous vein obtained from a nearby venous tributary.

When the stenosis occurs at the distal anastomosis, it is necessary to open the toe of the vein graft, as well as the adjacent distal host artery, to allow an oval-shaped venous patch to be placed with continuous 6-0 or 7-0 polypropylene. Naturally, this cuts the previous continuous suture, which must then be drawn out for several millimeters to enable a long enough end to be developed to be tied to the new suture and prevent the possibility of lateral unraveling and subsequent hemorrhage.

IMPROPER TENSION OF THE GRAFT

It is far better to place a vein which is too long, since the extra portion curves easily, than it is to place one which is too short, in which case the knee cannot be extended. Figure 12-3 shows successful correction of a vein graft which was originally too short to span the distance between the common femoral and popliteal arteries. The error was recognized at once, and the proximal anastomosis was shifted to a new position more inferior on the femoral artery.

Correct positioning is particularly important when a synthetic graft is used, particularly if polytetrafluoroethylene (PTFE) be the material, since the elasticity inherent in a crimped Dacron graft is not present in PTFE. The problem of a PTFE graft cut too short is so severe that particular attention should be paid to determining the site of the cut to be certain that the fit is accurate. The extremity should be extended and the graft held alongside the arteriotomy in the distal vessel while dye marks are placed on the PTFE graft prior to its precise cutting.

If a synthetic graft is cut too short, it may be possible to enlarge the arteriotomy proximally, to allow the anastomosis to be performed with a distal vein patch closure. However, it is probably wiser to select a new piece of synthetic graft for the distal anastomosis and then join the two pieces by a long ovoid anastomosis of the two grafts. Another solution is to change the proximal anastomosis to a more distal position.

It is uncommon to find that a synthetic graft has been cut too long. A small disproportion may be managed by some curvature of the graft within the wound. If the graft is considerably too long, the correction is by resection with anastomosis of the spatulated ends.

IMPROPER PATHWAY OF THE GRAFT

If, at completion of the anastomosis and release of the clamps, the graft is found to lie outside the skin rather than tunneled properly beneath it, the error is at once apparent. Since there is little practical value in discussing responsibility for this error, it is perhaps well to immediately assign a scapegoat, such as the anesthesiologist or the circulating nurse, and proceed to correct the situation by either dividing the skin bridge or cutting and reanastomosing the graft. The former is the better solution.

An even more glaring error once occurred when a completed vein graft was found to pass through the ring of a steel hemostat. Being unable to obtain a cutting instrument with sufficiently powerful jaws and leverage to cut this ring handle, the surgery team had to divide and reanastomose the graft itself. This rather ridiculous error does seem improbable in the presence of four team members, of which two were supposedly experienced in vascular surgery.

GRAFT-VESSEL DISPROPORTION

Luminal size differences between a large bypassing graft and a small host vessel lead to immediate irregularity of blood flow with eddying. There is a tendency to thrombosis as well as the later deposition of a thick neointima as the overly large graft becomes reduced in size to that of the run-off vessel.

Similarly dangerous are overly large patches (which are therefore aneurys-

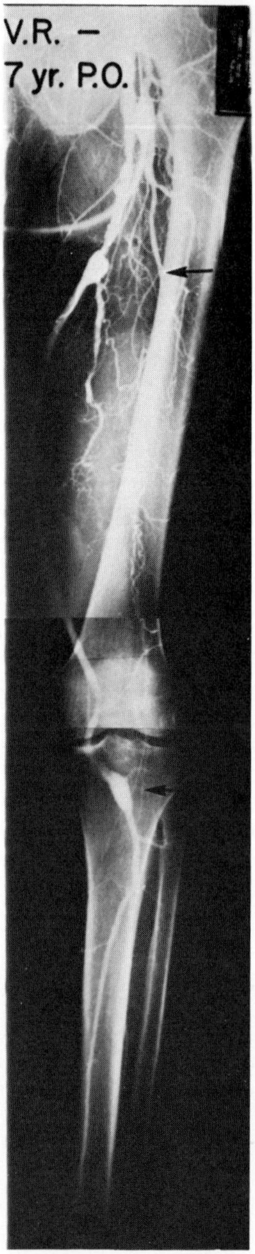

FIGURE 12-3 The vein graft was originally too short for the distance to be covered. The proximal anastomosis was at once shifted distally. This arteriogram, 7 years later, shows continued function.

mal) that tend to thrombosis. Our canine experiments showed that autogenous vein patches had a considerably higher success rate than did Dacron patches placed on dogs' femoral arteries. If either kind of patch graft was intentionally made too large (and thereby aneurysmal), the success rate was greatly diminished. As shown by Figure 12-4, 100 percent of 178 standard vein patches and 78 percent of 118 Dacron patches remained patent. The patency rates dropped precipitously when the same models were prepared with excessively large, aneurysmal patch grafts.[7] This explains why venous patch grafts placed on long femoral artery thromboendarterectomies had such a high failure rate in the past.[8]

Not many patients are good candidates for femoral or popliteal thromboendarterectomies. If they are done, most can be satisfactorily closed without patch grafting. If a long patch seems necessary, the tailoring is so critical that it may be better to change the entire procedure to a bypass graft.

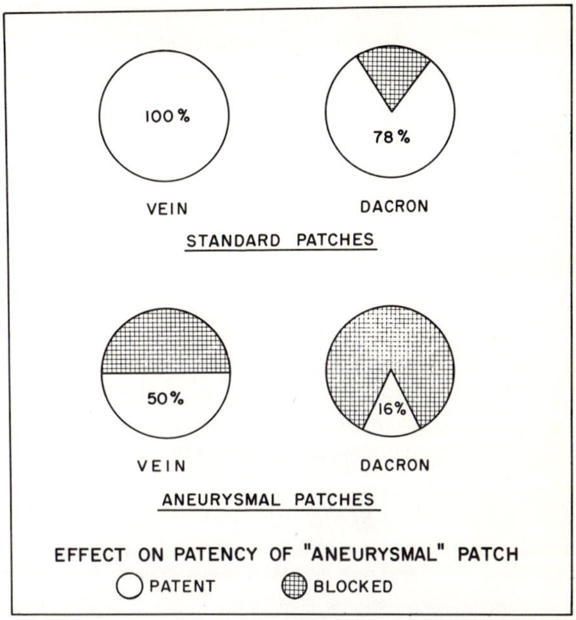

FIGURE 12-4 Summary of 296 lateral arterial patch grafts in dogs.[7] Well-fitted standard patches invariably remained patent, and 78 percent of Dacron patches remained patent in the dogs' superficial femoral arteries. When the patch grafts were placed loosely, the patency rates decreased precipitously.

DISTAL ANASTOMOSIS TO A VEIN

The inflammatory reaction about the popliteal vessels may make it difficult to differentiate the vein from the artery. The vein ordinarily lies medial and somewhat anterior to the artery and has visual and palpation characteristics which lead to its differentiation. Nevertheless, the graft can be incorrectly anastomosed to the vein. The use of routine completion angiography should reveal the situation and lead to immediate reanastomosis to the proper vessel.

PROBLEMS AT COMPLETION ANGIOGRAPHY

Various types of stenosis and intraluminal defects may be demonstrated by an arteriogram performed just after completion of the arterial reconstruction. These require immediate attention and are discussed further in Chapter 14.

MISCELLANEOUS

To the list of errors directly involving the arteries and the graft itself may be added mismanagement of the wound through which the operation is conducted. Perhaps the most common mismanagement is failure to achieve minute hemostasis, the sine qua non for the prevention of infection. Not only should every bleeding and oozing point be obliterated by tie, clip, or cautery prior to closure, but some consideration should be given to placement of a suction drain whenever the wound is extensive or undermined or when a secondary procedure has been done. It is probably better to provide a suction drain for every wound than to follow a policy of complete nonuse. Somewhere between these extremes lies the golden mean but, if in doubt, suction drainage should be implemented.

Fat and lymph nodes which are devitalized should be debrided prior to closure of the wound. Traumatized skin edges should be trimmed back prior to placement of the final sutures.

Excessive undermining of the skin edge should be avoided by placement of each of the incisions directly over the saphenous vein. The skin flap in Figure 12-5 required secondary removal and closure.

SUMMARY

Vascular surgery is an unforgiving and demanding discipline with little or no room for error, where mistakes are poorly tolerated and their resultant tragedies inexorable. Steady concentration is required from beginning to end. Physical stamina must allow for a needed secondary corrective procedure, even after previous hours of toil. Patience and persistence are necessary characteristics of the vascular surgeon. Imagination and innovative techniques must sometimes replace customary methods.

FIGURE 12-5 An ischemic skin flap was caused by excessive undermining during removal of the saphenous vein. It required secondary excision and closure.

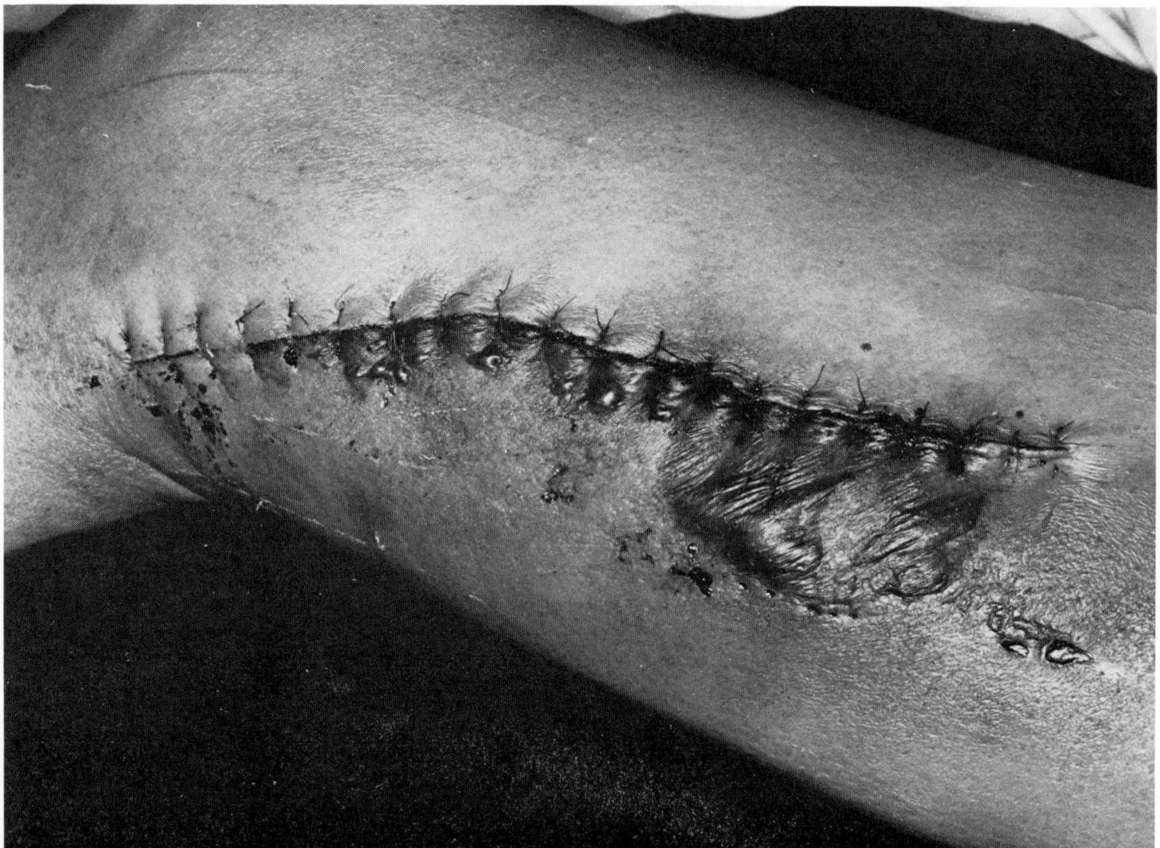

REFERENCES

1 Abbott WM, Wieland S, Austen WG: Structural changes during preparation of autogenous venous grafts. *Surgery* 1974, 76:1031.
2 Baumann PG, Catinella FP, Cunningham JN Jr, Spencer FC: Vein contraction and smooth muscle cell extensions as causes of endothelial damage during graft preparation. *Ann Surg* 1981, 194:199.
3 Krupski W, Thal E, Gewertz B, Buja L, Murphy M, Hagler H, Fry W: Endothelial response to venous injury. *Arch Surg* 1979, 114:1240.
4 LoGerfo F, Quist W, Crawshaw H, Haudenschild C: An improved technique for preservation of endothelial morphology in vein grafts. *Surgery* 1981, 90:1015.
5 Ramos JR, Berger K, Mansfield PB, Sauvage LR: Histologic fate and endothelial changes of distended and nondistended vein grafts. *Ann Surg* 1976, 183:205.
6 Dale WA: Holder to prepare vein grafts. *Surg Gynecol Obstet* 1978, 147:91.
7 Dale WA, Lewis MR, Cowden CM: Lateral vascular patch grafts. *Angiology* 1966, 17:229.
8 Edwards WS: Autogenous vein patch reconstruction of small leg arteries after endarterectomy. *J Cardiovasc Surg* (Torino) 1962, 3:106.

Invited Commentary

John Ochsner, M.D.
New Orleans, Louisiana

The most common error in femoropopliteal operations is improper selection of the patient. Rarely is a femoropopliteal bypass indicated for salvage of an extremity. Exceptions to this rule are the instances when there is absence of or an inadequate profunda femoris or when the bypass is to an isolated popliteal segment in which there is discontinuity between the isolated segment and the distal vessels. In my practice, femoropopliteal bypass operations are reserved for individuals desiring a better quality of life. Before 1970 femoropopliteal bypass was performed in 90 percent of our operations for revascularization of the lower extremity. Since then, less than 20 percent of these operations have been femoropopliteal bypasses, and most operations have been performed for salvage of the extremity in which the bypass needed to be extended to the tibial and peroneal arteries. It has been shown that the longevity of a viable extremity with a superficial femoral artery occlusion is greater in a patient who has not had a femoropopliteal bypass than in an individual who has had the operation.

Mention is made of a possible proximal obstruction to the femoral artery. It is helpful to thread a no. 5 or no. 8 infant feeding tube proximally into the aorta and measure pressures as one pulls back, to determine if there is a pressure gradient at any point. Isolated areas can be dilated, as mentioned, with an angioplasty catheter.

I prefer to do all distal anastomoses first, because one can properly determine the adequate length without undue sacrifice of graft and, more important, one is able to manipulate the graft during the anastomosis, to allow precise technique.

When there is inadequate length of vein and yet one desires autogenous tissue below the knee to the distal popliteal segment, one can perform either a composite graft or, in our preference, a bypass with a prosthesis to the proximal part of an isolated endarterectomized distal superficial femoral artery, and then use the limited length of autogenous vein to bypass from the distal part of this endarterectomized segment, down to the distal popliteal artery.

In the illustrated case of a twisted graft, I would prefer to perform an arteriogram to determine the cause than to blindly transect the graft and do an end-to-end anastomosis after realignment. The arteriogram can differentiate between twist and intraluminal obstruction by the typical hourglass or tapered appearance in a twisted vessel.

In regard to improper tension of the graft, it is important to remove any folded sheets or towels that are usually in place to flex the knees. The leg should be extended during measurement of the full length of vein required.

I don't believe that I have heard of running the graft outside the skin before; surely this is a unique error.

We have found it helpful, in performing a proper distal anastomosis, to place a Parsonnet dilator thru the graft and anastomotic site and use interrupted sutures at the toe of the anastomosis to ensure a patent lumen.

One of the most common errors in femoropopliteal bypass operations is injury to the saphenous nerve in procurement of the saphenous vein. This nerve runs adjacent to the artery, and extreme care should be taken not to sever or injure the nerve, because the paresthesia associated with this error can be very irritating to the patient.

13 EXTRAANATOMIC GRAFTS

Revascularizations performed outside the usual anatomic positions are useful in two circumstances: first, to avoid an infected field, and second, to limit the procedure to extracavitary soft tissues because of the higher mortality and complication rate associated with intrathoracic and intraabdominal operations.

Blaisdell is generally credited with developing extraanatomic techniques, but he modestly has traced the evolution of these operations back a decade earlier to Freeman and Leeds's use of the splenic artery to bypass an abdominal aortic aneurysm in 1952[1] and also to their transposition of a superficial femoral artery to form a femorofemoral bypass.[2] McCaughan and Kahn reported an external iliac artery used similarly in 1960.[3]

Blaisdell bypassed an infected aortic field in 1960 by attaching a Dacron graft to the thoracic aorta, "passing it down the lateral side of the abdomen to the groin and then [anastomosing it] to the left femoral artery" and performing a "crossover femoral-femoral graft." This established the concept that blood flow through a small conduit could support the lower half of the body.[4] Subsequent laboratory experience indicated that an artery smaller than the aorta, such as the axillary, could be used as the donor site without compromising the upper extremity. The first axillofemoral bypass was performed in 1962.[5] In the same year Vetto described 10 successful femorofemoral grafts.[6]

Since then these operations and their modifications have been practiced widely with general satisfaction. Let us examine some questions which arise in connection with them.

Hemodynamics and the Steal Phenomenon

The principles of blood flow through and beyond extraanatomic bypasses, which were learned from femoral crossover models and patients, are applicable to other such shunts. Thus, blood flow in a nonstenotic donor artery increases greatly to furnish blood to the new peripheral field, as shown by Ehrenfeld, Harris, and Wylie in 1968.[7] The change may be enormous—as much as 11-fold.[8]

If there is stenosis of the donor vessel, a "steal" from its ipsilateral peripheral field may occur, as blood is shunted to the contralateral limb.[9] Bergan, Yao, and Flinn concluded that the recipient limb rarely is returned to a normal hemodynamic status, although the clinical situation is improved.[10]

From such studies it is recognized that blood flow in the donor artery increases readily to provide enough blood for the arterial field supplied by the donor artery as well as enough blood for the newly opened field. However, if there is a significant stenosis in the donor artery, this increase may not occur and the distal flow and blood supply then depend on the respective peripheral resistances of the two peripheral arterial fields.

In properly chosen patients the hemodynamic changes which may be shown in the laboratory are rarely of clinical significance. None have occurred in my series of 90 femoral crossover grafts.

Progressive Atherosclerotic Disease

Brief and Parsonnet developed the idea that femorofemoral grafting diminished the progression of atherosclerosis in the donor iliac artery,[11] although a few did eventually develop lesions.[12] Leeds also noted less progression of disease among cross-femoral graft patients when compared with unilateral iliac-to-femoral graftees.[13] The reason for this is unknown.

Configuration and Anastomoses

Long arterial anastomoses provide protection against technical errors which may lead to later stenosis. The graft should therefore be brought alongside the native donor vessel to allow a spatulated end-to-side junction (Figure 13-1). "Plugging in" the graft to the artery by end-to-side "T" anastomosis should be avoided.

Proper anastomoses lead to a gentle curve as the graft departs the vicinity of the native vessel

FIGURE 13-1 A long anastomosis placed on the anteromedial aspect of the recipient common femoral artery prevents kinking and allows maximum blood flow through this Dacron femorofemoral crossover graft.

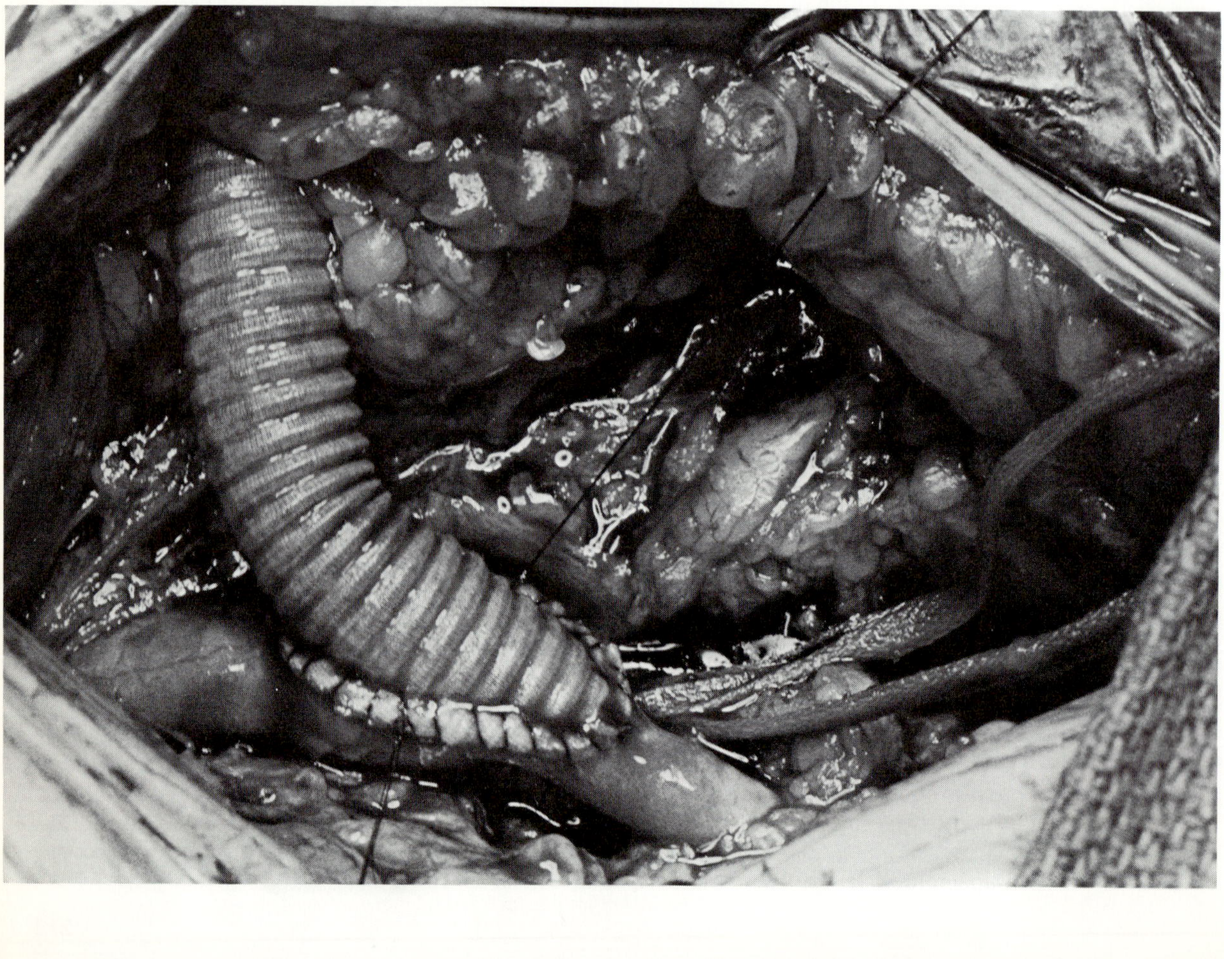

to course inferiorly along the chest wall (if it is an axillofemoral graft) or to lie as an "S" (if it is a crossover femoral graft). Grafts anastomosed to host vessels at a low angle (15°) provide better flow characteristics than those at a high angle (45 or 60°).[14]

Optimal Graft Material

To a considerable extent the material depends upon the length needed and to a lesser degree upon the position. Autogenous vein, usually the saphenous, may be chosen for a bypass between the axillary arteries, since the graft is relatively short (Figure 13-2). It is preferred to a synthetic for that position, although the latter has been used successfully many times, such as for the patient in Figure 13-3.

Similarly, saphenous vein may be placed between the femoral arteries, but that distance is short and little motion occurs. A synthetic tube performs as well and allows the saphenous vein to be reserved for other use.

Finally, a short segment of vein is quite useful in the several reconstructions which may be needed in the root of the neck between various segments of the carotid, subclavian, and vertebral arteries.

Long bypasses, specifically the axillary-to-femoral shunts, require synthetic tubes. Whether Dacron or polytetrafluoroethylene (PTFE) is better is not known;[15] both are presently acceptable. My preference for PTFE reflects its ease in suturing and lack of the need to preclot.

FIGURE 13-2 This autogenous saphenous vein graft was placed between the axillary arteries to bypass an innominate arterial occlusion.

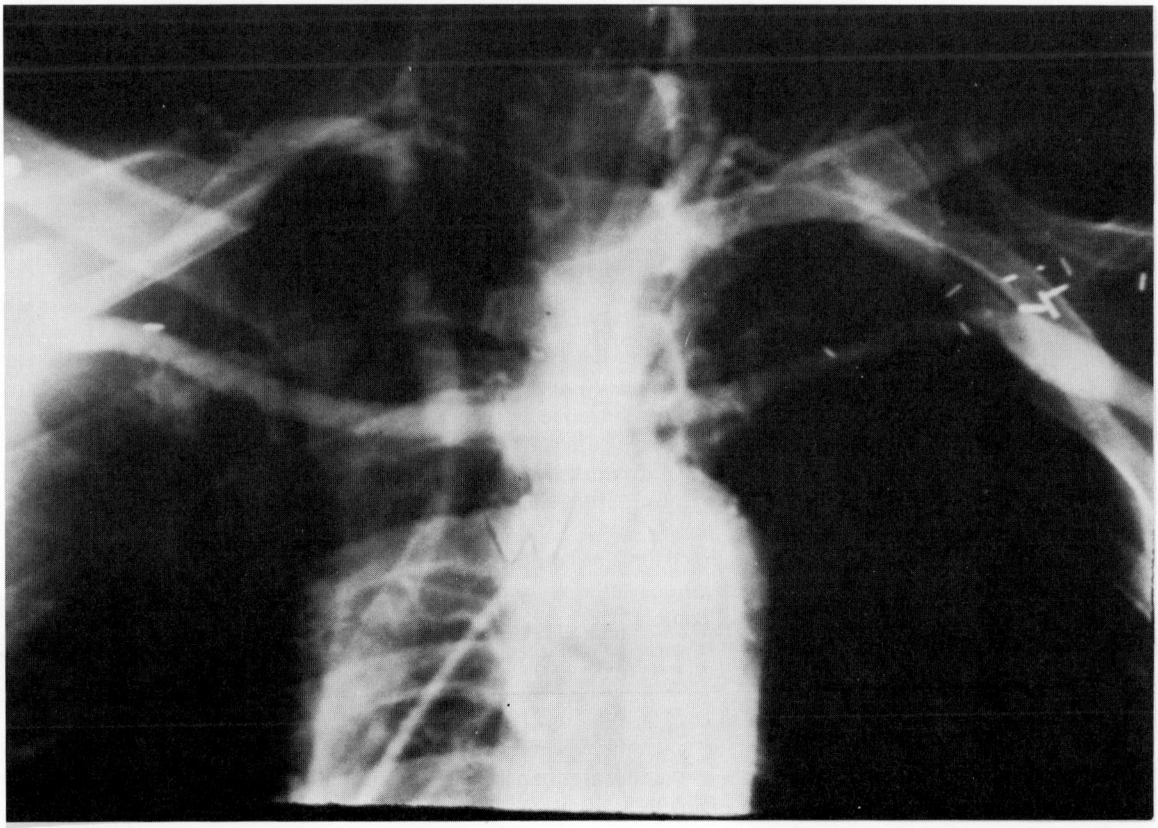

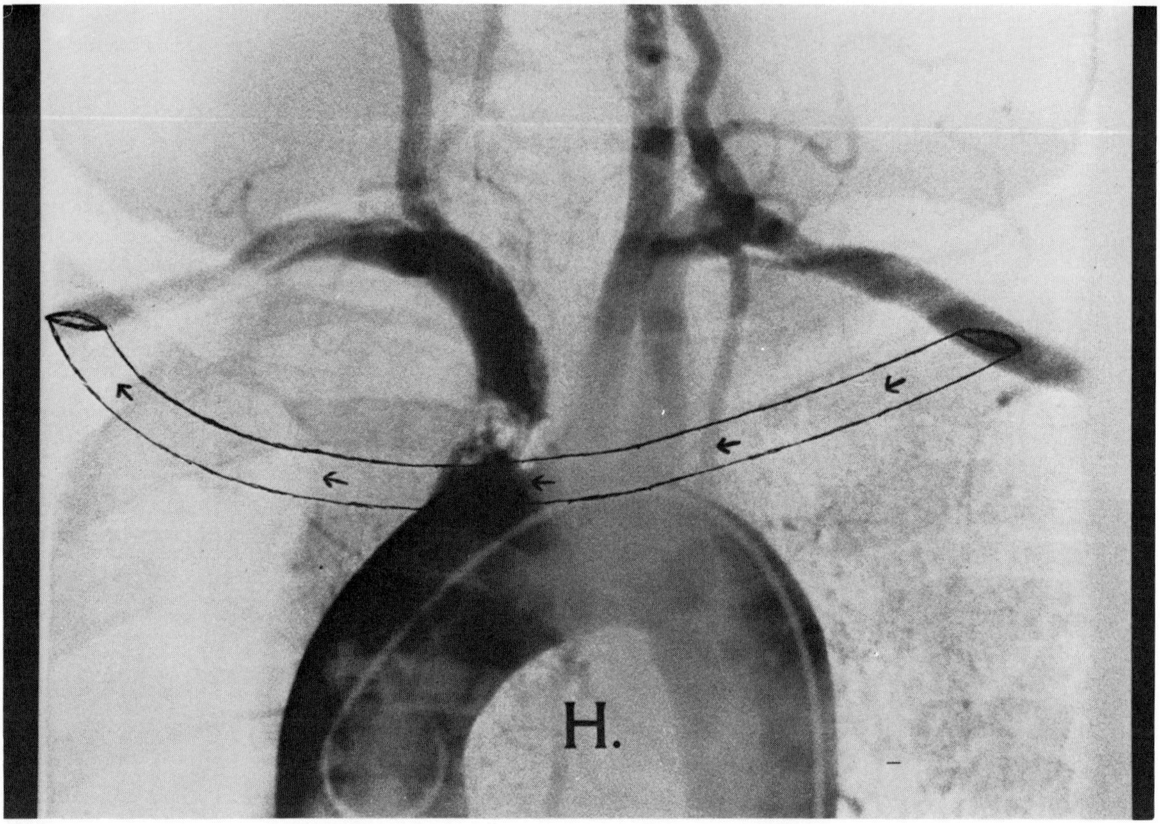

FIGURE 13-3 PTFE or a Dacron tube may be used as an axilloaxillary bypass around an occluded innominate artery.

The Risks of Extraanatomic and Direct Intracavitary Reconstructions

The trade-off is less risk versus somewhat lower long-term patency rates. In some situations, such as at the root of the neck, the patency rates are so favorable that intrathoracic procedures are essentially outmoded. In other areas, such as in the aortoiliac system, the 20 to 30 percent lesser long-term patency rate must be viewed against the greater hazards of placing an aortofemoral graft, whose risks vary with the individual. Another factor to be considered is the need for revascularization, which may be great if a limb is about to be lost but is often not needed for claudication alone.

It is well to view these procedures as complementary rather than as competitive, since each has somewhat different indications and risks to be fitted to the individual, and not to insist upon one way or the other for all comers.

Results of Extraanatomic Grafts

It would be informative to compare the results of various bypasses with those of direct revascularizations. Unfortunately, when the reported statistics were placed in tabular form, the complexity of the result was more confusing than helpful, so the table was deleted. (Rutherford's attempt at such a table, along with a discussion of these problems, will interest some readers.[16])

There were differences in the periods of time of the surveys, criteria of patency were not the same, selections of patients varied, and the indications for the several bypasses were different. It is currently impossible to predict the prognosis for any of the procedures from studying the published literature. Some general observations do appear valid.

It is fair to say that under the same conditions the patency rates of extraanatomic bypasses will not be as good as those for direct arterial reconstructions. Further, except for the relatively simple femorofemoral graft, the technical problems and time involved for the operation may be no less, although an extracavitary procedure should be less risky. The few axillofemoral grafts I have done parallel the paucity of these by other surgeons in our hospital during the last 10 years. The axillofemorofemoral graft is not often needed.

Failure of Extraanatomic Grafts

Low flow rates due to poor run-off, anastomotic errors, and intimal hyperplasia may singly or together account for most thromboses. Thus, of the 13 thromboses among 51 operations in Flanigan's group, 8 instances were ascribed to severe or progressive outflow disease and a single instance each was ascribed to infection and technical failure.[17]

Graft thrombosis due to external pressure may be a myth, since studies of six patients lying on their graft side showed no ill effects from body weight on the segmental Doppler pressure or on pulse volume.[18] On the other hand, Lee and associates recently doubted these conclusions. Their six patients showed "marked reduction in pulsatile blood flow" in several positions when compared with normal patients. They suggested tying a patient's wrist to the bedside to prevent lying on the graft side.[19] Their argument is not convincing, nor the method practical.

SPECIFIC PROCEDURES

Femorofemoral Grafts

Simplicity, low risk, and good patency rates recommend this reconstruction rather than an axillary-to-femoral one when possible. Poor-risk patients with unilateral iliac occlusion are notable candidates, although percutaneous transluminal dilation is an even simpler alternative if the lesion is short.

The clinical implication of the hemodynamic studies related above is that the iliac, as well as the femoropopliteal, run-off systems must be clearly visualized angiographically. This must be done to detect stenosis of the intended donor iliac system as well as occlusion of the run-off on that side, in which case worsening is possible. Hemodynamic study of the donor side's response to exercise may also provide a preoperative warning of a likely steal by a femorofemoral graft. Otherwise, a variety of noninvasive techniques have failed to predict more accurately than arteriograms and clinical examination the result of using the iliac artery as a donor.

If there is no stenosis in the donor iliac artery and both femoropopliteal systems are patent, the outlook for a crossover femoral arterial graft is excellent. A decade ago Plecha and Pories reported a 4- to 5-year cumulative patency rate of 87 percent in 75 patients.[20] The success rate in the Flanigan 51-patient series varied from 90 percent, when the donor artery was patent, to 41 percent, when there was recipient artery disease, to 21 percent, when there was less than 50 percent donor artery stenosis plus recipient outflow disease, to zero, when there was over 50 percent donor artery stenosis. Their cumulative patency rate at 5 years was 74 percent, and the 30-day mortality rate was 4 percent.[17] The Newark Beth Israel 154-patient series had an 81 percent 5-year and a 77 percent 10-year cumulative patency rate with 5 percent mortality.[21]

Femorofemoral bypass also averts the potential sexual dysfunction sometimes associated with aortoiliac dissection and in selected cases at once corrects extremity ischemia and erectile dysfunction. Thus Merchant and DePalma returned function to 17 of 23 preoperatively impotent patients.[22]

Indications Indications for cross-femoral grafting include (1) chronic unilateral iliac arterial occulsion which is not amenable to dilation, (2) occlusion of one limb of an aortobifemoral graft, and (3) fear of sexual dysfunction if an aortic operation is done for a male. Indications have been extended to include severe claudication. Cooley's 85-patient series showed an uncommonly high number of claudication corrections (62 percent) versus salvage procedures (38 percent).[23] The Northwestern group addressed this issue in 1981, reporting 44 claudicators, whose cumulative patency rate at 4 years was 85 percent. They found hemodynamic evidence of flow diversion from the lower limb in a significant number of patients, even though there were no symptoms of ischemia.[24] It was agreed by them and several discussants that there is not yet any preoperative test which will predetermine these donor limb changes. The results indicate that caution is needed in expanding indications to include claudication.

It appears reasonable to suggest that a disabled claudicator whose risk is too great for aorto-bifemoral grafting and whose disease is too severe for transluminal angioplasty should walk to the point of pain and accept that. If symptoms progress to rest pain or to threatened loss of tissue, the indications become different.

In view of the risk of sexual dysfunction it is difficult to justify an aortobifemoral graft for a potent male with any situation short of a salvage limb. Certainly most of these patients prefer claudication to the risk of sexual failure.

Technical Principles Bypass from the iliac arteries, using a retromuscular tunnel, is needlessly complex. It is simpler to place the graft subcutaneously between the common femoral arteries. Long anastomoses are performed with the graft in an "S" configuration, but not straight across as is the crossbar of an "H." The femoral arteriotomies to which the graft is attached should lie on the anteromedial (rather than directly anterior) aspect of the host vessels, to avoid kinking of the graft.

Dacron or PTFE may be preferred by the individual surgeon. Attachment of the donor side first, with precise tailoring of the recipient end, will prevent placing a graft whose length is incorrect.

Concomitant profundaplasty is mandatory if indicated (Figures 13-4 and 13-5).

If occlusion of the superficial femoral artery exists distally, there should be consideration of continuing the graft to another distal anastomosis to bypass that, in which event the graft has an "L" configuration with a side-to-side anastomosis in the groin. While the femoropopliteal component of the "L" has a lower patency rate than does the femorofemoral component (63 percent versus 91 percent at 42 months in the 13 patients of Schuler's group[25]), the latter's results are not diminished by the distal limb.

Occasionally a "U" configuration is used to provide a crossover limb to the contralateral femoral artery as well as bilateral femoropopliteal limbs (Figure 13-6).

Axillofemoral Grafts

Evolution of this long graft from a single limb to bilateral ones to the present axillobifemoral bypass has led to increased patency rates due to greater blood flow in the long segment of tubing which courses from shoulder to groin before supplying the ipsilateral femoral as well as the crossover tube to the contralateral femoral artery. The long-term results average about 20 percent less patency than aortobifemoral grafts and about 10 to 20 percent less then femoral crossover grafts.[1]

The high patency rates of Burrell, Wheeler, Gregory, Snyder, Gayle, and Mason of 1982 are difficult to interpret, since both unifemoral and bifemoral grafts were included, later successful thrombectomies were counted as patencies, and many of the grafts were done for claudication.[26] The 76 percent 5-year patency rate of Johnson and associates also suggested this bypass as competitive to aortofemoral grafts, particularly if the lesser initial risks are considered. In fact, there was a 5-year cumulative patency rate of 76 percent for both 88 aortobifemoral grafts and 56

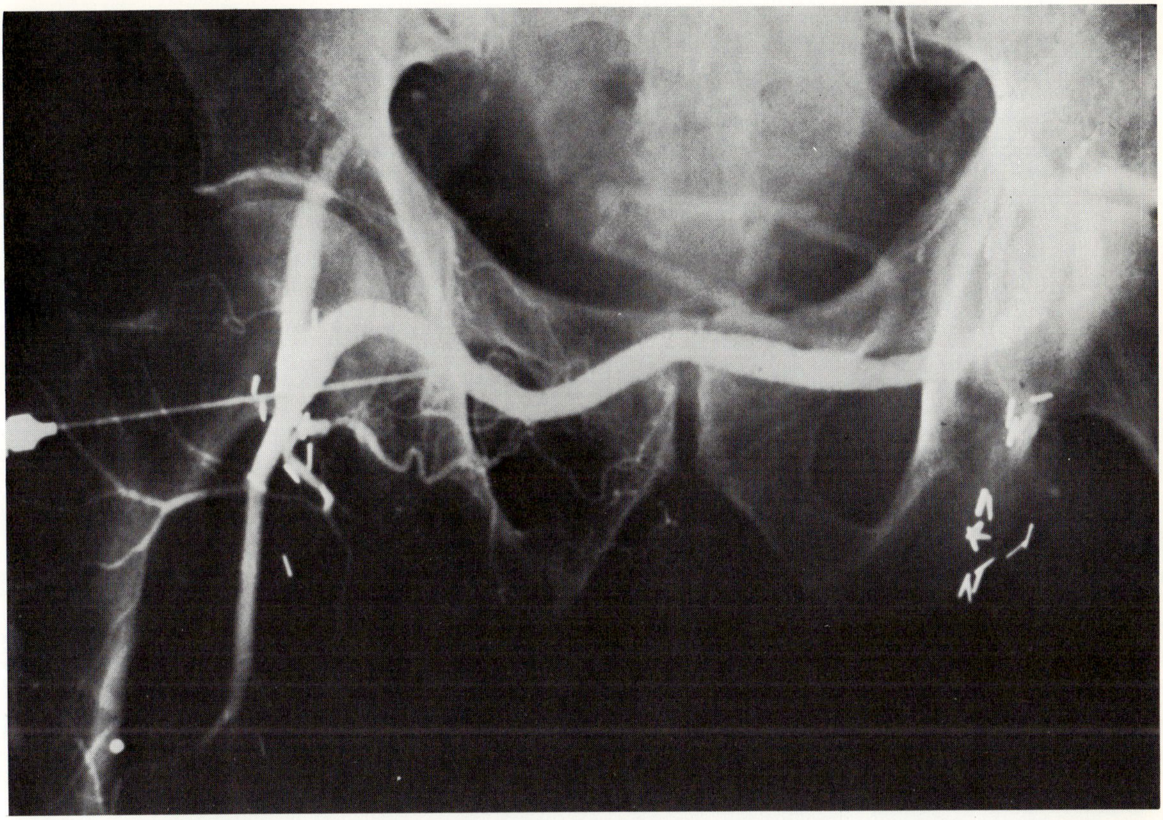

FIGURE 13-4 This 8-mm PTFE femorofemoral crossover graft flows into the endarterectomized profunda branch of the femoral artery.

axillobifemoral ones. To be noted, however, were restorations of patency by thrombectomy, which were counted as successes in the latter group.[27]

Indications Indications center around (1) infection of a previous aortofemoral graft, where an entirely new field is needed, and (2) an occasional patient with complete aortoiliac occlusion whose overall condition precludes aortobifemoral grafting.

Technical Principles The technical principles include the usual long anastomosis to the proximal portion of the axillary artery just after it emerges from beneath the clavicle. Whether the pectoralis minor muscle lies here or there (or is simply severed) is immaterial. The graft passes inferiorly in the subcutaneous tissue of the lateral chest and abdominal wall, and the tunnel is often interrupted by small midaxillary line incisions to allow the tunneling clamp to be guided properly.

Dacron or PTFE of 8- or 10-mm diameter may be used. It is cut accurately and anastomosed ipsilaterally. The crossing graft should be placed quite distal, to encourage flow through the entire length of the long tube. The anastomosis for the crossover graft may be just proximal to the ipsilateral anastomosis or to the hood of it (Figure 13-7), or even from the common femoral artery just distal to it, although the latter is unusual. Blaisdell's use of the distal divided end of the common femoral artery above the ipsilateral femoral anastomosis is another alternative, although that prevents any reflux of blood back into the pelvis.[1]

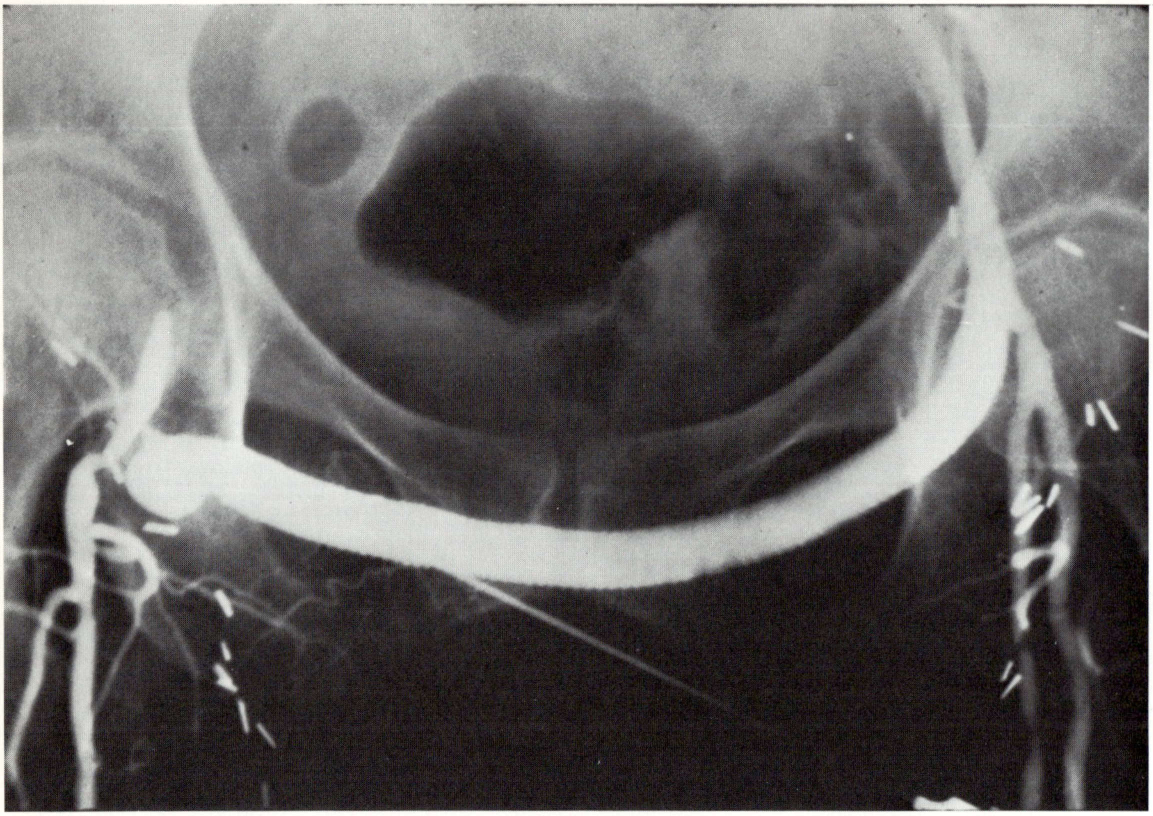

FIGURE 13-5 Anastomotic stenosis is uncommon but did occur in this PTFE femorofemoral graft to the profunda femoris. The stenosis was corrected by a secondary endarterectomy with replacement of the distal end of the synthetic tube.

An alternative method based the graft upon the aorta or a common iliac artery (via a retroperitoneal approach) instead of using the axillary artery as a donor in 75 patients, with an 87 percent 4- to 5-year cumulative patency rate.[20] No further development of this procedure has occurred.

Extraanatomic Splanchnic Bypasses

Conventional bypass grafting from the aorta to renal or mesenteric arteries may be difficult because of atherosclerotic disease. One solution is to replace the diseased aorta with a graft from which side arms originate to the kidney or mesenteric arteries. A simple alternative, particularly if there is no other reason to resect the aorta, is to base the graft, usually a saphenous vein, upon the iliac artery, which is often less diseased. The 10 cases of Wichterman and Stansel did well with several variations of this technique,[28] and personal experience also has been favorable in selected cases.

Obturator Bypass

This somewhat complicated extraanatomic shunt was originally described by Shaw and Baue in 1963.[29] It occasionally offers escape from a groin infection following a previous arterial recon-

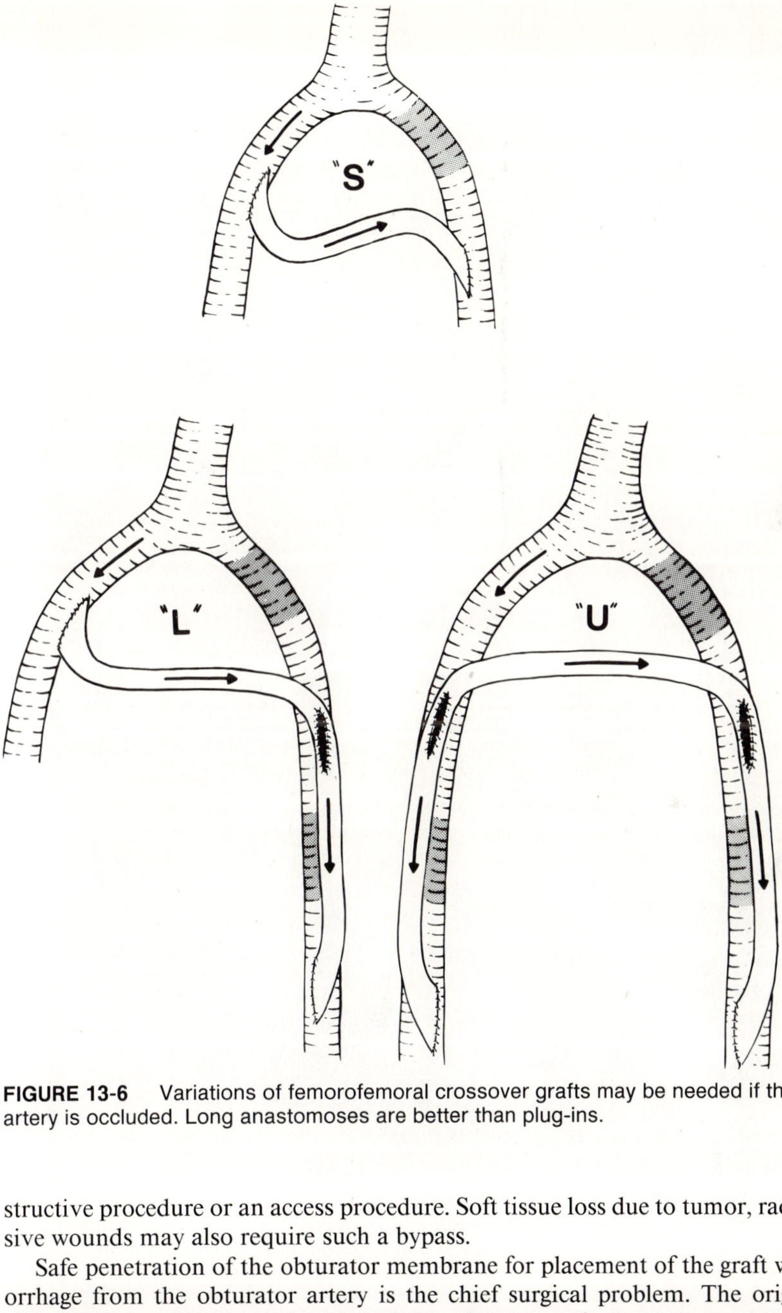

FIGURE 13-6 Variations of femorofemoral crossover grafts may be needed if the superficial femoral artery is occluded. Long anastomoses are better than plug-ins.

structive procedure or an access procedure. Soft tissue loss due to tumor, radionecrosis, or extensive wounds may also require such a bypass.

Safe penetration of the obturator membrane for placement of the graft without causing hemorrhage from the obturator artery is the chief surgical problem. The original approach from above has generally been altered in favor of passage of a long clamp or tunneler from a distal medial thigh incision, traversing the adductor magnus muscle. Through a lower abdominal extraperitoneal approach a hand is placed within the pelvis superior to the obturator membrane, to guide the tunneler or clamp from below upward. The penetrating pressure should be directed medially and anteriorly to avoid hemorrhage.

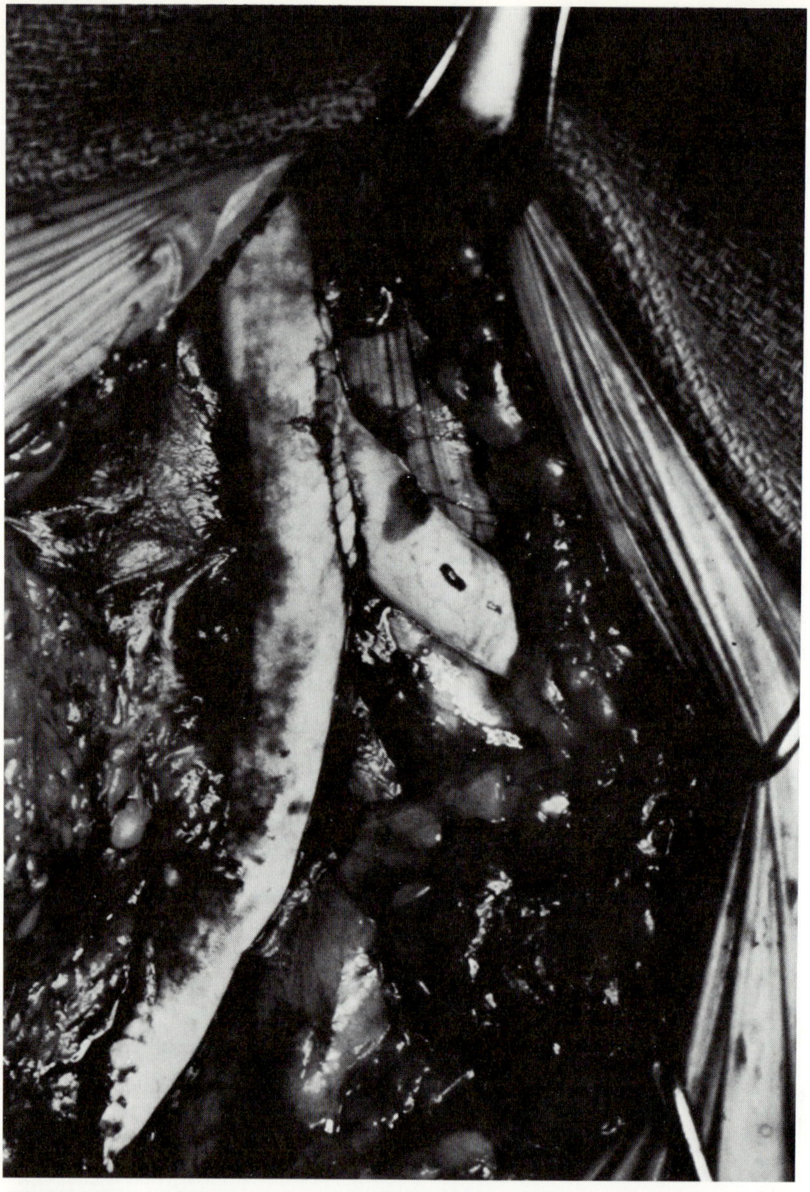

FIGURE 13-7 PTFE was used for this axillobifemoral bypass. More distal placement of the crossing portion of the graft would not have allowed a long anastomosis to be constructed but would have created more blood flow through the distal portion of the right limb of the graft.

The extraperitoneal route also allows easy access to the external iliac artery for early proximal control as well as formation of the proximal arterial anastomosis.

No one has extensive experience with this procedure, the largest number of reported cases being 13 by Van Det and Brands.[30] The excellent summary of the literature by Prenner and Rendl will be worthwhile reading for a surgeon contemplating this operation.[31]

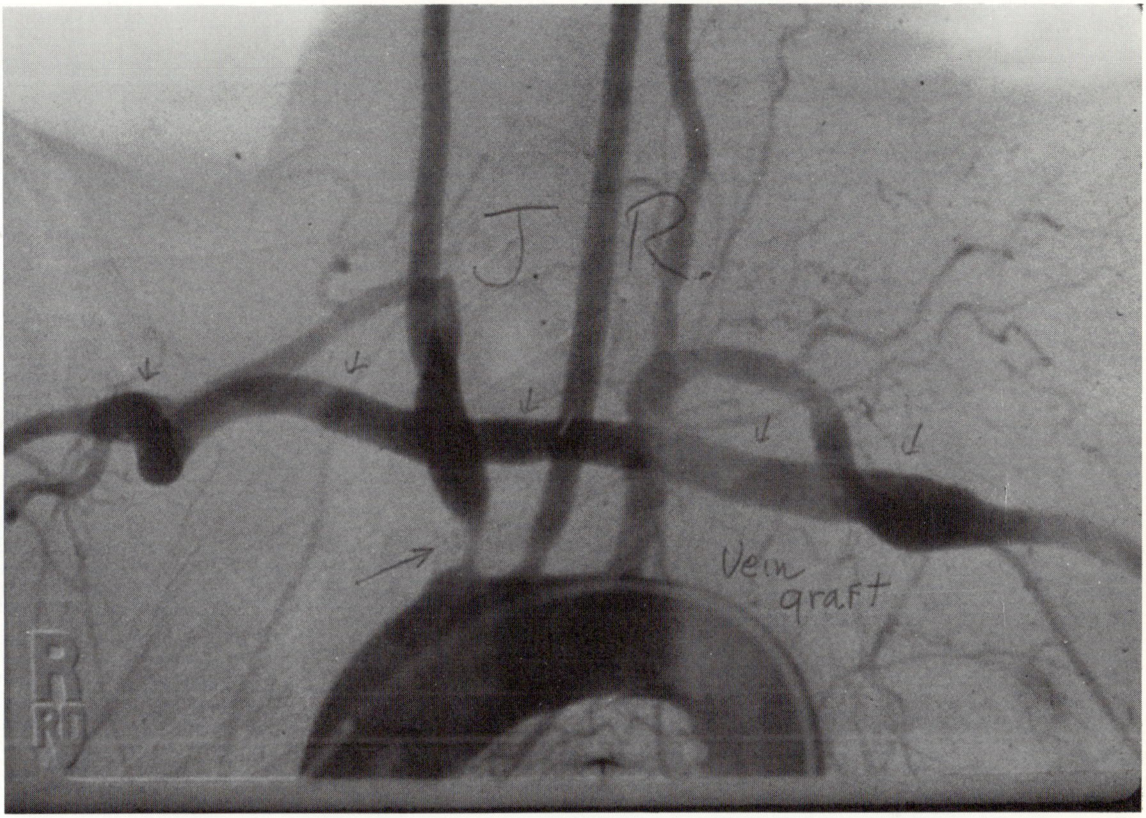

FIGURE 13-8 An autogenous vein graft placed between the axillary arteries bypasses a tight innominate arterial stenosis.

An alternative to this deep and generally unfamiliar route is to pass the graft laterally in the subcutaneous tissue. Another method is to place a crossover via the perineum.

Axilloaxillary Shunts

While subclavian-to-subclavian bypasses are possible, they require deeper dissection and the course of the graft is more convoluted. Despite earlier personal successes with these, using a saphenous vein graft, the simpler placement of a PTFE or saphenous vein graft between the axillary vessels is now recommended (Figure 13-8). Intrathoracic procedures can usually be avoided.

REFERENCES

1 Blaisdell FW, Holcroft JW, Ward RE: Axillo-femoral and femoro-femoral bypass: History and evolution of technique (Chapter 11), in Greenhalgh RM (ed); *Extra-Anatomic and Secondary Arterial Reconstruction.* Pitman, Bath 1982, p 84.

2 Freeman NE, Leeds FH: Operations on large arteries: Application of recent advances. *Calif Med* 1959, 77:229.

3 McCaughan JJ Jr, Kahn SF: Cross-over graft for unilateral occlusive disease of the iliofemoral arteries. *Ann Surg* 1960, 151:26.

4 Blaisdell FW, DeMattei GA, Gauder PJ: Extraperitoneal thoracic aorta to femoral bypass graft as replacement for infected aortic bifurcation prosthesis. *Am J Surg* 1961, 102:583.
5 Blaisdell FW, Hall AD: Axillary-femoral artery bypass for lower extremity ischemia. *Surgery* 1963, 54:563.
6 Vetto RM: The treatment of unilateral iliac artery obstruction with a transabdominal, subcutaneous femoro-femoral graft. *Surgery* 1962, 52:342.
7 Ehrenfeld WK, Harris JD, Wylie EW: Vascular steal phenomenon: An experimental study. *Am J Surg* 1968, 116:192.
8 Shin CS, Chaudhry AG: The hemodynamics of extra-anatomic bypass grafts. *Surg Gynecol Obstet* 1979, 148:567.
9 Trimble IR, Stonesifer GL Jr, Wilgis EFS, Montague AC: Criteria for femorofemoral bypass from clinical and hemodynamic studies. *Ann Surg* 1972, 175:985.
10 Bergan JJ, Yao JST, Flinn WR: Limitations of femoro-femoral bypass (Chapter 16), in Greenhalgh RM (ed): *Extra-Anatomic and Secondary Arterial Reconstruction.* Pitman, Bath 1982, p 131.
11 Brief DK, Alpert J, Parsonnet V: Crossover femorofemoral grafts. *Arch Surg* 1972, 105:889.
12 Dick LS, Brief DK, Alpert J, Brener BJ, Goldenkranz R, Parsonett V: A twelve year experience with femorofemoral crossover grafts. *Arch Surg* 1980, 115:1359.
13 Leeds FH: Discussion of Dick LS, Brief DK, Alpert J, Brener BJ, Goldenkrane R, Parsonett V: A twelve year experience with femorofemoral crossover grafts. *Arch Surg* 1980, 115:1364.
14 Crawshaw HE, Quist WC, LoFergo FW: Flow disturbances at the distal end-to-side anastomosis (Chapter 20), in Greenhalgh RM (ed): *Extra-Anatomic and Secondary Arterial Reconstruction.* Pitman, Bath 1982, p 177.
15 Courbier R, Jausseran JM, Bergeron P: Axillary femoral bypass: Material of choice (Chapter 15) in Greenhalgh RM (ed): *Extra-Anatomic and Secondary Arterial Reconstruction.* Pitman, Bath 1982, p 122.
16 Rutherford RB: Results of extra-anatomic bypass: Reasons for variance and relationship to indications (Chapter 13), in Greenhalgh RM (ed): *Extra-Anatomic and Secondary Arterial Reconstruction.* Pitman, Bath 1982, p 108.
17 Flanigan DP, Pratt DG, Goodreau JJ, Burnham SJ, Yao JST, Bergan JJ: Hemodynamic and angiographic guidelines in selection of patients for femorofemoral bypass. *Arch Surg* 1978, 113:1257.
18 Jarowenko MV, Buchbinder D, Shah DM: Effect of external pressure on axillofemoral bypass grafts. *Ann Surg* 1981, 193:274.
19 Lee BY, Thoden WR, McCann WJ, Madden JL: Effects of changes in body position on axillofemoral bypass. *Contemp Surg* 1984, 24:65.
20 Plecha FR, Pories WJ: Extra-anatomic bypasses for aorto-iliac disease in high risk patients. *Surgery* 1976, 80:480.
21 Brief DK, Brener BJ, Alpert J: Crossover femoro-femoral grafts: A 15 year experience. *J Cardiovasc Surg* (Torino) 1983, 24:381.
22 Merchant RF Jr, DePalma RG: Effects of femorofemoral grafts on postoperative sexual function: Correlation with penile pulse volume recordings. *Surgery* 1981, 90:962.
23 Subram AN, Urrutia-S CO, Ott DA, Cooley DA: Femorofemoral bypass: Prognostic factors. *J Tex Heart Inst* 1983, 10:257.
24 Harris JP, Flinn WR, Rudo ND, Bergan JJ, Yao JST: Assessment of donor limb hemodynamics in femorofemoral bypass for claudication. *Surgery* 1981, 90:764.
25 Schuler JJ, Flanigan DP, Ryan TJ, Buchbinder D, Castronuovo JJ: Crossover femorofemoropopliteal sequential bypass for combined ipsilateral iliac and femoropopliteal occlusive disease. *Arch Surg* 1984, 119:460.
26 Burrell MJ, Wheeler JR, Gregory RT, Snyder SO Jr, Gayle RG, Mason MS: Axillofemoral bypass: A ten-year review. *Ann Surg* 1982, 195:796.
27 Johnson WC, Lofergo FW, Vollman RW, Corson JO, O'Hara ET, Mannick JA, Nabseth DC: Is axillo-bilateral femoral graft an effective substitute for aortic-bilateral iliac-femoral graft? *Ann Surg* 1977, 186:123.
28 Wichterman HC, Stansel HC Jr: Simplified splanchnic artery revascularization using extra-anatomic bypass grafts: A report of ten cases. *Arch Surg* 1979, 114:1052.
29 Shaw RS, Baue AE: Management of sepsis complicating arterial reconstruction surgery. *Surgery* 1963, 53:75.

30 Van Det RJ, Brands LC: The obturator foramen bypass: An alternative procedure in ilio-femoral artery revascularization. *Surgery* 1981, 89:543.
31 Prenner KV, Rendl RH: Indications and technique of obturator bypass (Chapter 11), in Greenhalgh RM (ed): *Extra-Anatomic and Secondary Arterial Reconstruction.* Pitman, Bath 1982, p 201.

Invited Commentary

John A. Mannick, M.D.
Boston, Massachusetts

This chapter summarizes the pertinent literature on extraanatomic bypass grafts and offers the perspective of an experienced and thoughtful vascular surgeon. I have one philosophic difference, which has to do with the indications for femorofemoral grafts. A recent analysis of the results obtained on our service with conventional aortoiliac reconstruction and extraanatomic bypass grafts done for aortoiliac occlusive disease has shown that aortofemoral bypass grafts have a 5-year patency rate of 87 percent. Femorofemoral grafts have a cummulative 5-year patency rate of approximately 80 percent, and axillobifemoral grafts have a 5-year patency rate of 70 percent (when all grafts which require thrombectomy are considered as failures). The axillobifemoral grafts have statistically significantly inferior late results when compared with aortobifemoral grafts, and like Dr. Dale, we do not believe that the axillofemoral graft should be offered as an alternative to aortofemoral bypass grafting in any but poor-risk patients.

Femorofemoral grafts, on the other hand, have a 5-year patency rate not significantly different from aortobifemoral grafts, and we offer femorofemoral bypass grafting to selected patients with unilateral iliac occlusive disease who have disabling claudication and are in no danger of limb loss. We have so far not found that femorofemoral grafts cause any clinically evident deterioration of the circulation in the leg supplied by the donor femoral artery in such patients.

I also differ with respect to two technical points. It is simpler to construct a femorofemoral graft in a "C" configuration rather than the "S" configuration preferred by Dr. Dale. In the "C" configuration the graft arcs upward toward the suprapubic tunnel from both the donor and recipient femoral anastomoses. I find femorofemoral grafts performed in this fashion are less subject to the danger of kinking, which may occur if an "S" configuration of the graft is attempted.

I am also not convinced that the final word is in on compression of an axillofemoral graft by lying on the graft. While I am prepared to believe that very little compression of the graft can occur late in the postoperative period after a fibrous capsule forms around the prosthesis. I believe that early after grafting it is possible to occlude the graft by lying on the axillary limb, particularly if the elbow is compressed against the rib cage when the patient is lying on the graft side. It is our impression that the new externally supported grafts have all but eliminated this kind of early graft failure, and these grafts are now our choice for axillofemoral bypasses.

14 INTRAOPERATIVE COMPLETION ARTERIOGRAPHY

Intraoperative completion angiography is widely known[1-4] yet not always practiced, perhaps because of the fear that it will needlessly prolong the operation or because of unfamiliarity with the procedure or the belief that clinical observation makes it unnecessary.

Several years ago a policy of completion arteriography for cases in which the anastomosis appeared to be faulty or the distal pulse was inadequate or absent was changed; completion arteriography was made routine following reconstructive procedures in the femoral, popliteal, or more distal arterial system of the leg or in the arteries of the arm and forearm. Retrospective analysis of that policy indicates that it allows easy recognition and correction of problems and improvement in the patency results of small arterial reconstructions.

Illustrative Case

A 70-year-old male had a 2-cm excavated ulcer of the dorsum of the left foot, which was severely ischemic throughout, and associated cellulitis (Figure 14-1). The preoperative arteriogram showed scattered arterial lesions, including stenosis of the left common femoral artery with failure of opacification of the profunda femoris, stenoses as well as complete occlusions of the superficial femoral artery, and an isolated popliteal segment with reconstitution of the tibial arteries distally (Figure 14-2).

A long segment of saphenous vein was reversed and placed as a sequential graft from the common femoral artery (whose profunda orifice was cleaned out at the same time) to a side-to-side anastomosis to the isolated popliteal artery just below the knee. The vein segment was then carried onto an anastomosis to the posterior tibial artery just below the knee and then carried onto an anastomosis to the posterior tibial artery at midcalf. At conclusion there appeared to be excellent pulsation at all points. Completion angiography demonstrated a widely patent anastomosis to the isolated popliteal segment. The distal anastomosis was patent, but there was failure of opacification of the posterior tibial artery just distal to that (center section of Figure 14-2). A Fogarty catheter was placed through the hood of the graft. The hood of the graft was closed, and another arteriogram was made. This showed no change. The hood was reopened and a new segment of vein was placed as a patch from this to a more distal section of the posterior tibial artery. A third arteriogram then showed patency of the involved area (right section of Figure 14-2).

The foot became warm, cellulitus promptly subsided, and healing occurred rapidly on the dorsum of the foot.

The concise review of previous reports by Mannick's group in 1981 summarized the goals to be achieved by intraoperative arteriography, namely, examination of the graft, visualization of

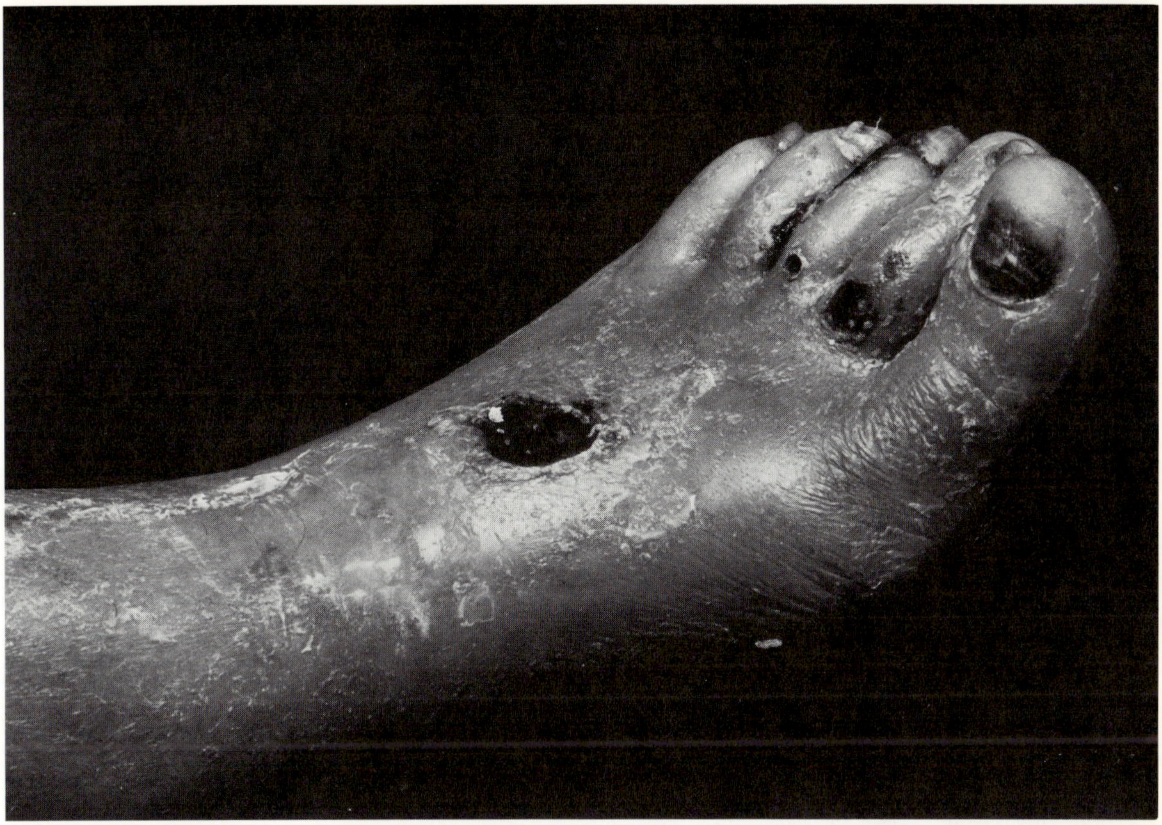

FIGURE 14-1 The severely ischemic foot of this 70-year-old male has cellulitis and ulcers of the second and third toes as well as the dorsum of the foot, along with interdigital ulceration.

the anastomoses, and simplicity.[5] To this may be added visualization of the distal run-off circulation.

TECHNIQUE

My earlier experience with injection of the contrast material above the proximal anastomosis indicated that the arteriogram did not often provide information about flow within the graft beyond what could be obtained by palpation and by observation of the blood flow prior to final closure of the distal anastomosis. At the same time, such proximal injections complicated the situation by requiring multiple cassettes to be placed and multiple exposures to be made. Too often there was poor visualization of the distal run-off arteries. For this reason the site of injection was changed to place the needle just proximal to the distal anastomosis (Figure 14-3).

Trial of both no. 19 and no. 21 needles indicate that the smaller size serves well. The needle may be pointed proximally or distally. The former position forces the contrast material against the blood stream, and it is gathered into a bolus, which then flows in a concentrated fashion distally. When the tip is pointed distally, the material tends to stream out and produce less visualization (Figure 14-4).

Heparinized saline solution is flushed through the tubing and needle to ensure its patency. Twenty-five milligrams of tolazoline (Priscoline) is then injected to reduce peripheral resistance and improve filling of the distal circulation.

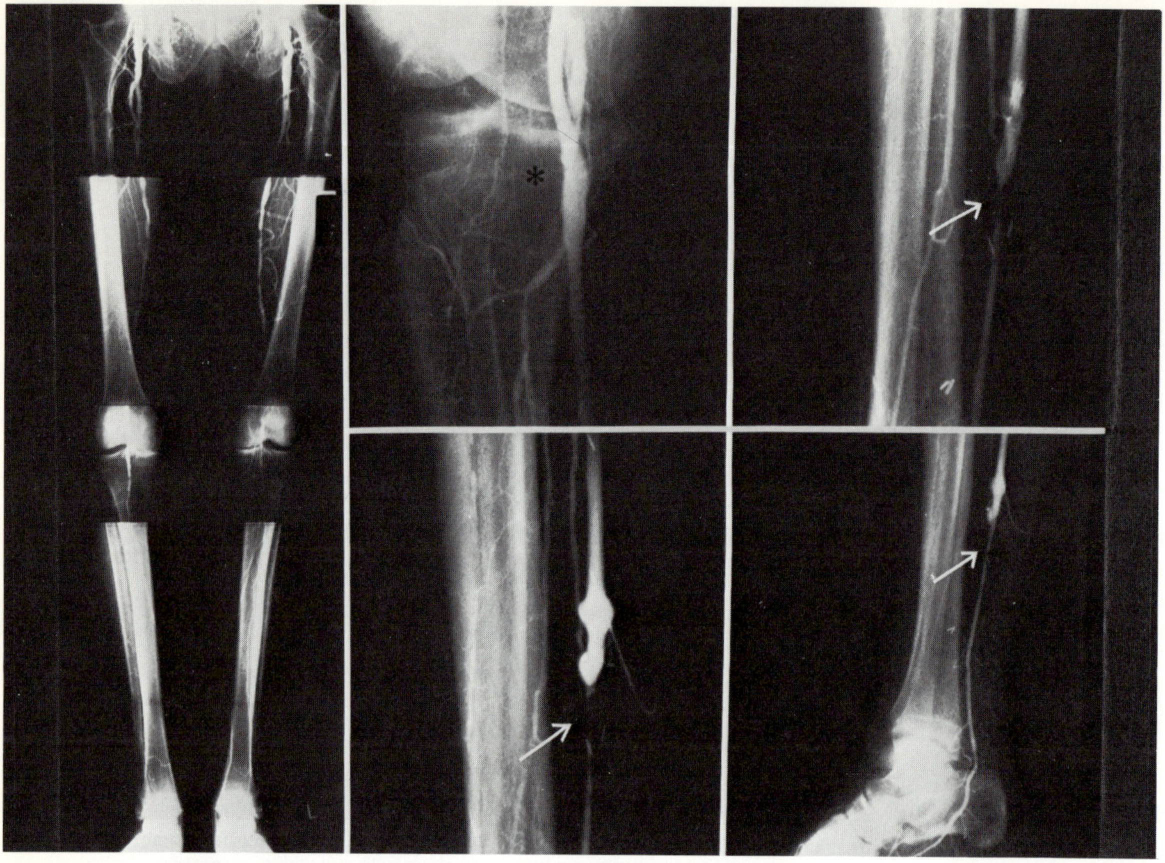

FIGURE 14-2 *Left,* a preoperative arteriogram shows scattered atherosclerotic stenoses and occlusions. The severely ischemic left foot was served by a common femoral artery with a large plaque causing proximal stenosis. The superficial artery ended at Hunter's canal with a reconstituted, isolated popliteal segment, beyond which was a patent posterior tibial artery in the lower third of the calf. *Upper middle,* a patent side-to-side anastomosis of the vein graft to the isolated popliteal segment at the *asterisk. Lower middle,* a bulbous end-to-side anastomosis of the autogenous vein graft to the posterior tibial artery in the distal calf. The *arrow* shows occlusion just distal to the anastomosis. *Upper right,* following passage of a Fogarty catheter through the hood of the graft, the lumen was still not restored. Closure of the hood of the graft reduced the previously bulbous venous hood. *Lower right,* a venous patch was placed to enlarge the posterior tibial artery just distal to the anastomosis, where patency is now shown at the *arrow* by dye streaming distally to the foot.

A sterilely draped portable shield is placed beside the operating table, behind which the injector stands for radiation protection while forcibly hand-pushing a plastic syringe containing 25 ml of meglumine iothalamate (Conray-60) (Figure 14-5). The call for exposure of the single film is made with 3 to 5 ml of contrast material remaining in the syringe, to allow for the latent period between the command and actual exposure of the film. If the exposure is incorrect for any reason, there is no hesitation in performing a second injection (Figure 14-6). The needle is left indwelling until the film is reviewed by the operating team. The protamine used to reverse intraoperative heparinization is delayed until the film is inspected.

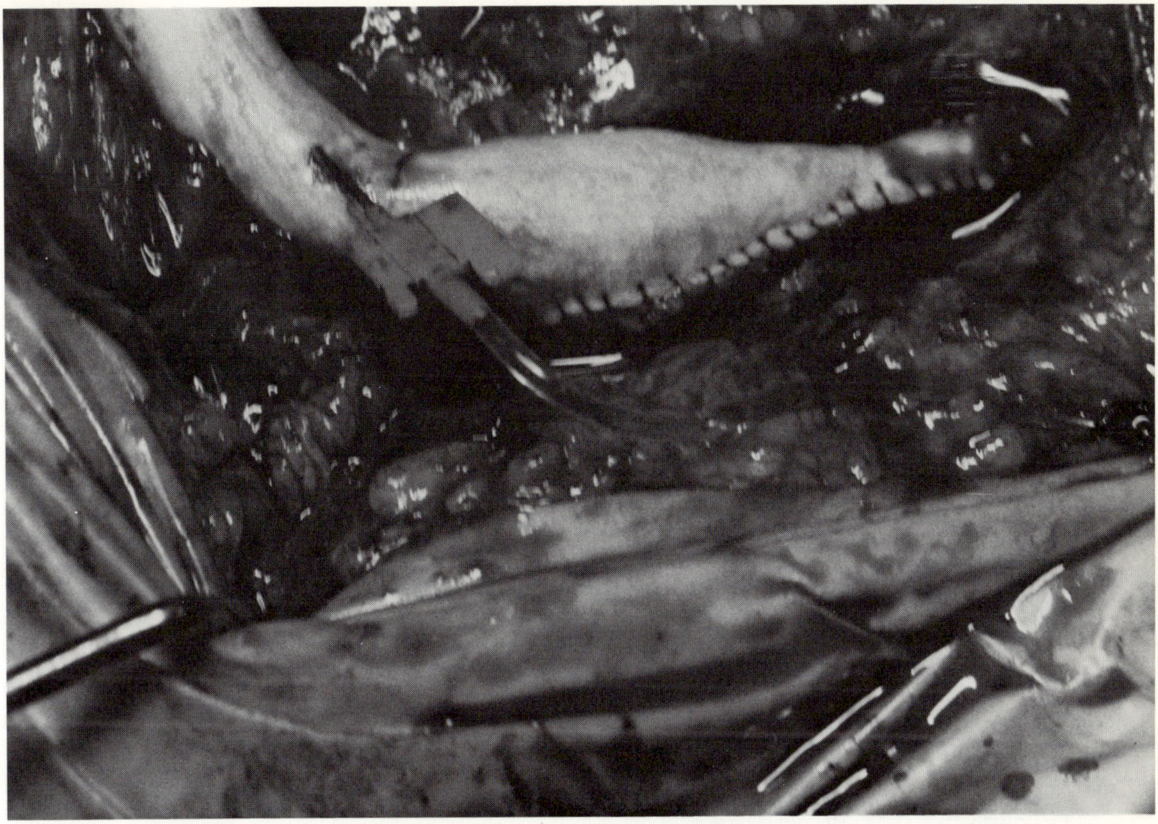

FIGURE 14-3 A no. 21 needle placed proximal to an anastomosis of PTFE to the popliteal artery.

TIME NEEDED

The key to efficient intraoperative arteriography is frequent use so that personnel from the departments of radiology as well as surgery are completely familiar with all aspects of the examination. In order to provide the radiologic technician some warning, preliminary calls are sent 30 minutes, 15 minutes, and 5 minutes before the estimated time of need. The last 5-minute call is actually a request for the immediate presence of the technician and the portable x-ray machine.

Familiarity with intraoperative arteriograms has developed, so the actual measured time recently has been 12 to 14 minutes from the completion of the distal anastomosis to the appearance of the dry film upon the viewing box in the operating room.

RESULTS

A recent retrospective analysis of 180 consecutive routine completion arteriograms documented the simplicity and lack of danger, the brief time required, and the improvement in patency rates which occurred.

There have been no operative complications due to completion arteriography in my experience. Bleeding from the needle hole in a vein graft usually stops with pressure maintained for several minutes, but it occasionally requires a 7-0 polypropylene suture. The hole in a synthetic tube almost always requires a suture for control.

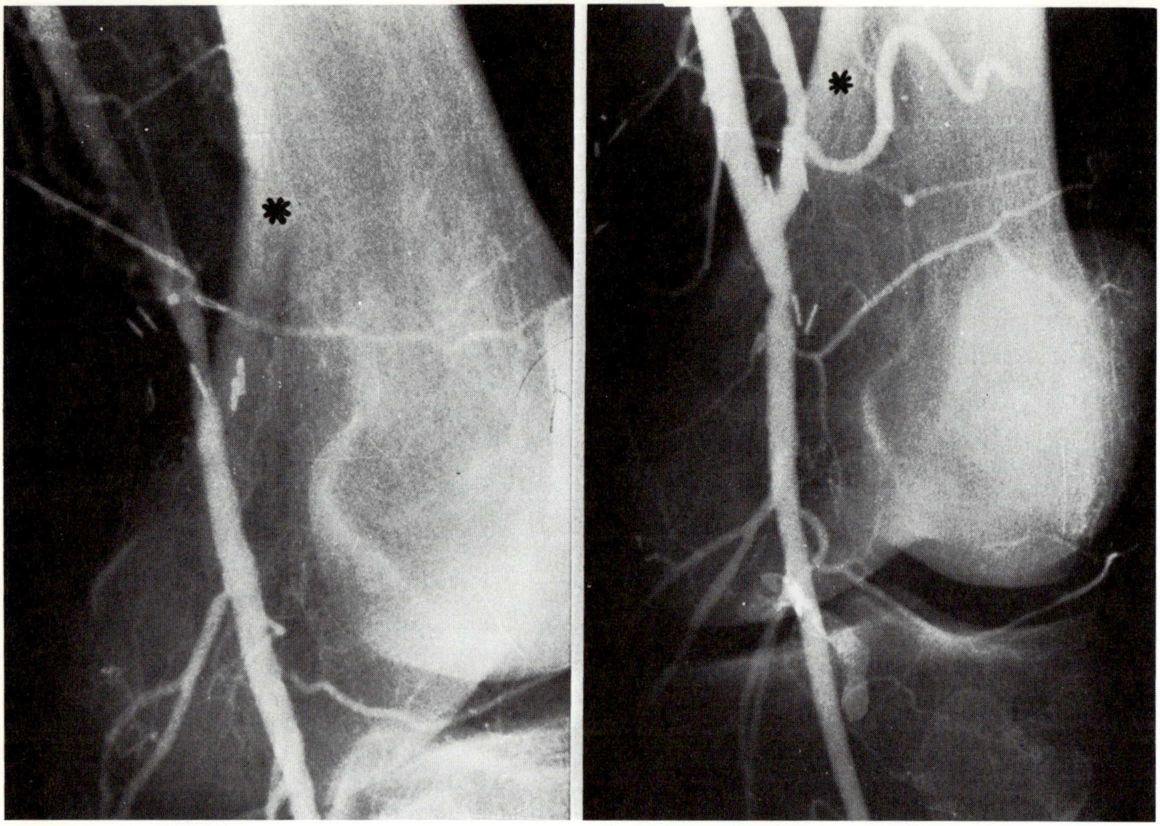

FIGURE 14-4 *Left,* a needle for a completion arteriogram is placed pointing distally at the *asterisk.* The radiopaque material streams and does not opacify the distal graft or the anastomosis. *Right,* the position of the needle is changed so that the tip points proximally as well as passing distally and opacifies the entire arterial network.

Table 14-1 indicates the results of 180 consecutive completion arteriograms. One hundred fifty (83 percent) showed normal anastomoses with run-off as good as or better than the preoperative arteriogram; those required no further attention.

Thirty (17 percent) showed some abnormality. Of these there were 14 where inspection indicated a minor degree of stenosis or irregularity, for which further procedure was not judged to be necessary. Of these 14 there were 10 which showed continued patency of the graft. Four of the fourteen patients had postoperative problems: One required an embolectomy the same night. Another occluded and required a new graft during the same hospitalization. A third occluded but the foot remained viable, so nothing further was done. A fourth occluded and had an early below-knee amputation.

Sixteen of the thirty patients with abnormal arteriograms had immediate further operative procedures: opening of the hood of the graft and removal of clot by Fogarty catheter, dilation of the distal vessel, or placement of a patch graft. All of these patients retained patency of the reconstruction during the hospital period.

This retrospective study therefore confirmed our clinical belief that the technique is simple, requires little additional time, encourages a high technical standard during operation, and discovers unrecognized correctable problems, whose alleviation leads to a higher early patency rate.

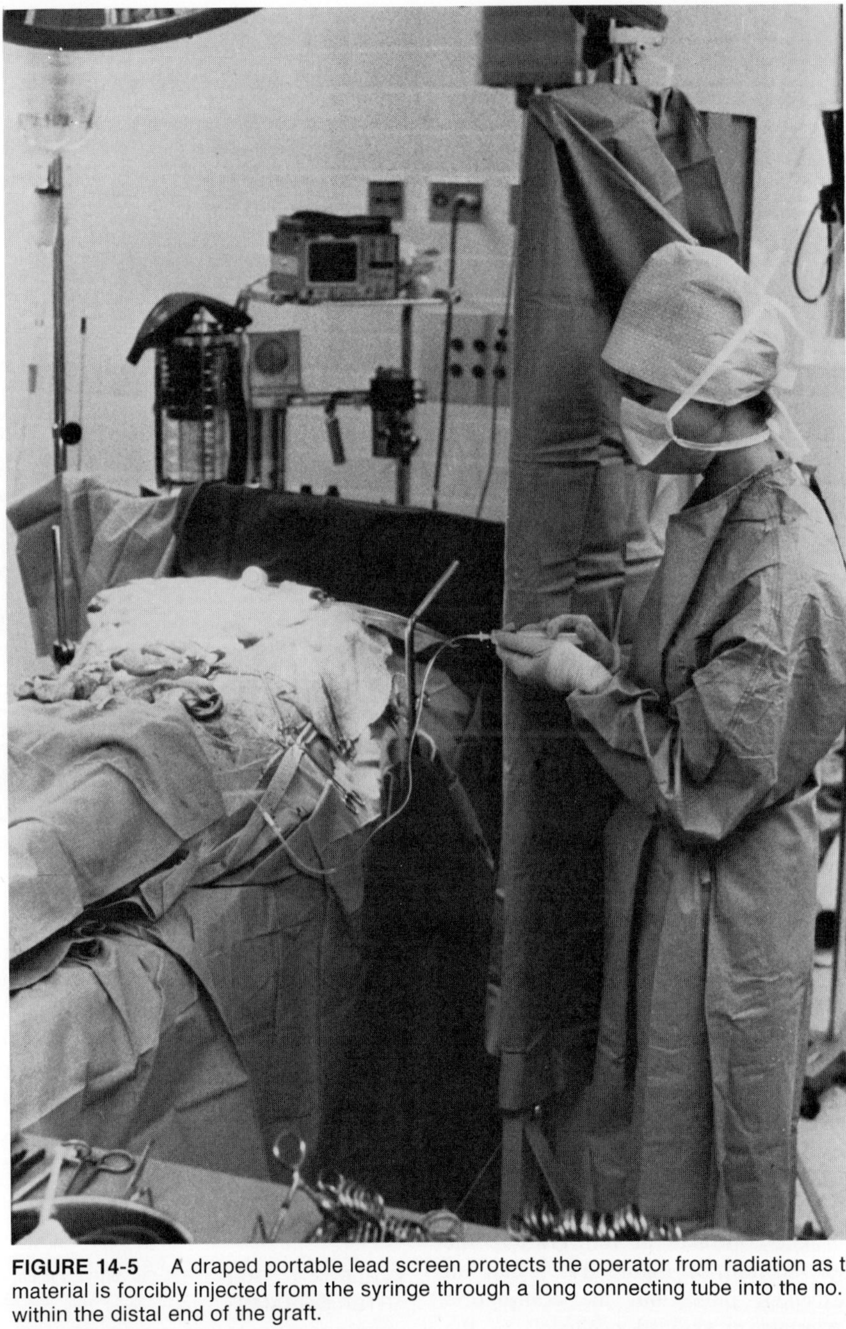

FIGURE 14-5 A draped portable lead screen protects the operator from radiation as the contrast material is forcibly injected from the syringe through a long connecting tube into the no. 21 needle lying within the distal end of the graft.

It suggests an aggressive policy of exploration if there is any evidence of abnormality. The procedure has no effect on late occlusions due to progression of atherosclerotic disease or to late deterioration of the graft.

A completion arteriogram which disclosed unsuspected distal run-off thrombosis is shown in

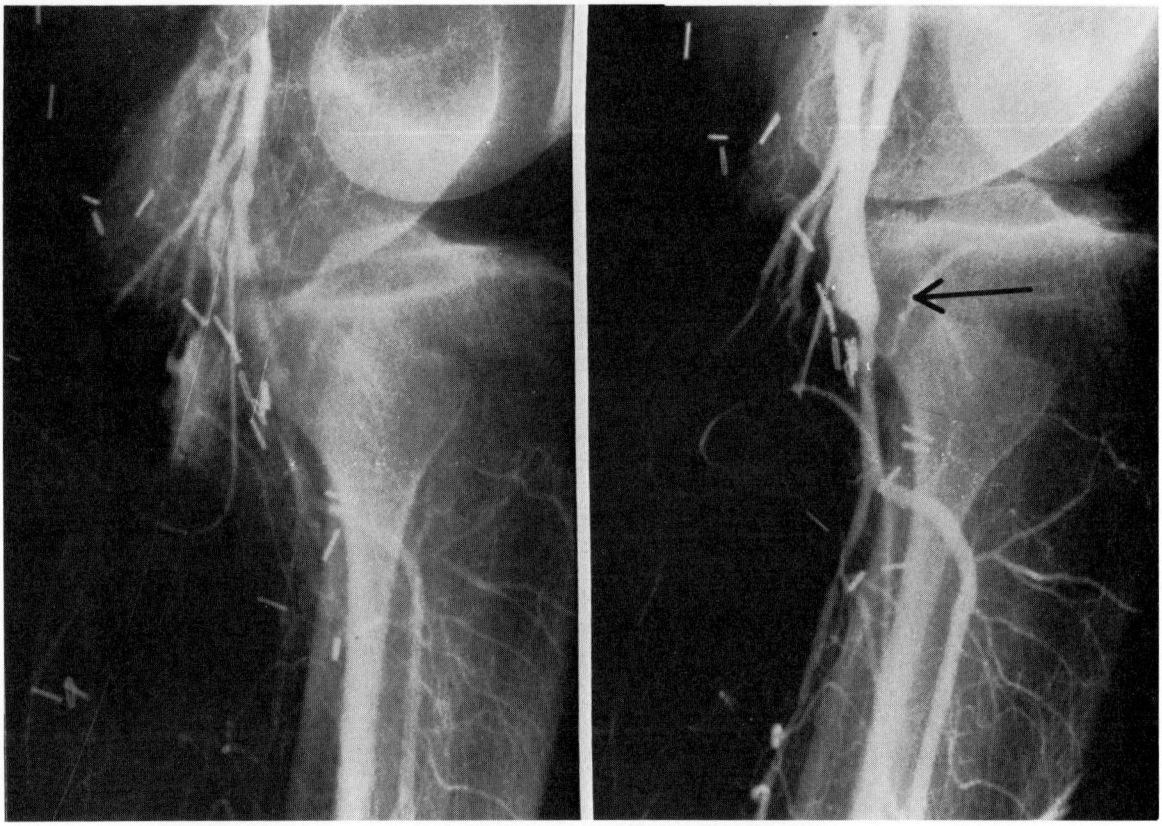

FIGURE 14-6 *Left,* film exposed too late. *Right,* film exposed earlier shows a patent graft and anastomosis.

Figure 14-7. The graft, its anastomosis, and the artery just distal to it appeared and felt pulsatile, yet the completion arteriogram (right section of Figure 14-7) clearly demonstrated an intraluminal thrombus. Following Fogarty catheter thrombectomy through an opening in the hood of the graft, a second arteriogram showed complete patency (left section of Figure 14-7).

Another example is shown in Figure 14-8, where the left side shows an apparently patent polytetrafluoroethylene (PTFE) graft and anastomosis to the popliteal artery below the knee. The pulse was good just beyond the graft. No foot pulse was present, or expected, since only the peroneal artery remained patent. Since the contrast material ceased abruptly and did not fill the run-off vessel shown preoperatively, a catheter thrombectomy was performed. It restored the run-off, as seen in the right side of the Figure 14-8.

The contralateral vein graft in the left section of Figure 14-9, had an excellent pulse, but the completion arteriogram showed occlusion of the artery distal to the anastomosis. Following catheter thrombectomy, there was patency (right section of Figure 14-9). Figures 14-10 to 14-12 show other examples.

TABLE 14-1 RESULTS OF 180 COMPLETION ARTERIOGRAMS

150	(83.3%): anastomosis and run-off good (no procedure needed)
30	(16.7%): abnormal arteriogram
	14: no further procedure (10 patent, 4 problems)
	16: further procedure (all patent)

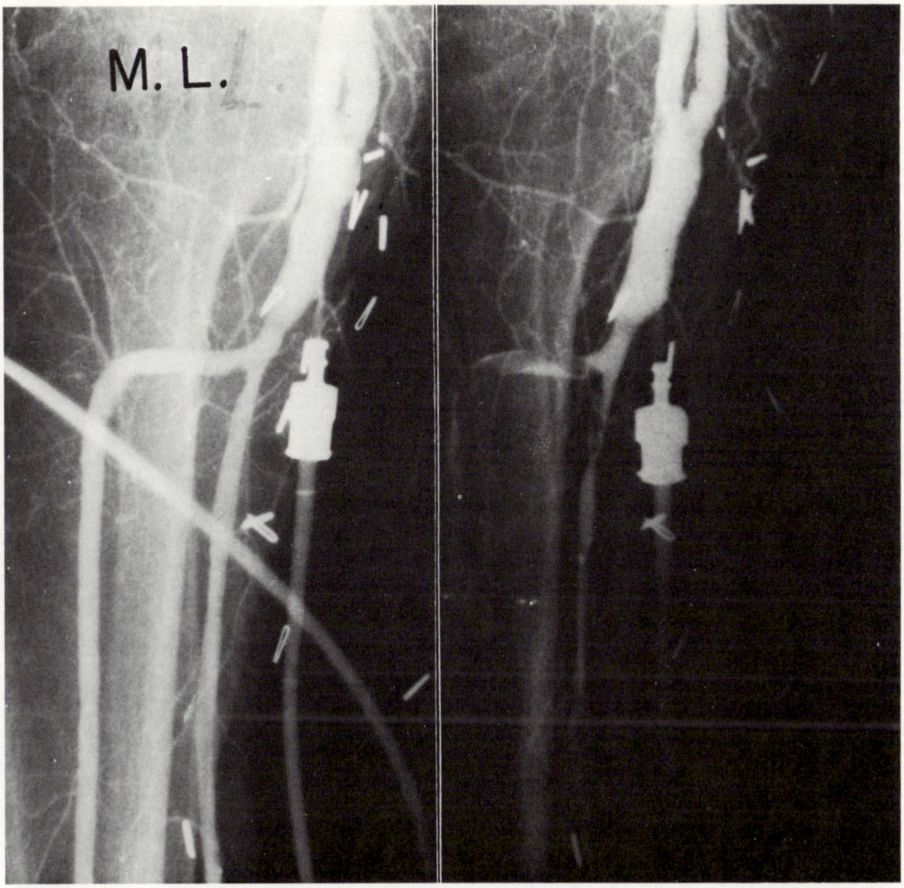

FIGURE 14-7 *Right,* a patent graft and anastomosis with an unsuspected intraluminal thrombus in the anterior tibial and posterior tibial arteries distal to a palpable pulse. *Left,* complete patency following Fogarty catheterization thrombectomy.

RESULTS OF OTHERS

The decreasing incidence of defects discovered by completion angiography during the last decade reflects greater expertise in reconstructive arterial surgery. Part of this is due to a greater insistence upon absolute technical accuracy in performance of the anastomoses, based upon their immediate radiographic inspection for the detection of unrecognized defects. Thus Dardik and associates' report of a 17 percent error rate found in 1975[6] had decreased to 3 percent by 1978.[7]

Another feature is the delineation of the run-off system so that early failure may be predicted on the basis of severe distal disease. This may suggest that the surgeon refrain from reoperation. In other words, the completion arteriogram assures a technically correct reconstruction. If the run-off is so poor that failure occurs, there is no need to perform another procedure.

NONINVASIVE PROCEDURES

A variety of techniques to study blood flow in the graft and distal to it have been reported. Several of these have been tried, but none have been found to be as predictable as physical exami-

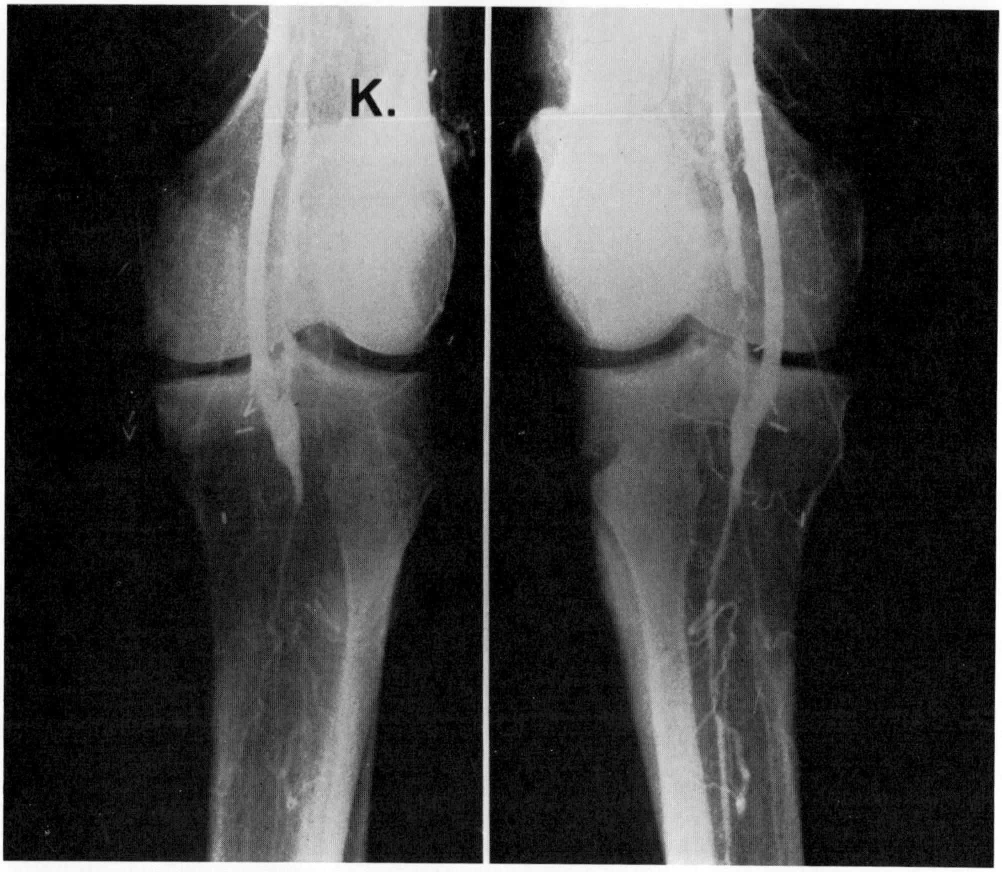

FIGURE 14-8 *Left,* a PTFE graft connected to the popliteal artery just distal to the knee joint appeared to be functioning satisfactorily, with a good pulse just distal to the anastomosis. No foot pulse was felt or expected, since the only run-off was the peroneal artery. *Right,* recognizing the failure of distal opacification prompted Fogarty catheter thrombectomy through the hood of the graft, resulting in patency of the run-off peroneal artery.

nation of the foot (with the drapes temporarily removed), complemented by the completion arteriogram.

Hackler and Bunt have recently presented a strong argument for completion Doppler study of the run-off, to allow a selective policy of completion arteriography. Among 35 cases they found 6 which had abnormal Doppler scans; these also had abnormal arteriograms and were at once corrected. The other 29, having normal Doppler studies, did not undergo angiography, and all remained patent.[8] Certainly, such experience requires consideration, and if accuracy is confirmed, Doppler study may lead to simplification and to a selective program of completion angiography. The matter requires further study.

At present the completion arteriogram allows rapid verification of a technically correct anastomosis as well as of the patency of the run-off. Physical examination complements but does not replace it.

If any question is raised by the arteriogram, an aggressive approach to correction of the defect is indicated.

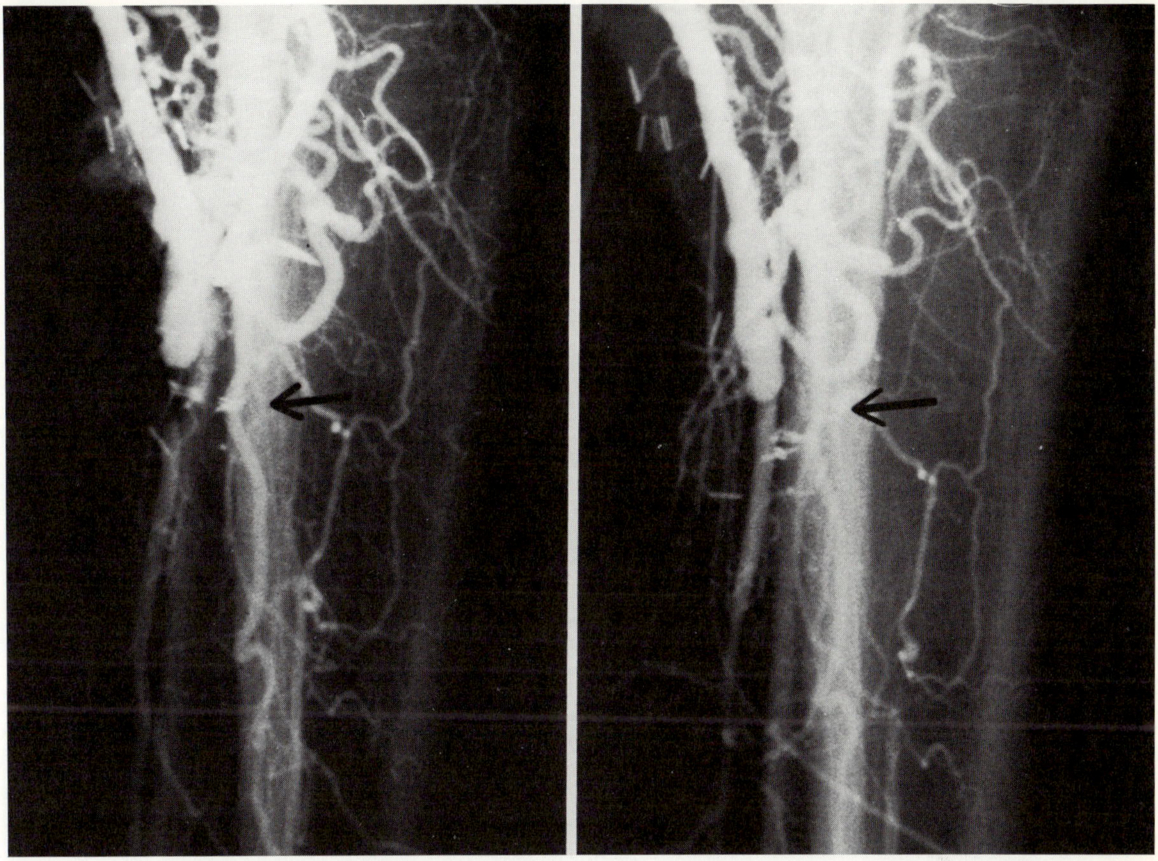

FIGURE 14-9 *Left,* a thrombus occludes the artery distal to a vein graft anastomosis. *Right,* after thrombectomy the tibial artery is patent.

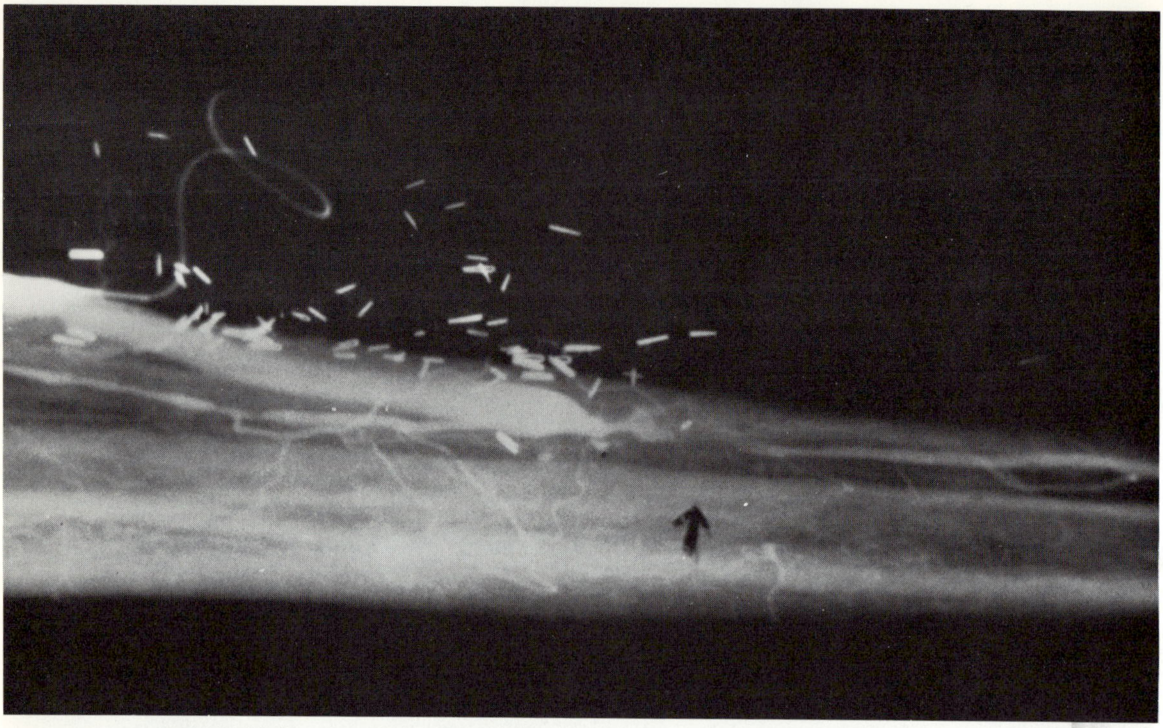

FIGURE 14-10 A patent anastomosis with an occlusion distal to it.

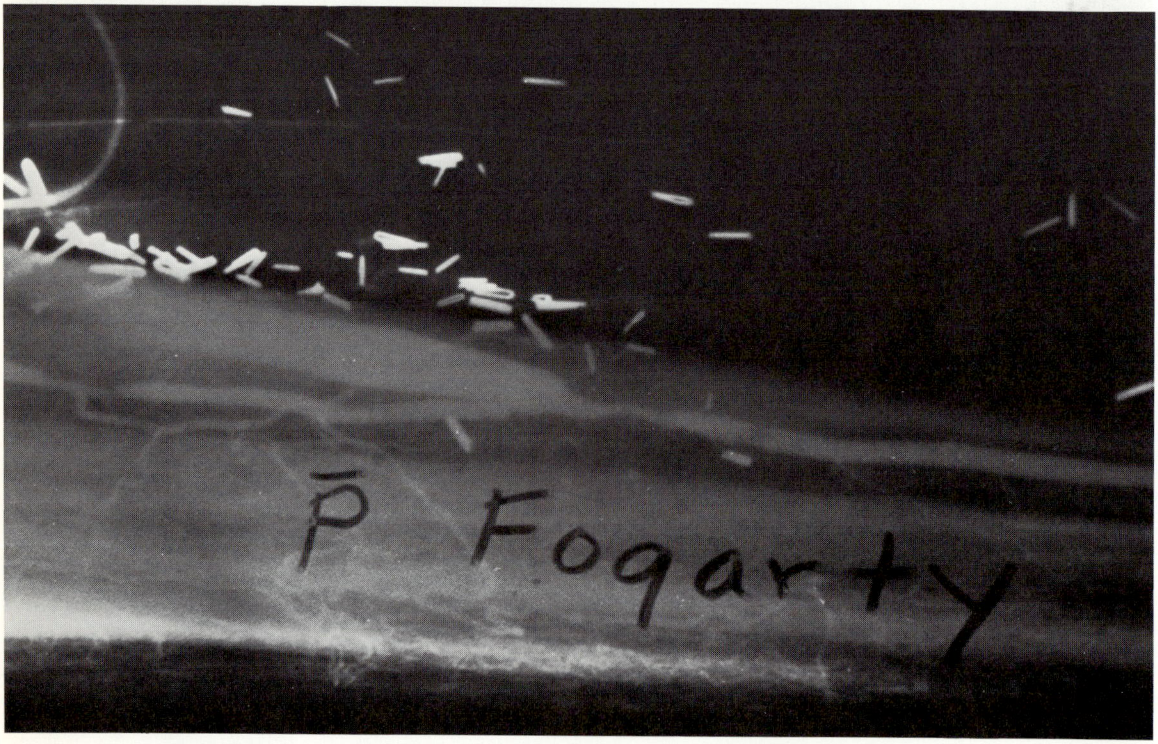

FIGURE 14-11 Distal patency was restored by catheter thrombectomy.

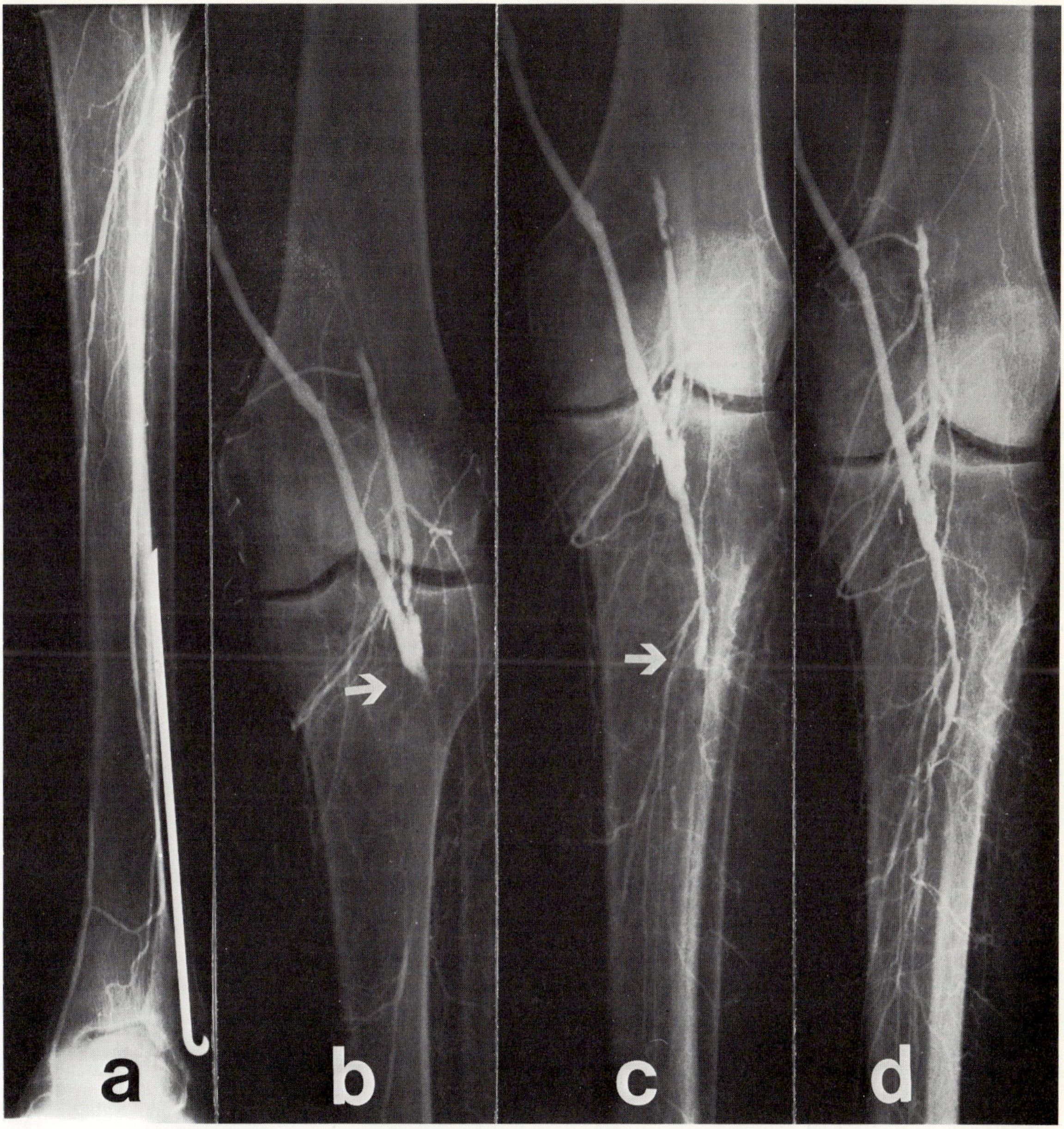

FIGURE 14-12 Two repetitive procedures were required to obtain a good result. (*a*) Preoperative run-off. (*b*) The anastomosis seemed correct, but there was no outflow. (*c*) After Fogarty thrombectomy there was persistent distal occlusion. (*d*) After another Fogarty thrombectomy the run-off was satisfactory.

REFERENCES

1 Johnson WC: Operative angiography for femoro-popliteal vein by-pass reconstruction. *Am J Surg* 1973, 16:120.
2 Liddicoat JE, Bekassy SM, DeBakey ME: Intraoperative arteriography during femoro-popliteal by-pass. *Arch Surg* 1975, 110:839.
3 Pinkerton JA Jr: Operative arteriography: A new variation. *Arch Surg* 1975, 110:841.
4 Plecha FR, Pories WJ: Intraoperative angiography in the immediate assessment of arterial reconstruction. *Arch Surg* 1972, 105:902.
5 Liebman PR, Menzoian JO, Mannick JA, Lowney BW, LoGerfo FW: Intraoperative arteriography in femoropopliteal and femorotibial bypass grafts. *Arch Surg* 1981, 116:1019.
6 Dardik II, Ibrahim IM, Sprayregen S, Veith F, Dardik H: Routine intraoperative angiography. *Arch Surg* 1975, 110:184.
7 Dardik H: Evaluation of intraoperative arteriography as a routine for vascular reconstructions. *Surg Gynecol Obstet* 1978, 147:853.
8 Hackler MT, Bunt TJ: Negative impact of routine post-reconstructive intraoperative angiography in lower extremity revascularization. *Am Surg* 1983, 49:15.

Invited Commentary

Herbert Dardik, M.D.
Englewood, New Jersey

Intraoperative arteriography performed immediately after arterial reconstruction provides valuable information with regard to technical adequacy of the operation and prognosis for the durability of graft function. The derived information is, in fact, usually more accurate than that provided by the preoperative arteriogram and may thus alter the prognosis for the particular reconstruction performed. Despite these favorable aspects, including the advantage of simplicity of performance, completion arteriography has failed to achieve universal popularity. It is tempting at the conclusion of a long and tedious operation to get the patient "off the table." In fact, completion arteriograhy requires but a fraction of the overall surgical time, is easy to perform, and is inexpensive. Surgeons must adjust their attitudes to this procedure, which, with critical analysis of the findings, will improve results and, ultimately, the fate of their patients. Dr. Dale has addressed all these points and documented the usefulness of completion arteriography.

The primary reason for performing a completion arteriogram is to visualize any potential mechanism for graft closure that would then enable either prophylactic correction or prompt revision after graft closure, depending upon individual clinical circumstances. Other benefits that have accrued from the routine performance of completion arteriography include refinements in technique which, in turn, have significantly decreased the incidence of surgical errors. Many of these technical faults would not have been otherwise appreciated, even by sophisticated noninvasive methods. In cases of severe distal atherosclerosis, the discovery of run-off vessels not previously appreciated or visualized by preoperative arteriography is both joyous and reassuring. If necessary, a synchronous sequential bypass can be constructed or bypass can be considered for a later date (Figure 14-A).

Routine intraoperative completion arteriography for revascularization procedures of the lower extremity has enabled us to classify the run-off and correlate these findings with subsequent

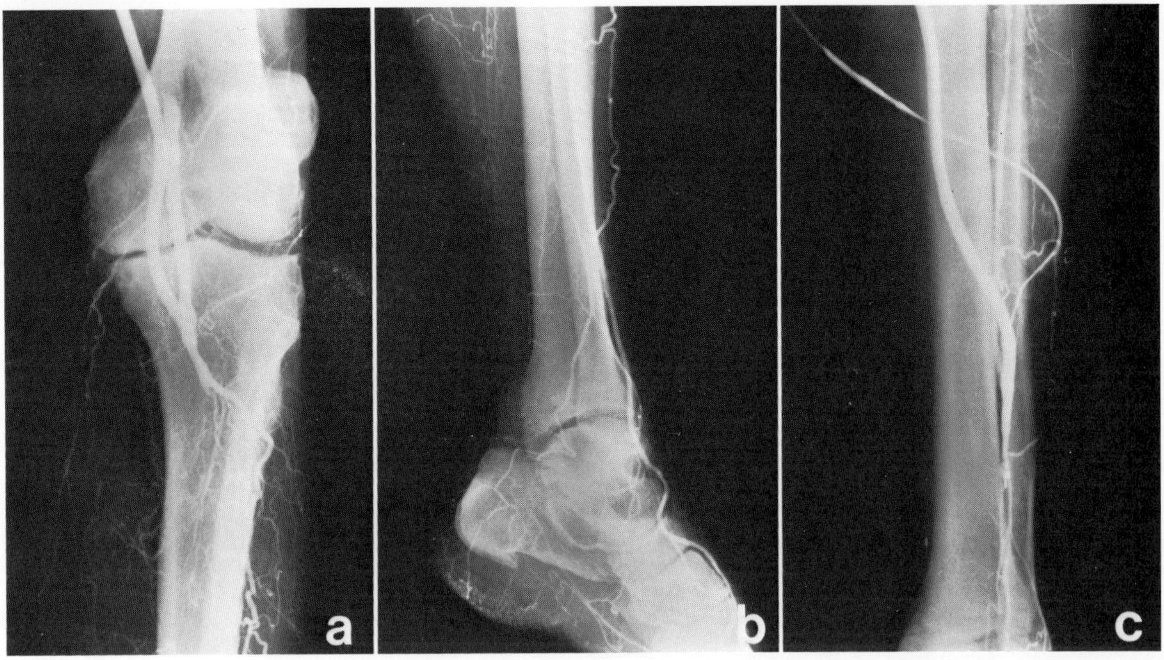

FIGURE 14-A Intraoperative arteriograms depicting (*a*) a femoral popliteal bypass to a blind segment and (*b*) visualization of a distal anterior tibial artery on a second intraoperative completion arteriogram. Subsequent closure of the femoral popliteal bypass enabled the performance of a thrombectomy and a sequential jump bypass (*c*) to the anterior tibial artery.

graft patency. In instances of the most advanced obliterative disease, fruitless and potentially harmful reoperative vascular procedures may be obviated. Delayed graft closure due to progressive or accelerated obliterating atherosclerosis in the distal circulation occurs frequently in patients showing poor run-off by completion arteriography. This group, in particular, should be closely monitored by noninvasive testing and even postoperative digital or standard contrast arteriography, to enable thoughtful consideration of either prophylactic or therapeutic correction.

A simple device to perform intraoperative arteriography has been developed to enable remote injection of contrast (Figure 14-B). It includes two disposable plastic syringes (50 mL) coupled with plastic tubing. One syringe is filled with water and purged of air. A second component of the device consists of a holding fixture that permits the empty syringe of the coupled system to be aligned with a third syringe, filled with contrast medium. The latter is, in turn, attached to the patient via standard intravenous tubing and the butterfly needle. When the water-filled syringe is brought out of the operating room area and depressed from this point, the previously empty syringe in the holder fills and depresses the barrel of the final syringe, which contains contrast, and allows for direct infusion of the contrast into the site to be visualized. This technique is simple and rapid and provides for excellent arteriograms at minimal cost. Most important, it avoids exposure to radiation of all operating room personnel. The exact timing of film exposure depends on the location of the cassette and field to be visualized with respect to the site of the butterfly needle in the artery or graft. Normally, this occurs at 4 to 6 s after the injection is initiated and when the contrast-filled syringe is half to two-thirds depressed. Repeat injections may be required and are routine for obtaining foot films and for visualization of a distal anastomotic area at a higher point such as at the popliteal artery.

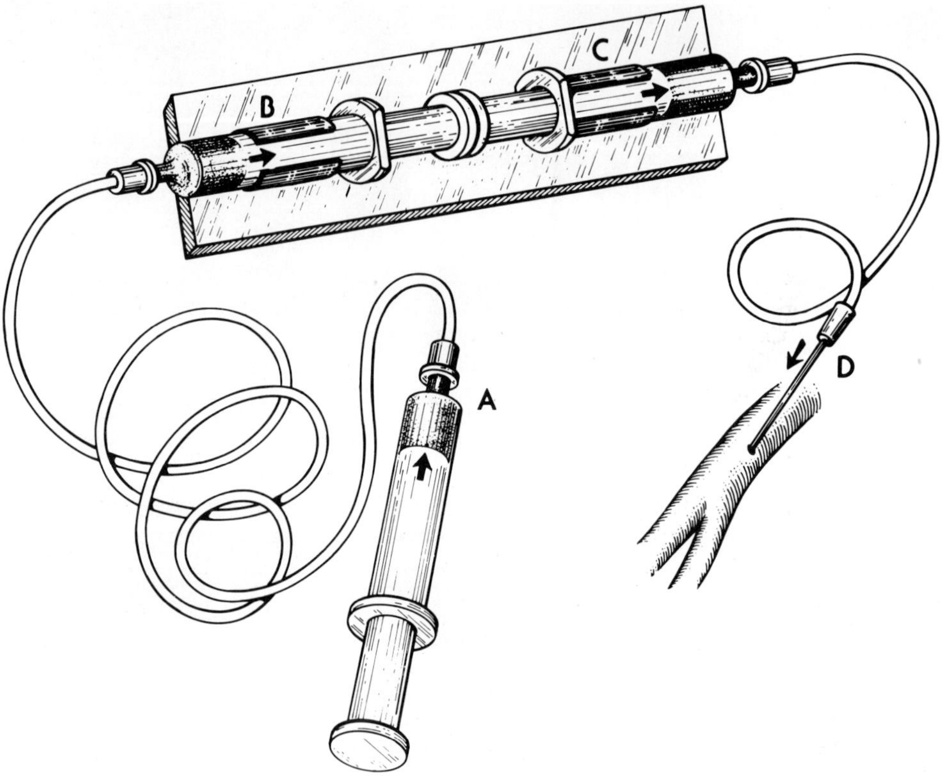

FIGURE 14-B The schema of apparatus employed to perform intraoperative arteriography. (*a*) A syringe filled with saline is depressed in order to fill (*b*) a second syringe in a holder. (*c*) The barrel of the latter enables the syringe filled with contrast to be depressed. That, in turn, then permits (*d*) direct infusion of contrast into the area of interest.

The advantages of performing completion arteriography far outweigh the disadvantages and punctuate the need for all vascular surgeons to include this procedure as a routine component of lower-extremity revascularization operations (Table 14-A).

TABLE 14-A INTRAOPERATIVE COMPLETION ARTERIOGRAPHY

Advantages	Disadvantages
Detection of technical defects	Time
Surgical quality control	Radiation
Definitive view of run-off	Contrast sensitivity
Learning device	Cost
Prognosis	Renal insufficiency
Permanent record	Iatrogenic trauma
Availability for review	Vasodilator hypotension

15 RENOVASCULAR DISEASE

Hypertension occurs in a large number of Americans, perhaps on the order of 60 million,[1] of which approximately 10 percent are severe hypertensives. Arbitrarily, adult diastolic blood pressure between 90 and 104 mmHg has been labeled *mild,* between 105 and 114 *moderate,* and greater than 115 *severe.*[2] A sizable amount of hypertension is caused by the renovascular lesions of either atherosclerosis or fibrous dysplasia or a few other odd entities (Table 15-1). Identification and treatment of these are important issues, since renovascular ischemia tends to produce severe, rather than minor, degrees of hypertension and is usually surgically correctable.

HISTORICAL BACKGROUND

In 1898 Tigerstedt and Bergman discovered the renal pressor substance *renin* in the kidneys of rabbits.[3] Thirty-six years later Goldblatt reversed the traditional idea that renal arterial disease and arteriosclerosis were caused by hypertension, by demonstrating in dogs that renal arterial constriction produced hypertension.[4]

Recognition of Goldblatt kidney hypertension soon led to large numbers of nephrectomies in hypertensive patients with small kidneys. This trend was sharply checked in 1956 by the critical analysis of Homer Smith,* who, after reviewing 575 such cases with only 26 percent relief of hypertension, suggested that nephrectomy was not proper for such indications and should be limited to urologic ones alone.[5]

Surgical management of hypertension by bilateral ablation of the thoracolumbar sympathetic chains was tried extensively during the 1940s. There was variable success for this severe two-stage procedure. I can testify that it was severe for the surgeon and assistants also, having completed a residency program during the peak of its popularity. Its use ended rather abruptly with the explosive development of antihypertensive drug therapy in the 1950s. By that time the first surgical cure of renovascular hypertension had already been done by Norman Freeman in 1954[8] and was soon followed by increasingly large numbers of such operative procedures by others.

The coexistence of renal artery stenosis and hypertension does not necessarily establish a causal relationship; again, increasing numbers of operations were often unsuccessful in relieving hypertension. In the late 1960s and 1970s critical diagnostic studies were developed, so today as much as 95 percent success can be achieved in properly selected hypertensive patients. Among the leaders in this progressive and productive investigation of clinical patients were John Foster, who was important in establishing the investigative and therapeutic program at Vanderbilt University, and later Richard Dean, who continued as an important contributor to renovascular study programs.

*Renal physiologist Smith became well-known to the lay population after publication of his popular accounts of evolution in *From Fish to Philosopher*[6] and of comparative religions in *Man and His Gods.*[7]

PATHOPHYSIOLOGY

The intermediate metabolic pathways following the release of renin by the juxtaglomerular cells about the afferent renal arterioles are too complex for detailed description here. Interested readers may consult the splendid papers of Brown and Laragh[9] and of Vaughan.[10] Briefly, when the juxtaglomerular apparatus senses a low perfusion pressure, there is release of the proteolytic enzyme renin, which converts angiotensinogen to angiotensin I, which is thereafter changed to angiotensin II via a plasmolytic enzyme found predominantly in the lung. This potent pressor affects arterioles, promotes sodium retention, and increases the secretion of aldosterone, all of which elevate the blood pressure. In simple terms, when the kidney senses low perfusion pressure, it reacts in several ways to raise the blood pressure. The end result of the release of renin is to produce generalized arteriolar vasoconstriction with hypertension. Increased volume in the arterial system may also be an important factor under some circumstances.

TABLE 15-1 CAUSES OF HYPERTENSION

Primary
Essential
Secondary
Renovascular disease
Renal parenchymal disease
Primary aldosteronism
Pheochromocytoma
Cushing's syndrome
Coarctation of the aorta
Drugs
Hypercalcemic states

TABLE 15-2 ETIOLOGY OF RENOVASCULAR HYPERTENSION

Intrinsic arterial lesions
Arteriosclerosis
Fibromuscular dysplasia
Embolism
Dissection
Trauma
Arteritis
Aneurysm
Extrinsic lesions
Pressure (retroperitoneal fibrosis)
Tumor
Congenital band
Scarring

The two common lesions which cause renal arterial stenosis are arteriosclerosis (70 percent) and fibromuscular dysplasia (30 percent) (Table 15-2). As in other vessels the atherosclerotic lesions leave skip areas of patency. The stenotic lesions do not always cause hypertension—many occur in normotensive people (Figure 15-1) or coincidentally in hypertensives—hence the importance of establishing a causal relationship prior to advising surgical repair.[11,12] Atherosclerotic lesions tend to be orificial in a third and are bilateral in a third of patients.[13]

The etiology of fibromuscular dysplasia continues to be unknown. It more often occurs in females, is frequently bilateral, and may extend into the distal renal arterial tree. It is progressive in about a third of patients.[13]

Other, less frequent, causes of renovascular hypertension (Figure 15-2) are listed in Table 15-2.

DIAGNOSIS OF RENOVASCULAR HYPERTENSION

There are three important diagnostic questions for those managing hypertensive patients: First, who should be studied for the possibility of a renovascular cause of hypertension? Second, what screening tests should be used? Finally, what diagnostic studies are critical for the decision between nonoperative and surgical management?

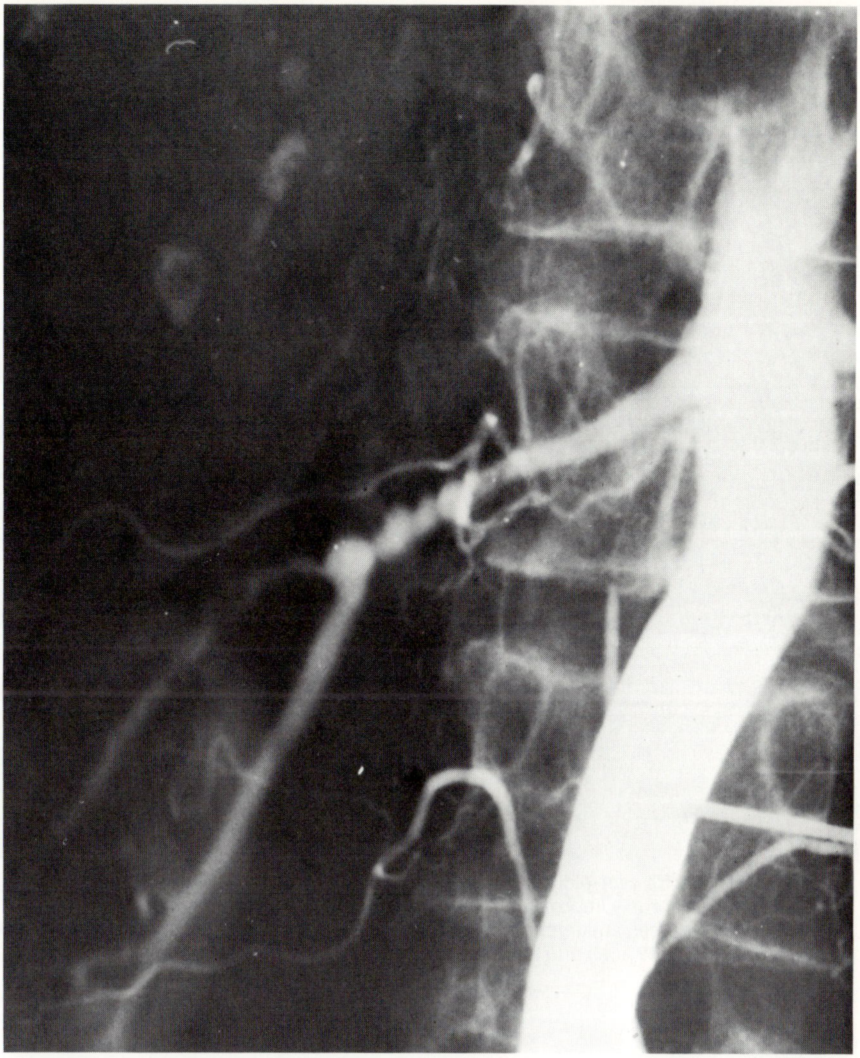

FIGURE 15-1 A 48-year-old female with typical renal fibromuscular dysplasia, who was normotensive.

Which Hypertensive Patients Should Be Studied?

Richard Dean recently discussed demographic factors, in the light of his experience with large groups of patients in the Renal Vascular Center here, and concluded that "one should base a decision for diagnostic study on the severity of the hypertension." While renovascular hypertension is certainly more likely in the nonblack population, at the extremes of life, in patients with the recent onset of hypertension, and in those with an upper-abdominal bruit, limitation to patients with the recent onset of hypertension and to those with an upper-abdominal bruit or limitation to patients with any one or any combination of those factors would inappropriately exclude some patients with renovascular hypertension from further study. He therefore recommended that all patients with a diastolic pressure above 110 who would be acceptable operative candidates be evaluated.[14] Individualization beyond this is obviously needed for some others.

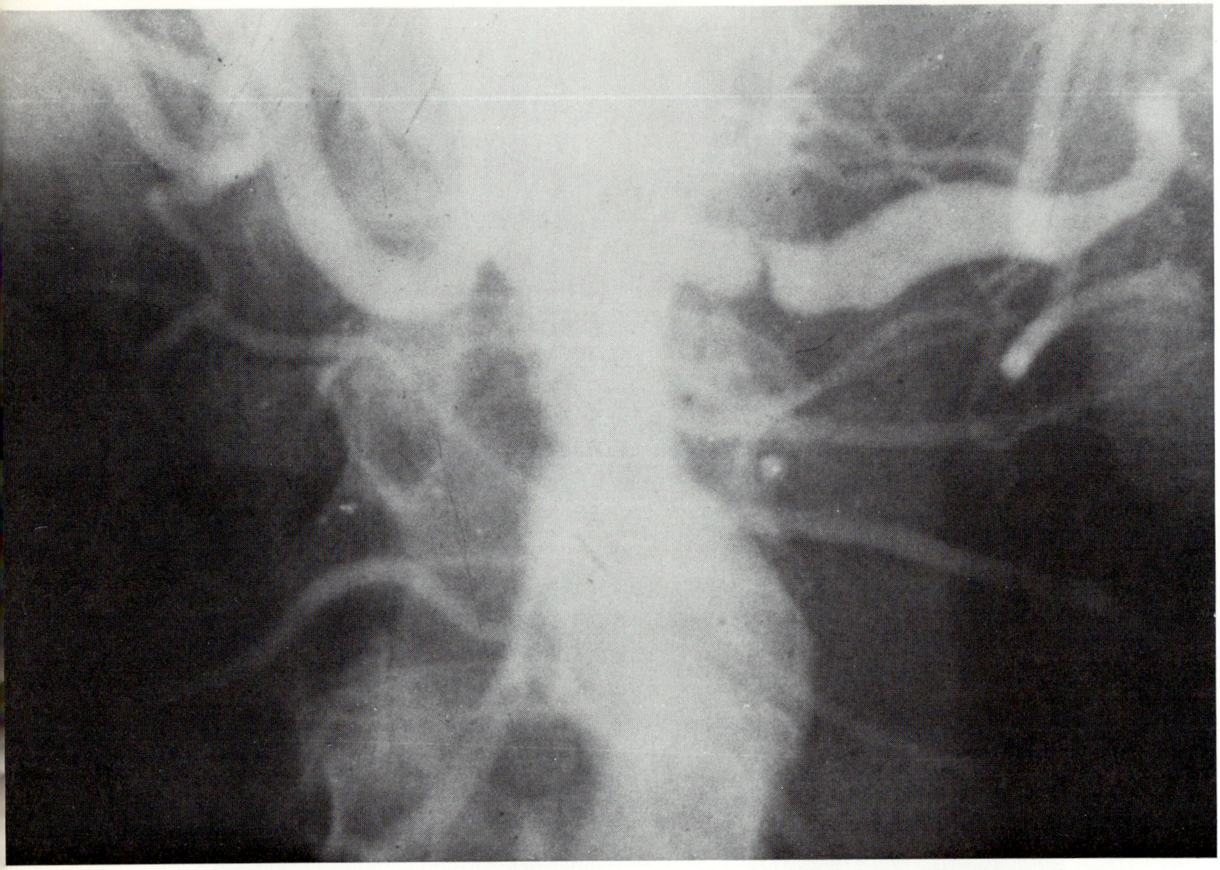

FIGURE 15-2 A 57-year-old male with left renal stenosis due to retroperitoneal fibrosis. His hypertension temporarily improved following dissection relief of the extrinsic pressure on the renal artery. The small aortic aneurysm embedded in the fibrotic tissue was not distrubed. Later the left kidney did not opacify at all and hypertension recurred. Further treatment was refused.

Screening Studies

Primary aldosteronism can be excluded by measurement of a serum electrolyte if the potassium level is greater than 3 mEq/L, recognizing instances of hypokalemia due to diet and diuretic therapy. A hypertension-producing pheochromocytoma or adrenal cortical tumor should be ruled out by study of the urinary excretion of 17-hydroxy and 17-ketosteroids and by vanillylmandelic acid levels.

Rapid Intravenous Pyelography

Intravenous pyelography may be suggestive of unilateral renovascular disease if the renal size is 1.5 to 2 cm different from the size of the contralateral kidney, if the contrast material is delayed in appearance time on one side, or if there is ureteral notching or a defect in the renal appearance suggesting infarction. However, Foster, Dean, Pinkerton, and Rhamy found a positive intravenous pyelogram in only 69 percent of 122 proven cases of renovascular hypertension.[15] The test was even less reliable among 21 children, where only 42 percent were positive.[16]

The intravenous pyelogram alone therefore has many false negatives but does furnish information about other lesions, and when positive it strongly suggests angiography. It is widely available and is better than nothing: if it is positive, there is a strong indication for further definitive study; if negative, it should be ignored and the severe hypertensive should be studied further. This comes down, then, to using it to convince the patient and family in either event to have further studies done.

Peripheral Plasma Renin

The necessity to establish a sodium balance using a calculated sodium diet, the frequent inability to stop all hypertensive medications prior to the test, and the variability of this study make it too inaccurate to use as a screening test. Thus, Melman's team found that a program designed to suppress or to stimulate peripheral plasma renin activity in 19 patients was not helpful in identifying those with renovascular hypertension.[17]

Response to Angiotensin Inhibitors

The degree of response to pharmacologic agents such as saralasin[18] and captopril, which block the renin-angiotensin-aldosterone system, has not proved particularly helpful in detecting which hypertensives are of renovascular origin.[19]

Isotope Renogram

Despite modern modifications of the original 131-I-hippuran test the 25 percent incidence of false negatives is too high to allow this to serve as a single screening test.[14]

Renal Angiography

There is increasing agreement that in the absence of simple screening tests which are accurate, renal arteriograms are indicated for hypertensives of severe degree whose general status would allow reconstructive surgery if needed. Dean has long since taken this position,[14] and Black in 1983 advised angiography for "all patients in whom I seriously suspect renal artery stenosis."[20]

Angiographic visualization of the renal arterial systems is not only the most accurate screening technique but also the necessary road map to successful surgical revascularization of the kidney (Figure 15-3). Intravenous and translumbar needle techniques used in the past have now been completely superseded by the injection of radiopaque material through a catheter lying in the aorta to produce a "flush" arteriogram in one or more projections, followed by selective views made in the several different projections which may be necessary to visualize the entire renal arterial system (Figures 15-4 to 15-6). Bear in mind that the curved course of the arteries may require repeated injections and several positions to accurately determine the situtation.

Modern angiography is a relatively safe procedure when performed by an experienced person. In Chapter 6 this was discussed fully, including the complication rate of below 2.9 percent and mortality rate of 0.05 percent or less among 118,591 examinations in 514 U.S. hospitals, for both the translumbar and transfemoral techniques. Only 13 patients (0.01 percent) developed renal failure, with 2 deaths.[21]

Reports such as that of Swartz and associates of renal failure in 12 percent of 109 patients[22] and the report from the University of California at Los Angeles of 11 percent among 400 patients, including some with normal renal function who later required permanent dialysis, are difficult to understand. Talner discussed these differences editorially, including variation in the definition of acute renal insufficiency, failure of some authors to follow their patients beyond 24 hours, and differences in the amount of injected contrast material.[23] Perhaps better hydration with crystalloid solutions (not D_5W), less contrast material, and other safer methods are involved.[24] Eisenberg's group suggested that their emphasis on improved hydration had significant results on conducting 537 major angiographies without a single instance of acute renal failure.[25]

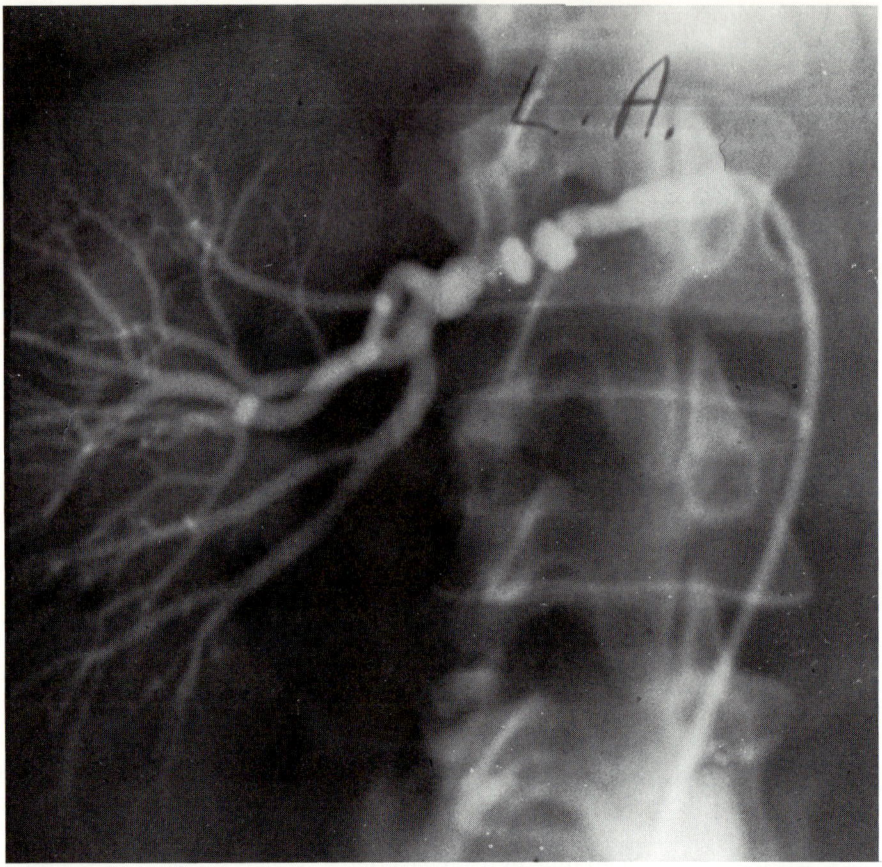

FIGURE 15-3 Right renal fibromuscular dysplasia in a hypertensive 50-year-old male.

Our results with angiography done by experienced radiologists indicate that procedure is relatively safe if high-risk patients (with renal problems, heart failure, or diabetes) are recognized and managed with care; if hydration is stressed before, during, and after the procedure; and if the amount of injected material is reduced to the lowest volume needed to make the diagnosis and map the indicated vessels. Competent radiologists avoid injections for "publishable" radiographs.

Surgical procedures should be delayed 24 to 48 hours after angiography, to allow complete renal clearance of the contrast material as well as to evaluate the renal function by observation of the urea nitrogen and creatinine levels.

Reactions to the contrast medium are infrequent when it is injected intraarterially, as opposed to a higher incidence of reactions following intravenous injection. Patients with a prior history of a reaction to contrast material should be pretreated with intravenous corticoids and diphenhydramine (Benadryl) and should have an anesthesia standby team present at the time of injection. No serious problems have been encountered personally after such prophylaxis.

Properly conducted renal angiograms are highly diagnostic and are the best screening for patients with severe hypertension, as well as the necessary map to allow planning of successful revascularization.

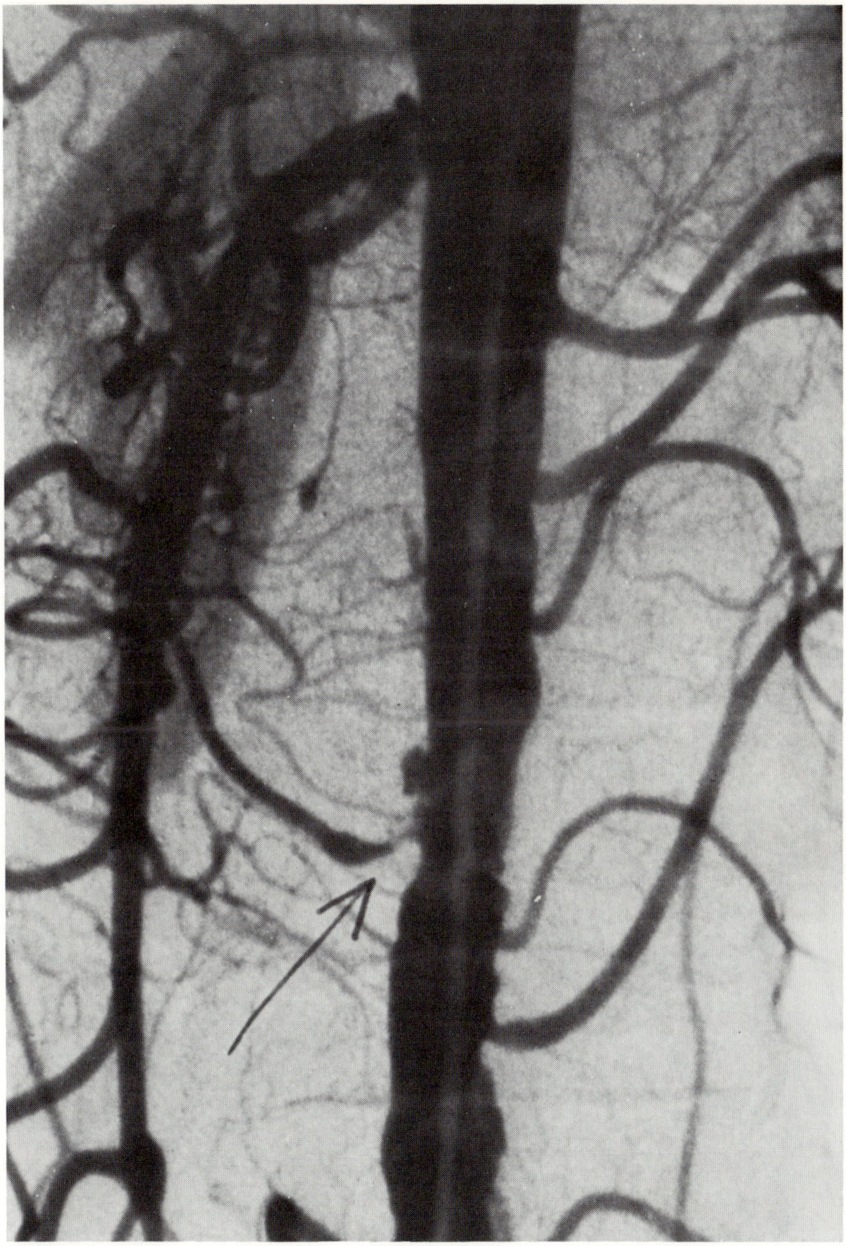

FIGURE 15-4 A secondary right renal artery with orificial stenosis supplied the lower pole of the kidney in a hypertensive 52-year-old female.

Computer-Assisted Subtraction Angiography

Computer-assisted subtraction angiography via an intravenous injection[26] has not yet replaced conventional angiography, because of false negatives which result from inadequate contrast visu-

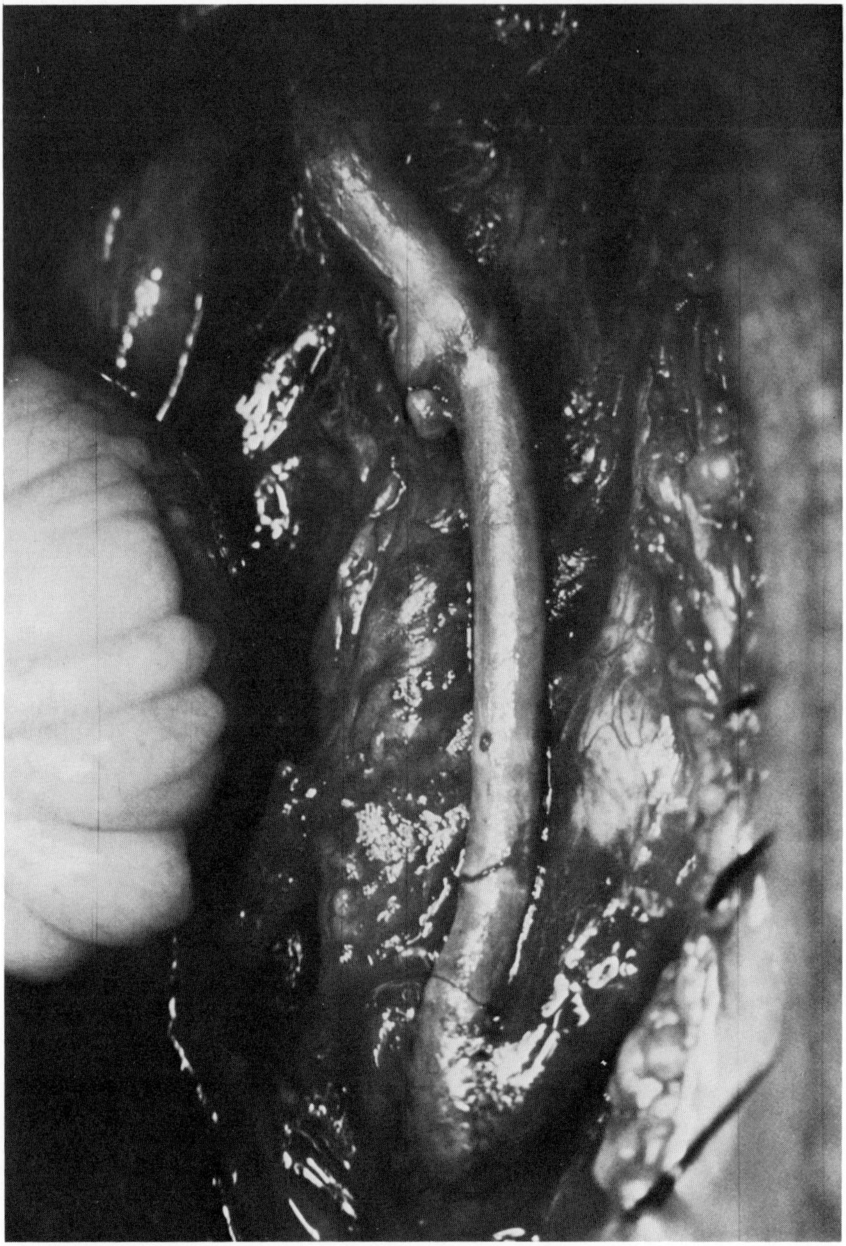

FIGURE 15-5 The lower pole of the right kidney was revascularized by a saphenous vein graft from the right common iliac artery.

alization of the renal arteries and their branches. However, the recent plan to pass a catheter via an arm vein into the inferior vena cava to obtain renal vein renins (RVRs), followed by withdrawal to an intracardiac position for injection of radiopaque material for such angiography, may prove to be worthwhile. This technique allows smaller amounts to be injected intravenously, thus reducing the risk of toxicity.

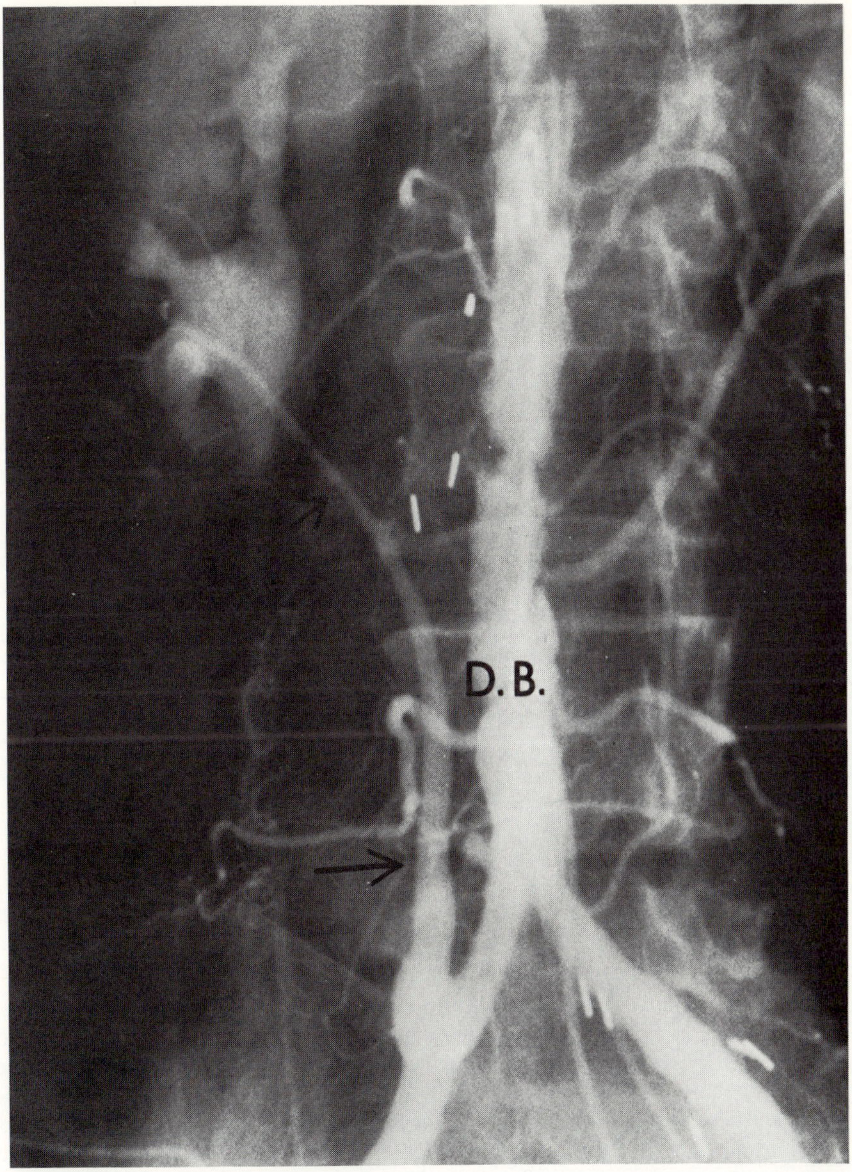

FIGURE 15-6 This postoperative aortogram demonstrates a patent vein graft from the right common iliac artery.

Renal Vein Renin

Assay of the levels of RVR in blood samples withdrawn by catheter from the renal veins is widely recognized as a critical predictor of hypertension due to renovascular lesions; a ratio greater than 1.5:1 between the two sides is the usually accepted minimum (Figure 15-7). If the ratio for diagnosis is raised to 2:1, the accuracy will be increased but more potentially curable patients will be denied operation.

A variety of factors influence the RVR level, including variations in sodium intake, medica-

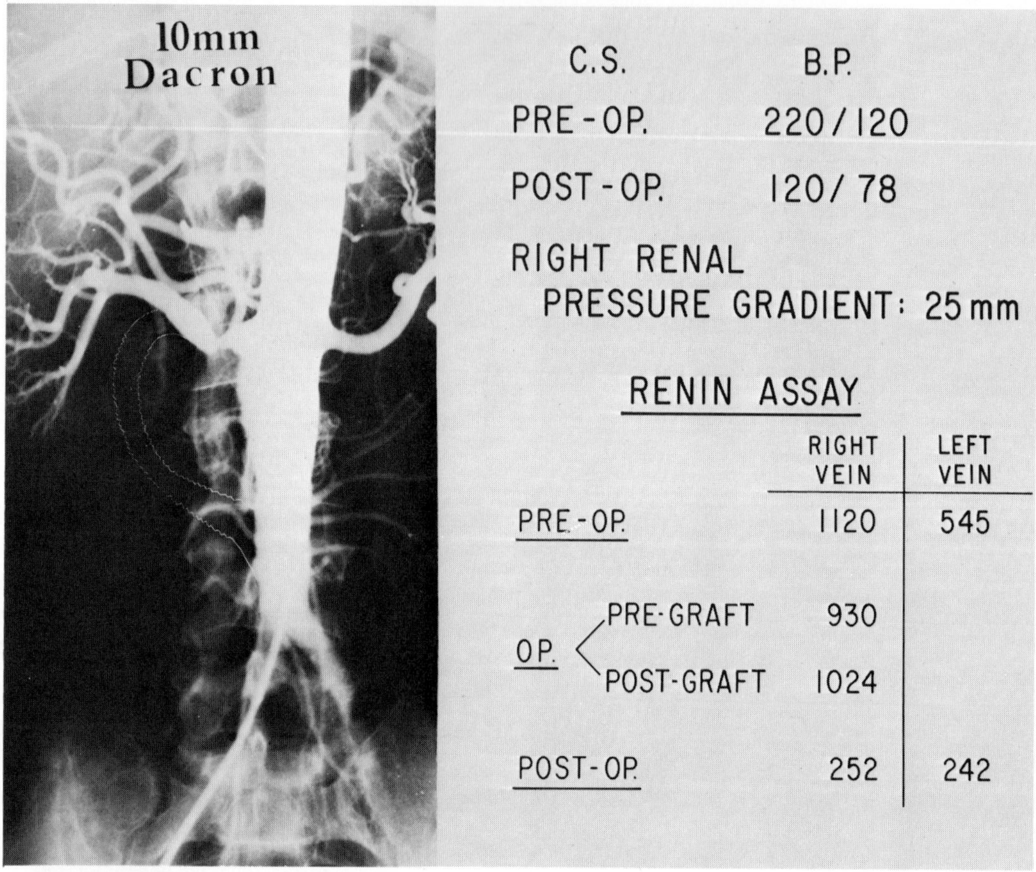

FIGURE 15-7 A 58-year-old male had relief of renovascular hypertension by a 10-mm Dacron bypass graft. The increased right RVR with a ratio of 1120:545 changed to normal, with a ratio 252:242, following the reconstructive operation.

tions, posture, and the technique employed. The effect of sodium depletion was demonstrated by Melman and associates in six patients who were studied with and without depletion, with only the latter condition resulting in renin increases. Increases were also shown when the patient's position was changed from recumbency to elevation on a tilt-table.[17] Hietala and associates studied 20 patients to determine the effects upon RVR assays of injecting sodium-containing contrast material during arteriography, concluding that the values changed but usually remained within the preinjection normal or abnormal range, so there was no consistent change due to the injection.[27]

The details of methodology are not yet completely determined. False positives were found in 24 percent of RVR assays when a single catheter was moved from one to the other renal vein in Dean's series.[14] Whelton's group similarly reported 22 percent false positives,[28] On the other hand, Harrington's team documented that results obtained by a single-catheter sequential technique did not differ significantly from those obtained simultaneously with two catheters among 65 patients.[29]

Recognizing the uncertainties and the variables in renin sampling but attempting to place it in a real world where hospital time, costs, and patient acceptance must be balanced against the importance of the information obtained, the suggested protocol of Table 15-3 has been developed. The RVR study may be done just prior to the renal arteriogram, if intravenous hydration is performed, or on the next day, to allow oral hydration.

Despite these recognized problems the RVR assay is at present the most valuable available predictor of a causal relationship between the renal arterial lesion and hypertension. If the patient has bilateral renal lesions, the likelihood of obtaining meaningful results is small, but sometimes the assay points to one rather than the other artery. In such a situation further study by split renal function testing may be helpful.

TABLE 15-3 SUGGESTED PREPARATION FOR RENAL VEIN RENIN STUDY

1 Diet
 - 2 g of sodium for 72 hours
 - Nothing by mouth for 8 hours pretest

2 Medication
 - No beta-blockers for 48 hours
 - No sympatholytics for 48 hours
 - Preferably no methyldopa (Aldomet), clonidine hydrochloride (Catapres), or prazosin (Minipress) for 48 hours
 - Captopril, hydralazine, and diuretics allowed (last dose 12 hours before the test)
 - Intramuscular atropine prior to the test to decrease vasovagal response
 - Parenteral diazepam (Valium) for pretest sedation

3 Sodium and volume depletion
 - 40 to 80 mg of furosemide from 6 P.M. the night before

4 Posture
 - Recumbent after 6 A.M.

Split Renal Function Studies

Comparison of the urine volume, creatinine concentration, and other parameters of function of the two kidneys obtained via bilateral ureteral catheterization may provide information which is not obtained from RVR assays. The involved kidney resorbs a larger volume of water and sodium and concentrates solutes such as creatinine, urea, or paraaminophippurate. Sometimes split renal function studies lateralize the functional lesion when RVRs fail to do so. Split function studies are not recommended routinely but are used as an additional diagnostic tool when needed.[30]

Is Functional Testing Mandatory?

In North America there is the general opinion that functional localization is important, since there are many renal stenoses which are not the cause of hypertension and whose correction will therefore not reduce the blood pressure. The Vanderbilt team has especially advocated this concept,[14] and it is also widely accepted elsewhere. Brewster, for example, has stated that "the functional significance of an arteriosclerotic lesion should be established . . . to allow reliable diagnosis."[31]

The 1983 report of Eigler's group from Essen, Germany, contradicts this opinion. Their hypertension cure and modification rates (Table 15-4) were quite similar to the American ones, yet they found that "functional tests, especially renal vein renin assay . . . were not considered necessary" and used angiographic indications primarily.[32] There obviously are enormous implications of this seeming heresy, in terms of time, cost, and patient discomfort. The matter does require further study.

INDICATIONS FOR SURGERY

Many physicians are reluctant to refer hypertensive patients for surgical management so long as their pressure can be controlled reasonably well by drugs. This attitude has been fostered by failures of operations to correct the hypertension, which reflect incorrect preoperative evaluation of angiographic lesions, as well as by failures of the revascularized arteries to remain patent. It is also widely believed that effective drug therapy is as protective to the patient's organs and life as is a successful operation. This latter concept is incorrect.

Several studies now support the concept of better organ and life results after a correctly indi-

TABLE 15-4 RESULTS OF RENAL REVASCULARIZATION PROCEDURES FOR HYPERTENSION

Researcher	Year	Ref no.	Total no. of patients	Normal, %			Improved, %			Failure, %			Mortality
				AS†	FMD§	All	AS	FMD	All	AS	FMD	All	
Vollmar	1970–1974	48	63			54			23			23	13
Stanley	1977	46	164			49			41			10	1.1
Buda	1976	18	116			66			19			15	1
Brewster	1980	31	NA*	32	60	58	32			10	6		3
Lawrie	1980	49	505	46	43		27	24		22	38		1.8
Von Schilfgaarde	1961–1981	35	148						70			30	8
Novick	1981	50	78		40				51		9		2
Dean	1982	14	182	31	77							6	0.5
Eigler	1983	32	242	36	70								4.1

*Not available.
†Arteriosclerosis.
§Fibromuscular Dysplasia.

cated operation, as opposed to drug therapy. Comparison of 100 surgical patients with 114 drug therapy patients by Hunt and Strong showed that 7 to 14 years later 84 percent of the surgical group were alive versus 66 percent of the drug groups (who also had other bad sequelae).[33] Deterioration of renal function during drug therapy has been further documented by serial renal function studies on 41 random patients with arteriosclerotic renal artery disease. Some 37 percent had loss of over 10 percent of renal size, while 12 percent had stenosis which progressed to total occlusion, and another 41 percent required later operations because of the deterioration of function.[34] These considerations lead to the recommendation for a revascularization operation for all severely hypertensive patients (1) who have reconstructible lesion, (2) whose functional studies are positive, and (3) who are reasonable operative risks. *Drug control is not as conservative of function and life as is a complete surgical cure.*

Hypertensives who have other intraabdominal arterial lesions which require operation should have preoperative renal evaluation to determine whether simultaneous renal revascularization is indicated. Patients with aortic aneurysms, aortic occlusive disease, and/or other visceral lesions do not always require concomitant renal artery repairs, since many are merely ateriographic visualizations of incidental nonfunctional lesions, but some patients do need it (Figure 15-8). It may be a close call in an individual case, but in general the addition of bilateral aortorenal bypasses for patients with aterioscierotic plaques but without either hypertention or renal dysfunction adds unnecessary risk to an aortic graft for either aneurysm or aortic occlusion.[35] The Everest syndrome (page 24) is not a proper indication for an operation.

Another situation which merits discussion is the one of a hypertensive patient with bilateral lesions in whom the functional studies point to one side. Since the diagnostic studies are not infallible and operation must be performed on at least one side, it is reasonable to correct the other side at the time rather than hope it does not already (or will not in the future) hypersecrete renin.

SURGICAL PROCEDURES

Exposure

Renal arterial procedures are often approached through a long midline incision. Better exposure may be obtained through a "bucket handle" upper-abdominal incision, i.e., a bilateral subcostal one which transects both rectus muscles and opens the oblique muscles laterally (Figure 15-9). This affords better lateral exposure and centers in the upper abdomen rather than the midabdomen. It requires a bit more time than the midline incision, but that is regained by an easier overall procedure. The closure is as strong as, or even more certain than, in the midline. The distal aorta is readily available by retraction of the abdominal wall flap inferiorly. If only one renal artery requires repair, the contralateral portion of the incision is not carried far laterally.

Endarterectomy

Over the years a number of operative procedures have been used to revascularize the kidneys. Present-day alternatives essentially consist of aortorenal bypass grafting or direct open endarterectomy. The latter is attractive in terms of theoretic simplicity but in practice requires a more difficult dissection and is therefore infrequently used.

In the past, endarterectomy was performed on the left with complete exposure of the renal artery along with the adjacent portion of the aorta. The aorta was "side-clamped" during the endarterectomy. This sometimes resulted in such limited aortic exposure that a clean internal dissection was not possible. Modern endarterectomy requires aortic cross-clamping above and below the renal arteries and a wide opening of the aorta and renal artery to allow a complete removal of the atherosclerotic material under direct vision.

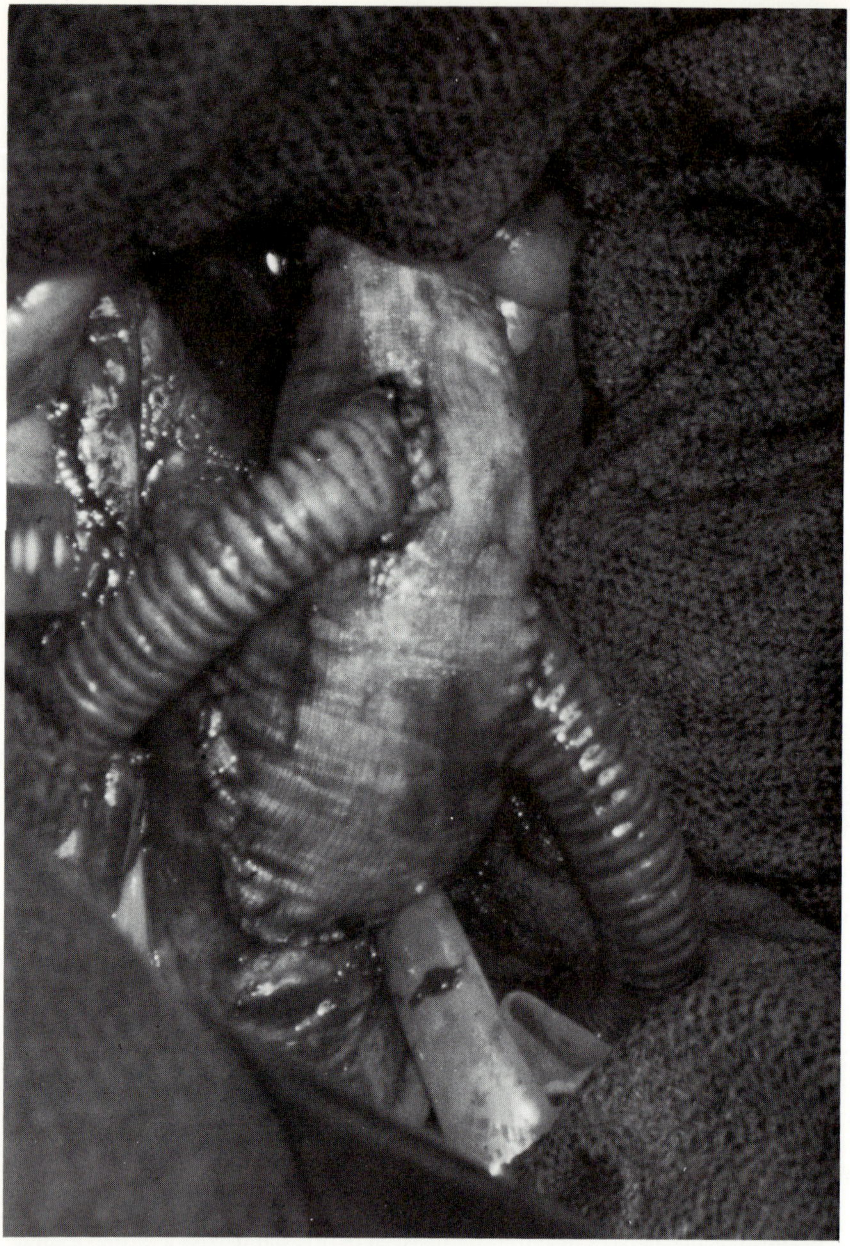

FIGURE 15-8 A 55-year-old required an aortobifemoral graft for atherosclerotic disease. Bilateral aortorenal shunts of knitted Dacron relieved the renovascular hypertension at a simultaneous operation.

Endarterectomy is now commonly used for bilateral orificial lesions. The proximal aorta is dissected and cross-clamped between the celiac axis and the superior mesenteric artery, along with infrarenal cross-clamping. A transverse opening in the aorta is carried into each renal artery so that complete endarterectomy can be performed. The closure may be with or without a patch

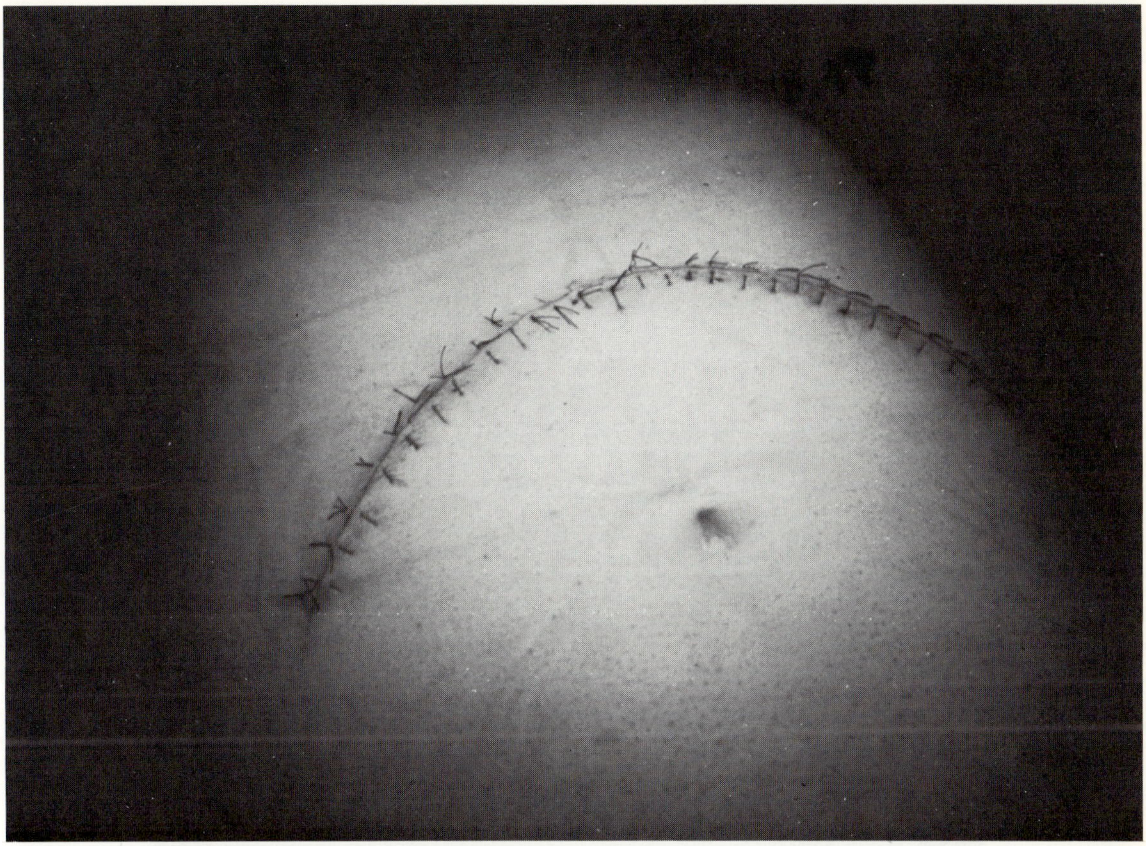

FIGURE 15-9 A high transverse incision for bilateral renal artery repair.

graft (Figure 15-10). An orificial lesion of an accessory but more distal renal artery is similarly performed under direct vision, but it more often requires a patch graft to prevent stenosis at the site of closure. Ideally, the patch should consist of a segment of autogenous vein, but in practice there is little difference between this and a small polytetrafluoroethylene (PTFE) patch. The latter is simpler.

Alternatively, if an aortic graft is also to be placed, the aorta may be divided just below the renal arteries, which allows the renal endarterectomy to be done through the opened end of the proximal aorta. If additional exposure is needed, this end may be split in order that the operator can more clearly see the renal orifices. The longitudinal split may be either oversewn or patched with a tongue of the graft as it is attached to the aorta.

Aortorenal Bypass

Autogenous saphenous vein is the material of choice, even though late postoperative angiograms sometimes show dilatation or even aneurysm formation (Figure 15-11). Among 93 vein grafts studied by the Vanderbilt group, there were 30 dilatations, 20 stenoses, and 2 aneurysms, but the x-ray findings did not usually indicate poor clinical results.[36]

Synthetic tubes have not been widely used as aortorenal bypasses, although the reported

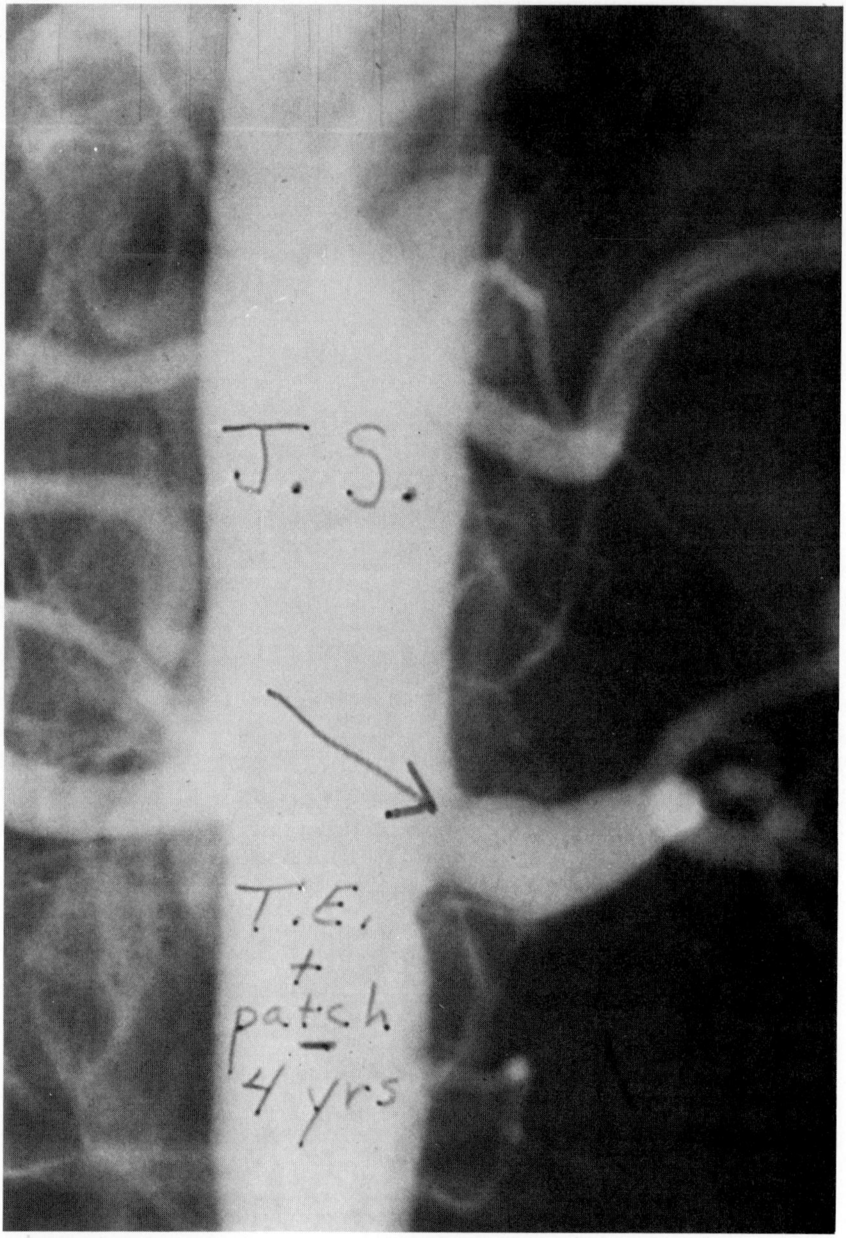

FIGURE 15-10 A 61-year-old male had continued relief of hypertension 4 years following left renal thromboendarterectomy with a venous patch graft.

results for these short, nonmoving retroperitoneal grafts are good (Figures 15-12 to 15-14). Kaufman noted favorable outcomes of 13 among 15 patients followed 6 to 11 years.[37] Sometimes Dacron tubes, like vein grafts, show long-term postoperative stenoses (4 among 19 in the Vanderbilt series), which again are not necessarily clinically significant.[36] One disadvantage of a syn-

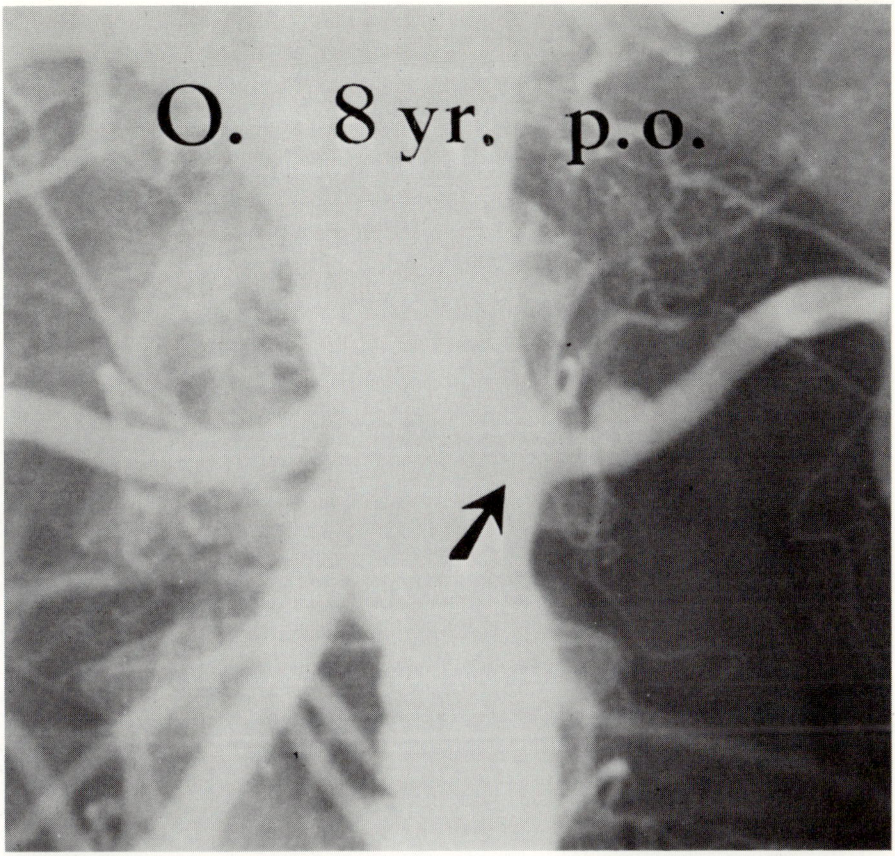

FIGURE 15-11 A 54-year-old male continued to be normotensive 8 years following left renal thromboendarterectomy and a venous patch graft. The arteriograms suggest dilatation or even aneurysm at follow-up 8 years after the operation.

thetic tube is the late development of a false aneurysm at a suture line, which is not a problem after use of vein grafts.[38]

There has not yet been a comparison of PTFE to Dacron tubes in this position. PTFE is easy to use, and I prefer it rather than vein if the aortorenal graft is to be based upon a replacement synthetic graft of the aorta.

The autogenous hypogastric artery may be useful, especially in a child, since its size increases with age.[39]

The pathway of the aortorenal graft should allow an easy "S" or "C" curve. Although this appears to reverse the flow of blood as it passes into the graft, there have occurred no particular problems with it, since the pulsatile flow pursues the course of least resistance in whatever direction it may be (Figure 15-15).

It is usually easier to perform the anastomosis to the renal artery first, since the graft can be held in any desired position during the process of suturing. If the graft is placed end to side, there remains some flow through the stenotic area. If the renal artery is divided near the aorta, this flow does not compete with flow through the graft and may allow the position of the graft to be more appropriate. Sometimes it is easier to begin the anastomosis at the toe of the graft in the

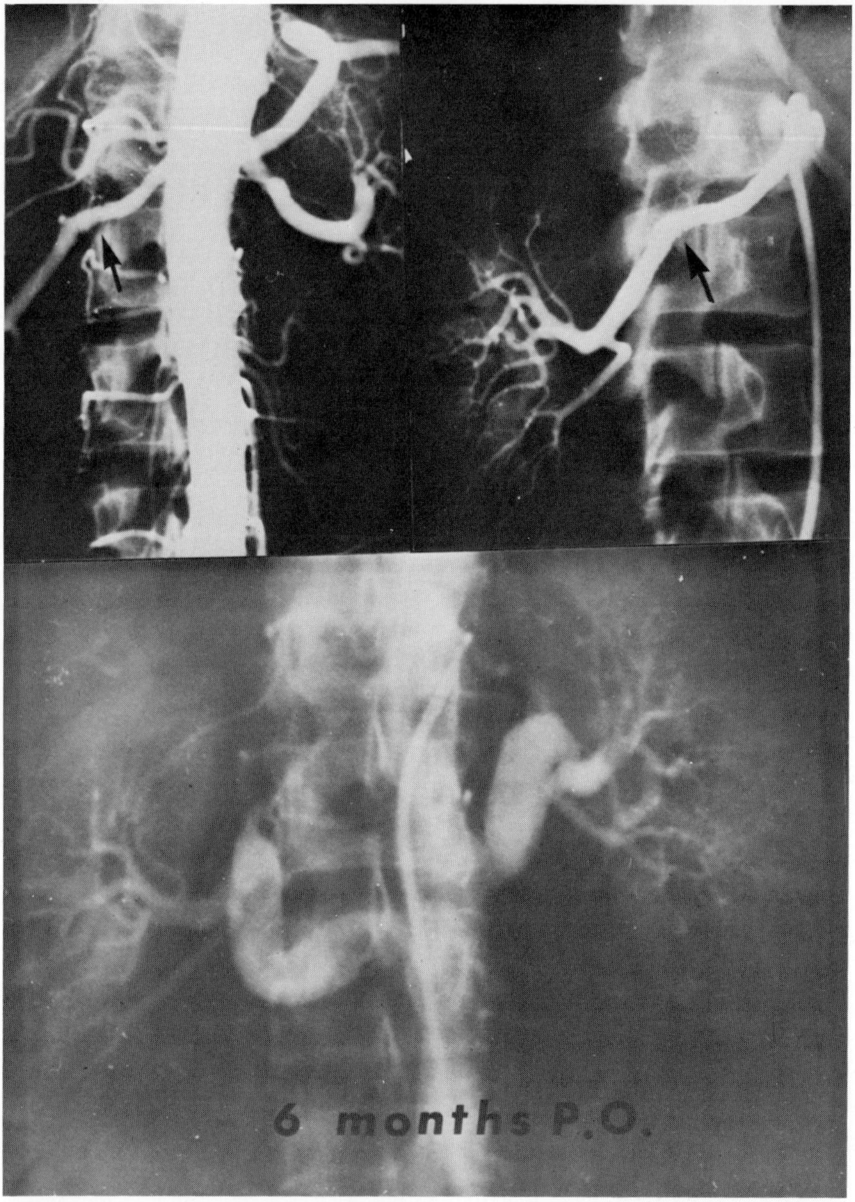

FIGURE 15-12 A 49-year-old female with bilateral fibromuscular dysplasia has patent knit Dacron bypass grafts 6 months following operation.

distal renal artery before dividing the proximal renal artery. The artery later may be divided proximally so that the end result is a long ovoid end-to-end anastomosis. In any event, the anastomosis should be approximately three times the diameter of the renal artery. The other end of the renal artery may then be applied to the aorta in whatever fashion seems most appropriate.

The few surgeons who prefer to anastomose the aortic end to that vessel proximal to the

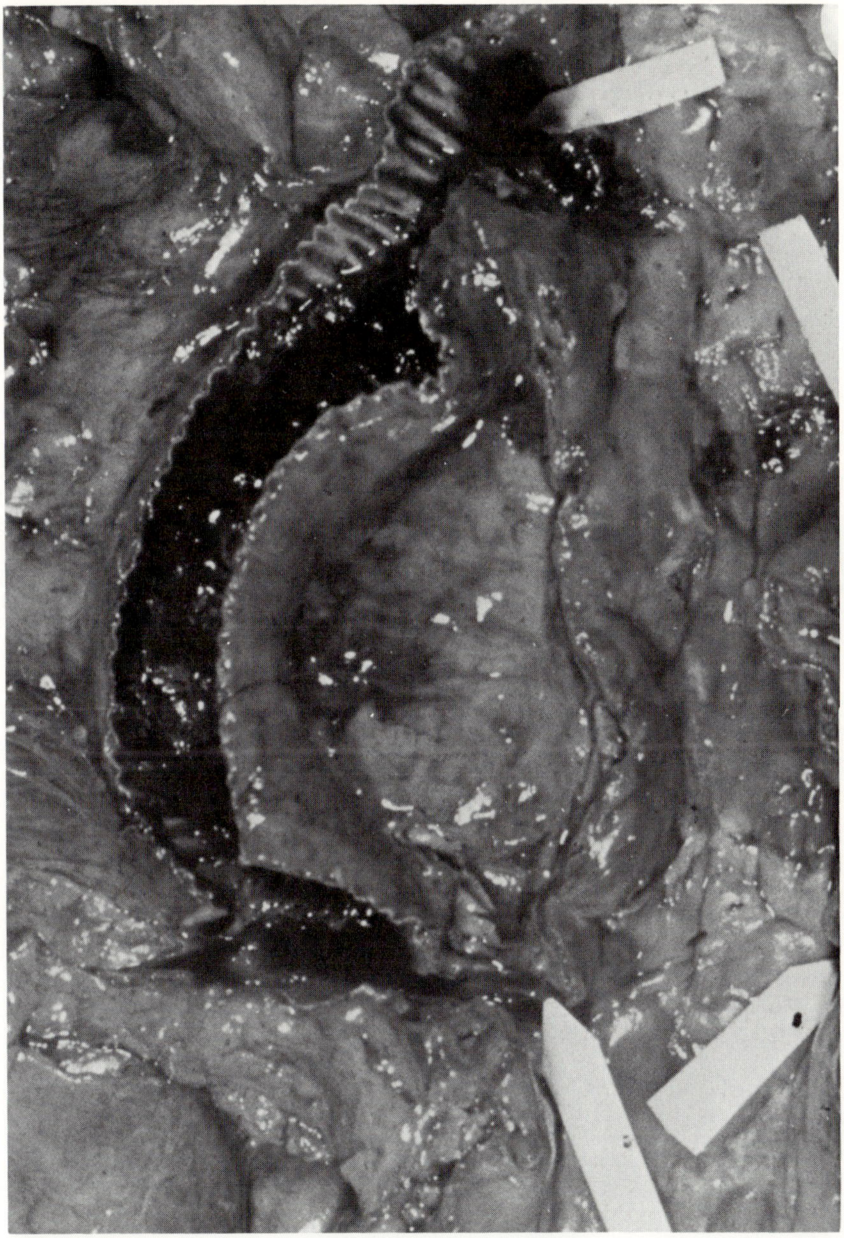

FIGURE 15-13 A 38-year-old male died of ruptured diverticulitis with generalized peritonitis 4 months following placment of bilateral aortorenal tube Dacron bypass grafts. At autopsy both grafts were widely patent, with fresh postmorten clot lying within the opened autopsy specimen.

visceral vessels must perform considerably more dissection to free the prerenal aorta and avoid the celiac and mesenteric arteries. Most place the aortic anastomosis distal to the renal arteries.

A complicating factor occurs when the infrarenal aorta is so atherosclerotic that the anastomosis of a small graft to it is difficult and may not remain patent. This problem can be solved

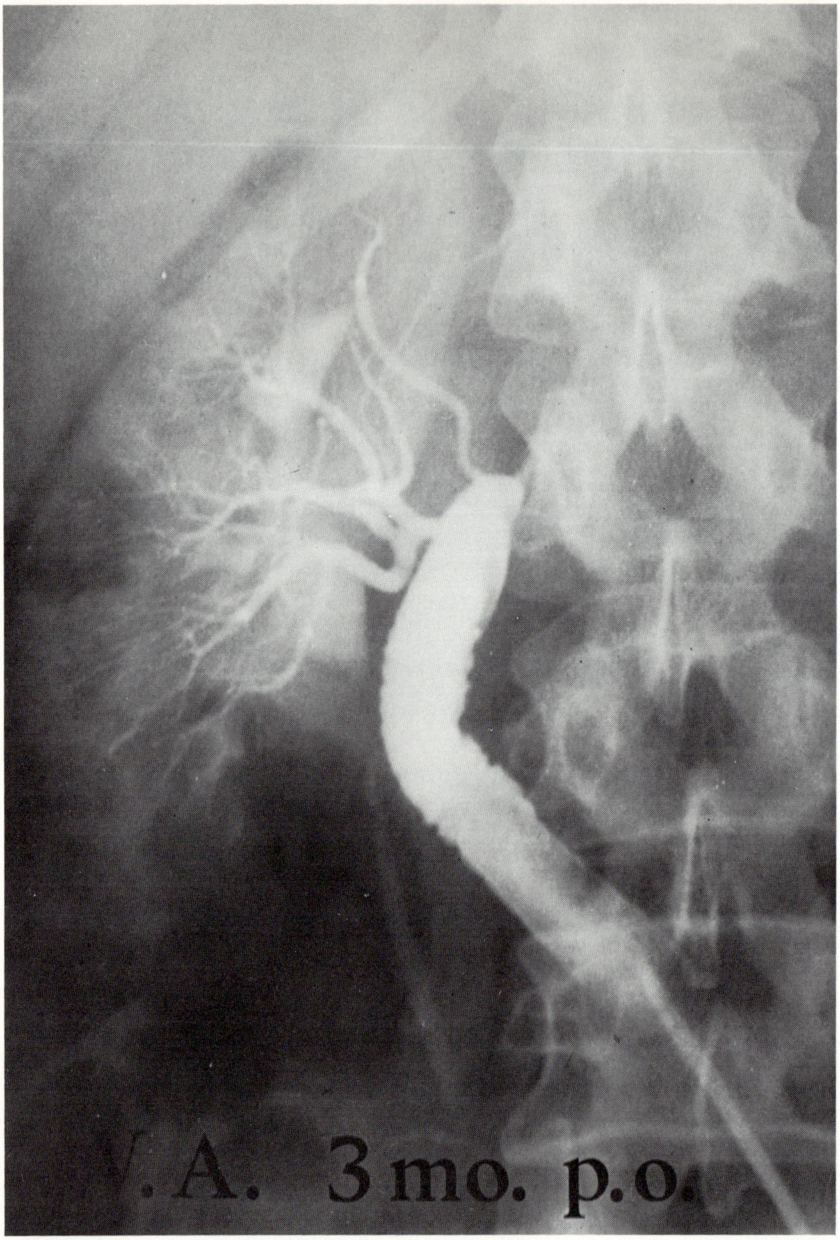

FIGURE 15-14 A 43-year-old female with a patent tube Dacron graft to the right renal artery 3 months postoperative.

by resection of the aorta and replacement with a synthetic tube or by use of a longer graft whose origin is iliac artery, which may be free of the severe atherosclerotic process (Figure 15-5).

In the event that the aortic end of the bypass graft is placed to a replacement synthetic tube, the alternative of using a synthetic graft rather than a vein is attractive, since the latter is smaller and its orifice may be more easily occluded by proliferating new intima. Certainly, it is widely

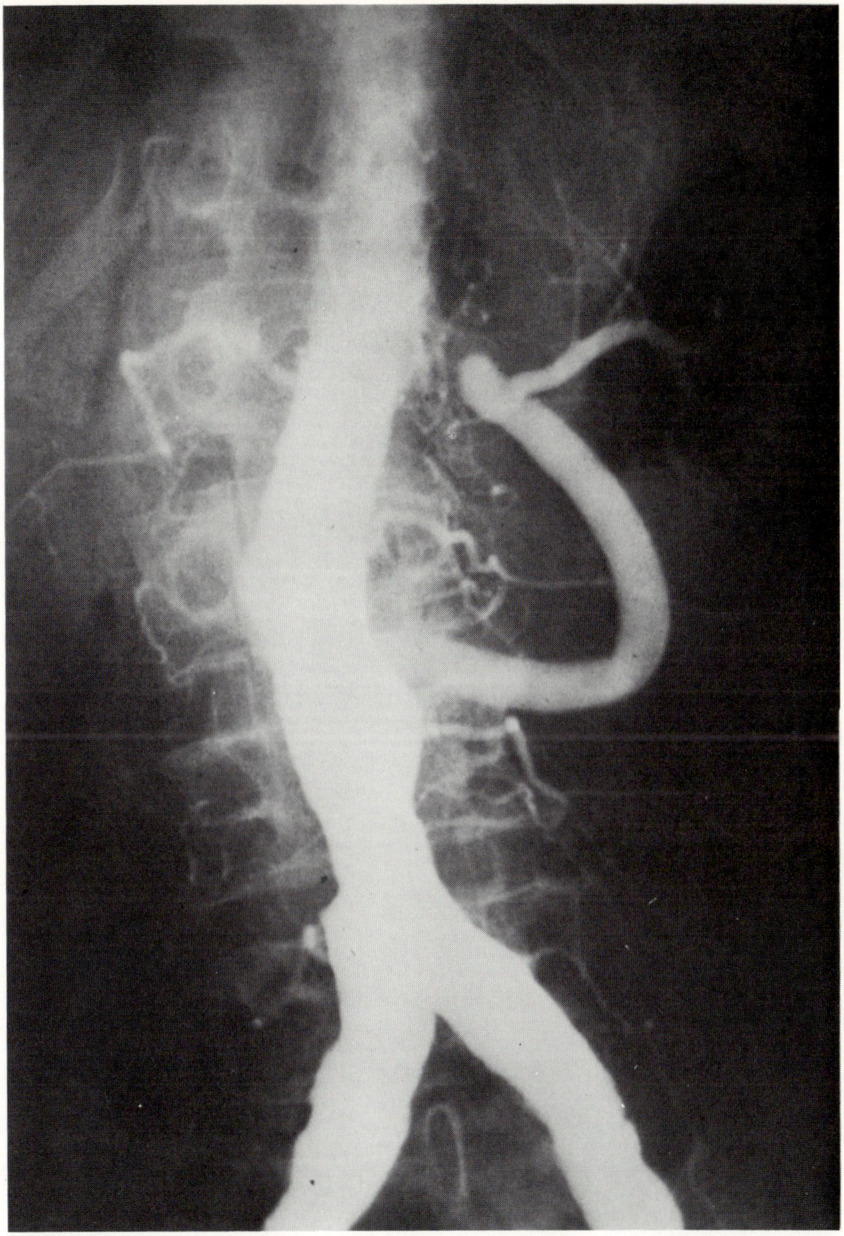

FIGURE 15-15 A 54-year-old female whose hypertension was relieved by this 8-mm Dacron graft placed in a "C" curve to the left renal artery.

believed that a saphenous vein graft is preferable, but personal experience with Dacron bypasses reflects the good patency reports of others.[37] For this reason I prefer to attach a synthetic side-arm graft to the aortic graft (Figure 15-16).

Revascularization of each kidney should be carried out efficiently so that the total ischemia time is as short as is consistent with a well-done anastomosis. Most of these anastomoses can be

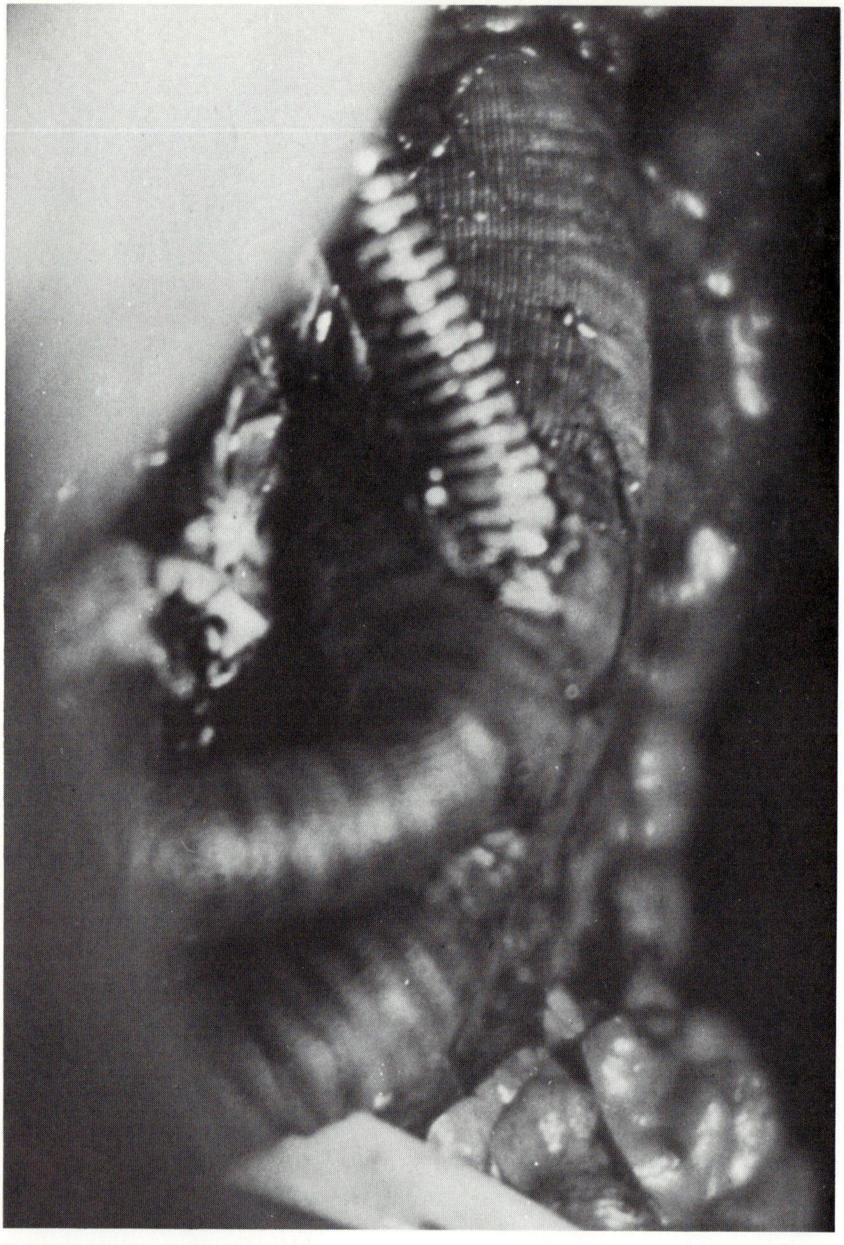

FIGURE 15-16 A 73-year-old female had an aorto-bi-iliac graft for an aneurysm, to which was added a right aortorenal 8-mm Dacron graft.

completed within 20 minutes; 30 minutes is always tolerated well, and the kidney will probably survive an hour of ischemia. If the graft is connected end-to-side to the renal artery, it may thereafter be temporarily cross-clamped so that blood will continue to flow through the stenotic portion while the other end of the graft is anastomosed to the aorta. Another technique for decreasing ischemic time is to attach the side graft to the main aortic graft prior to its placement so that only one anastomosis is necessary after the renal artery is clamped. Complicated techniques of hypothermia are not ordinarily necessary.

Splenic and Hepatic Bypass

These require a more extensive exposure and dissection but can be used to supply blood to one of the renal arteries. The splenic artery itself can be directed inferiorly. The hepatic vessel may be used as the origin for a vein graft.[40]

Bilateral Operation

In the past some surgeons avoided bilateral renal arterial repairs for fear that excessive blood loss and longer anesthesia time would result in an increased morbidity rate. Against those considerations must be assessed the risk of two different anesthesias, the necessity to deal with intraperitoneal adhesions with scar tissue about the aorta the second time, and the possible complications of the continued hypertension during the time period while one side remains stenotic.

Once experience has been acquired with exposing the renal arteries and with the general techniques of small-vessel anastomoses, there need be no hestitation to perform simultaneously both left and right renal revascularizations (Figure 15-8). This course has always been followed personally without any known complication or bad result for the patient and with the considerable advantage that a secondary procedure is not necessary.

Percutaneous Transluminal Angioplasty

The development of percutaneous transluminal dilation of arteries has recently been extended to the renal vessels, but further elapsed time is needed for final evaluation of this technique. Certainly a nonoperative method is appealing, especially for poor-risk patients. At present (January 1985), while early success rates are favorable, there are conflicting reports regarding indications and long-term results. Luft's group retrospectively studied 12 such problem patients, finding that only 3 were improved, while 4 suffered oliguric renal failure. On the other hand, among 12 operations, there were 10 improvements and 2 deaths.[41] Kaufman commented editorially that these results "underscore the opinion held by the majority that . . . PTA occasionally may open a renal artery . . . but is rarely of lasting value."[42]

The experience of others is more optimistic. Tegtmeyer's group reported 100 percent initial technical success, with intermediate-term (1 to 30 months) cures in 62 percent and improvement in 38 percent of 21 cases.[43] Sos and associates recently discussed renal angioplasty in 89 patients, with 87 percent early technical success in fibrous dysplasia (with 93 percent continued success at 16 months) and 57 percent early success in unilateral atherosclerotic stenoses (with 82 percent continued success at 16 months) but only 10 percent early success in bilateral arteriosclerotic stenoses. They concluded that "partial" technical successes usually failed later, that ostial lesions responded poorly, and that advanced bilateral lesions were not often helped. There were no angioplasty-related deaths, and only one patient lost a kidney.[44]

Schwarten's 70-patient series had 93 percent early success, with 90 percent of their first group cured or improved at 6 months.[45]

It appears that angioplasty is still in the developing stage, so there is not yet any standardization of technique (e.g., balloon size or amount of tension) or of results. There is promise of widespread usefulness, however, as its indications are clarified and as expertise develops (Figures 15-17 and 15-18).

Fibrodysplastic lesions are better candidates than are atherosclerotic ones. Among the latter, orificial lesions are particularly to be avoided, along with bilateral and widespread atherosclerotic stenoses.

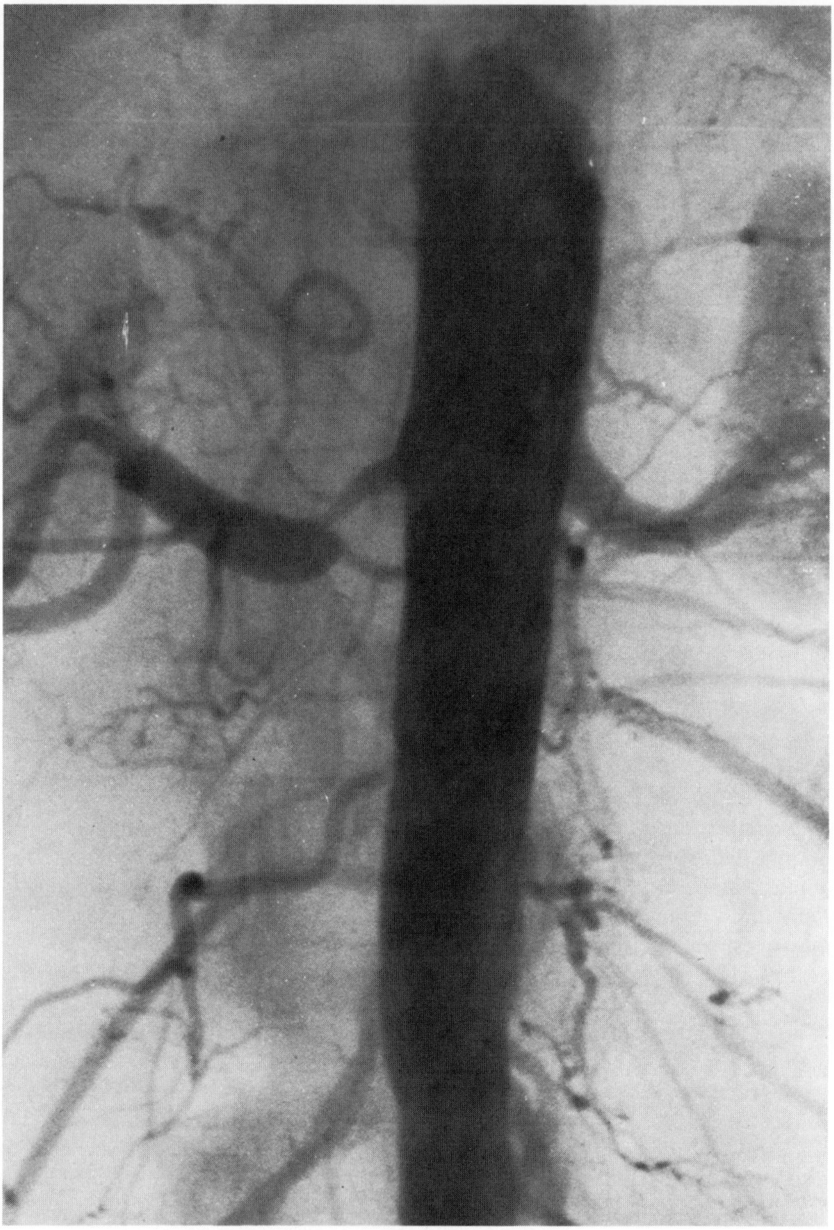

FIGURE 15-17 Tight stenosis of the right renal artery.

Nephrectomy

Occasionally a hypertensive patient has a kidney with multiple stenotic renal vessels which appear virtually impossible to repair successfully, so ablation of the kidney must be considered. If a nonreconstructible situation is accompanied by severe loss of function, there is little doubt that nephrectomy is indicated. If residual function is reasonable and the hypertension can be

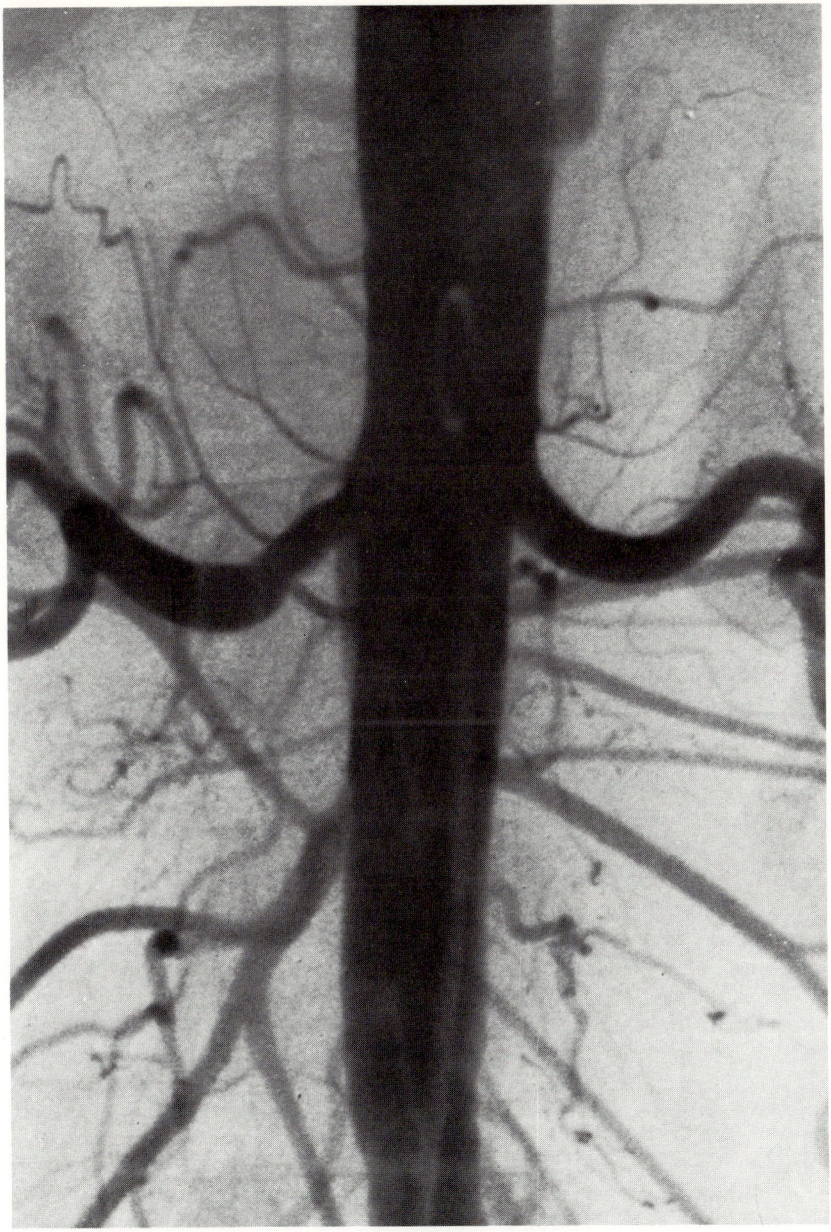

FIGURE 15-18 Relief of renovascular hypertension was achieved by percutaneous balloon dilation of the right renal artery.

controlled with suitable medication, the kidney should probably be preserved, particularly if the patient is young. Certainly maximum efforts to avoid nephrectomy are in order.

Release of Extrinsic Pressure

Two of my patients have been successfully operated upon for the relief of extrinsic pressure causing localized renal arteriostenosis. A 45-year-old female had a sharply demarcated stenosis near the origin of the left renal artery , which was completely relieved by freeing up the artery, without any specific etiology being discovered. The other patient was a 57-year-old male with stenosis secondary to retroperitoneal fibrosis (Figure 15-2).

RESULTS OF SURGERY

The cure or amelioration of renovascular hypertension depends upon proper selection of patients so that operations are performed only upon patients with functionally significant lesions, as well as upon the technical success of the procedure. Successes therefore reflect accurate diagnosis as well as surgical prowess.

Good success rates have been achieved in several series. Melman, Donohue, Weinberger, and Grim reported 81 percent success among unilateral and 91 percent among bilateral atherosclerotic renovascular lesions.[17] Dean reported a good blood pressure response after successful operation in 94 percent of 182 cases followed 6 months or longer. The complete cure rate was better in fibromuscular disease (77 percent) than in atherosclerotic disease (31 percent).[14] Stanley's summary of the results of six series of renal revascularizations in 200 or more patients showed that all groups except one "cured" or "improved" 81 to 89 percent of all those operated upon, with a risk of death of 1.8 to 3.1 percent.[46]

The statistics shown in Table 15-4 were collected from the recent literature as representative of large series. Variations in criteria of success and failure to differentiate the results of treatment of different causes, make overall conclusions shaky, to say the least. It does, however, appear (1) that fibromuscular disease offers a better outlook for reconstruction than do atherosclerotic lesions, (2) that complete failure rates may be reduced below 10 percent by proper case selection, and (3) that mortality rates of 0.5 to 3 percent may be expected among patients managed by experienced teams.

Approximately 3 percent of renovascular hypertensives are children under 18 years of age. Novick's group cured 59 percent of 27 children, with 19 percent improvement and 22 percent failure.[39]

IMPROVEMENT OF RENAL FUNCTION

There is no doubt now that revascularization often improves renal function as well as reduces blood pressure. Sicard and associates reported a reduction of creatinine from a mean of 5.0 to 2.4 mg in 12 of 18 patients, while 2 others survived but without reduction of creatinine. Four who were at first improved died later.[47] Novick's group reduced the creatinine levels in 86 percent of 22 patients, with no change in 2 and an increase in 1 other, concluding that renal revascularization to improve function was quite worthwhile for selected patients.[39]

RISKS

Complication and mortality rates have become a bit difficult to assess, since it is becoming fashionable to show "operation-related" morbidity and mortality. The figures in Table 15-4 are therefore suspect, in some instances, as representing the most optimistic view possible. It is hard to assign the death of a patient by myocardial infarction 10 days after an operation as either operation-related or not. In the past, deaths in the hospital were considered as related to the operation. But what of the patient who was discharged in good condition and died of pulmonary embolism at home on the following day? Survival-against-time curves will reflect such but require longer periods of time for their construction. In any event, statistics must be judged with care.

REFERENCES

1 *Health U.S. 1980 with Prevention Profile.* US Department of Health and Human Services, Public Health Service pub no (PHS) 81-121. Washington, 1981.

2 Black HR: Evaluation and treatment of the hypertensive patient. *Primary Care* 1983, 10:3.
3 Tigerstedt R, Bergman PG: Niere und Kreislauf. *Scand Arch Physiol* 1909, 8:223.
4 Goldblatt H, Lynch J, Hanzal RF, Summerville WW: Studies on experimental hypertension. I The production of persistent evaluation of systolic blood pressure by means of renal ischemia. *J Exp Med* 1934, 59:347.
5 Smith HW: Unilateral nephrectomy in hypertensive disease. *J Urol* 1956, 76:685.
6 Smith HW: *From Fish to Philosopher.* Little, Brown, Boston, 1953.
7 Smith HW: *Man and His Gods.* Grosset & Dunlap, New York, 1952.
8 Freeman NE, Leeds FH, Elliott WC, Roland SI: Thromboendarterectomy for hypertension due to renal artery occlusion. *JAMA* 1954, 156:1077.
9 Brown LED, Laragh JH: New concepts of renin system and of vasoconstriction volume mechanisms: Diagnosis and treatment. *Urol Clin Am* 1975, 2:237.
10 Vaughan ED Jr: Pathophysiology of renovascular hypertension, in Rutherford RB (ed): *Vascular Surgery.* WB Saunders, Philadelphia, 1977, p 979.
11 Holley KE, Hunt JC, Brown AL Jr, Kincaid OW, Sheps SG: Renal artery stenosis: A clinical-pathologic study in normotensive and hypertensive patients. *Am J Med* 1964, 37:14.
12 Eyler WR, Clark MD, Garman JE, Rian RL, Meininger DE: Angiography of the renal areas including comparative study of renal artery stenoses in patients with or without hypertension. *Radiology* 1962, 78:879.
13 Gaspar MR: Renovascular hypertension. *Major Probl Clin Surg* 1981, 4:383.
14 Dean RH: Renovascular hypertension (Chapter 16), in Moore WS (ed): *Vascular Surgery: A Comprehensive Review.* Grune & Stratton, New York, 1983, p 433.
15 Foster JH, Dean RH, Pinkerton JA, Rhamy RK: Ten years experience with the surgical management of renovascular hypertension. *Ann Surg* 1973, 177:755.
16 Lawson, JD, Boerth R, Foster JH, Dean RH: Diagnosis and management of renovascular hypertension in children. *Arch Surg* 1977, 112:1307.
17 Melman A, Donohue JP, Weinberger MH, Grim CE: Improved diagnostic accuracy of renal venous renin ratios with stimulation of renin release. *J Urol* 1977, 117:145.
18 Buda JA, Baer L, Parra-Carrillo JZ, Kashef MM, McAllister FF, Voorhees AB Jr, Pirani CL: Predictability of surgical response in renovascular hypertension. *Arch Surg* 1976, 111:1243.
19 Arendell R, Lawson JD, Petracek MR, Meacham PW, Hollifield JW, Dean RH: Study of Sar-1–Ala-8 angiotensin II responsiveness in hypertension of renal origin. *J Surg Res* 1978, 24:284.
20 Black HR: Renovascular hypertension: Detection evaluation and management. *Primary Care* 1983, 10:63.
21 Hessel SJ, Adams DF, Abrams HL: Complications of angiography. *Diagn Radiol* 1981, 138:273.
22 Swartz FD, Rubin J, Lemming BW, Silva P: Renal failure following major angiography. *Am J Med* 1978, 65:31.
23 Talner LB: Editorial. Does hydration prevent contrast material injury? *Am J Radiol* 1981, 136:1021.
24 Martin-Paredero V, Dixon SM, Baker JD, Takiff H, Gomes AS, Busuttil RW, Moore WS: Risk of renal failure after major angiography. *Arch Surg* 1983, 118:1417.
25 Eisenberg RL, Bank WO, Hedgock MW: Renal failure after major angiography can be avoided with hydration. *Am J Radiol* 1981, 136:859.
26 Gomes AS, Pais SO, Barbaric ZL: Digital subtraction angiography in the evaluation of hypertension. *Am J Radiol* 1983, 140:783.
27 Hietala SO, Zelenak JJ, Beachley MC, Tisnado J: Influence of contrast material on renal venous renin activity. *Am Roent Ray Soc* 1979, 132:429.
28 Whelton PK, Harrington DP, Russel RP, et al: Renal vein renin activity: A prospective study of sampling techniques and methods of interpretation. *John Hopkins Med J* 1977, 141:112.
29 Harrington DP, Whelton PK, Mackenzie EJ, Russell RP, Kaufman SL, Barth KH, White RI Jr, Walker WG: Renal venous renin sampling: Prospective study of techniques and methods. *Diagn Radiol* 1981, 138:571.
30 Schaeffer AJ, Starney TA: Ureteral catheterization studies. *Urol Clin N Am* 1975, 2:327.
31 Brewster D: Surgical management of renovascular disease. *AJR* 1980, 135:963.
32 Eigler HR, Dostal G, Montag H, Jakubowski HD: Results of a ten year period of reconstructive surgery for renovascular disease. *Thorac Cardiovasc Surg* 1983, 37:45.
33 Hunt JC, Strong CG: Renovascular hypertension: Mechanisms, natural history and treatment. *Am J Cardiol* 1973, 32:562.

34 Dean RH, Kieffer RW, Smith BM, Oates JA, Nadau JHJ, Hoolliefield JW, DuPont WD: Renovascular hypertension. *Arch Surg* 1981, 116:1408.

35 Von Schilfgaarde R, Von Bockel JH, Felthuis W, Terpstra JL: Clinical results of surgical therapy for renovascular hypertension (Chapter 12), in Von Schilfgaarde R, Stanley JC, Turmmelen P, Overbosch EH: *Clinical Aspects of Renovascular Hypertension.* Martinus Nijhoff, Boston, 1983.

36 Ekelund L, Gerlock J, Gonchaneku V, Foster JH: Angiographic findings following surgical treatment. *Radiology* 1978, 126:345.

37 Kaufman JJ: Dacron grafts and splenorenal by-pass in the surgical treatment of stenosing lesions of the renal artery. *Urol Clin N Am* 1975, 2:356.

38 Dean R, Krueger T, Whiteneck J, Dupont B, Foster J, Smith B, Hollifield J, Oates J: Operative management of renovascular hypertension. *J Vasc Surg* 1984, 1:234.

39 Novick AC, Straffon RA, Stewart BH, Benjamin S: Surgical treatment of renovascular hypertension in the pediatric patient. *J Urol* 1978, 119:794.

40 Chibraro EA, Libertino JA, Novick AC: Use of the hepatic circulation for renal revascularization. *Ann Surg* 1984, 199:406.

41 Luft FC, Grim CE, Weinberger MH: Intervention in patients with renovascular hypertension and renal insufficiency. *J Urol* 1983, 130:654.

42 Kaufman JJ: Editorial comment. *J Urol* 1983, 130:656.

43 Tegtmeyer CJ, Elson J, Glass TA, Ayers CR, Chevalier RL, Wellons HA, Studdard WE: Percutaneous transluminal angioplasty: Treatment of choice for renovascular hypertension due to fibromuscular dysplasia. *Radiology* 1982, 143:631.

44 Sos TA, Pickering TG, Phil D, Sniderman K, Saddekni S, Case DB, Silane MF, Vaughan ED Jr, Larah JH: Percutaneous transluminal renal angioplasty in renovascular hypertension due to atheroma or fibromuscular dysplasia. *N Engl J Med* 1983,309:274.

45 Schwarten DE: Transluminal angioplasty of renal artery stenosis: 70 experiences. *Am J Radiol* 1980, 135:969.

46 Stanley JC: Renovascular hypertension: The surgical point of view (Chapter 19), in Von Schilfgaarde R, Stanley JC, Brimmelen P, Overbosch EH: *Clinical Aspects of Renovascular Hypertension.* Martinus Nijhoff, Boston, 1983, p 259.

47 Sicard GA, Anderson CB, Maeser MBN: Improved renal function after renal revascularization. *J Cardiovasc Surg* (Torino) 1983, 24:383.

48 Vollmar J, Nadjafi S, Rosenthal J: Surgical consideration in the treatment of renovascular hypertension. *Surg Gynecol Obstet* 1977, 144:553.

49 Lawrie GM, Morris CC, Soossou ID, Starr DM, Silvers A, Glaeser DS, DeBakey ME: Later results of reconstructive surgery for renovascular disease. *Ann Surg* 1980, 191:528.

50 Novick AC, Stratton RA, Steward BH, Gifford RW, Vidt D: Diminished operative morbidity and mortality in renal revascularization. *JAMA* 1981, 749:53.

Invited Commentary

Richard H. Dean, M.D.
Nashville, Tennessee

This chapter is an inclusive survey of the current knowledge of the evaluation and management of renovascular disease.

The nondiscriminating results of rapid intravenous pyelography, peripheral plasma renin assays, response to angiotensin inhibitors, and isotopic renography are underscored, as is the necessity for anatomic assessment prior to excluding the patient from further diagnostic study. Although there is recognition of the potential role of computer-assisted subtraction angiography, its value probably will be in the limitation of contrast material injected in the intraarterial route of catheterization. The bolus technique of intravenous injection requires essentially the same volume of contrast material as does routine aortography. However, a small catheter placed intraarterially, used in conjunction with the computer-assisted subtraction technique, allows anatomic delineation with as little as 5 mL of contrast material. Its use will be more prevalent as technology advances and availability increases.

Discussion of the controversy regarding the actual use of functional studies in the diagnostic evaluation is quite pertinent. Renal vein renin assays are common although there is infrequent use of split renal function studies. Published reports strongly advocate the establishment of a functional relationship between anatomic stenosis and hypertension; nevertheless, throughout the United States and other countries there are a significant number of operations performed on the basis of anatomic study alone. Reports such as Eigler's[32] suggest intervention without functional assessment. These underscore the limitations of current studies and argue for further investigation to increase their sensitivity and specificity. When an anatomic lesion alone is the reason for operation, there is a significantly higher incidence of functional failure. Current attitudes on cost tend to support fewer studies and reduce the precision of diagnosis and patient selection. Such economic pressures should be an impetus to develop more precise and cost-effective means of evaluation and management.

The author's resume of indications for operation reflect current attitudes in patient selection. Certainly for atherosclerotic lesions the concept of bilateral simultaneous correction of anatomically severe lesions, even in the face of lateralizing functional studies, is soundly accepted. In contrast, however, the liberal use of bilateral branch renal artery reconstructions for bilateral diffuse fibromuscular dysplastic lesions is less widely accepted. In my institution such lesions are only corrected when functional studies are positive and the procedure is limited to the side to which functional studies are positive. Although current proof of the value of such potentially staged procedures is not definitive, our concern is over the potentially increased risk of technical error when such small vessel procedures requiring extensive dissection are employed bilaterally. Prior to accepting such a liberal approach to management of complicated branch lesions in the contralateral kidney, we need to be certain that there is no increased risk.

Finally, a resume of currently published results is provided in this chapter as well as a brief resume of the results of percutaneous transluminal angioplasty. The controversy regarding primary use of percutaneous transluminal angioplasty versus operative intervention will continue for some time. It requires a carefully controlled prospective study. Only thus will clarity be introduced into an area where results from either technique appear to be heterogeneous and in which multiple factors influence patient selection and the outcome of an intervention.

This chapter is timely and well written. It gives the reader a clear synopsis of currently accepted principles and areas of controversy in the management of renovascular disease in hypertensive patients.

16 SMALL-AORTA SYNDROME

Vascular surgeons and angiographers recognize a small group of patients, usually female and often middle-aged, whose abdominal aortas are smaller than expected. These patients are in a clinical category commonly termed small-aorta syndrome, or hypoplastic aortoiliac sydrome (HAIS). They develop ischemic problems due to atherosclerosis at a relatively early age.

ILLUSTRATIVE CASE

Over 18 months a 49-year-old female developed claudication which steadily progressed and became disabling. Angiography demonstrated a quite small aorta (10 mm at the bifurcation and 12 mm at the third lumbar vertebra), occlusion of both iliac arteries, and patency of small femoral arteries. In 1975 an onlay aortobifemoral graft was placed (Figure 16-1). Concomitant bilateral sympathectomy was performed.

Eighteen months later, in December 1976, acute thrombosis of the left limb of the graft required thromboendarterectomy of the femoral artery at the anastomosis and replacement of the distal end of the graft.

Some 3½ years later, in October 1980, because of chest pain cardiac angiograms were performed and small areas of irregularity were discovered in the coronary vessels.

In May 1983, 6½ years after the original operation, a considerable portion of the small intestine was removed because of infarction secondary to intraabdominal adhesions. In the postoperative period pulmonary embolization was successfully treated with heparin. Shortly after discharge the right limb of the old Dacron graft thrombosed, but collateral circulation maintained viability, although claudication returned. Over the next 6 months there was little or no change in symptoms.

Comment

This began as a typical small-aorta syndrome. During the ensuing 8 years the patient's course was typical of the slow progression of atherosclerotic disease with complications due to that and to intraabdominal adhesions. Small arteries were originally suggested by the occurrence of severe disease in a young female and were later proved by the angiogram and operation.

ETIOLOGY

A variety of explanations of small arterial size have been proposed (Table 16-1). The hypothesis that excessive fusion of the embryonic dorsal aortas occurs around the twenty-fifth day of fetal

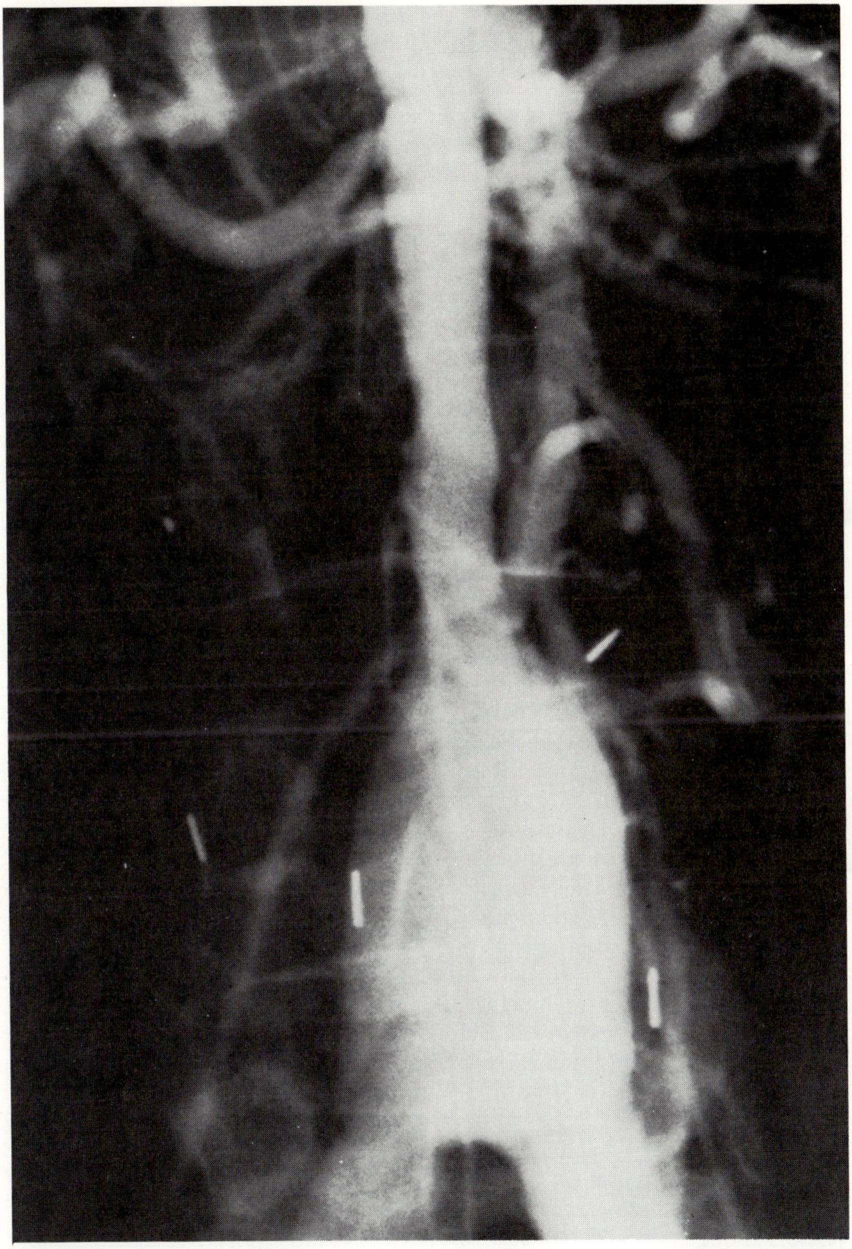

FIGURE 16-1 An onlay graft of a small aorta 3 years after operation. The size of the hood would be made smaller today.

life does not explain the predominance in females.[1] Rubella during pregnancy is recognized as a cause of various congenital anomalies, among which are three reported cases of hypoplastic aorta,[2] and the effect of therapeutic radiation upon the growing aorta has been documented in two cases.[3]

Despite these and other theories the most likely explanation is that atherosclerotic lesions cause considerably more trouble in smaller arteries than they do in large vessels. Why a few women have hypoplastic aortoiliac arteries remains unknown.

TABLE 16-1 SUGGESTED ETIOLOGY OF SMALL ARTERIES

1	Embryonic anomaly
2	Fetal rubella
3	Radiation during infancy
4	Drugs—oral contraceptives
5	Hormonal imbalance

PATHOLOGY

Womersley showed in a series of mathematical calculations that the reflection of pressure pulse waves vary according to the ratio of the sum of the areas of bifurcation vessels to the area of the vessel above the split.[4] Gosling and associates extended this theory; measured aortic bifurcations in the cockerel, dog, and human; and concluded that the area ratios correspond to that which produces minimal reflection of the pressure pulse—but in humans only in infancy.[5]* Beyond that age the aortic bifurcation becomes progressively mismatched. In six women between 45 and 51 years of age with ischemia of the leg, Lallemand, Brown, and Boulter found an abnormal ratio in five[7] and suggested that this might be the major factor inducing premature atheromas of the aorta. Additionally, one of the patients had a hypoplastic aorta (8 mm at the bifurcation). They suggested that increased oscillatory pressures in the aorta might be the cause of abnormal endothelial mitosis.[8]

INCIDENCE

DeLaurentis in 1978 reported that 9 percent of 204 patients with symptomatic aortoiliac disease had hypoplastic aortoiliac arterial systems.[9] These figures were updated in 1982 to 7 percent of 369 patients—23 percent of the 107 females and 0.7 percent of the 262 males. The average age at time of operation for HAIS patients was 47 years, while that of all patients was 60 years. All were smokers. None were diabetic.[10]

In a Veterans Administration hospital series of 408 male patients 4.4 percent had aortic bifurcations of 12.5 mm or less. No details of the clinical situations of these patients were given.[11]

Intending to publish the results of a series study, during the past 20 years I have collected data on 47 patients with small aortas. Unfortunately, during a recent period of turmoil in which the hospital moved its location, films were destroyed to the extent that only a few aortograms are now available for measurements. Of the 47 charts 30 are available in sufficient detail for analysis, and these are summarized in Tables 16-2 and 16-3.

Hypoplastic aortoiliac syndrome occurred in relatively young females (90 percent), while only a few males (10 percent) were discovered to have HAIS. Among these 30 patients 33 percent were initially found to have clinically significant disease in arteries outside the aortoiliac system; another 17 percent later developed extraaortic disease, so to date half the total have had

TABLE 16-2 30 PATIENTS WITH HYPOPLASTIC AORTOILIAC SYNDROME

Age, yr	No. of males	No. of females
30 to 40	1	5
41 to 50	0	10
51 to 60	1	4
61 to 70	0	7
71 to 80	1	1
Total	3	27

Other arteries involved

Type	Initially	Later
Femoropopliteal	9	2
Carotid	0	3
Hand	1	0

*Apropos this discussion is the suggestion of Longo and Santa that the ideal synthetic graft should have a bifurcation ratio of 0.65 to 0.70:1 rather than the usual 0.5:1 which is currently available.[6]

TABLE 16-3 OPERATIONS PERFORMED

Type of operation	No.	Results: Good	Limb loss	Later operation
None	2	2	0	0
Aortofemoral graft and sympathectomy	12	11	1	3
Femorofemoral graft	4	3	1	1
Femoropopliteal graft	6	6	0	0
Aortoiliac thromboendarterectomy	2	2	0	0
Iliac transluminal angioplasty	2	2	0	0
Primary below-knee amputation	1	0	1	0
Lumbar sympathectomy	1	1	0	0
Total	28	25	3	4

involvement of other arteries. It is suspected that with the passage of time this incidence will increase.

Six of these patients had no operation because their symptoms were not judged significant enough to warrant a major vascular procedure. They had varying degrees of nondisabling claudication and/or coolness and color changes distally. Eight other patients did not require an operation upon the aorta or iliac arteries. One had immediate below-knee amputation, another was treated by unilateral lumbar sympathectomy, and six had successful femoropopliteal grafting procedures. Sixteen (59 percent) required operation upon the aorta and/or iliac arteries. Two of these were treated by transluminal iliac angioplasty, with satisfactory results to date. Four patients had femorofemoral grafts placed, and twelve patients had aortobifemoral grafts with concomitant lumbar sympathectomy.

The summarized results indicate satisfactory relief of symptoms following 25 of the 28 (89 percent) operative procedures. Three limbs (10 percent) were lost. Four of the patients (14 percent) required later vascular operations of one sort or another. There were no deaths. Thus, the surgical results have been rewarding. Perhaps their occurrence in relatively young patients explains the general lack of morbidity and mortality.

OTHER ARTERIES

Some authors have concentrated so heavily upon the aortoiliac involvement that atherosclerosis of other vessels has been deemphasized or ignored to the point that the disease has appeared to be limited to the aorta and iliac arteries alone (Figure 16-2). DeLaurentis's group noted only 1 renal and 3 femoral arterial lesions among their original 18 patients.[9] Callow, however, pointed out the occurrence of lesions in other arteries.[12]

The recent analysis of 19 women with HAIS by Jernigan, Fallat, and Hatfield showed 4 with concomitant renal artery stenosis and 7 with lesions of one or more of the large arteries of the neck.[13] The atherosclerotic process in these patients followed the usual widespread stenosis and occlusions with skip areas of complete patency.

AORTIC SIZE

The extensive measurements of aortic size by Cronenwett and Garrett were uninodal and distributed as a single group. When body surface area was taken into account, there was a significant difference between "normal" and "small" aortas but not in the iliac or femoral arteries. Small aortas were defined as those less than one standard deviation below the mean: 18.8 mm above the renal arteries, 13.2 mm below the renals, and 10.3 mm at the bifurcation. They thus discov-

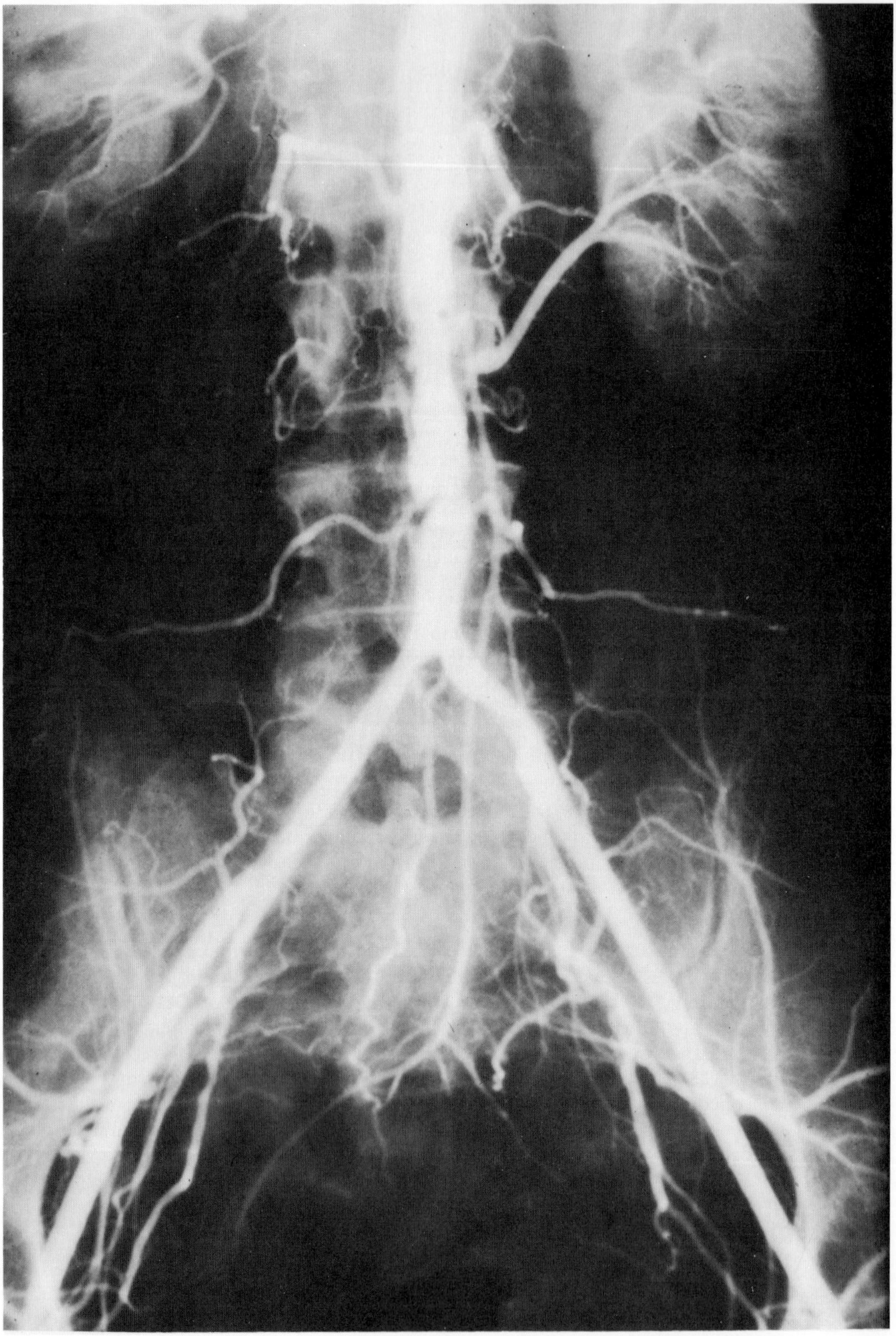

TABLE 16-4 AORTA SIZE MEASUREMENTS

Ref no.	First author	No.	Suprarenal, mm	Infrarenal, mm	Bifurcation, mm
14	Steinberg	NA* (male)	23.9	21.4	18.7
		NA* (female)	21.6	18.7	27.5
9	DeLaurentis	NA*			11.3
15	Johnson	21	18	15	12
16	Holmes	31		13.9	10.7
17	Cronenwett	73 normal	23.6	17.3	14.4
		17 small	18.8	13.2	10.3
		(Suggested definition of HAIS)	18	14	11

*Not available.

ered that 17 (23 percent) of the 73 women operated upon had small aortas. These measurements match other reports of expected aortic size fairly well (Table 16-4).[9,14–17]

It is obvious that if the diagnosis of HAIS is dependent upon size alone, there will be some patients who are borderline. Jernigan's group has suggested the additional criterion of a "high" bifurcation of the aorta with straighter course of the iliac arteries distally.[13]

Small-aorta patients should be differentiated from those with isolated atherosclerotic lesions in larger aortas, such as the six reported by Raaf and Shannon.[18]

CLINICAL SYNDROME

A female with lower-extremity ischemic symptoms who is under 50 years of age should be suspected of having a small aorta. Beyond this the manifestations are those of atherosclerotic ischemia in all its variant forms.

The absence of systemic hypertension rules out congenital coarctation of the aorta.

SURGICAL TREATMENT

Because of the small size it is particularly important to provide adequate reconstructions. Thromboendarterectomy of small arteries is prone to early failure because of operative errors and later failure because of recurrence of disease. DeLaurentis commented upon abandoning attempted thromboendarterectomies and resorting to grafts in several cases.[9] Clean-out procedures may be useful but their hazards must be recalled.

The usual end-to-end anastomosis of an aortic graft should often be changed to an end-to-side technique. I am reluctant to bypass the distal aorta and iliac arteries in these patients, who often do not have well-developed collaterals. For this reason onlay grafts are used.

Concomitant lumbar sympathectomy to reduce the peripheral resistance is a rational concomitant procedure. It can be done in 5 or 10 minutes after the aorta is dissected.

SUMMARY

Hypoplastic aortoiliac syndrome is not a pathologic entity but a convenient clinical description of young patients, chiefly female, who develop ischemic symptoms early in life because a small amount of atherosclerotic disease is clinically significant in their undersized aortas and arterial systems. The size cannot be explained except as a variation from the average. Those who require operation ordinarily respond well to revascularization procedures based on the usual indications.

FIGURE 16-2 Normal size terminal arteries associated with a small aorta.

REFERENCES

1 Arnot RS, Louw JH: The anatomy of the posterior wall of the aorta. *S Afr Med J* 1975, 47:899.
2 Siassi B, Klyman G, Emmanouilides GC: Hypoplasia of the abdominal aorta associated with the rubella syndrome. *Am J Dis Child* 1920, 120:476.
3 Colquhoun J: Hypoplasia of the abdominal aorta following therapeutic irradiation in infancy. *J Radio* 1966, 86:454.
4 Womersley JR: Oscillatory flow in arteries: The reflection of the pulse waves at junctions and rigid inserts in the arterial system. *Phys Med Biol* 1958, 2:313.
5 Gosling RG, Newman DL, Bowden NLR, Twinn KW: The area ratio or normal aortic junctions: Aortic configuration and pulsewave reflection. *Br J Radiol* 1971, 44:850.
6 Longo T, Santa A: A study of the ideal geometric properties of an aorta-iliac Y graft. *J Cardiovasc Surg* 1971, 12:52.
7 Lallemand RC, Brown KGE, Boulter PS: Vessel dimensions in premature atheromatous disease of aortic bifurcation. *Br Med J* 1972, 2:255.
8 Wright HP: Endothelial mitosis around aortic branches in normal guinea pigs. *Nature* 1968, 220:78.
9 DeLaurentis DA, Friedmann P, Wolferth CC Jr, Wilson A, Naide D: Atherosclerosis and the hypoplastic aortoiliac system. *Surgery* 1978, 83:27.
10 DeLaurentis DA: The hypoplastic aortoiliac syndrome, in Veith FA (ed): *Critical Problems in Vascular Surgery.* Appleton-Century-Crofts, New York, 1982, pp 411–428.
11 Palmaz JC, Carson SN, Hunter G: Male hypoplastic infrarenal aorta and premature atherosclerosis. *Surgery* 1983, 94:91.
12 Callow AD: Discussion of DeLaurentis DA, Friedman P, Wolferth CC Jr, Wilson A, Naide D: Atherosclerosis and the hypoplastic aortoiliac system. *Surgery* 1978, 83:36.
13 Jernigan WR, Fallat ME, Hatfield DR: Hypoplastic aortoiliac syndrome: An entity peculiar to women. *Surgery* 1983, 94:752.
14 Steinberg CR, Archer M, Steinberg I: Measurement of the abdominal aorta after intravenous aortography in health and arteriosclerotic peripheral vascular disease. *AJR* 1965, 95:703.
15 Johnson TE: Small vessel syndrome: Constitutional arterial narrowing. *Minn Med* 1969, 52:1903.
16 Holmes DR Jr, Burbank MK, Fulton RE, Bernatz PE: Arteriosclerosis obliterans in young women. *Am J Med* 1979, 66:997.
17 Cronenwett JL, Garrett HE: Arteriographic measurement of the abdominal aorta, iliac and femoral arteries in women with atherosclerotic occlusive disease. *Radiology* 1983, 148:389.
18 Raaf JH, Shannon J: Atherosclerotic coarctation of the abdominal aorta in women. *Surg Gynecol Obstet* 1980, 150:715.

Invited Commentary

Dominic A. DeLaurentis, M.D.
Philadelphia, Pennsylvania

Small-aorta syndrome is a commonly used phrase to describe this entity; however, in these patients not only the aorta, but the iliac and femoropopliteal segments are hypoplastic. Also, it seems that the progression of atherosclerosis is closely related to cigarette smoking. The illustrative case demonstrates that often an occluded limb of an aortofemoral bypass does not lead to limb loss, and recurrent claudication is preferable to the hazards of redo surgery.

I do not believe this syndrome merely represents small aortas in small women. With the recent recognition of the inflammatory abdominal aortic aneurysm, one wonders whether this diminutive aortoiliac system may not be the result (shrinkage) of an inflammatory type of atherosclerosis. In our series, the hypoplastic aortas had a reflection coefficient of over two times that of the 20 normal aortas. This hemodynamic stress may help explain the tendency to atherosclerosis in the abdominal aorta; however, it does not explain the etiology of the small vessels.

The incidence of hypoplasia in our patients with aortoiliac occlusive disease remains at about 7 percent. However, it is a rather common scenario in women with atherosclerosis, where it occurs 25 percent of the time. The incidence in males continues to be quite low (under 2 percent). Because of the age of onset of symptoms, most surgeons are inclined to reconstruct these young patients in order to allow regular, full activity.

Two-thirds of our patients have had occlusive disease in the carotid bifurcation or the subclavian artery. The incidence of concomitant renal artery disease has remained low (as has that of hypertension). Superficial femoral artery occlusion at the time of operation has occurred in 15 percent, and it has usually indicated a late stage of this syndrome. We originally noted a paucity of coronary artery disease, but in our follow-up at least four patients required coronary artery bypass surgery. The descending order of involvement for our group has been the aortoiliac, the brachiocephalic, the coronary, and the superficial femoral arteries.

What size constitutes a hypoplastic aortoiliac system? We analyzed arteriograms of 20 normal aortoiliac segments (from renal donors) and compared that group to our small-aortic group (Figure 16-A). We concluded that to be considered small, the infrarenal aorta must measure under 15 mm, the common iliac artery under 8 mm, and the external iliac artery under 4 mm

FIGURE 16-A Average measurements of 20 normal segments and 27 hypoplastic aortas.

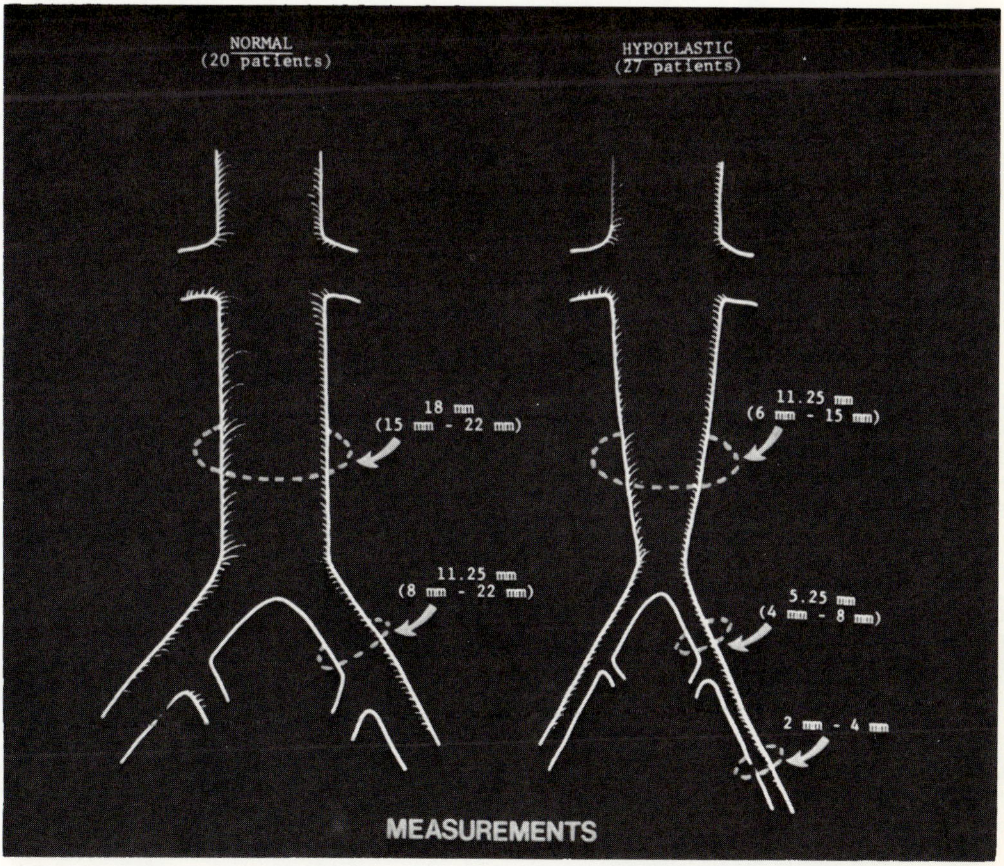

(i.e., none of the normal arteries' measurements were below these values, and none of the hypoplastic arteries' measurements were above these values).

Transluminal angioplasty is used sparingly because of the small femoral arteries. Indeed, some early problems with retrograde aortography led us to recommend translumbar aortography. I, too, use the bypass technique with an end-to-side anastomosis in the aorta and distally in the external iliac or femoral area. If the disease is limited to the aortoiliac segment, I prefer an intraabdominal long anastomosis to the external iliac artery. If there is superficial femoral artery occlusion, then I do an onlay to the profunda femoris and, often, a concomitant femoral popliteal bypass. A small aortic graft (10 to 12 mm) must be available at the time of surgery. I also continue to do a concomitant bilateral lumbar sympathectomy, and the "hot foot" postoperatively is reassuring. However, there are no data that support the efficacy of bilateral lumbar sympathectomy, with regard to long-term patency rates.

We have had no operative deaths, and morbidity has been low and related to pulmonary toilet. Recently, I have been advising these patients to take antiplatelet medication (aspirin and dipyridamole). They are examined at least every 6 months, at which time Doppler ankle pressures or pulse volume recordings are carried out. Often, superficial femoral artery disease can be detected, and reconstruction will avert graft thrombosis.

17 BUERGER'S THROMBOANGIITIS OBLITERANS

Whether Buerger's thromboangiitis obliterans (TAO) is a distinct pathologic entity[1] or an unusual variation of the arteriosclerotic progress, the term does serve to delineate a subgroup of patients with periphereal vascular disease who present a similar and recognizable clinical pattern.* Doubts regarding TAO's separation from other atherosclerotic lesions soon created the controversy which to some extent still persists.

Undoubtedly the diagnosis was made too often prior to the widespread use of angiography—males under 50 were usually termed TAO patients, and females and older men were thought to be arteriosclerotics.

The astute vascular clinician Geza de Takats discussed the matter thoroughly in 1959 on the basis of his experience with 200 patients believed to have TAO; he characterized it as invariably starting prior to age 45, affecting males in 97 percent of cases, and always being found in tobacco smokers.[5] Other experienced clinicians have agreed,[6] yet it is recognized that the course, angiographic pattern, and pathologic lesions blend into those of other disease processes, especially atherosclerosis. Thus Welling in 1982 stated that there are "no specific clinical, radiologic or pathologic features."[7]

In 1970 the problem was discussed in Warsaw at the nineteenth congress of the European Society of Cardiovascular Surgery, where most of the speakers favored the idea that the process was a distinct entity.[8–14] Nielubowicz and his colleagues thereafter studied 102 patients in Poland, concluding also that the process was different from arteriosclerosis. Of special interest were their conclusions that these patients did not die young, that visceral and cerebral arteries were not involved, and that no form of treatment was beneficial.[15]

ETIOLOGY

The cause of TAO remains unknown. Its common association with tobacco smoking and frequent remission after cessation strongly suggest a direct relationship, but the pathogenesis is unclear. Perhaps smoking is only an aggravating factor, since the occurrence of TAO among millions of smokers is uncommon.

PATHOLOGIC FEATURES

The sequential nature of the inflammatory matting of small arteries and veins is well known, along with the often accompanying migratory phlebitis. However, there are no specific features

*Leo Buerger, 1879–1943, born in Vienna, was a urologist in New York and later in Los Angeles who devised many instruments[2] and in 1908 published his first account of the disease[3] which had originally been described by von Winiwater in 1879.[4]

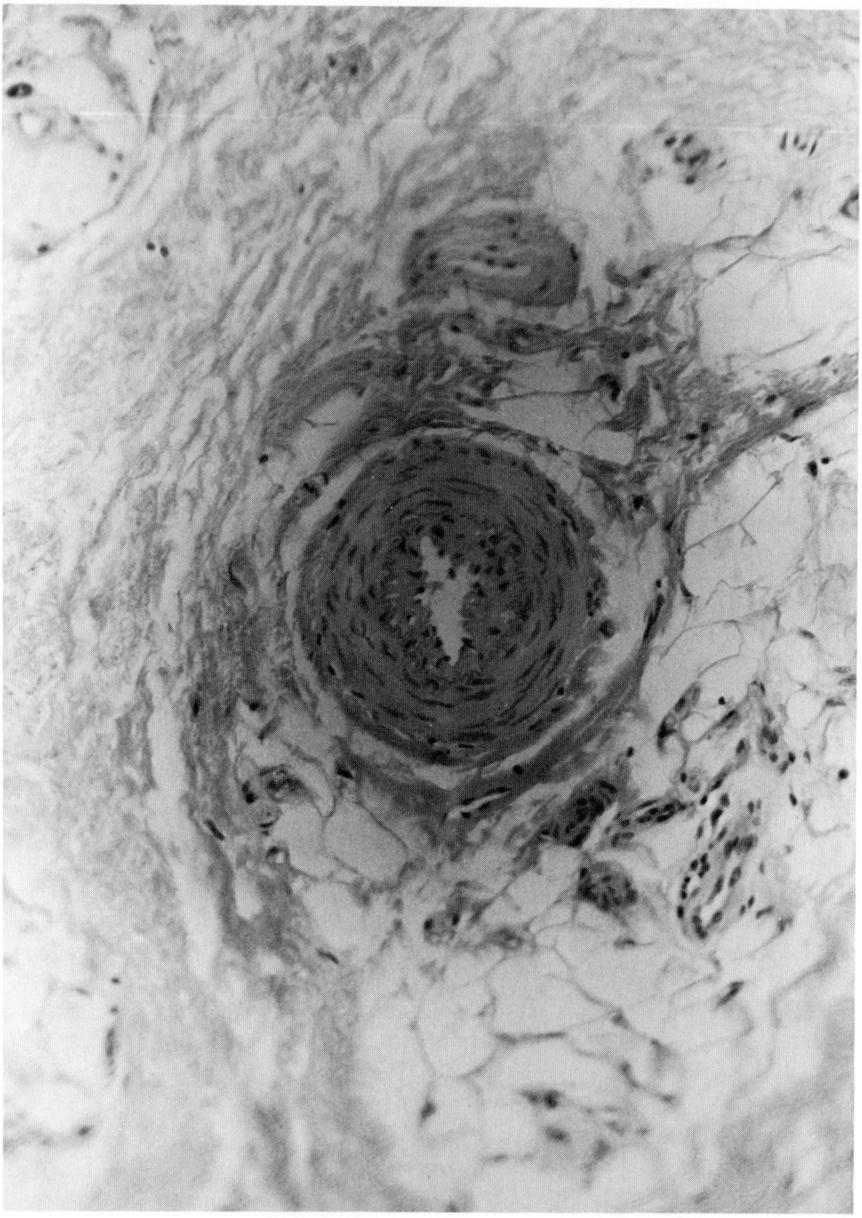

FIGURE 17-1 Concentric thickening of a digital arteriole representing Buerger's thromboangiitis obliterans.

to differentiate TAO from atherosclerotic lesions. Inflammation is common to both. Occasionally microabscesses within luminal thrombi have been reported, but again these may not be specific. Lack of vascular wall calcification is notable, yet this may only indicate lack of time for degeneration to occur.

Dietch and Sikkema recently noted that the TAO lesion consists of a concentric thickening of the intima with intact media, associated with a transmural vascular inflammation, often with fibrosis of the nearby veins and nerves. In contrast, arteriosclerotic lesions feature eccentric luminal narrowing with medial degeneration.[16]

These lesions commonly occur in small distal vessels (Figure 17-1), which is certainly different from the occurrence of atherosclerotic ones, which stenose and occlude medium and larger arteries while allowing distal patency (and the possiblity of bypass grafting). Whether the distal lesions of TAO progress to later involvement of larger vessels (i.e., foot and tibials to popliteal) or whether atherosclerotic lesions are overlaid as a second disease upon the earlier-occurring TAO is not clear. De Takats certainly suggested such proximal progression.[5]

CLINICAL PATTERNS

The syndrome is variable yet centers upon young males who smoke. Females occasionally fit the pattern, usually as small subgroups but sometimes in groups as large as 10 percent (in the Mayo Clinic series).[17]

Shionoya's 1983 analysis of 115 Japanese patients allows a modern view of the clinical pattern of TAO.[18] His diagnostic criteria—smokers below age 50 with below-knee arterial occlusion plus either phlebitis or upper-limb involvement and absence of atherogenic risk factors—do appear to rule out patients with early-onset atherosclerotic lesions.

Some features of Shionoya's series (Table 17-1) are of particular interest. The patients who had above-knee arterial lesions (46 percent), and in particular the 11 percent in whom the iliac artery was involved, were said to have skip lesions, yet the thought that perhaps there is a concomitant (or even an entire) arteriosclerosis problem lingers. TAO therefore continues as a clinically recognizable entity whose exact etiology remains unclear 76 years after Buerger's original description.

The Early Phase There are minimal symptoms of peripheral ischemia, such as numbness, coldness, excessive sweating, and pain in the presence of normal pulses. Often a single toe or finger is alone symptomatic.

Progression Progression usually occurs, symptoms accelerate, and signs of ischemia increase to discoloration or ulceration. Migratory thrombophlebitis is sometimes present. Medium-size vessels may become occluded.

Visceral Lesions Rarely arteries of the brain, eyes, heart, and mesentery may be involved. Mesenteric arterial thromboses causing intestinal infarction probably occur more often than reported.

Buerger first reported one such in 1924,[19] but by 1981 Deitch and Sikkema found only six others and added a seventh who had required intestinal resection.[16] De Takats indicated that 26 percent of his patients had such, but by his own admission the high figure probably represented "over-diagnosis" on a clinical basis.[5] Shionoya reported none among his 115 patients.[18]

Unusual Manifestations These include the early occurrence of TAO in a 17-year-old female who required a

TABLE 17-1 SHIONOYA'S CLINICAL SUMMARY
Data on 115 Japanese Patients

Sex	
male 98%	
female 2%	
Clinical diagnosis	
Tissue necrosis	74%
Phlebitis	45%
Upper extremity TAO	84%
Multiple-limb TAO	98%
Angiography results	
Above-knee occlusion	46%
Iliac artery occlusion	11%
Treatment	
Bypass grafts	18%

Source: Shionoya S: What is Buerger's disease? *World J Surg* 1983, 7:544.

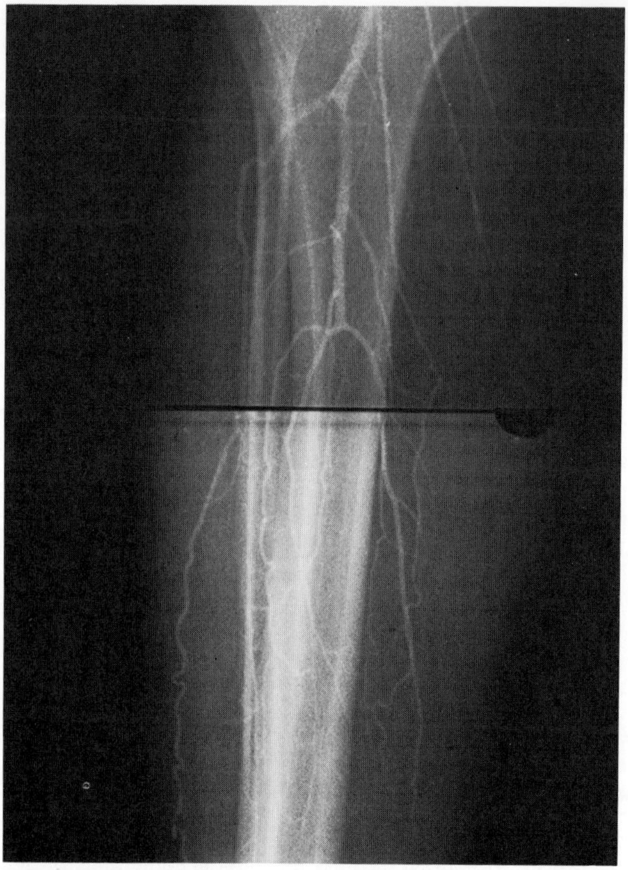

FIGURE 17-2 An arteriogram showing patency of the femoropopliteal system and occlusion of the arteries of the distal two-thirds of the calf.

femoropopliteal bypass for occlusion with strong pathologic documentation of TAO.[20] Neither youth nor sex are completely protective.

Twenty years ago it was shown that the survival curve of TAO patients differed little from the normal population's, while the arteriosclerotic death rate was distinctly higher.[17] In 1980 the Polish investigator Nielubowicz reaffirmed this concept.[15]

DIFFERENTIAL DIAGNOSIS

The age and sex at onset of symptoms, along with signs of acute peripheral arterial disease, suggest TAO (Figure 17-2). The history of presence of thrombophlebitis adds weight to the diagnosis (Figure 17-3).

Arteriograms which show distal small-artery disease without large-vessel disease lend further weight to the diagnosis. It must, however, be admitted that there will be some patients whose exact diagnosis will remain unclear. Time will allow some of these to be sorted out.

TREATMENT

Cessation of smoking is widely recognized as beneficial for most patients. It must be absolute, since decreasing the amount is worthless.

The thesis of Nielubowicz[15] that no presently known treatment is worthwhile is a bit strong, although vasodilator drugs, anti-inflammatory agents, and corticoids have not proved to be useful.

Long-term anticoagulants such as warfarin probably carry a greater risk in terms of bleeding complications than benefit to the thrombotic process.

Bypass Grafting Bypasses for lesions of the large and medium-size arteries have the usual indications: an isolated occlusion with a patent artery proximal and distal to the lesion. Shionoya recounted 21 such operations among 115 patients (18 percent), with patency of 8 months to 5 years.[18] Whether the progression of TAO is more or less likely to cause late graft failure than is atherosclerosis is not known. It does not presently seem that TAO should alter the usual indications for peripheral bypass grafts.

Since sympathectomy alone is expected to benefit TAO, it is logical to recommend it as a concomitant procedure with a shunt operation. Shionoya did such in 75 percent of his graft cases.

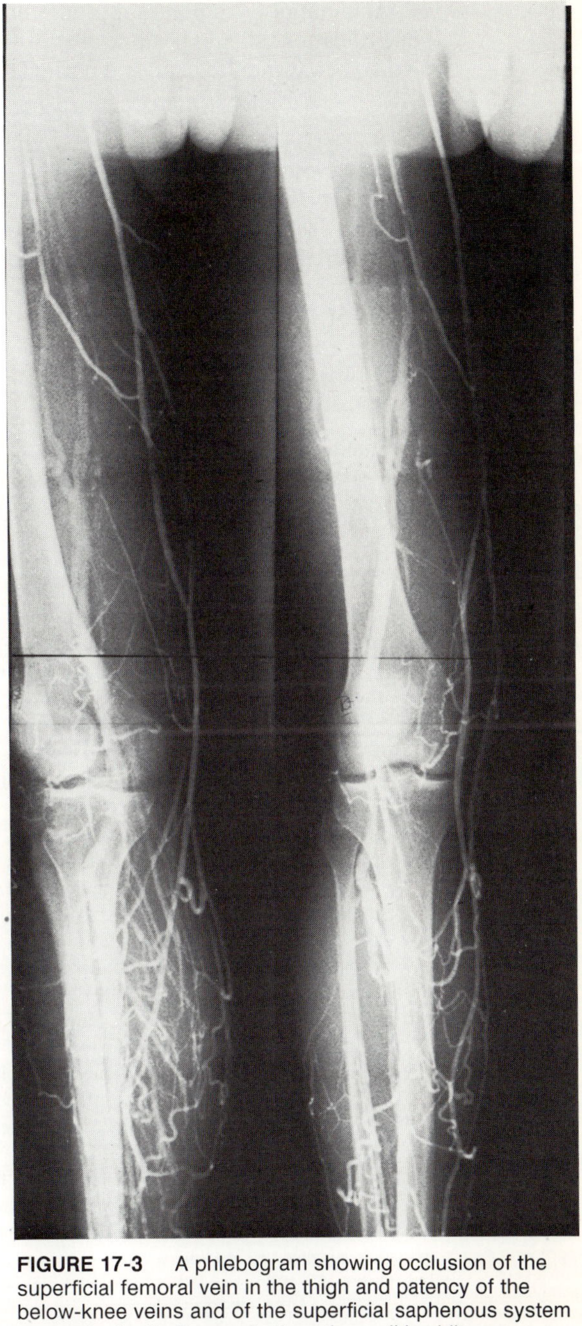

FIGURE 17-3 A phlebogram showing occlusion of the superficial femoral vein in the thigh and patency of the below-knee veins and of the superficial saphenous system in a patient with Buerger's thromboangiitis obliterans.

Sympathectomy The common occurrence of skin necroses and ulcers in TAO strongly suggests the value of sympathectomy, which increases blood flow in the skin considerably more than it does in the muscle. Thus sympathectomy and cessation of smoking have long been regarded as cornerstones of therapy.

My experience with thoracic sympathectomy led to the conclusion that it is quite beneficial for skin lesions due to organic occlusion of the wrist, hand, and finger arteries, many of which are due to TAO. The excellent results among such patients are discussed in Chapter 21, where it is also noted that histologic confirmation of the diagnosis was not obtained because of the fear of making even a small biopsy incision on an ischemic finger.

Lumbar sympathetic ablations are better known and are discussed in Chapter 20.

Amputation Amputation of toes or fingers or at more proximal sites is necessary at times. Such ablations should be done at as distal a site of election as possible. Loss of the upper extremity or even the entire hand is not usual, and amputations above the calf level are rarely required.

Illustrative Case

A 30-year-old male developed throbbing pain in the right ankle and numbness of the foot, which he thought were related to a tennis injury. An osteochondroma of the femur was found and surgically excised, but there was no improvement.

An arteriogram showed a normal femoropopliteal system with distal occlusion of all three below-knee vessels (Figure 17-2), which explained the absence of foot pulses. A phlebogram (Figure 17-3) showed occlusion of the superficial femoral vein and other abnormalities of the deep venous system of the calf.

Lumbar sympathectomy increased the warmth of the foot, but the patient continued to have some pain.

Comment This occurrence of distal arterial occlusion with venous thrombosis in a young male smoker provides a classic example of thromboangiitis obliterans with a response to lumbar sympathectomy.

REFERENCES

1 McKusick VA, Harris WS, Ottesen OE, Goodwin RM, Shelley WM, Bloodwell RD: Buerger's disease: A distinct clinical and pathologic entity. *JAMA* 1962, 181:5.
2 Winsor T: *Peripheral Vascular Diseases.* Charles C Thomas, Springfield, Illinois, 1959.
3 Buerger L: Thromboangiitis obliterans: A study of the vascular lesions leading to presenile spontaneous gangrene. *Am J M Sci* 136: 567, 1908.
4 von Winiwater F: Neber eime eigentoemliche Form von Endarteritis und Endophlebitis mit Gangrean des Fusses. *Arch Klin Chir* 1879, 23:207.
5 de Takats G: *Vascular Surgery.* Saunders, Philadelphia, 1959.
6 Strandness DE: *Peripheral Arterial Disease.* Little, Brown, Boston, 1962.
7 Welling RE: Buerger's disease revisited. *Angiology* 1982, 33:239.
8 Stojanovic VK, Marcovic A, Arsov V, Bujanic J, Lotina S: Clinical course and therapy of Buerger's disease. *J Cardiovasc Surg (Torino)* 1973, 14:5.
9 Zannini G, Cotrufo M: Epidemiological, angiographic and clinical aspects of Buerger's disease. *J Cardiovasc Surg (Torino)* 1973, 14:17.
10 Kunlin J, Lengua F, Testart J, Pagot A: Thromboangiosis or thromboangiitis treated by adrenalectomy and sympathectomy from 1942 to 1962. *J Cardiovasc Surg (Torino)* 1973, 14:21.
11 Corelli F: Buerger's disease: Cigarette smoker disease may not always be cured by medical therapy alone; usefulness of operative treatment. *J Cardiovasc Surg (Torino)* 1973, 14:28.
12 Vollmar J: Surgical considerations on the terminology and treatment of so-called Buerger's disease, *J Cardiovasc Surg (Torino)* 1973, 14:37.
13 Rivera R: Roentgenographic diagnosis of Buerger's disease. *J Cardiovasc Surg (Torino)* 1973, 14:40.
14 Symposium on Buerger's disease: Discussion. *J Cardiovasc Surg (Torino)* 1973, 14:47.
15 Nielubowicz J, Rosnowski A, Pruszynski B, Preztakiewics Z, Potemkowski A: Natural history of Buerger's disease. *J Cardiovasc Surg (Torino)* 1980, 21:529.
16 Deitch EA, Sikkema WW: Intestinal manifestation of Buerger's disease: Case report and literature review. *Am Surg* 1981, 47:326.
17 Fairbairn JF, Jurgens JL, Spittell JA: *Peripheral Vascular Disease.* 4th ed. Saunders, Philadelphia, 1972.
18 Shionoya S: What is Buerger's disease? *World J Surg* 1983, 7:544.
19 Buerger L: *The Circulatory Disturbances of the Extremities Including Gangrene, Vasomotor and Trophic Disorders.* Saunders, Philadelphia, 1924.
20 Laslett LJ, Ikeda RM, Mason DT: Female adolescent Buerger's disease: Objective documentation and therapeutic remission. *Am Heart J* 1981, 102:452.

INVITED COMMENTARY

D. Eugene Strandness, Jr., M.D.
Seattle, Washington

Buerger's disease remains a source of considerable confusion and controversy. After its description by Leo Buerger in 1908,[1] it remained an accepted entity until 1960, when a report by Wessler, Ming, Gurewich, and Freiman sparked renewed interest in the disease.[2] They reexamined the entire issue and concluded that Buerger's disease probably never existed as originally described. This report resulted in an outpouring of communications that documented once again that it was a specific disorder which could be recognized if certain diagnostic criteria were followed. In fact, not a single paper appeared that supported those conclusions. An excellent case for the retention of Buerger's disease as originally described was made by McKusick's team.[3]

What then is this disorder, and how can it be recognized? Students of peripheral vascular diseases will accept the diagnosis if certain criteria are met in terms of both clinical presentation and pathologic findings. Most of these have already been covered in the chapter, but those not listed will be highlighted, since this reviewer feels they are important in reaching a diagnosis.

One of the symptoms that is peculiar to Buerger's disease is instep claudication; i.e., the pain which develops with walking is in the instep. While it may occur in patients with atherosclerosis, it is rare. This may be the only symptom early in the disease and is very useful in supporting the diagnosis. It probably develops because of the distal location of the lesions within the plantar arteries, an uncommon site for atherosclerotic lesions to occur.

The coincidence of hand involvement is another important clue. In fact, about one-half of patients with Buerger's disease will develop occlusive lesions in the hand which are responsible for the development of cold sensitivity of the Raynaud's type. The presence of such lesions can be suspected from the measurement of finger blood pressures or by anteriography.

Another, very peculiar aspect of this disease is its association with cigarette smoking. While it is clearly true that only a small percentage of smokers will ever develop this disease, it is rarely if ever seen in the nonsmoker. In fact, these patients have a very strong addiction to cigarette smoking and will rarely stop even when faced with the reality of limb loss involving both lower extremities and, in some cases, fingers as well. The phenomenon is seen not only in the western world but also in southeast Asia, where Buerger's disease remains one of the most common causes of limb ischemia.

Finally, when tissue becomes available, the diagnosis can be verified with certainty. The essential tissue features include both arterial and venous occlusion by organized material with occasional giant cells present, preservation of arterial wall architecture, and fibrous encasement of the neurovascular bundle. In addition, no atheromas are to be found in association with the area of occlusion.

For the reader who is interested in a lucid description of this entity, the original report by Buerger must be read.[1] This work remains a classic and should be reviewed by those students interested in the field of vascular diseases.

COMMENTARY REFERENCES

1 Buerger L: Thromboangiitis obliterans: Study of vascular lesions leading to presenile spontaneous gangrene. *Am J Med Sci* 1908, 136:567.

2 Wessler S, Ming SD, Gurewich V, Freiman DG: A critical evaluation of thromboangiitis obliterans: The case against Buerger's disease. *N Engl J Med* 1960, 262:1149.

3 McKusick VA, Harris WS, Otteson OE, Goodwin RM, Shelley WM, Bloodwell RD: Buerger's disease: A distinct clinical and pathologic entity. *JAMA* 1962, 181:5.

18 THE ARTERIAL EFFECTS OF ERGOTISM

The symptoms of ergot intoxication, due to the ingestion of wheat or rye infested with the fungus *Claviceps purpurea,* were well known in the Middle Ages as St. Anthony's Fire. This problem is rare today, but peripheral arterial problems which may follow the medicinal use of ergot now sometimes cause severe unrecognized ischemic manifestions. Four recent patients with severe arterial vasospasm that threatened or caused small-artery thrombosis and subsequent tissue necrosis or gangrene suggest that this intoxication may be more common than is currently supposed.[1] Since recognition and cessation of medication at once reverses the process (unless there is actual tissue necrosis), it is important that the syndrome be widely recognized.

ILLUSTRATIVE CASE

A 43-year-old woman presented with wet gangrene of the great toe and foot and ascending cellulitis and lymphangitis. Both femoral pulses were diminished. No pedal pulses were palpable (Figure 18-1).

She admitted to occasional headaches, for which several medications had been taken, but denied any ergot preparation. However, it was later learned that she had been using ergotamine in unknown quantities. Angiography (Figure 18-2) showed diffusely small femoral, popliteal, and tibial arteries with localized areas of severe constriction.

No arterial reconstruction was possible, and the advanced gangrene necessitated below-knee amputation on the second hospital day. Another arteriogram done on the sixteenth postoperative day (Figure 18-3) showed significant increases in the arterial luminal diameter of all the vessels. The amputation healed without difficulty, and when seen 6 months later, the patient had no other unusual findings.

Comment

Persistent questioning is sometimes needed to detect the use of ergot medication, since the patient thinks of the drug as a painkiller only.

HISTORY

Ergot intoxication has been known as a clinical entity for hundreds of years.[2] Epidemics of the disease periodically swept across Europe and Asia in the Middle Ages; in the present era occasional outbreaks have been reported. These ancient epidemics were called St. Anthony's fire because of the fiery feeling of burning of the extremities. Actual gangrene sometimes occurred.[3–6]

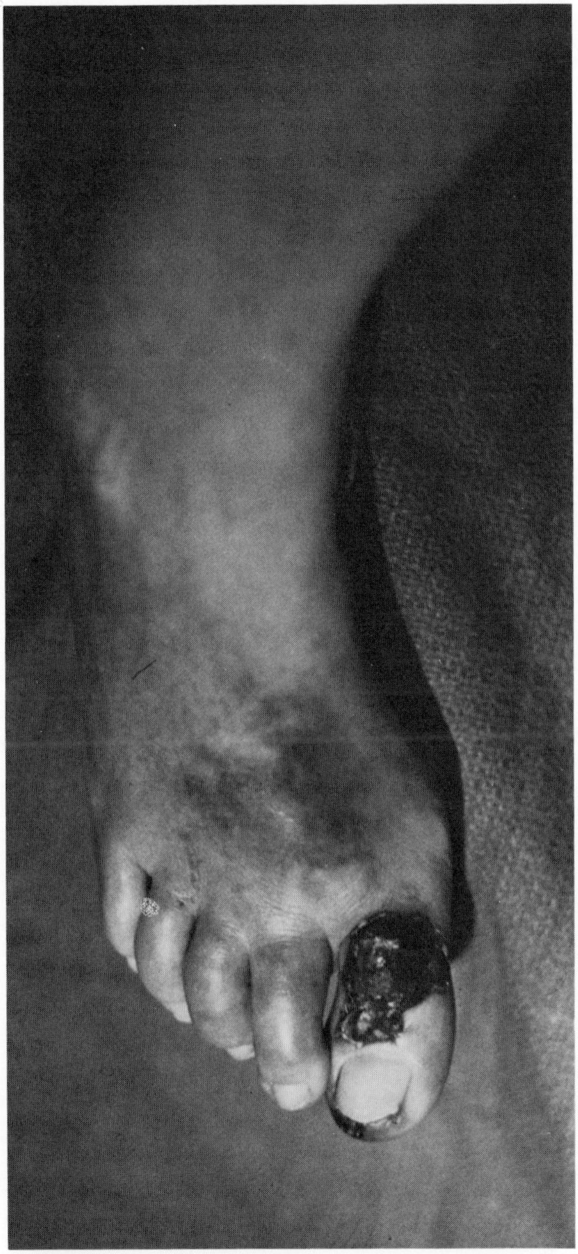

FIGURE 18-1 The right great toe shows an ischemic ulcer, and the dorsum of the foot is ecchymotic. No arterial reconstruction was possible for the diffuse distal below-knee arterial lesions. The advanced ischemia associated with ascending cellulitis and lymphangitis and septicemia forced a below-knee amputation 48 hours after admission. *(Reprinted courtesy of Maples M, Mulherin JL, Harris J, Dale WA: Am Surg 1981, 47:224.)*

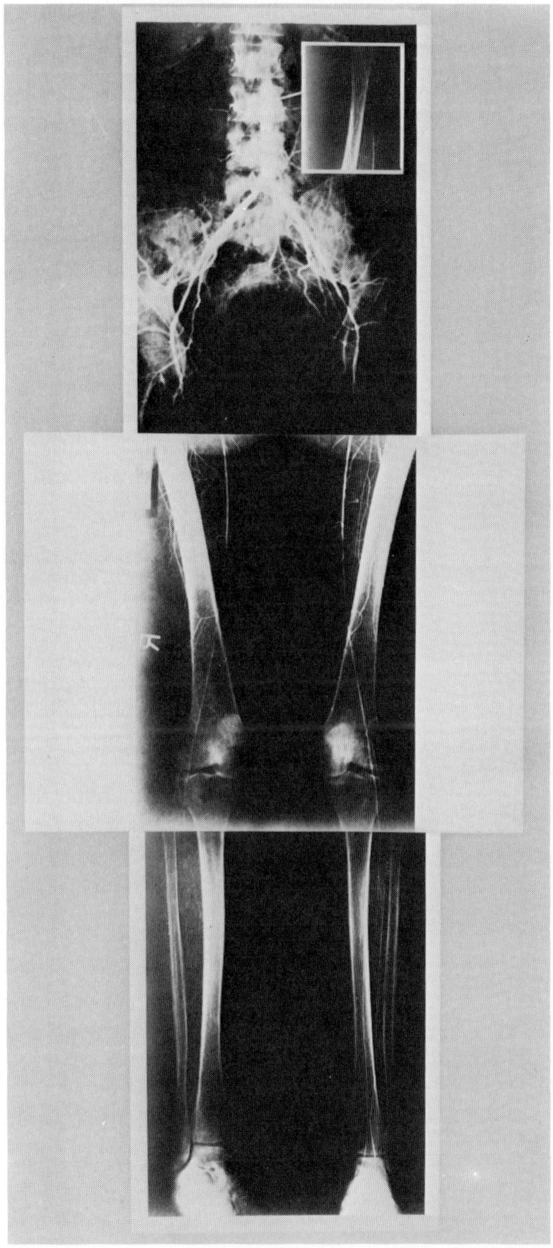

FIGURE 18-2 An arteriogram shows the classic arterial lesions of diffuse arteriospasm associated with segmental areas of more-pronounced narrowing. Eventually this severe ischemia with cyanosis, anesthesia, and absence of foot pulses cleared after cessation of ergot ingestion and lumbar sympathectomy. *(Reprinted courtesy of Maples M, Mulherin JL, Harris J, Dale WA: Am Surg 1981, 47:224.)*

During the Middle Ages ergotism was usually experienced by the peasants, since the aristocracy used clean grains sorted from those blighted by the rust-purple fungus, the latter providing bread for the serfs.[7]

The ingestion of wheat or rye contaminated by the fungus *Claviceps purpurea* produces the clinical syndrome known as ergotism, which centers about intense vasoconstriction of the arteries of the brain, alimentary canal, or limbs.[3,4,8–14]

After the ergot alkaloids were identified early in this century, it was recognized that ergotism is produced by ergotamine's effects on the arteries (Table 18-1.)[4,9,15–17] When the brain vessels are primarily involved, there are visual disturbances, headaches, psychosis, and convulsions.[14,17] Gastrointestinal symptoms include cramping, emesis, and diarrhea.[4,13,18] Peripheral vascular involvement produces pain and burning. Severe ischemia sometimes ends in gangrene.[4,8,11,14,19–22] The reason for geographic variation in the clinical syndrome has never been discovered. Thus, ergotism in France was often associated with peripheral vascular symptoms, whereas central nervous symptoms were common in Germany. Perhaps this reflected a difference in the fungus.[5]

Ergotism from grain ingestion has not been reported in the United States, but the therapeutic overuse of ergotamine for migraine has occasionally produced similar poisoning, as in our patients.[9,14,24–27]

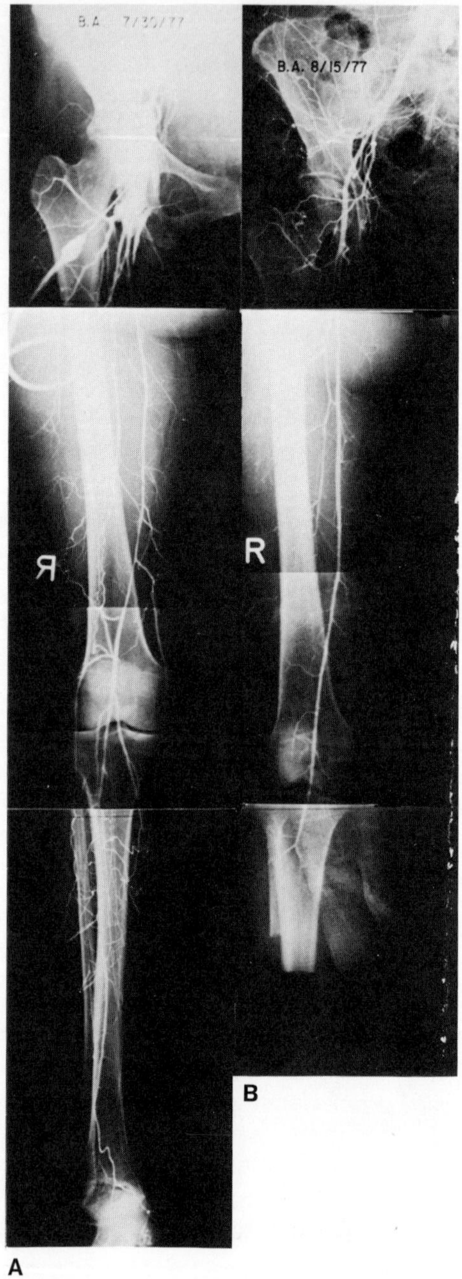

FIGURE 18-3 Arteriogram shows the patient's admission arteriogram (*A*) and an arteriogram done 16 days later (*B*). The marked narrowing of the distal right superficial femoral artery in the earlier film can be appreciated and compared to the later film.

PHARMACOLOGIC ACTIVITY OF ERGOT ALKALOIDS

The overuse of ergot alkaloids for migraine or uterine bleeding may produce symptoms. All of the three forms of ergot alkaloids have vasoconstrictive, oxytocic, and adrenergic blockade properties. The amine alkaloids (ergonovine) and dehydrogenated alkaloids are not as active on the cardiovascular system as are the naturally occurring amino acid alkaloids (ergotamine). Ergotamine is a potent peripheral vasoconstrictor and may cause capillary endothelial damage. Whether the mechanism is direct vasoconstriction of the vascular smooth muscle or whether ergotamine acts as an alpha-adrenergic blocker, the overall effect is vasoconstrictive and the action is peripherally and not centrally mediated.[3,15,22,28] Ergotamine tartrate has become widely used for the relief of migraine headaches.

TABLE 18-1 EFFECTS OF ERGOT POISONING ON ARTERIES

Central nervous system effects
Headaches
Visual disturbances
Unconsciousness
Convulsions
Gastrointestinal system effects
Nausea and emesis
Cramps
Diarrhea
Peripheral artery effects
Cold or hot feelings
Ischemia progressing to gangrene

Ergotamine administered orally is erratically absorbed from the gut, so that the magnitude of effect is unpredictable. Intramuscular injection of 0.25 to 1.0 mg is useful for migraine, but 24-hour dosage should not exceed 1.0 mg and should not be repeated over twice per week.[15] Patients rather understandably tend to overuse the drug because of the severe pain and disability of migraine.

DIAGNOSIS

Insistent questioning should occur whenever there is a history of medication for headaches, since patients may forget or deemphasize their use of ergotamine. The illustrative case includes an example of this. Central nervous system, gastrointestinal, and/or peripheral arterial manifestations following use of the drug should arouse suspicion and lead to immediate cessation of use, since that in itself relieves the syndrome unless ischemic necrosis has already occurred.[15,22]

Angiography shows arteries with general or segmental decrease in size.[3,19,29,30] There may be secondary arterial thrombosis. Venous thrombosis may occur.[23] All these changes (except actual thrombotic occlusion) regress after cessation of the drug.[22,31]

Our four recent cases are summarized in Table 18-2.

TABLE 18-2 RECENT CASES OF ERGOTISM CAUSING ARTERIAL PROBLEMS

Age/sex	Clinical problem	Ergotamine history	Treatment	Result
1 56/F	Ischemia of a foot	Unknown duration of use; for headache	Epidural block, sympathectomy	Causalgia relief at 5 months
2 50/F	Claudication in an arm	Unknown duration of use; for headache	Exploration of brachial artery	Normalcy
3 53/M	Ischemia of the feet	10-year use; for headache	Below-knee amputation at age 47; above-knee amputation at age 53	Loss of both legs
4 43/F	Gangrene of a toe	Unknown duration of use; for headache	Below-knee amputation	Loss of a leg

Source: Maples M, Mulherin JL, Harris J, Dale WA: Arterial complications of ergotism. *Am Surg* 1981, 47:224.

TREATMENT

Ergot intoxication is most effectively treated by withdrawal of the offending agent. Arteriographic and physical findings in acute ergotism may revert in 24 to 48 hours. However, in the cases presented here and in cases of chronic ergot abuse with advanced symptomatology, remission is slow.[15,17,22]

As yet no specific treatment has become standard. A variety of vasodilators as well as local anesthesia, low-molecular-weight dextran, and anticoagulants have been used unsuccessfully. Sympathectomy has been of little value.[4,15,31]

Carliner, Denune, Finch, and Goldberg in 1974 reported the successful treatment of ergotism with a sodium nitroprusside infusion.[32] Anderson, Christensen, and Hole tried this and in two cases compared it to continuous epidural blockade. They could not demonstrate any significant vasodilatory effects of epidural anesthesia but obtained excellent results with sodium nitroprusside infusions in dosages ranging up from 25 mg/min.[28]

Failure of sodium nitroprusside to improve perfusion of the feet was reported in a single case by Husum, Berthelsen, Metz, and Rasmussen.[33] They achieved good results in one case by infusing nitroglycerine (10 mg of glyceryl nitrate 0.5% in ethanol added to 500 mL of 5.5% glucose at 3.2 μg per kilogram of body weight per minute).

Surgical procedures to remove clots, to bypass occlusions, or to amputate necrotic tissue may be needed.

RISK OF HEPARIN-ERGOTAMINE FOR PROPHYLAXIS

Surgeons should be especially aware of the risk of an occasional arterial complication and even death following the administration of a heparin–dihydroergotamine mesylate combination for prophylaxis of deep venous thrombosis, as proposed by Kakkar's group recently.[34] While the incidence of peripheral arterial complications is low (estimated at 1 percent by Bhuta[35]), they are severe for the individual patient.

This risk, even though unusual, contraindicates the combination drugs, especially since their usefulness is not established.

SUMMARY

Overuse of ergot alkaloids may produce severe lesions. Oral ingestion may produce symptoms; parenteral injection is not mandatory.

Angiography may show either diffuse or localized arterial or venous constriction.

Although the lower extremity is the usual site, the arm and/or hand may be involved.

The arterial changes are reversible by cessation of alkaloid use unless actual tissue necrosis has occurred.

Ancillary measures to combat ischemia and infection should be used simultaneously.

The necessity for a tenacious search into the patient's history is emphasized, since initial questioning may fail to identify the drug.

Our recognition of four such cases suggests that the problem is actually more common than is currently suspected.

REFERENCES

1 Maples M, Mulherin JL, Harris J, Dale WA: Arterial complications of ergotism. *Am Surg* 1981, 47:224.
2 Matossian MK: Mold poisoning: An unrecognized English health problem, 1550–1800. *Med Hist* 1981, 25:73.

3 Bagby RJ, Cooper ED: Angiography in ergotism. *AJR* 1972, 166:179.
4 Greene FL, Ariyan S, Stansel HC Jr: Mesenteric and peripheral vascular ischemia secondary to ergotism. *Surgery* 1977, 81:176.
5 London M, Magora F, Rogel S: Acute ergot poisoning. *Angiology* 1970, 21:565.
6 Dotz W: St. Anthony's fire. *Am J Dermatopathol* 1980, 2:249.
7 Levin S: Ergot poisoning (letter). *S Afr Med J* 1980, 58:629.
8 Ahlgren I, Hager K, Nylander L, Wehlin L: Imminent gangrene of the leg after ergot poisoning. *Angiology* 1968, 13:354.
9 Allen EV, Barker NW, Hines EA Jr: *Peripheral Vascular Diseases.* 3d ed. Saunders, Philadelphia, 1962, pp 145–149.
10 Ancalmo N, Ochsner JL: Peripheral ischemia secondary to ergotamine intoxication. *Arch Surg* 1974, 109:832.
11 Cranley JJ, Krause RJ, Strasser ES, Hafner CD: Impending gangrene of four extremities secondary to ergotism. *N Engl J Med* 1963, 269:727.
12 Felix RH, Carroll JD: Upper limb ischemia due to ergotamine tartrate. *Practitioner* 1970, 205:71.
13 Katz J: Abdominal angina as a complication of methysergide maleate therapy. *JAMA* 1967, 199:124.
14 Merhoff GC: Ergot intoxication: Historical review and description of unusual clinical manifestations. *Ann Surg* 1974, 180:773.
15 Goodman LS, Gilman A: *The Pharmacological Basis of Therapeutics.* 4th ed. Macmillan, New York, 1970.
16 Imui C: Arterial spasm associated with oral ergotamine therapy. *Br J Clin Pract* 1973, 27:457.
17 London M, Magora F, Rogel S: Acute ergot posioning. *Angiology* 1970, 21:565.
18 Buenger RE, Hunter JA: Reversible mesenteric artery stenosis due to methysergide maleate. *JAMA* 1966, 198: 144.
19 Fairbairn JF: Severe arteriospastic disease secondary to use of ergot preparation. *Med Clin North Am* 1958, 42:971.
20 Henry, LG, Blackwood JS, Conley JE, Bernhard VM: Ergotism. *Arch Surg* 1975, 110:929.
21 Iuel J, Mune O: Peripheral arterial insufficiency in ergotism. *Vasc Dis* 1967, 4:159.
22 Kempezinski RF, Buckley CJ, Darling RC: Vascular insufficiency secondary to ergotism. *Surgery* 1976, 79:597.
23 Mintz US, Bar-Meier S, DeVries A: Ergotamine induced venous thrombosis. *Postgrad Med J* 1974, 50:244.
24 Cameron EA, French EB: St. Anthony's fire rekindled: Gangrene due to therapeutic dose of ergotamine. *Br Med J* 1960, 2:28.
25 Byrne-Quinn E: Prolonged arteriospasm after overdose of oral ergotamine tartrate in migraine. *Br Med J* 1964, 2:552.
26 Engle I, Sivertssen E: Ergotism due to therapeutic doses of ergotamine tartrate. *Am Heart J* 1965, 70:665.
27 Richter AM, Banker VP: Carotid ergotism, a complication of migraine therapy. *Radiology* 1973, 106:399.
28 Andersen PK, Christensen KN, Hole P, Bent J, Rosendal T, Sokke DB: Sodium nitroprusside and epidural blockade in the treatment of ergotism. *N Engl J Med* 1977, 296:1271.
29 Haynes CA, Davis ME: Ergotism: Report of a case with localized arteriographic changes in the femoral vessel. *Angiology* 1968, 19:199.
30 Moir JC: Ergot: From "St Anthony's fire" to the isolation of its active principle, ergometrine (ergonovine). *Am J Obstet Gynecol* 1974, 120:291.
31 Herlache J, Hoskins P, Schmidt CM: Ergotism: Unilateral brachial artery thrombosis secondary to ergotamine tartrate. *Angiology* 1973, 24:369.
32 Carliner NJ, Denune DP, Finch CS Jr, Goldberg LI: Sodium nitroprusside treatment of ergotamine induced peripheral ischemia. *JAMA* 1974, 227:308.
33 Husum B, Berthelsen P, Metz P, Rasmussen JP: Different approaches to the treatment of ergotism: A review of three cases. *Angiology* 1980, 31:650.
34 Kakkar VV, Stamatakis JD, Bentley PG, Lawrence D, deHaas, HA, Ward VP: Prophylaxis for postoperative deep vein thrombosis. *JAMA* 1979, 241:39.
35 Bhuta I: Acute lower extremity ischemia due to ergotism. *J Med Assoc State Ala* 1982, 28:34.

INVITED COMMENTARY

Joseph L. Mulherin, Jr., M.D.
Nashville, Tennessee

The rare sporadic nature of ergot intoxication makes controlled clinical trials of various therapeutic alternatives difficult, if not impossible. The rarity of the problem is indicated by the fact that we have been able to find only four instances of the disorder in the records of two major hospitals with busy vascular services.

Recognition of the nature of the problem is of paramount importance, since cessation of the causative medication may be the only therapeutic action needed. This may be difficult, since the drug history may be inaccurate and angiographic studies in patients with ergotism may at times show segmental involvement mimicking atherosclerosis.

Since the etiology is pharmacologic, then the treatment is also, unless complications of vascular thrombosis or tissue gangrene have developed. Spinal or epidural anesthesia and sympathectomy probably have little place in treatment because the effects of the ergot drugs are not mediated by the sympathetic pathways. While good results with intraarterial injection of vasodilators have been reported, the most consistently favorable results seem to have been obtained with continuous intravenous infusion of sodium nitroprusside. Nitroglycerin has also been used favorably in this fashion. The role of calcium channel blockers awaits further investigation.

While ergot intoxication continues to be a rare phenomenon, the increased use of the pharmacologic support of the potent vasoconstrictors in the perioperative period, especially in those patients with low cardiac output, has made the problem of dealing with arterial vasoconstriction of an iatrogenic nature fairly commonplace. When manifested in the extremities, ergot intoxication is easily recognizable and seldom in itself leads to tissue loss. Diminished renal or mesenteric perfusion, however, may be more subtle initially but may lead to catastrophic results.

19 PERIGRAFT LYMPHOCELES AND SEROMAS

Occasionally sterile fluid persistently accumulates around an arterial graft. Usually it occurs immediately following the operation and consists of lymph draining from unhealed severed lymphatics. This may be termed *lymphocele.* Less commonly, the fluid occurs after a delay of weeks or even months and is due to serum filtered through the wall of the graft, causing a *seroma.*

It is important to differentiate the two entities: the cause, prognosis, and treatment are quite different.

LYMPH COLLECTIONS

The continuous accumulation of clear fluid in the wound surrounding a fresh arterial graft is uncommon but nevertheless frequent enough to be well known to vascular surgeons. Kwaan, Bernstein, and Connolly reported that 1.8 percent of 634 arterial reconstructions involving the femoral vessels developed such lymph collections.[1]

Illustrative Case

R.T., a 66-year-old female, had resection of an aortic abdominal aneurysm with a woven Dacron replacement as well as a side limb to the left renal artery. Postoperatively 70 to 100 mL of straw-color fluid drained daily from the left groin suction tube, and a lesser amount drained from the right. On the eighth postoperative day both wounds were explored. Several points of lymph drainage were secured with Dexon sutures; new suction drains were placed in the depths of the wounds, and they were closed in four layers. Uneventful healing followed.

Comment Whether lymph drains from unhealed lymphatics or from the nodes themselves has never been determined; whichever, large nodes should be excised rather than split and recognizable lymphatics should be ligated or cauterized prior to their division.

Management of lymph collections in the past usually consisted of repeated needle aspirations, pressure dressings, and antibiotic prophylaxis. This was often successful after a period of days or weeks. Occasionally the lymphocele became infected, with secondary involvement of the vascular anastomosis, the necessity for removal of the graft, and sometimes subsequent loss of the limb. Kwann, Bernstein, and Connolly described this in their seven patients, of whom three developed positive wound cultures and one ended with infection and an amputation. At the same time they documented their later experience with five additional patients, all of whom were treated by early exploration of the wound and direct ligation of the lymph leak, followed by immediate secondary closure of the wound. They had no complications.[1] My own experience parallels theirs.

Optimal treatment presently consists of a return to the sterile environment of the operating room as soon as such a lymphatic leak is recognized. Using appropriate antibiotic prophylaxis systemically and careful wound preparation and draping, the entire wound should be explored for the lymphatic leak (or leaks). Each of these must be ligated.

The wound is then immediately closed in layers to achieve close approximation to the graft. While most of these would probably heal without drainage, it is safer to place a suction drain through an independent stab wound for 1 or 2 days.

Immediate recognition and surgical treatment of lymphorrhea has thus not only prevented infections but also decreased the hospital time, since it is no longer necessary to hold the patient in the hospital on antibiotics awaiting spontaneous or aspiration-aided resolution of the problem.

PERIGRAFT SEROMAS

The delayed accumulation of sterile fluid about vascular grafts after several weeks or months was initially reported by Harry A. Kaupp and his associates in 1979. Their five patients all had Dacron arterial grafts which were well-incorporated until the development of fluid later.[2] Other similar cases have been recognized since then.[3–5]

Illustrative Case

L.S., a 53-year-old female, was first examined at age 48 in 1972 and was found to have disabling claudication, for which an aortoiliac thromboendarterectomy was performed. During the next 9 years she had 13 different arterial operations as well as 3 nonvascular procedures.

Her subsequent operations included transfer of the left subclavian artery to the carotid to relieve subclavian steal made manifest by arm claudication and mental disorientation, patch grafting of the left iliac repair, placement of a Mobin-Uddin filter for pulmonary embolism, and an aortobifemoral Dacron graft 39 months after thromboendarterectomy.

Three months later there was a right nephrectomy for ureteral entrapment and hydronephrosis; 6 weeks after this she required lateral femoral neurectomy for meralgia paresthetica.

Later operations included replacement of a thrombosed iliac limb of the Dacron graft, another femoral thrombectomy, and finally a femorofemoral crossover knitted Dacron graft for tertiary thrombosis of the iliac limb of the graft.

The complication of perigraft fluid was first noted 28 months after placement of the femorofemoral Dacron graft. Despite weekly aspirations and pressure dressings the clear yellow fluid persisted. Twenty cultures were negative.

Because the grafts and anastomoses were functioning well and the patient was asymptomatic except for the presence of fluid, nonoperative therapy was continued, although the patient increasingly reported discomfort. Five months after the initial development of fluid her case was presented to the surgical vascular conference, where there was uniform agreement that a nonoperative course should be followed.

Nevertheless, the fluid continued to form, so a month later the knitted Dacron crossover graft was removed (Figure 19-1) and replaced with an 8-mm polytetrafluoroethylene (PTFE) graft (Figure 19-2). The wound healed but fluid recurred almost immediately. Eight weeks later the new PTFE crossover graft was removed. Revascularization was achieved by placement of an 8-mm PTFE graft from the right axillary artery to the superficial femoral artery halfway down the right thigh. This healed well but within a short time fluid began to surround the new axillofemoral graft and eventually formed a boggy mass extending from the midthigh to the axilla at the attachment of the graft.

Five months after it was placed, the axillofemoral graft was removed and replaced by an 8-mm woven Dacron graft taking its origin from the left limb of the old Dacron graft within the pelvic cavity and coursing retroperitoneally across to the right side to the right superficial femoral

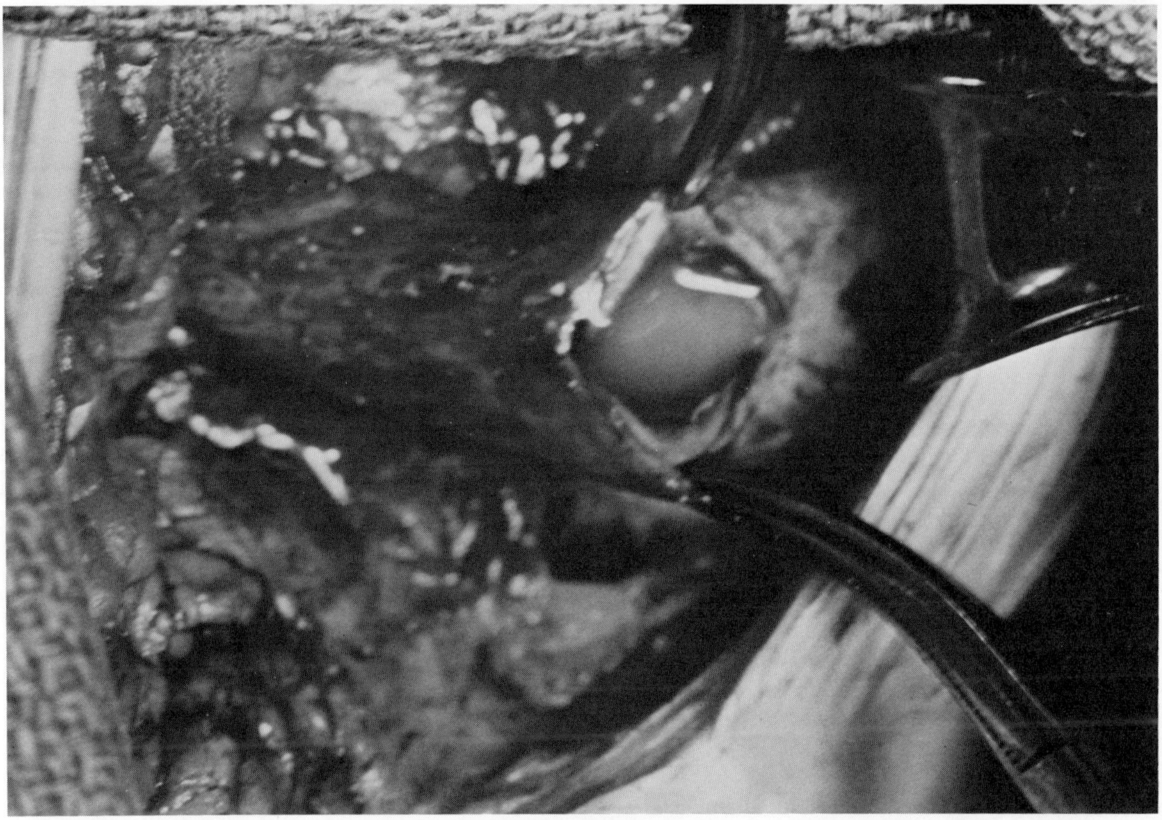

FIGURE 19-1 The perigraft seroma has been exposed in the left groin and its capsule opened anteriorly. The previously placed knit Dacron is seen lying within a pool of straw-color serum. The capsule is well-formed. *(Reprinted courtesy of Dale WA, Blumenberg RM, Gelfand ML, in Greenhalgh RM (ed): Extra-anatomic and Secondary Arterial Reconstruction. Pitman, Bath, 1981, pp 35–40.)*

artery in midthigh. This operation was complicated by the development of sudden contralateral ischemia on the left side, requiring thrombectomy. Fortunately, the limb was salvaged.

Five weeks later fluid recurred in the right groin and upper thigh. The portion of the Dacron tube lying in the groin and thigh was removed and replaced with an umbilical cord graft. This healed promptly and there has been no recurrence of fluid.

All wounds have continued to be healed. The patient has pulses at all points in her extremities and is functioning in a completely normal fashion 12 years after her first operation and 54 months after the synthetic was replaced with an umbilical cord vein graft. Despite these vicissitudes she is presently completely rehabilitated physically and emotionally.

Comment Personal inquiry showed that similar late fluid accumulations had occurred in other patients. This led to a national inquiry among members of the North American Chapter of the International Cardiovascular Society by Blumenberg, Gelfand, and myself.[6] The initial letter of inquiry mailed to approximately 1000 vascular surgeons brought 300 responses, with 159 surgeons documenting 269 cases, as shown in Table 19-1. The collected cases were divided among grafts in a variety of positions, 94 percent of which were outside the cavities of the body so that they were easily palpable. Furthermore, 95 percent occurred in connection with synthetic

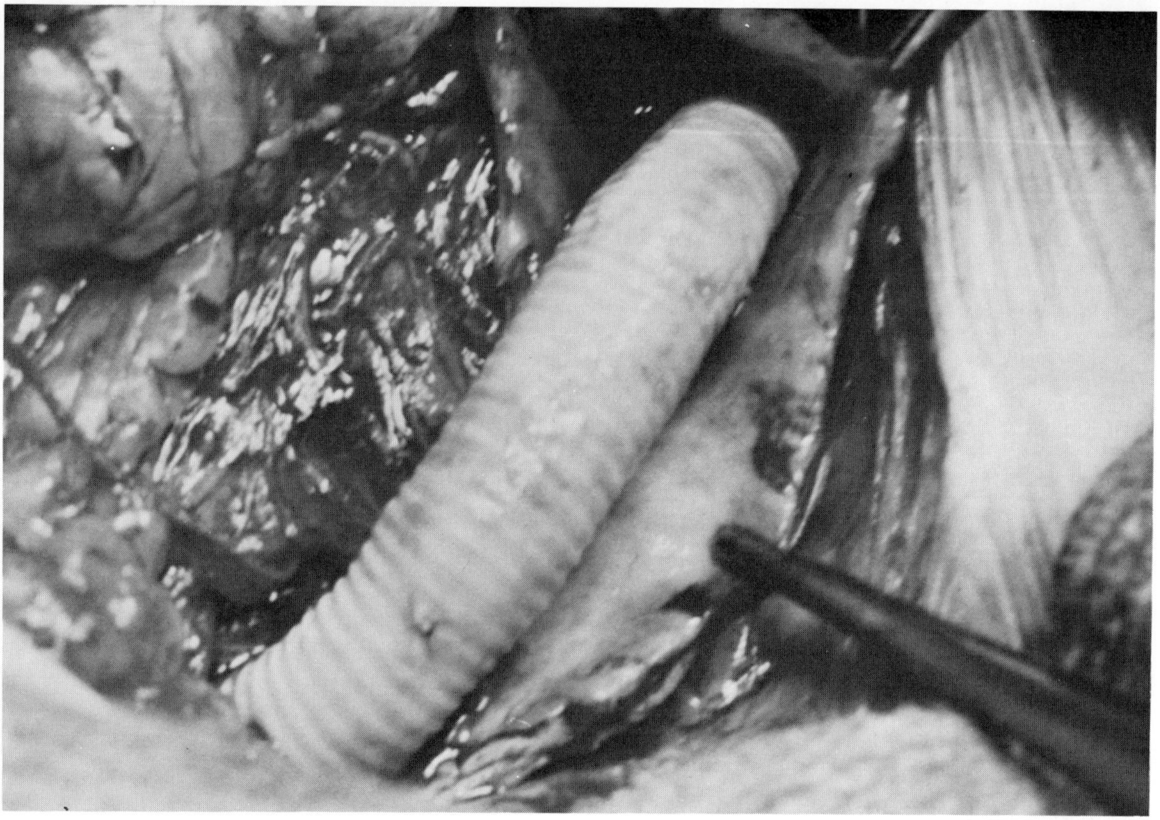

FIGURE 19-2 The original femorofemoral Dacron graft was replaced with PTFE. It is patent within the perigraft seroma.

tubes with more or less porosity, while only 5 percent occurred with nonporous grafts such as autogenous vein or heterologous bovine grafts. Actually, the chief difficulty in assessing the reports was in attempting to be certain that lymphatic collections were not confused with the late occurrence of perigraft collections of serum, and it is likely that this separation was not completely achieved.

Pathogenesis In an effort to understand the origin of late fluid accumulations in 20 patients with arteriovenous access shunts of PTFE, Bolton studied the flow of blood through such grafts in dogs both in vivo and in vitro. Transudation of serum through the graft appeared to be affected by several factors, including bends in the graft, the velocity of blood flow, and the presence of uremia. Why this occurred only occasionally and not commonly is not

TABLE 19-1 RESULTS OF INQUIRY ON PERIGRAFT SEROMAS

Graft types used	
Knit Dacron	54%
PTFE	34%
Woven Dacron	7%
Autogenous vein	3%
Bovine heterograft	2%
Graft positions	
Axillofemoral	49%
Femorofemoral	22%
Femoropopliteal	11%
Aortofemoral	6%
Axilloaxillary	4%
Other	8%

Note: We received responses from 300 vascular surgeons; 159 surgeons reported 269 cases.

clear. Bolton suggested that faulty formation of fibrin in the graft pores may have been the actual cause, although this hypothesis was unproven.[7]

The question of an immunologic reaction has been suggested by several authors,[3] but to date no proof of such a hypothesis has occurred.

Must the Graft Be Replaced? It is a serious matter to remove a functioning bypass graft and subject the patient not only to the risk of perioperative thrombosis but also to the possibility of infection. The patient discussed herein was treated by aspiration for many weeks prior to the final decision to replace the material. Current information indicates that lymph collections frequently tend to heal following aspirations, while seromas do not.

Changes from one synthetic graft to another solved the problem in many of the collected cases, yet it did not in the instance herein presented, where the seroma recurred after the Dacron graft was changed to PTFE. Recurrence ceased in this particular case only after the permeable graft was changed to a nonpermeable one so that transudation of serum through the graft wall was impossible.

Is It Important to Reroute the New Graft? Changing the pathway did not solve the problem in the illustrated case, while changing to a nonpermeable graft in the same bed did; thus the importance of the route itself is uncertain. However, if a new anatomic pathway is readily available, it should be used.

It should also be noted that only partial excision of inflammatory tissue was done and most was left in situ, without subsequent difficulty. On the other hand, a considerable number of the collected cases did well after removal of the fibrous pseudomembrane; perhaps that should be done during the reoperation, to prevent further difficulty.

Must the Pseudocapsule Be Removed? My coauthor and colleague, Robert Blumenberg, stresses the importance of removing the capsular fibrous tissue, but since the difficult case cited above was successful without that, I doubt the importance of the bloody technique needed to remove all the fibrous tissue about the seroma. However, the matter has not yet been finally settled.

RECOMMENDED TREATMENT

The optimal management of the late perigraft seroma is not yet completely clear, but the collected cases and the meager experience reported in the literature suggest that if the graft is a permeable one, it should be completely removed and replaced with a nonpermeable tube. This might be an autogenous artery, an autogenous vein, or an umbilical vein graft. It should definitely be recalled that the PTFE graft is somewhat permeable, even though it does not transmit blood readily, and therefore is contraindicated as a replacement material. Whether a new pathway enhances the chances for cure is not yet certain, but that should be considered if available.

REFERENCES

1 Kwann JH, Bernstein JM, Connolly JE: Management of lymph fistula in the groin after arterial reconstruction. *Arch Surg* 1979, 114:1416.

2 Kaupp HA, Matulexis TH, Lattimer GL, Kremen JE, Celani VH: Graft infection or reaction. *Arch Surg* 1979, 114:1419.

3 Szilagyi DE: Discussion of Celani VH: Graft infection or reaction. *Arch Surg* 1979, 114:1419.

4 Bhuta EB, Dorrough R: Non-infectious fluid collection around velour Dacron graft: Possible allergic reaction. *South Med J* 1981, 74:870.

5 Burnham SJ: Letter, December 1980.

6 Dale WA, Blumenberg RM, Gelfand ML: Peri-graft seromas complicating arterial grafts, in Greenhalgh RM (ed): *Extra-anatomic and Secondary Arterial Reconstruction.* Pitman, Bath, 1981, pp 35–40.

7 Bolton W, Cannon JA: Seroma formation associated with PTFE vascular graft used as arterial venous fistula. *Dialysis Transplant.* 1981, 10:60.

INVITED COMMENTARY

Robert M. Blumenberg, M.D.
Schenectady, New York

The differential diagnosis of perigraft seroma from lymphorrhea or lymphocele formation is predominantly based on the nature of the fluid obtained from either aspirations or reoperation. The fluid is clear, similar to dilute urine in gross appearance, and is distinguished from lymph by protein electrophoretic and biochemical studies. At reoperation the graft is found to be "floating" within a nonsecretory fibrous pseudomembrane and most commonly involves prostheses placed in the subcutaneous position. In 60 percent of the cases, the initial clinical appearance occurs between 1 and 6 months after surgery, and the mid and distal portions of the graft are involved most frequently.

Our data suggest that the perigraft fluid is an ultrafiltrate of serum, and the gross and histologic findings incriminate faulty incorporation of the outer graft wall by surrounding tissues as the major cause of transudation of serum through the graft wall into the surrounding tissues, especially near the anastomoses. The graft wall at its ends is noted to be poorly incorporated by surrounding fibrous tissue, and the interstices of the graft wall are filled with an acellular, sparse fibrin-protein matrix. The body of the graft is encompassed by firmly adherent fibrous tissue along its outer surface and has a healthy interstitial graft wall matrix and inner lining.

Graft soilage by organic solvents, such as alcohol and povidone-iodine, as well as by tissue fluids and blood can "wet" a PTFE graft, causing increased porosity and permeability to serum. The hydrophobic nature of the PTFE is rendered hydrophylic by the wetting agent. Meticulous tunneling techniques are helpful in avoiding this problem. Histopathologic examination of the material in our studies failed to confirm inflammation as a significant causal factor in the etiology of perigraft seromas.

The spectrum of successful treatment can vary from ultraconservative (watchful waiting only) to radical (removal of the graft and the pseudocyst membrane and rerouting via a new anatomic route). Multiple aspirations as the sole mode of therapy achieved seroma resolution in 70 percent of the cases so treated, 80 percent of which became infected. This is a reasonable therapeutic alternative in an elderly or poor-risk patient. The seroma can be monitored by serial computerized tomography (CT) scanning.

Although removal of the pseudocyst without graft replacement was successful in 72 percent of cases treated in this manner, 12 percent of the grafts became infected. If surgery is to be undertaken, both graft and pseudomembrane should be excised. In 63 cases, graft replacement achieved a 92 percent cure rate. The removed graft should be replaced with a material dissimilar to the original, either PTFE or a velour knitted Dacron. An impermeable substitute, such as an autogenous vein or umbilical vein graft, is a prime choice if available and of the proper size. Rerouting of the graft through a new anatomic pathway completes the radical surgical approach to the problem. Areas of cyst excision are drained with soft pump–type drains; prophylactic antibiotics are routinely used; and prosthetic angulation, especially near the anastomosis, should be avoided.

20 THE ROLE OF LUMBAR SYMPATHECTOMY

Since Julio Diez of Argentina introduced sympathectomy for limb ischemia in 1924,[1] there have been recurring cycles of enthusiasm and disenchantment with its results in peripheral arterial disease.

Some of the difficulty has been because of misunderstanding of the peripheral vasomotor mechanism and its effect upon the different tissues of the extremities. Even more important has been inability to predict the results of sympathectomy by any objective test. There also has been no standard for measurement of the postoperative condition. For years viewpoints have been defended with noncontrolled data; clinical impressions rather than objective facts have dominated the field.

Prior to the development of reconstructive vascular surgery, when sympathectomy was the only procedure available, master surgeons such as Alton Ochsner and Michael DeBakey naturally promulgated its virtues. Their 1940 review is still informative.[2]

In the mid-1950s my attempts to use venous occlusion plethysmography and skin temperatures to evaluate the indications for and results of lumbar sympathectomies over a period of 3 years only caused confusion and frustration. The results of over 300 such studies could not be understood and correlated well enough to produce a publication!

Little progress has occurred in the 30 following years, as attested by the inability of James Yao, an experienced as well as candid clinical investigator, to provide any better answer in 1982.[3]

FUNCTIONAL ANATOMY

A brief review of the sympathetic nervous system may be worthwhile, since many of us do not now often perform the procedure.

The autonomic nervous system consists of two anatomically and functionally separate components, namely, the parasympathetic (craniosacral) nerves and the sympathetic (thoracolumbar) outflow. The sympathetic, or thoracolumbar, segment is composed of bilateral chains of nerves and their ganglia which parallel the spine and adhere closely to the fascia covering the vertebrae.

Preganglionic neurons course down in the gray matter of the spinal cord, emerge through the anterior roots as white rami communicantes, and terminate in the sympathetic ganglia (Figure 20-1). Here originate postganglionic neurons which run through the gray rami from the sympathetic ganglia to join various spinal nerves, passing peripherally through these to the distal vessels, sweat glands, and arrector pili muscles.

The sympathetic portion of the nerves of the leg leaves the spinal cord from the tenth thoracic segment (T10) through the second lumbar (L2) (or occasionally through the third) and enters the

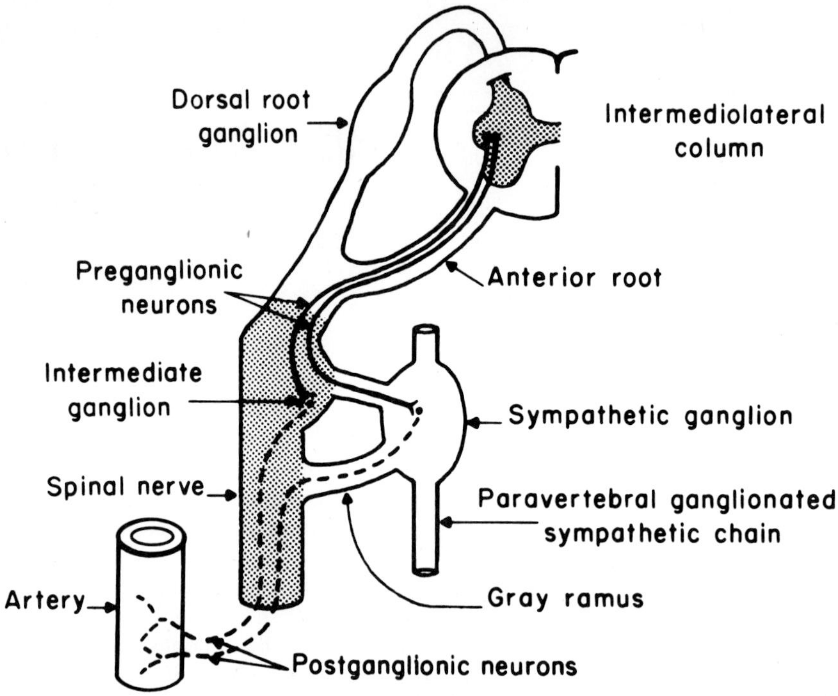

FIGURE 20-1 The complicated arrangement of the autonomic nerves. Notice the preganglionic neurons which bypass the ganglionated chain via intermediate ganglia.

ganglionated chains. Postganglionic neurons from the ganglionated chains enter the lumbosacral nerve plexus in the lumbar and sacral regions. If the chain is removed (by the usual sympathectomy) from L2 through L4, there is interruption of most of the vasoconstriction fibers to the periphery, although further release of vasoconstriction by nerve block can often be demonstrated even after bilateral surgical sympathectomy.

This failure of sympathectomy to completely eliminate peripheral vasoconstriction is often noted and may be due to preganglionic neurons which connect with postganglionic ones in the intermediate ganglia of the spinal nerves without passing through the ganglionated chain (Figure 20-1), or it may be due to intraspinal pathways which are not disturbed by sympathectomy.[4] Surgical ablation completely misses this latter pathway.

The "high" sympathectomy recommended in the past, whereby the chain was excised along the L1 ganglia downward,[5] is not necessary, and its potential sexual complications contraindicate this radical ablation. Removal of both L1 ganglia in the male prevents closure of the internal vesicle sphincter, so sexual ejaculation becomes retrograde into the bladder rather than external as is usual. Perhaps this complication has been overstated,[6] but such high proximal sympathetic ablations are not useful, so the point is made.[7]

Vasoconstriction mediated by the sympathetic nervous system can be blocked at the level of its root outlets from the cord by epidural or spinal anesthesia, at the ganglionated chain level by anesthetic block or by surgical sympathectomy, and at the level of the peripheral nerves by an anesthetic nerve block, such as to the posterior tibial nerve at the ankle.

It is now generally agreed that the differences in sensitivity of the effector organs caused by preganglionic rather than postganglionic sympathectomy are not of clinical significance.

THE EFFECTS OF SYMPATHECTOMY

Lumbar sympathectomy prevents vasoconstriction in response to thermal, pharmacologic, and stress stimulation in patients with significant degrees of vasomotor activity. The effect is more pronounced in the skin than in muscle, whose response to exercise and to ischemia is not greatly affected by sympathectomy.[8] Additionally, sympathectomy prevents the sweating which is sometimes detrimental to ischemic extremities.[9]

The immediate decrease in vasomotor tone in the legs and feet which follows sympathectomy is partially lost in the following days but persists to some extent for years. The reason for some return of vascular tone is not clear, although it has been supposed that nerve regeneration slowly occurs. Goetz has suggested automaticity of vascular small muscle cells, which produces an inherent basal tone.[4]

Removal of the lumbar sympathetic vasoconstrictive influence not only allows maximal distention of the arterial system by the intravascular pressure but also prevents vasoconstriction in response to cold, smoking, and stress. While the vessels may be too fixed by disease to allow enlargement when their muscle tone is released, the sympathectomy may still be protective against any vasoconstrictive response and allow distal tissue perfusion to continue in situations where vasoconstriction might restrict this.

Shifts in the effective circulation to different organs and different parts allow maximal flow to different regions as the demand varies. This borrowing-lending phenomenon was originally termed hemometakinesia by DeBakey, Burch, Ray, and Ochsner in 1947 to indicate the shift in blood flow to a part of the body engaged in activity by decreased vascular resistance or to a part whose resistance had been decreased by sympathectomy.[10] Further documentation of this effect of unilateral lumbar sympathectomy has been provided by May, DeWeese, and Rob, who studied the effects of sympathectomy upon the iliac blood flow in dogs. There was a large increase in ipsilateral flow at the same time that a smaller diminution of contralateral flow occurred. The effect was less when arterial stenosis was present, but relief of the stenosis again allowed a greatly augmented blood flow. This suggests that direct arterial surgery should be preferred to sympathectomy and that the latter should be tailored to denervate only the ischemic area.[11]

It has been estimated that about 80 percent of the blood flow through the feet goes to the skin and is therefore under vasomotor control while about 20 percent goes to muscle, where it is not. This may explain why lumbar sympathectomy ablation favorably affects ischemia of the skin but does not usually influence muscle claudication. Strandness and Bell reported that only 13 percent of 39 extremities studied experienced any significant improvement in claudication after sympathetic denervation.[12]

The failure of benefit to a leg whose large vessels are occluded is probably related to the fixed resistance of the collateral bed, which prevents much flow increase from diminution of the tone of the distal arterioles. Thus the majority of the 23 legs with femoropopliteal disease whose blood flow was studied by Folse, Mack, and Cantrell showed no significant increase, while the 9 without major vascular occlusion responded well to epidural block.[13]

PREDICTION OF THE RESULT OF SYMPATHECTOMY

Prior to the widespread use of angiography it was recognized by experienced clinicians that sympathectomy would produce better results for patients meeting certain criteria. Thus Smithwick in 1957 indicated that a flushing time (return of color to a dependent foot after elevation) of over 20 seconds predicted a "questionable or hopeless outlook" for the patient after sympathectomy.[14] Correlation of flushing times with angiograms has indicated that the shorter times are associated not only with collateral vessels but, of more importance, with main vessels which are still patent distal to an occlusion. These patients are also the best candidates for arterial repair and in addition have a better chance of spontaneous improvement as the collateral circulation builds if nothing is done.

INDICATIONS FOR LUMBAR SYMPATHECTOMY

It should at once be recognized that sophisticated peripheral angiography to find still-patent distal arteries, skilled surgical techniques, and an aggressive philosophy of salvage instead of amputation have led to our present situation, where reconstructive procedures vastly outnumber sympathectomies, perhaps in the order of 500 to 1.

Yet there are occasional sound indications for sympathectomy (Table 20-1), and the procedure should not be completely relegated to history.

TABLE 20-1 INDICATIONS FOR LUMBAR SYMPATHECTOMY

1 Arteriosclerotic arterial disease
  a Small skin lesions without extensive gangrene
  b Impossible or failed arterial repair
  c Continued vasoconstriction after arterial repair
  d Prominent hyperhidrosis
  e Concomitant aortic reconstruction
2 Buerger's thromboangiitis
3 Hyperhidrosis
4 Acrocyanosis
5 Causalgia

If arterial reconstruction is possible, there is no reason to delay it to observe the results of sympathectomy.

Lumbar sympathectomy is considerably more effective in the relief of small areas of pregangrene or actual gangrene of the skin than it is in the treatment of established rest pain or claudication, because it redirects blood flow to the skin rather than to muscle tissue. The best indication for sympathectomy, therefore, is a limited area of pregangrene or actual gangrene of the skin of the foot or toes without extensive gangrene; the patient should have no established rest pain, and direct arterial repair should be impossible or should already have failed.

ILLUSTRATIVE CASE

A 67-year-old diabetic female developed pregangrenous skin changes of the heel and toes in her pulseless right foot over a period of 3 years. Angiography showed complete occlusion of the right common iliac artery but patency of the left as well as of the femoral and popliteal arteries. An 8-mm polytetrafluoroethylene (PTFE) femoral-to-femoral graft was placed, which produced a good dorsalis pedis pulse. However, as time passed, the foot pulse disappeared and she increasingly complained of discomfort.

Six months later a new aortogram confirmed patency of the crossover graft (Figure 20-2) along with the femoropopliteal segment but increasing failure of the distal calf arteries. The foot continued to be discolored laterally (Figure 20-3).

Lumbar sympathectomy was performed. The foot immediately became warmer, and the dark discoloration turned to rubor. Pain ceased.

Comment

Slow progression of obliteration of the arteries of the calf is common in diabetic patients. Correction of the large-vessel lesion failed to overcome this problem. There appeared to be the best indication for relief by lumbar sympathectomy, namely, ischemia of the distal skin more than of the muscle; the results confirm this.

If the patient does not have sufficient distal circulation remaining to allow reconstruction of the arteries and has the typical painful, reddened foot which threatens early loss by spreading gangrene, it is reasonable to offer a lumbar sympathectomy rather than simply await demarcation for amputation. Because younger patients can ordinarily be expected to have relatively more vasoconstriction, sympathectomy is more favored for them.

If concomitant sympathectomy is to accompany a femoropopliteal graft, it should be done quickly, removing only one or two ganglia. A moist pack should then be placed within the wound and allowed to remain during the period of intraoperative heparinization, and wound closure

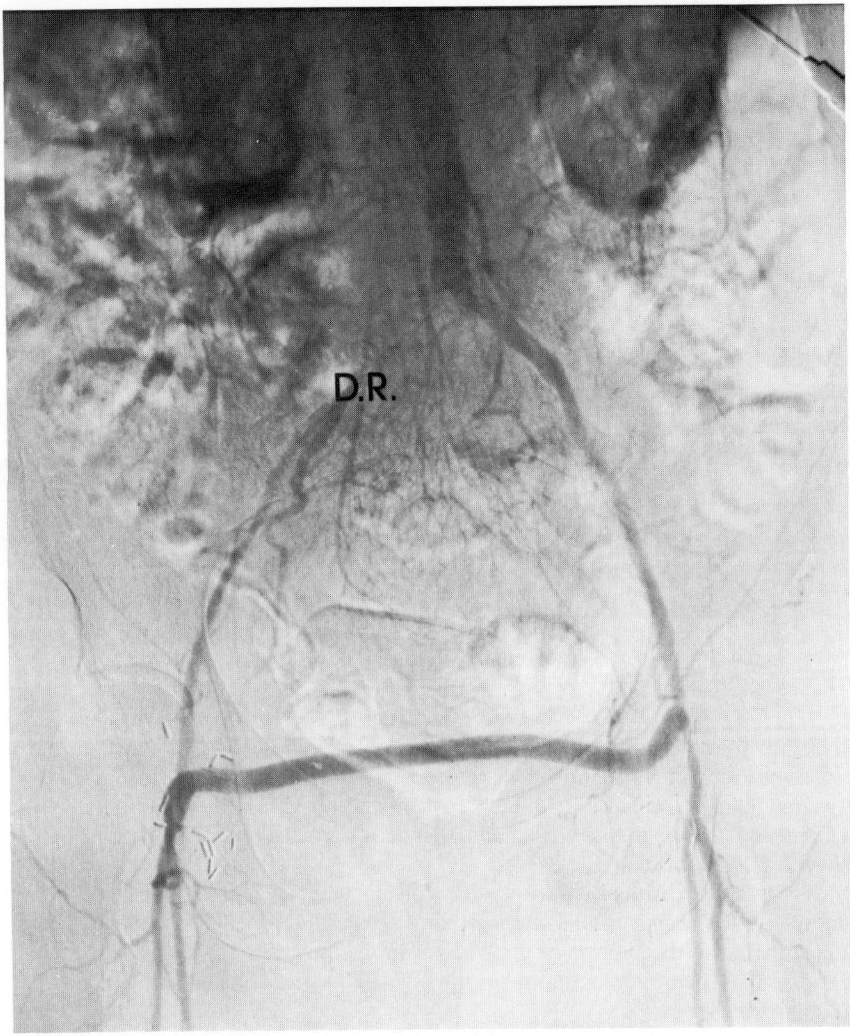

FIGURE 20-2 This patent femorofemoral graft bypasses the right iliac arterial occlusion but did not relieve foot symptoms, which were due to distal small-arterial disease.

should be performed simultaneously with closure of the wounds of the extremity. Thus, only 15 to 20 minutes need be added to the total operative time period.

It must be stressed that the chief effort should be devoted to a first-rate repair of the diseased artery, whose reconstruction is often time-consuming, frustrating, and demanding of patience; a concomitant sympathectomy should be efficient and quick.

Occasional patients show clear evidence postoperatively of vasoconstriction and require secondary sympathectomy for its relief.

Bilateral lumbar sympathectomy at the time of aortic reconstruction may be done just prior to heparinization and clamping of the vessels. Removal of a 3-cm segment of the ganglionated chain requires about 5 minutes for each side. No complications have been observed personally, although occasionally the dissection of one side has been abandoned due to local bleeding prior

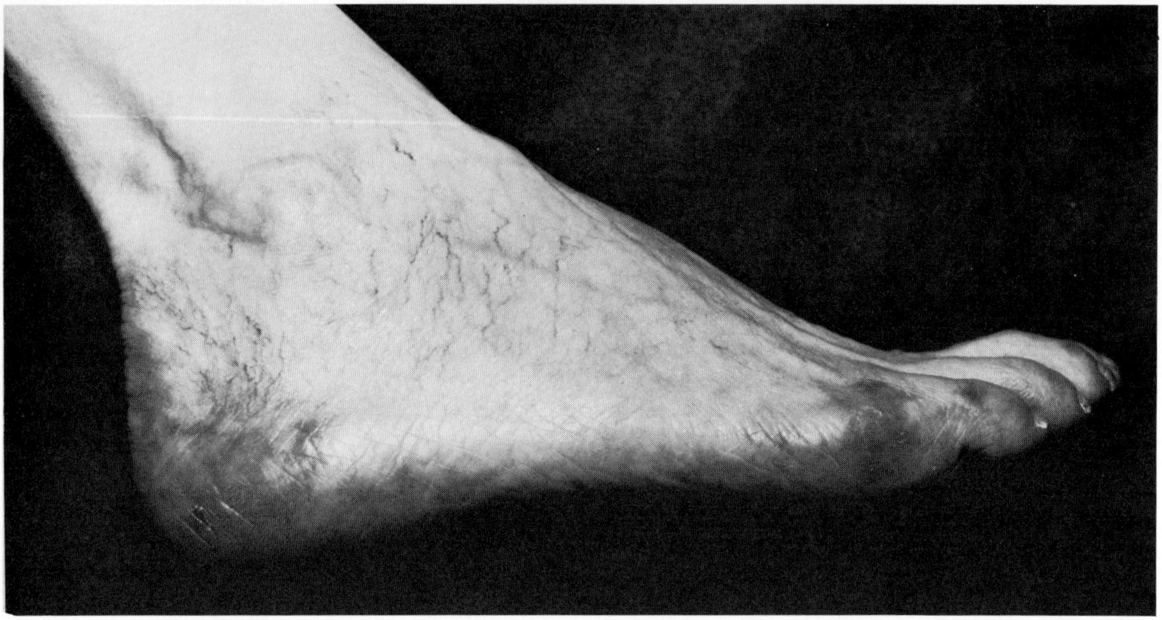

FIGURE 20-3 The discolored, painful foot of the patient whose bypass is shown in Figure 20-2. Lumbar sympathectomy increased the skin circulation and relieved symptoms.

to removal of the chain. Such bleeding has never been persistent or serious but should warn the operator to avoid getting into a large problem while dealing with a side issue.

The value of lumbar sympathectomy for Buerger's thromboangiitis obliterans is discussed in Chapter 17. Such patients are usually younger than arteriosclerotics and benefit greatly, provided they also cease smoking.

There are occasionally patients with primary hyperhidrosis whose extremities can be dried completely by appropriate sympathectomy. It should, however, be recalled that sweating of the unsympathectomized parts of the body or limbs may then increase and become a real problem. Preoperative planning should take this possibility into consideration. This is discussed further in Chapter 21.

Lumbar sympathectomy may be used to dry previously hyperhidrotic skin near a *chronic ankle ulcer*. Patman has suggested an even more specific effect in healing the ulcers of 23 patients who had not responded to other measures.[15]

Whether or not there is a curative effect, it is worthwhile at least to consider the procedure for a chronic leg ulcer which has been refractory to vein operations and grafts, because I have observed remarkable healing of a few.

The purplish cyanotic color of the extremities in acrocyanosis may be changed to pink by sympathectomy. This indication is rare and is largely a psychological or cosmetic one, but the effect has been much appreciated by two young females who have been treated by me.

Causalgic states (reflex sympathetic dystrophy) are generally said to be relieved by appropriate sympathectomy. Thus, Rutherford states "this probably is the most gratifying application of sympathectomy today,"[16] and Owens reports complete relief for 82 of 94 patients.[17] Patman says "sympathectomy can be counted on to relieve the pain of most patients with true causalgia."[18]

My own experience with 12 sympathectomies for such patients has been quite different; in fact, the relief of only 3 of these has led to my conclusion that sympathectomies often fail to relieve these patients. A guarded prognosis should be recognized if operation appears to be necessary. The matter is discussed further in Chapter 21.

CONTRAINDICATION TO SYMPATHECTOMY

TABLE 20-2 CONTRAINDICATIONS TO LUMBAR SYMPATHECTOMY

1	Claudication
2	Rest pain
3	Extensive gangrene
4	Possible arterial repair*

*If the repair fails or is unfeasible, sympathectomy should be considered before amputation.

Claudication and/or rest pain do not respond well to sympathectomy (Table 20-2). Cuthbert Owens reviewed various reports of sympathectomy for claudication, as well as his own experience, and concluded that "objective studies have not shown the procedure is warranted."[17]* For example Shaw, Austen, and Stiga demonstrated that a control group showed "the same improvement over the same period . . . without sympathectomy."[19]

Extensive areas of gangrene are clearly beyond its scope.

The earlier concept that sympathectomy should be done prior to an arterial reconstruction has been abandoned as results of arterial repairs have improved and their indications have become recognized.

If the repair fails or is not feasible and amputation is threatened, but not certain, there should be consideration of sympathectomy prior to loss of the limb. There is no absolute method of prediction of the result, but remarkable improvement sometimes occurs, even in elderly patients.

CHEMICAL SYMPATHECTOMY

I have had no personal experience with chemical sympathectomy by injection of phenol into the L2 to L4 area under fluoroscopic control. Its proponents report good results with low risk.[20]

OPERATIVE TECHNIQUE

High proximal sympathectomy to include the L1 ganglion, as recommended in the past,[5] is not necessary, since removal of L2 through L4 ordinarily produces complete denervation of the lower leg and foot, where the real problem lies.[7]

Anatomic regeneration is probably not of practical importance for lumbar sympathectomy.[21]

The anterior extraperitoneal approach to the ganglionated chain allows good visualization through an incision which heals well. A constant effort is made to obtain medial exposure in order to look "down" (from anterior to posterior) on the chain rather than "in" from a lateral position, because this diminishes the depth of the field.

Because lumbar sympathectomy has now become unusual and many surgeons are not familiar with it, certain details of the operative plan follow:

1 The patient's *position* is supine. No pads or propping are needed, since the modern operating table is easily tilted. Following the older advice to flex the thigh to relax the iliopsoas muscle is unnecessary.

2 The transverse *incision* resembles that of Flothow's original technique[22] more than the long oblique incision of Pearl.[23] It is carried an inch over the lateral rectus muscle edge to allow medial mobilization of that muscle.

3 The *muscles* are cut in the line of the incision. The older technique of splitting the external oblique muscle tends to limit exposure. The cut muscle heals well. The internal oblique and the underlying transversus abdominis muscles are then split in the direction of their fibers. After the

*Owens's complete discussion and list of 152 references will interest some readers.

transversalis fascia is split, the peritoneal sac is mobilized from the lateral to the medial aspect to allow entry into the retroperitoneal space.

4 The *retroperitoneal dissection* is begun laterally into the extraperitoneal fat rather than medially over the peritoneal sac itself, which is easily torn if initially dissected. Careful stripping of the peritoneal sac toward the midline is important in order to allow the approach to be as anterior as possible (rather than lateral).

5 The *peritoneal sac* is retracted medially with the ureter clinging to it. A self-containing retractor is placed to hold apart the abdominal muscles, and the hand is moved extraperitoneally anterior to the iliopsoas muscle until the vena cava (on the right) or aorta (on the left) is reached. A retractor is placed to hold the peritoneal sac medially. The old Royle spade retractor is too bulky; a smaller malleable Zalkind retractor is easier to use.

6 *Dissection of the aorta or cava* is done under direct vision. It is lifted off the ganglionated chain, which feels like a firm cord when it is palpated; the finger is rolled over it as it lies on the anterior surface of the vertebral bodies.

7 The overlying fascia is opened, and the *chain is elevated* on a nerve hook and gently dissected in both directions. Lumbar veins may cross anterior to the chain itself. Bleeding may be controlled by placement of clips or by the electrocautery. Better, it may be avoided. Clips need not be placed upon the rami but are put upon the proximal and distal ends of the chain as it is resected, since this will aid later exact localization of the ganglia which have been removed. If 3 cm of ganglionated chain to a point opposite the vascular bifurcation is removed, the foot and lower leg are denervated. Higher resection of the ganglia is not necessary.

The gross appearance of the nerve tissue is typical. If there is doubt, a frozen section may be examined microscopically to be certain.

When difficulty occurs in locating the chain, look medially well up under the great vessel, feel for the chain there, then clean off the areolar tissue until the vertebral body is well seen, looking at any small strands coursing longitudinally to see if one leads to the enlargement of a ganglion. If this fails, change the dissection to a more proximal area, where the chain may be larger and easier to find. Keep the field dry of blood, and strive for exposure from the anterior (not lateral) position to enable a more shallow and direct approach.

Torn veins cause troublesome bleeding which may be difficult to control. Pack the field while securing proper suction equipment, instruments, and vascular sutures. Veins torn flush with the inferior vena cava are better sutured, perhaps after further exposure of the vessel is secured by additional dissection.

POSTOPERATIVE COMPLICATIONS

Ileus Postoperative adynamic ileus is occasionally severe. Prophylaxis is begun the day after operation by administration of $\frac{1}{2}$ mL of 1:2000 neostigmine (Prostigmin) intramuscularly every 2 hours for 6 doses to encourage the return of peristalsis. This may be repeated daily as needed.

Postoperative Neuritis This condition is common, being manifested by pain with skin sensitivity of the thigh. Its cause is unclear. Relief of pain by medication may be necessary for 4 to 6 weeks. Spontaneous recovery is the rule.

Gangrene The "paradoxical gangrene" described by earlier authors is probably due either to embolism or to acute thrombosis. Such acute distal ischemia should at once suggest angiography to determine suitable treatment.[24]

Unusual Complications Complications such as a ventral hernia which followed one procedure and the temporary (but discouraging) fecal fistula which followed another may occur. The latter patient discharged fecal material through his incision for 10 days prior to ultimate healing, probably because of injury to the posterior aspect of the cecum as it was elevated from the retroperitoneal approach. Previous ruptured appendicitis with posterior adhesions no doubt predisposed the patient to the injury.

RESULTS

The results of sympathectomy are difficult to determine because of the many variables encountered. Reports in the literature vary with the enthusiasm and the particular viewpoint of the writer. Efforts to document the good results of sympathectomy have failed, despite the scores of reports of surgical experience.[25–28] Today the procedure must be limited to occasional patients.

TABLE 20-3 LUMBAR SYMPATHECTOMIES AT VANDERBILT UNIVERSITY AFFILIATED HOSPITALS

Type	No.
For arteriosclerosis	
With vascular repair	135
Without vascular repair	106
Total	241
Nonarteriosclerotic	30
Total	271

The five-year experience at the Vanderbilt University Affiliated Hospitals, 1969–1973, was summarized by Terry Allen, as shown in Table 20-3. Among the 106 cases where a concomitant vascular repair was not performed, the improvement rate was judged to be 59 percent. This figure should not be considered exact, because adjuvant measures undoubtedly influenced the outcome. This difficulty in evaluating our own results of the operation is discouraging but representative.

Still, lumbar sympathectomy for the properly selected patient may produce an outstanding result with little risk.

REFERENCES

1 Diez J: Un nuevo metodo de simpatectomia perfiferica para el tratamiento de las afecciones troficas y gangrenous de los miembros. *Bulll Soc Circ B. Aires* 1924, 8:792.

2 Ochsner A, DeBakey M: Peripheral vascular disease. *Surg Gynecol Obstet* 1940, 70:1058.

3 Yao JST, Flinn WR: The present role of lumbar sympathectomy in the treatment of lower limb ischemia, in Veith JJ (ed): *Critical Problems in Vascular Surgery.* Appleton-Century Crofts, New York, 1982, chap 18, pp 263–75.

4 Goetz RH: Clinical aspects of vascular reactivity. *Surg Gynecol Obstet* 1959, 109:209.

5 Lilly GD, Smith DW, Biggane CF Jr, Jana JT Jr: An evaluation of "high" lumbar sympathectomy in arteriosclerotic circulatory insufficiency of the lower extremities. *Surgery* 1954, 35:1.

6 Rutherford RB: Lumbar sympathectomy: Indications and technique, in Rutherford RB (ed): *Vascular Surgery.* Saunders, Philadelphia, 1977, chap 63, p 560.

7 Simeone FA: The anatomy of the lumbar sympathetic trunks in man. *J Cardiovasc Surg* (Torino) 1979, 20:283.

8 Beaconsfield P: Effect of exercise on muscle blood flow in normal and sympathectomized limbs: Collateral circulation before and after sympathectomy. *Ann Surg* 1954, 140:786.

9 Clement DL: Sympathetic nervous control of muscle and skin circulation. *J Cardiovasc Surg* (Torino) 1979, 20:291.

10 DeBakey ME, Burch G, Ray T, Ochsner A: The "borrowing-lending" hemyodynamic phenomenon (hemoketakinesia) and its therapeutic application in peripheral vascular disturbances. *Ann Surg* 1947, 129:850.

11 May A, DeWeese J, Rob CG: The effect of sympathectomy on blood flow in arterial stenosis. *Ann Surg* 1963, 158:182.

12 Strandness DE, Bell JW: Critical evaluation of the results of lumbar sympathectomy. *Ann Surg* 1964, 160:1021.

13 Folse R, Mack RM, Cantrell JR: Alterations in femoral blood flow and resistance following sympathetic blockade. *Ann Surg* 1965, 162:873.

14 Smithwick RH: Lumbar sympathectomy in treatment of obliterative vascular disease of lower extremities. *Surgery* 1957, 42:415.
15 Patman RD: Sympathectomy in the treatment of chronic venous leg ulcers. *Arch Surg* 1982, 117:1561.
16 Rutherford RB: Lumbar sympathectomy: Indications and technique, in Rutherford RB (ed): *Vascular Surgery*. Saunders, Philadelphia, 1977, 557.
17 Owens JC: Indications for lumbar sympathectomy, in Dat WA (ed): *Management of Arterial Occlusive Disease*. Year Book, Chicago, 1972, chap 24, pp 399–425.
18 Patman RD: Post-traumatic pain symdromes: Recognition and management, in Rutherford RB (ed): *Vascular Surgery*. Saunders, Philadelphia, 1977, chap 52, p 481.
19 Shaw RS, Austen WG, Stiga S: A ten year study of the effect of lumbar sympathectomy on the peripheral circulation of patients with arteriosclerotic occlusive disease. *Surg Gynecol Obstet* 1964, 119:486.
20 Walker PM, Johnston KW: predicting the success of a sympathectomy: A prospective study using discriminant function and multiple regression analysis. *Surgery* 1980, 87:216.
21 Callow A: Discussion of Simeone FA: The anatomy of the lumbar sympathetic trunks in man. J Cardiovasc Surg (Torino) 1979, 20:283.
22 Flothow PG: Anterior extraperitoneal approach to the lumbar sympathetic nerves. *Am J Surg* 1935, 20:23.
23 Pearl FL: Muscle splitting extraperitoneal lumbar ganglionectomy. *Surg Gynecol Obstet* 1937, 65:107.
24 Bergan JJ, Trippel OH: Arteriograms in ischemic limbs worsened after lumbar sympathectomy. *Arch Surg* 1962, 85:643.
25 Szilagyi DE, Smith RF, Scerpella JR, Hoffman K: Lumber sympathectomy: Current role in the treatment of arteriosclerotic occlusive disease. *Arch Surg* 1967, 95:753.
26 Edwards EA, Crane C: Ten-year status after sympathectomy for arteriosclerosis. *JAMA* 1961, 175:677.
27 Haimovici H, Steinman C, Karson H: Evaluation of lumbar sympathectomy: Advanced occlusive arterial disease. *Arch Surg* 1964, 89:1089.
28 King RD, Kaiser GC, Lempke RE, Shumacker HB Jr: Evaluation of lumbar sympathetic denervation. *Arch Surg* 1964, 88:36.

INVITED COMMENTARY

Geza de Takats, M.D.,
Chicago, Illinois

Reading this concise, clear-cut description of the present role of lumbar sympathectomy evokes a nostalgic feeling for our efforts in the forties. At that time, the vascular surgeon did his or her own arteriogram, and paravertebral block and even used paraverine or procaine hydrochloride (Novocain) intraarterially to learn how the terminal vascular bed would respond to the release of vasoconstrictor impulses.

Certain facts emphasized in this chapter were obvious even 40 to 50 years ago. Thus, the initial rise in temperature and other signs of increased flow lasted only 1 or 2 weeks; the rise in venous oxygen saturation was interpreted as being due to increased flow through arteriovenous shunts and did not increase nutritional flow. Some pregangrenous areas quickly became gangrenous and well-demarcated because blood was diverted to better-vascularized areas. Removal of the second and third lumbar sympathetic ganglia was the standard procedure, but in cases of causalgia or sympathetic reflex dystrophy affecting the thigh or inguinal region, the sympathectomy was extended to the level of the tenth thoracic ganglion.

It was also obvious that sympathetic denervation affected primarily the skin and not the muscle; intermittent claudication could not be expected to improve, but the level of amputation, determined by histamine flares before and after paravertebral, spinal, or epidural block, could be carefully lowered.

Certain questions raised in our early activities are still with us now. What is the role of the sympathetic afferent fibers? Do their sections relieve rest pain so that the patient can bear weight on his or her foot and begin to walk, thus diminishing claudication? What about cholinergic impulses causing more vasodilatation in the sympathectomized extremity? As far back as 1938, Gellhorn and Steck found on our sympathetomized patients that low oxygen and high carbon dioxide inhalation produced vasodilatation instead of vasoconstriction in the sympathectomized limb.[1] Did this mean that the confirmed smoker would have less ischemia in the sympathectomized extremity? And the individual standing up would not get postural vasoconstriction in the sympathectomized limb? Or the homemaker overstepping the family budget would not get cold feet on being confronted by a spouse?

In review of the autonomic balance rationalizing sympathetic blockade, I pointed out that simple cholinergic stimulants like neostigmine have a great effect on the sympathectomized extremity.[2]

I fully agree that sympathectomy today has limited indications. Certainly, when the abdomen is already open, it takes but a few minutes to remove both chains, but the average endarterectomy, bypass, or in situ venous anastomosis hardly needs a sympathectomy. Excessive hyperhidrosis, thromboangiitis obliterans, and causalgia (but not collagen disease) respond to sympathectomy. Remarkable effects can be produced by tolazoline (Priscoline) and lidocaine given intraarterially, and many of us have seen remarkable responses to a few intermittent doses.

Proper selection of cases has been stressed in this chapter, and that message should highly limit, but not cause abandonment of, denervation by sympathectomy.

COMMENTARY REFERENCES

1 Gellhorn E, Steck IE: The effect of gases with low oxygen and increased carbon dioxide-tension on the peripheral blood flow of man, *Am J Physiol* 1938, 124:735.

2 de Takats G: Autonomic nervous balance: A rationale for sympathetic blockade. *Curr Surg* 1978, 35:226.

21 THORACIC SYMPATHECTOMY

Ablation of the sympathetic nerve supply of the upper extremity has limited indications, but its results are rewarding for properly selected patients.

The indications listed in Table 21-1 may be surprising, since Raynaud's syndrome does not appear as such. Actually, some secondary forms of Raynaud's syndrome do benefit from sympathectomy, but the old idea that primary Raynaud's disease is a proper surgical indication must be abandoned.

RAYNAUD'S SYNDROME

The symptom complex of coldness, color changes, and pain known as Raynaud's phenomenon occurs as episodes due to cold or to stress or sometimes without a trigger event and commonly involves the hands (Figure 21-1), but also occasionally the feet. The diagnostic points outlined in Table 21-2 are clinically useful in differentiating other causes of hand and finger symptoms.

A clear distinction between primary disease showing Raynaud's phenomenon and the same phenomenon secondary to other processes is important (Table 21-3). Primary Raynaud's disease is uncommon, is usually seen in women, and is most often bilateral. Experience with large numbers of these cases has led to the recommendation that cases not be classified as primary until all studies have been accomplished and a considerable period (approximately 2 years) of careful follow-up has passed,[1] because as time passes, more and more patients are found to have another primary cause which allows differentiation from primary Raynaud's disease. Usually the typical history and examination allow a reasonable estimate of the cause of the hand symptoms.

BLOOD TESTS

A long list of studies which may aid in detecting rheumatoid states, connective tissue disease, and other systemic problems may be developed,[2] most of which lie in the realm of the internist rather than the vascular surgeon, who should of course be generally if not specifically aware of them.

Arteriograms have been thought

TABLE 21-1 INDICATIONS FOR THORACIC SYMPATHECTOMY

1 Arterial occlusive disease of distal arteries not suitable for reconstruction
  - Trauma
  - Arteriosclerosis
  - Thromboangiitis obliterans

2 Reflex sympathetic dystrophy
3 Cold injury
4 Hyperhidrosis

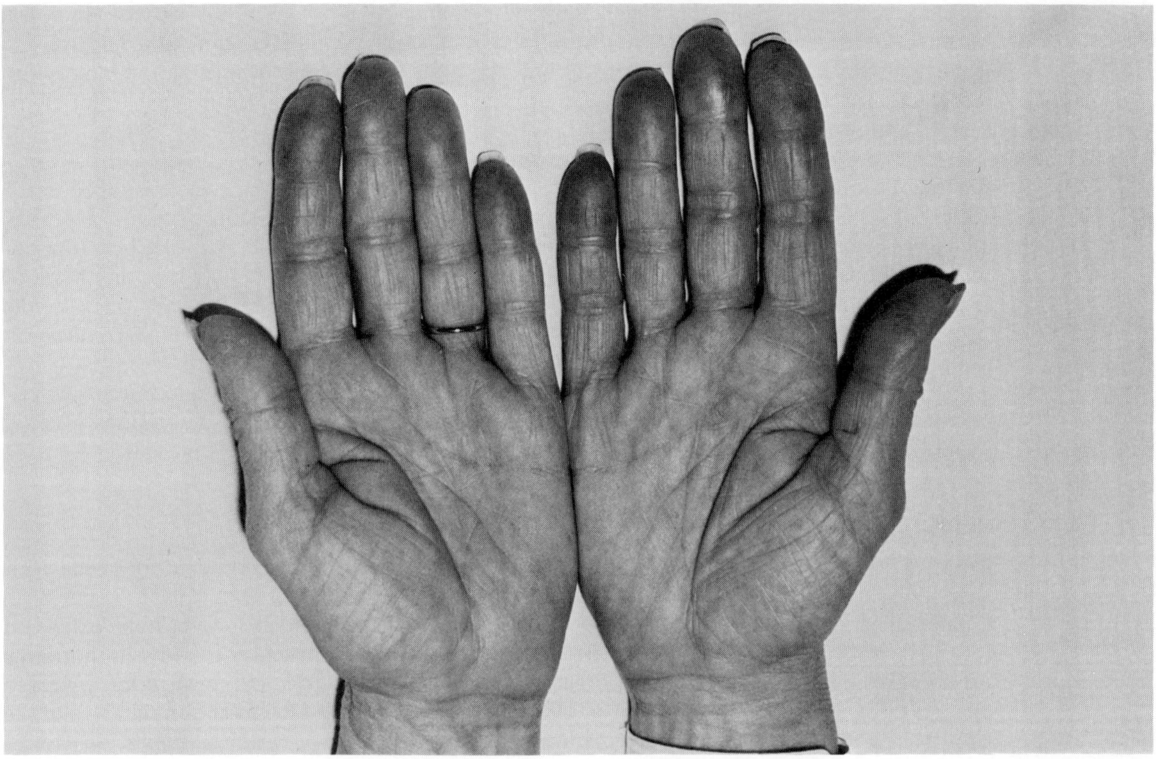

FIGURE 21-1 Primary Raynaud's disease in an acute phase with pain, cyanosis, and sweating of the fingertips.

TABLE 21-2 DIFFERENTIAL DIAGNOSIS OF HAND AND FINGER SYMPTOMS

Raynaud's disease: usually in females, episodic, bilateral; has minimal tissue necrosis, absence of a primary cause, of a long duration; triggered by cold and emotion
Arterial embolism: has an acute onset; accompanies recent cardiac arrhythmia or myocardial infarction; has uniform tissue ischemia
Arterial thrombosis: slow onset, minimal cyanosis, irregular distal distribution of tissue necrosis or gangrene with local pain
Acrocyanosis: painless cyanosis of the tips of appendages
Reflex sympathetic dystrophy (causalgia): posttraumatic; has decreased motion of joints, skin atrophy, prominent pain
Thoracic outlet syndrome: pain due to nerve compression, no arterial signs usually, no tissue necrosis

TABLE 21-3 CAUSES OF RAYNAUD'S SYNDROME

1 Primary Raynaud's disease
2 Raynaud's phenomenon due to
- *a* Arterial occlusion (arteriosclerosis, thromboangiitis obliterans, embolism, injury)
- *b* Nerve lesions (thoracic outlet syndrome, causalgia)
- *c* Intoxication (ergot, heavy metals)
- *d* Miscellaneous (scleroderma, disseminated lupus, rheumatoid arthritis, dermatomyositis, leukemia, myeloma)

unnecessary by some,[3,4] but this visualization allows an early estimate of the cause of the symptoms and, of more importance, of the likelihood of benefit from thoracic sympathectomy.

Angiography via the femoral-to-arm-to-brachial route is a bit complicated and often provides poor digital vascular visualization. Direct injection by needle into the brachial artery at the elbow is easier and produces splendid films.

A no. 18 Cournand needle is passed through a bleb of local anesthesia in the skin directly into the brachial artery just proximal to the antecubital fossa. The head of the needle is taped to the forearm, and a connecting tube is placed between the needle and a stopcock with a syringe attached. Twenty milliliters of Conray-60 is injected through the needle pointing in a superior direction. Blood flow from this point near the elbow to the distal fingers may be either rapid or slower than is usually anticipated, and the multiple-cassette changer should be set to expose the early films rapidly and the latter ones at slower, 2-second intervals. Figure 21-2 shows an occluded ulnar artery as well as multiple digital arterial blocks.

After the first set of films is inspected, 25 mg of tolazoline (Priscoline) is injected intraarterially and a second series is exposed (Figure 21-3). The total examination determines whether organic occlusion of one or more of the wrist, hand, and/or finger arteries is present.

STELLATE GANGLION BLOCK

Stellate ganglion block with 1% lidocaine may allow prediction of a good result following sympathectomy, but its failure does not necessarily rule out benefit.

With the patient lying supine, a pillow is placed beneath the shoulders to force hyperextension of the cervical spine. The head of the bed is elevated 30°. A skin wheal is raised with lidocaine just lateral to the trachea and a finger breadth superior to the clavicle, and through this is passed a long no. 22 needle directly posteriorly. The needle passes between the trachea medially and the carotid sheath laterally. After the needle impinges upon the bone or cartilage, aspiration assures that it does not lie within any large blood vessel. As the needle is slightly withdrawn from the bony contact, 5 ml of 1% lidocaine is placed. Then another 5 ml is placed as the needle is slowly withdrawn another centimeter. This places a sufficient amount of lidocaine within the proper fascial space to ensure prompt blockade of the lower cervical ganglia and the proximal thoracic ones, since the anesthetic solution spreads widely following its depositon. The needle is immediately withdrawn, and the patient is observed for development of a Horner's syndrome within a few minutes. The anterior approach is technically easier than any other.

After the block the patient is questioned in regard to improvement of pain or feeling of warmth, and objective measurements may be made of the skin temperature of the fingers. Figure 21-4 shows the results of such a study, where general body warming released vasoconstriction to some extent but full vasodilatation was achieved only after stellate block was performed. The ensuing sympathectomy was quite successful.

BIOPSY

Only a few biopsies have been done, because of fear of failure of healing of the distal tissues as well as the knowledge that the biopsy has often failed to aid diagnosis. If it is done, the most rational approach is a lateral or medial incision over the proximal portion of the distal phalanx to find the neurovascular bundle and actually remove a small portion. Biopsy is not recommended.

NONSURGICAL TREATMENT

There is no specific therapy presently available for primary idiopathic Raynaud's disease. Its natural history of remission and exacerbations lends to anecdotal triumphs for a variety of med-

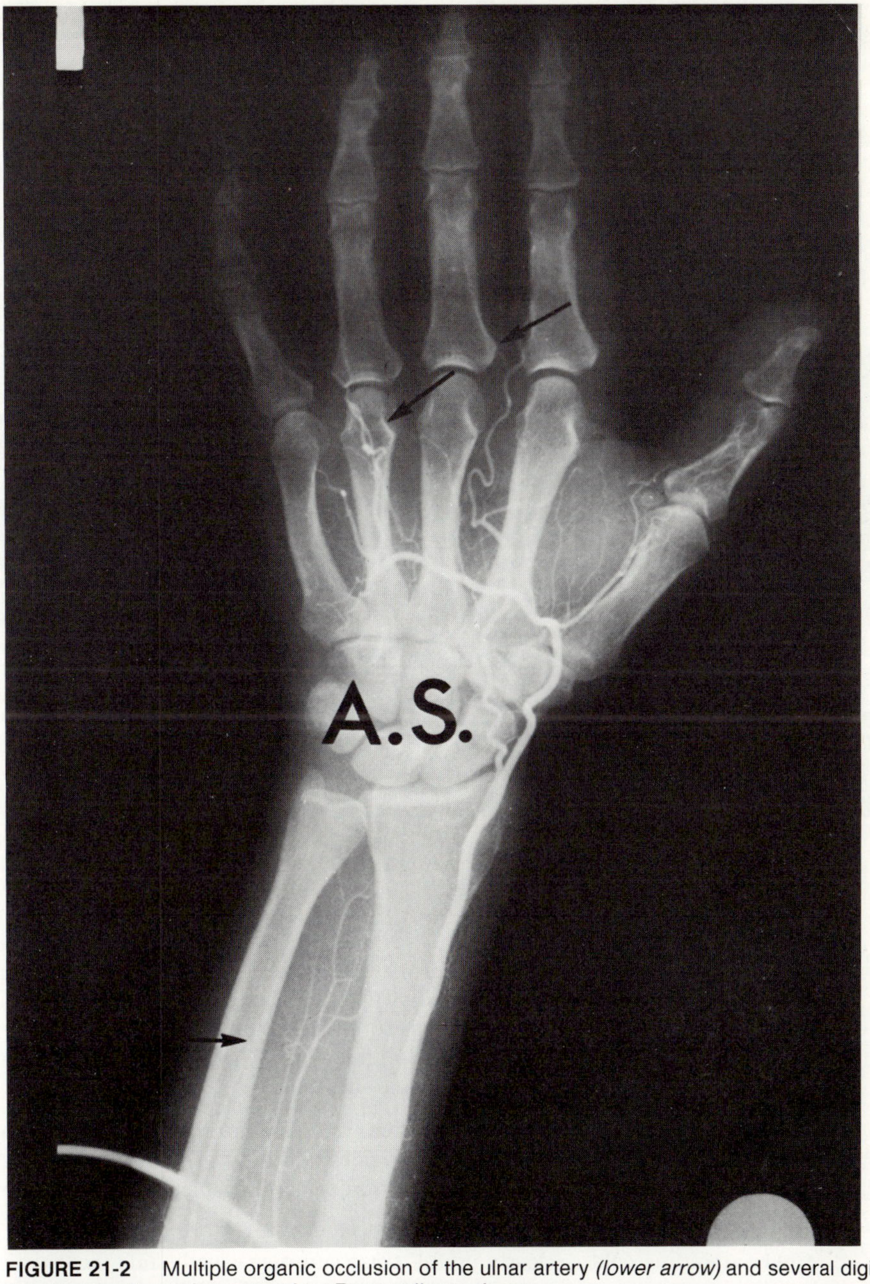

FIGURE 21-2 Multiple organic occlusion of the ulnar artery *(lower arrow)* and several digital arteries *(upper arrow)*, causing secondary Raynaud's syndrome.

ications which do not pass muster when used as a routine standard treatment for one patient after another.

The continuing serach for relief of vasospasm and impaired skin circulation leads to recurring reports of empirical trials of various drugs, while the real problem of basic investigation of the pathogenesis of the local arterial sensitivity is avoided. Thus, in a double-blind trial of nifedipine

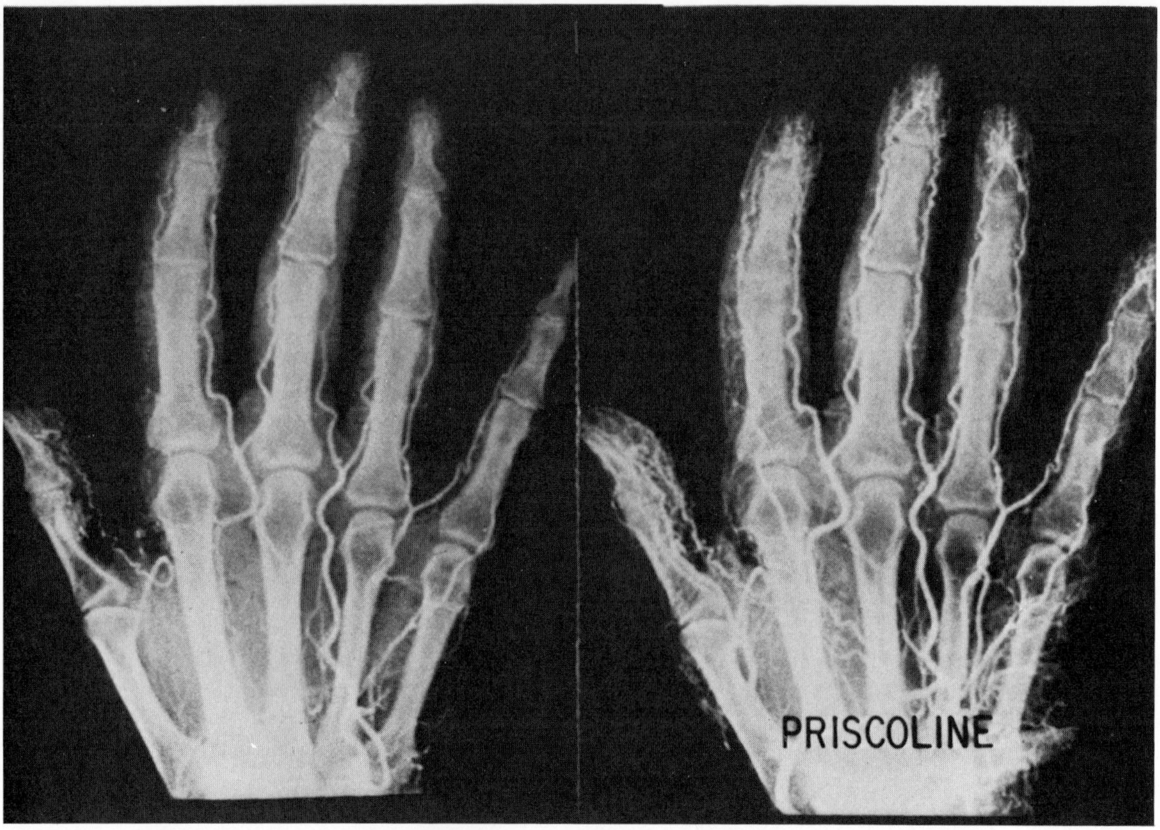

FIGURE 21-3 *Left,* an arteriogram made by injecting 20 mL of Conray-60 into the brachial artery at the elbow. *Right,* the same hand 1 minute after intraarterial injection of 25 mg of tolazoline. The terminal digital arteries are now well-filled and clearly opacified in areas not visualized on the previous series of films.

among a miserably few 15 patients (10 with systemic disease and 4 with primary Raynaud's disease) some clinical effectiveness was shown, although it clearly was not a final answer.[5] Nevertheless some therapy must be attempted, so a succession of *vasodilators* or *receptor-blocking drugs* may be used. These include guanethidine (10 to 20 mg daily), phenoxybenzamine (10 mg daily), prazosin (2 mg daily), and reserpine (1 mg daily).

Smoking Smoking is generally forbidden, yet there are no hard data to support this usual advice. My own observation is that tobacco does not affect primary Raynaud's disease, in contradistinction to its severe effects in the organic occlusive problems posed by arteriosclerosis and thromboangiitis obliterans.

Cold Avoiding cold is clearly useful, since summer usually aids these patients while cold weather or extreme air-conditioning causes symptoms. Not only must local cooling be avoided by gloves, but the entire body should be insulated with a cap, warm socks, dry shoes, and suitable outer clothing.

The occasional patient who can change residence to the tropics will benefit. Florida and the western desert are often not consistently warm enough, and it may be necessary to go to 18 to 20° latitude (Caribbean islands, Acapulco, Tahiti, Hawaii, and similar areas).

Rapid spinning of the arms (the McIntyre maneuver) may aid acute episodes by forcing blood to distal sites.

Local Treatment Local treatment of finger lesions may not be needed, since there is the increasing opinion that arterial occlusions and resultant tissue necroses do not occur in primary Raynaud's disease.

Thoracic Sympathectomy This is not useful in the primary form of Raynaud's disease. It has been difficult to correct the earlier belief that operation was useful, but there have now accumulated numbers of experienced vascular surgeons who deny the value of sympathectomy for such.

Thus Geza de Takats long ago stated that "lack of organic obstruction in the presence of clear-cut Raynaud's phenomenon is a warning signal of the first order,"[6] and in 1967 Edwards remarked that recurrence of symptoms was so common in primary Raynaud's disease that he found the operation inadvisable "except as a last-ditch effort."[7]

Birnstingl stated that "it is doubtful if sympathectomy should ever be advised in Raynaud's disease,"[8] and Porter has decried the operation for any form of Raynaud's syndrome.[3]

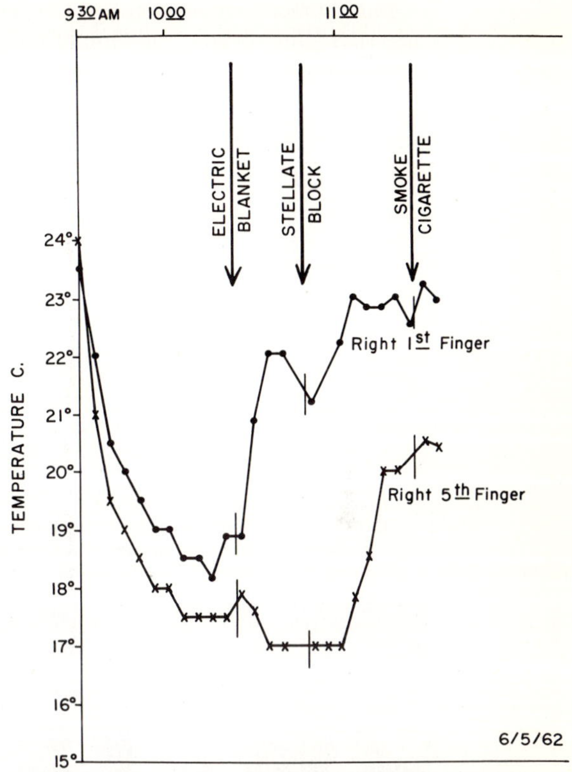

FIGURE 21-4 Skin temperatures of the first and fifth fingers of a patient with Raynaud's phenomenon due to multiple organic occlusions. In the constant-temperature room the temperature gradually stabilized. An electric blanket placed upon the abdomen and chest relieved vasoconstriction considerably in the first finger but not at all in the fifth finger. Stellate block thereafter achieved release of vasoconstriction in the fifth finger. Cigarette smoking had no discernible effect.

SURGICAL TREATMENT

Arterial Occlusion In this chapter we are not primarily concerned with stenoses and occlusion of the large arteries of the neck, shoulder, and arm, so we will pass on with acknowledgement of the value of embolectomies and bypasses there as needed.

The pathologic diagnosis of occlusion of the wrist, hand, and finger vessels often remains unproven, since biopsies are dangerously prone to poor healing and amputations are not often necessary. Rather than attempt to classify these lesions as arteriosclerosis or thromboangiitis obliterans, I simply call them organic occlusions, as differentiated from vasospasm.

The value of an operation for distal arterial lesions of the wrist, hand, and digital arteries has been decried by John Porter, who believes there is "no benefit from the use of cervicothoracic sympathectomy in the treatment of . . . severe hand artery occlusion without any associated systemic disease."[2] He describes invariable healing of small ulcers and necroses of the fingertip by simple hygienic care and minor debridement.

This doctrine of conservatism based upon simple wound care is useful and largely correct. Yet there are patients with multiple distal hand and finger arterial occlusions who do benefit from thoracic sympathectomy. Results include prevention of vasoconstriction due to cold and to stress, improved circulation of the skin of the fingers, and prompt healing of finger necroses before they progress to the need for amputation of a phalanx, which even Porter finds sometimes necessary.

Figure 21-5 illustrates multiple arterial blocks of ulnar and digital arteries and resultant ischemic necrosis of the tip of a ring finger. Prompt healing after thoracic sympathectomy in this patient has persisted for 15 years.

Another good result for an ischemic necrosis with severe pain in the fifth finger is shown in Figure 21-6.

Tissue loss with exposure of the bone of the distal phalanx (Figure 21-7) obviously requires terminal digital amputation.

Posttraumatic Pain Syndrome Occasionally an injury of an extremity, often minor but sometimes major, is followed by chronic pain and vasoconstriction manifested by coolness, sweating, and color changes. This failure of functional recovery may lead to severe disability. Confusion has arisen from the many terms used to describe variations of this symptom complex.

FIGURE 21-5 Multiple organic occlusions of the ulnar artery in the palm and of several digital arteries produced Raynaud's phenomenon with severe pain and ulceration of the tip of the ring finger, which responded to thoracic sympathectomy.

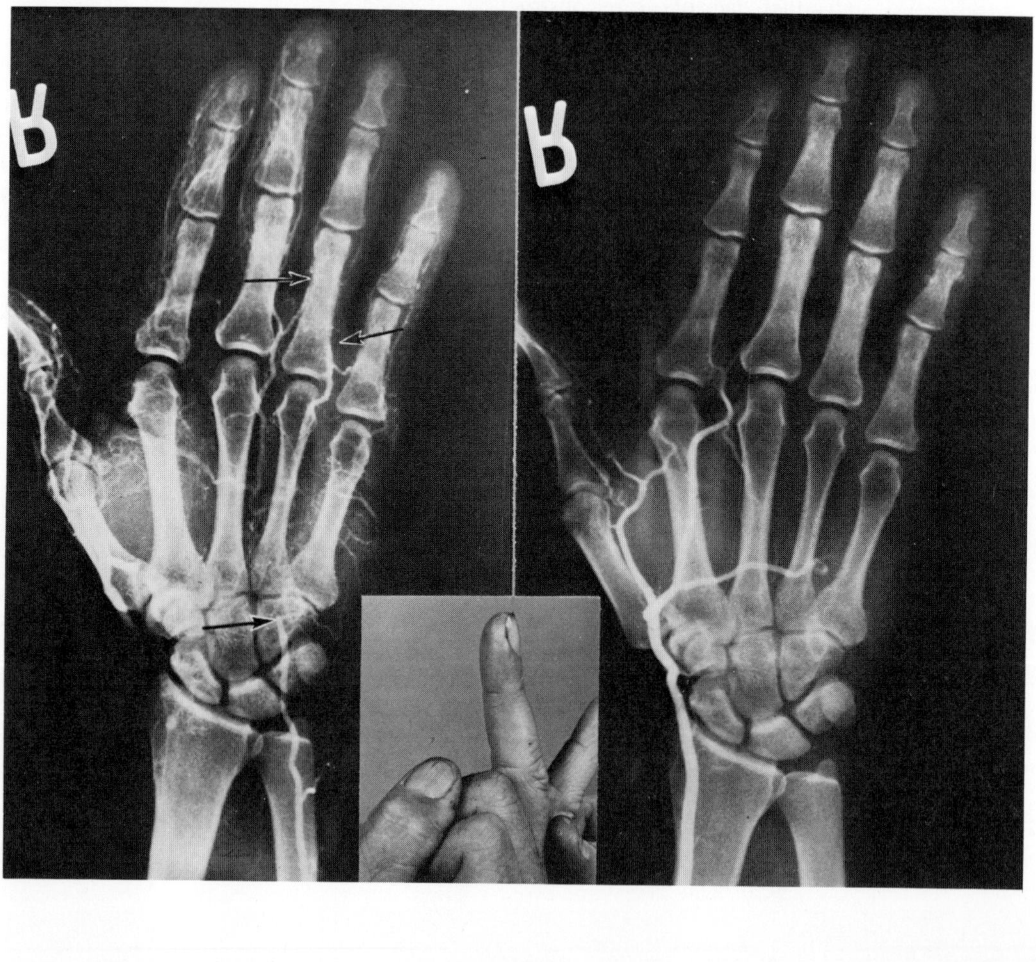

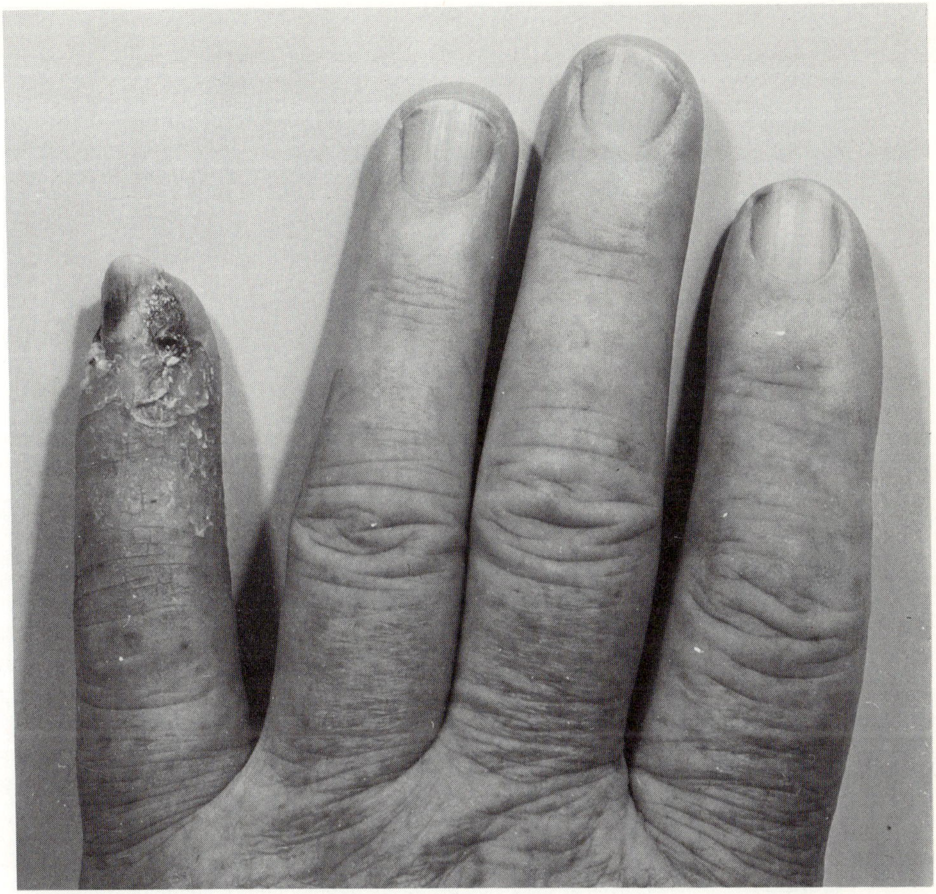

FIGURE 21-6 This painful, superficially ulcerated fifth finger responded to thoracic sympathectomy.

Patman listed over 30 of these and classified them as either causalgia or mimo-causalgia states, a differentiation which is often difficult.

A variety of nonsurgical treatments have in the past failed to relieve these causalgic states. During and following World War II, sympathectomy became popular, particularly when performed in the early posttraumatic period. It has since become commonplace for surgical texts to state that "sympathectomy can be counted on to relieve the pain of most patients with true causalgia,"[9] "a cure results after surgical sympathectomy," and "surgical sympathectomy may be curative."[10]

It is difficult to document the enthusiasm of surgeons who so strongly support sympathectomy for causalgic states. Welch and Geary recently discussed the results of transcervical sympathectomy for pain syndromes in 12 patients. They cited "a good response in four of five" with causalgia but warned of "a high degree of psychogenic and emotional dissatisfaction in four of six patients classed reflex sympathetic dystrophy."[11]

It is also difficult to understand how Thompson, Talkington, and Garrett have supported the operation so fully.[12] Their 1983 article recorded excellent results among 89 percent of 27 causalgic patients, yet at the same time they stated that 33 percent had residual symptoms. Also, among 120 patients classified as mimo-causalgia, 81 percent were said to have had an excellent result,

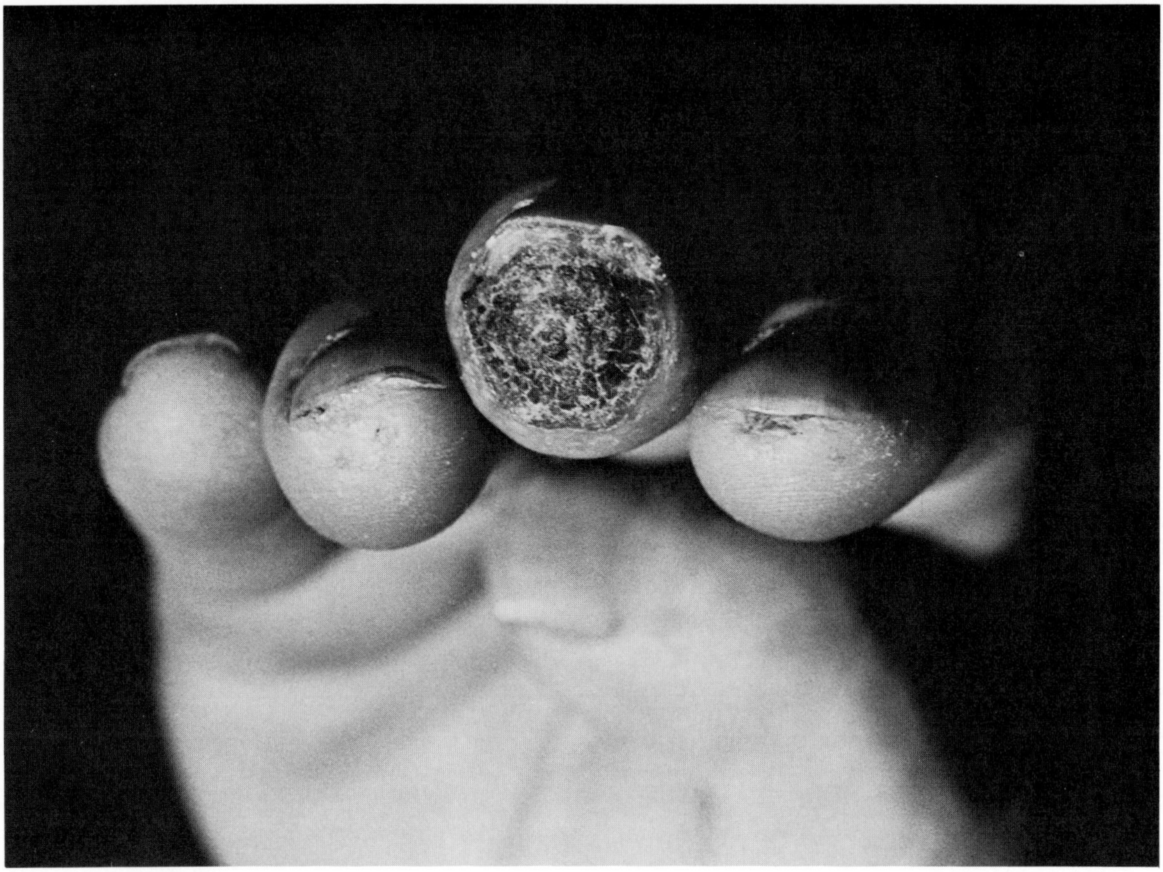

FIGURE 21-7 Distal vascular occulsion produced spontaneous amputation of the tip of the middle finger; it was treated by proximal amputation and closure.

yet 30 percent of these had residual symptoms. It is not clear how many of these latter had sympathectomies since it is uncertain how the clinicians differentiated causalgia and mimocausalgia.

My own experience with 18 such patients during the last 16 years is less optimistic than is generally reported and in fact is dismal. Among the 12 patients undergoing either thoracic or lumbar sympathectomy for reflex sympathetic dystrophy syndrome, there have been only 3 complete successes, while 9 (75 percent) must be classed as failures, since they continued to have more or less disabling symptoms. Whatever the cause may be, I no longer recommend sympathectomy to such patients except as an extreme last resort. However, if the procedure is to be done, it should not be delayed.

In summary, it appears that new, properly documented appraisal of sympathectomy for causalgic syndromes is badly needed.

Hyperhidrosis Occasionally there occurs unusual bodily sweating, particularly of the palms and/or soles, whose surfaces may literally drip sweat. The problem is severe for the unfortunate patient, especially since stress often accentuates the sweating.

Living in a cool climate may be helpful and should be suggested as a trial measure for such patients.

Since the pathogenesis of the hyperhidrosis is unknown, it is not surprising that pharmacologic control may be difficult, yet it should be tried fully prior to sympathectomy.

Sympathectomy will stop sweating from the denervated portion of the body but may shift it so that other areas produce more sweat. This hazard should be understood prior to the operation. Further, four-quadrant sympathectomy may interfere with heat control.

The excellent results reported by Stenberg and his colleagues from Tel Aviv were that 94 percent of their patients had completely dry hands. Of the 54 patients 86 percent were fully satisfied, and another 10 percent were partially satisfied, despite the compensatory sweating which occurred after 29 percent of the operations.[13] Bogokowsky and his associates in 1983 similarly reported good results among 42 patients treated by the supraclavicular removal of the T2 and T3 ganglia bilaterally at one operation. Their lower recurrence rate (7 percent), acceptable compensatory hyperhidosis in other areas (30 percent), and lack of Horner's syndrome suggest their mastery of this surgical technique.[14] These two large series from Israel outnumber other experiences to date.

Evaluation of the Modern Operation

The sympathetic innervation of the upper extremity originates in preganglionic nerve cells whose bodies lie in the corresponding lateral horns of the gray matter of the spinal cord. The dendrites pass out with the anterior nerve roots into the paravertebral sympathetic chain and synapse there with postganglionic neurons. Dendrites from the latter pass through the rami into the peripheral nerves of the brachial plexus and then down the arm to supply the skin and vessels of the head, neck, and upper extremity.

There has been continuing difficulty in defining the proper nervous elements for ablation to denervate completely the vessels of the fingers and hand. Not only are there anatomic varations, but also surgical failures have occurred because of inaccurate localization. While it was earlier believed that postganglionic sympathectomy caused hypersensitivity of the vessels to circulating epinephrine, it now appears that those poor results after upper-extremity denervations were the results of inadequate localization of the nerves or of incomplete operation.[15]

The preganglionic nerves enter the chain from the T1 through T10 segments of the cord, so the T1 through T5 resection should effectively sever the pathways. The occurrence of miosis, narrowing of the palpebral fissure, and enophthalmos (Horner's syndrome) if the sympathectomy disturbs the pupillociliary nerve pathway limits the superior extent of resection of the chain. Sympathectomy of T1 through T5 fulfills the criteria of denervation without a high incidence of Horner's syndrome and is the preferred ablation.

The deep anatomic position of the nerves serving the upper extremity has resulted in a succession of favored surgical approaches. The earlier use of the transcervical route did not allow sufficiently low resection of the ganglionated chain for complete denervation and produced Horner's syndrome frequently by damaging the sympathetic pathways to the eye.

Recently Welch and Geary reported their experience using the anterior route for 46 patients. "Only nine of 68 procedures (13 percent) were free of any untoward effects," including 67 percent resulting in permanent lid drop or Horner's syndrome and 26 percent resulting in permanent neuralgia. These problems reinforce my bias toward the transaxillary approach as less likely to produce such complications.[11]

A more limited sympathectomy via a posterior thoracic approach was next popularized. After resecting a portion of the posterior third rib, the operator could disconnect from the spinal cord a short length of the thoracic ganglionated chain (T2 and T3) by severing the rami and cutting the chain below T3. This resulted in a preganglionic form of sympathectomy, since the postganglionic fibers were left intact in the disconnected but nonresected trunk. This retropleural approach was somewhat complicated, did not allow wide denervation of the upper extremity, and soon began to be changed by several variations to a wider transpleural approach.

Louis T. Palumbo in 1957 asserted that, previous authorities notwithstanding, the usual description of the anatomic pathway of the pupillociliary mechanism was incorrect. He showed that it did not traverse the first ramus to the first thoracic ganglion but passed into the upper aspect of the stellate ganglion (Figure 21-8). This allowed resection of the distal portion of the stellate ganglion T1 without production of Horner's syndrome in most patients.[16] His and Lulu's experience was a significant contribution to proper denervation of the upper extremity.[17]

I have followed his technique in general but have now changed from the anterior approach to the axillary route (Figure 21-9). This transaxillary incision does not cut muscles, allows better direct vision of the nerve chain, and heals with less pain and a more acceptable scar.

Technique The patient is positioned laterally, and the arm is supported on the anesthesia screen. The table may later be rolled to either side to improve exposure. An incision 4 to 5 inches long is made in the axilla in the line of the third intercostal space and carried through the fat. The medial pectoralis major and the lateral latissimus dorsi muscles are mobilized underneath to allow placement of retractors. The third interspace is entered, and the intercostal incision is carried somewhat underneath the undermined pectoralis major and latissimus dorsi muscles to allow better spreading of the ribs by the thoracic retractor.

Exposure is obtained by slow opening of the self-retaining retractor. The apex of the lung is held inferiorly by a malleable retractor placed over a gauze pad. The ganglionated chain is seen as it lies on the rib ends adjacent to the transverse processes of the thoracic vertebrae. The pleura

FIGURE 21-8 Palumbo's scheme of the thoracic ganglia, as described in the text.[17]

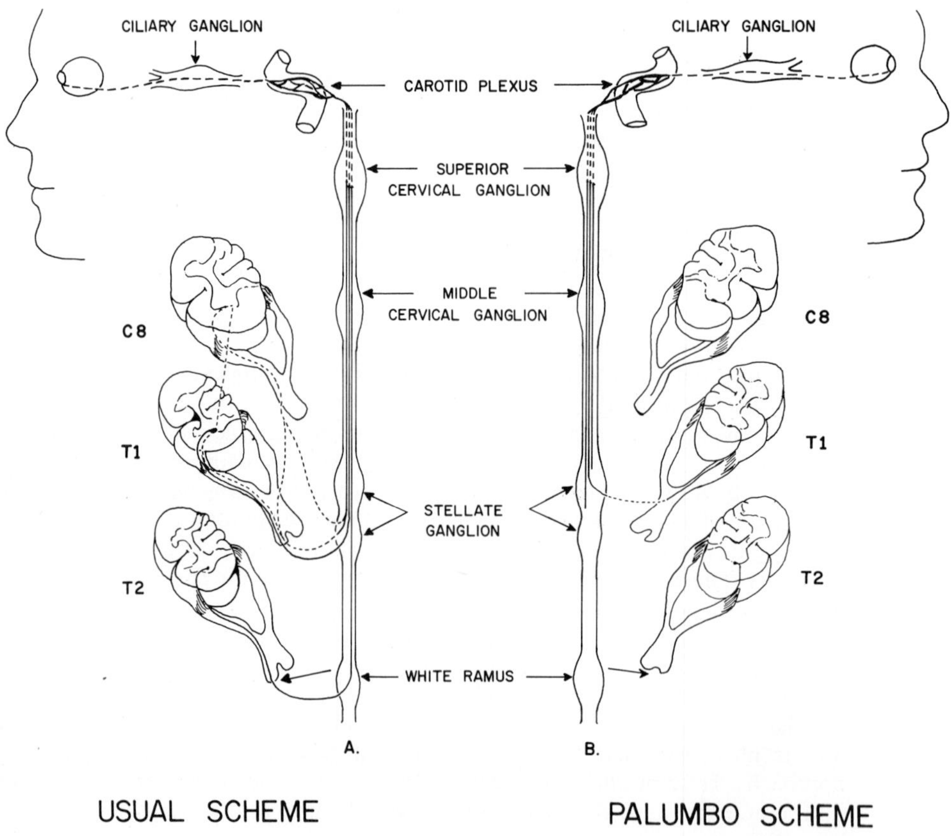

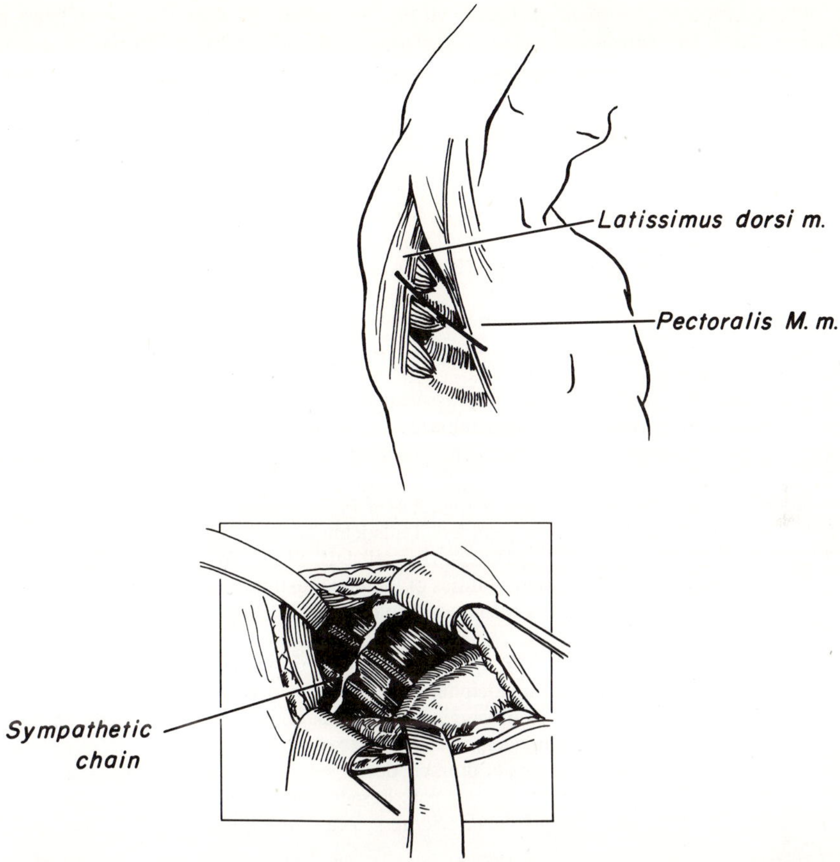

FIGURE 21-9 Transaxillary thoracic sympathectomy is begun by incision through the skin over the third interspace between the pectoralis major and latissimus dorsi muscles, undermining both these to allow extension of the intercostal incision. In the *box insert,* the retractor pressing the right upper lobe inferiorly allows visualization of the ganglionated chain lying beneath the pleura on the necks of the upper ribs.

is opened directly over the nerve chain to allow its dissection upward to the inferior border of the first rib, where a clip is placed transversely and the chain is cut across. The chain is then elevated with a clamp and similarly dissected down to the lower border of the fifth rib, where it is again clipped. No special attention need be made to clipping every attachment of the ganglionated chain, and the clips are primarily used for control of bleeding. The electrocautery also is useful for hemostasis. Particularly careful preservation of the azygos vein at the inferior aspect of the exposure (on the right) is in order.

If the apical pleural space is obliterated by adhesions, these may require lysis. In this event it may be difficult to visualize the chain through the scarred parietal pleura. The pleura should simply be opened at the approximate location, and a search should be made for the nerve trunk in the extrapleural tissue.

At conclusion the lung is reexpanded, the ribs are closed with no. 2 Dexon sutures placed pericostally, and the soft tissues are closed in layers.

While it may be unnecessary to provide tube drainage through a low lateral intercostal space, this has no particular disadvantage, and it offers protection against the accumulation of fluid and a warning of intrapleural bleeding, should that occur in the postoperative period.

The endoscopic thoracic sympathectomy described by Kux[18] has not been personally performed. That procedure denervated D1 through D6 and achieved 93 percent satisfaction in terms of relief of sweating. Compensatory sweating in 50 percent of the patients was not a major problem. No complications occurred. Malone, Duigan, and Hederman have more recently reported 54 such cases without complications.[19] The technique is indeed promising and indeed may replace open transthoracic techniques.

REFERENCES

1 Juergens JL, Spittell JA, Fairbairn JF (eds): *Allen-Barker-Hines Peripheral Vascular Disease.* 5th ed. Saunders, Philadelphia, 1980, p. 911.

2 Porter JM: Upper extremity ischemia: Role of the vascular surgeon in Raynaud's syndrome and finger gangrene, in Veith FJ (ed): *Critical Problems in Vascular Surgery.* Appleton-Century-Crofts, New York, 1982, chap 19.

3 Porter JM: Raynaud's syndrome and assoicated conditions of the extremities, in Rutherford RB (ed): *Vascular Surgery.* Saunders, Philadelphia, 1977, chap 69.

4 Birnstingl M: Results of sympathectomy in digital artery disease. *Br Med J* 1967, 2:601.

5 Rodeheffer RJ, Rommer JA, Wigley F, Smith CR: Controlled double-blind trial of nifedipine in the treatment of Raynaud's phenomenon. *N Engl J Med* 1983, 308:880.

6 de Takats G: *Vascular Surgery.* Saunders, Philadelphia, 1959.

7 Edwards WS: Discussion of Kirtley JA, Riddell DH, Stoney WS, Wright JK: Cervicothoracic sympathectomy in neurovascular abnormalities of the upper extremities. *Ann Surg* 1967, 165:878.

8 Birnstingl M: The Raynaud's syndrome and cold injury, in *Peripheral Vascular Surgery.* Lippincott, Philadelphia, 1973, chap 16.

9 Patman RD: Post-traumatic pain symdromes: Recognition and management, in Rutherford RB (ed): *Vascular Surgery.* Saunders, Philadelphia, 1977, chap 52, p 477.

10 Nashold BS, Friedman HR: Neurosurgical relief of pain, in Sabiston DC (ed): *Davis-Christopher Textbook of Surgery.* Saunders, Philadelphia, 1981, p 1510.

11 Welch E, Geary J: Current status of thoracic dorsal sympathectomy. *J Vasc Surg* 1984, 1:202.

12 Thompson JE, Talkington CM, Garrett WV: Post-traumatic pain syndromes: Causalgia, in Najarian JS, Delaney JP (eds): *Advances in Vascular Surgery.* Year Book Medical Publishers, Chicago, 1983, pp 255–262.

13 Sternberg A, Brickman S, Kott I, Reiss R: Transaxillary thoracic sympathectomy for primary hyperhidrosis of the upper limbs. *World J Surg* 1982, 6:458.

14 Bogokowsky H, Slutski S, Bacalu L, Abramsohn R, Negri M: Surgical treatment of primary hyperhidrosis: A report of 42 cases. *Arch Surg* 1983, 118:1065.

15 Dale WA, Lewis MR: Management of ischemia of the hand and fingers. 1970, 42:740.

16 Palumbo LT: A new concept of the sympathetic pathways to the eye. *Surgery* 1957, 42:740.

17 Palumbo LT, Lulu DJ: Transthoracic upper dorsal sympathectomy, *Surgery* 1963, 53:563.

18 Kux M: Thoracic endoscopic sympathectomy in palmar and axillary hyperhidrosis. *Arch Surg* 1978, 113:264.

19 Malone PS, Duignan JP, Hederman WP: Transthoracic electrocoagulation (TTEC)—a new and simple approach to upper limb sympathectomy. *Irish Med J* 1982, 75:20.

20 Wilgis EFS: Evaluation and treatment of chronic digital ischemia. *Ann Surg* 1981, 193:693.

The treatment of chronic ischemia of the fingers by *digital sympathectomy* is intentionally omitted, as it is outside of both the scope of this chapter and my experience.[20]

INVITED COMMENTARY

James S. T. Yao, M.D.
Chicago, Illinois

In the early development of vascular surgery, sympathectomy played an important role in the treatment of finger and hand ischemia.[1] Since the advent of vascular reconstructive surgery, however, sympathectomy has received less attention. For properly selected patients sympathectomy offers an alternative procedure for the relief of ischemia. Several points require clarification.

First, the widely available noninvasive tests, such as the recording of the systolic pressure of the finger, with or without cold stimulation, may help to detect organic arterial occlusion, thus separating Raynaud's phenomenon from Raynaud's disease instantly.[2–5] Measurement of pressure after local cooling gives further information regarding the severity of the disease, i.e., the temperature at which closure of the digital arteries occurs in these patients.[6] These tests may also provide an objective assessment of the result of various therapeutic measures, including sympathectomy.

In our institution, we use the Doppler technique to record finger systolic pressure and to assess the patency of the palmar arch. We add temperature response to local cooling, as suggested by Porter, [7] to evaluate the vasospastic reaction. If both tests are negative, this establishes the presence of normal vasculature in the upper extremity. In the presence of a normal Doppler examination and a positive cold response (prolonged temperature-recovery time), Raynaud's disease is suspected. In these patients, a workup for collagen disease is performed. If there is no evidence of collagen disease on the initial examination, the patient is observed for a 2-year period, with repeat testing as needed, prior to consideration of a final diagnosis of Raynaud's disease.

Second, we do not believe that brachial arteriography is a proper procedure in the evaluation of hand ischemia. Brachial arteriography is more hazardous than the Seldinger technique, and lesions proximal to the site of puncture will not be detected by this technique. Emboli to the hands from lesions in the subclavian or innominate artery, especially in thoracic outlet syndrome, are well known,[8,9] and such lesions will be missed if a brachial arteriogram is performed. We advocate retrograde femoral catheter arteriography for patients with hand ischemia, and the examination must include the subclavian artery and the entire hand. In selected instances, we have found that pharmacoangiography offers further information.

From the surgical point of view, the number of ganglia that need to be removed in order to achieve complete denervation is open to argument. Dr. Dale has suggested removal of T1 to T5, which includes part of the stellate ganglion. In order to avoid untoward effects, such as Horner's syndrome, a limited sympathectomy (T2 to T3) through an axillar approach, including the lower third of the stellate ganglion, may be sufficient to denervate the upper extremity. For palmar hyperhidrosis, interruption of the T2 to T3 ganglia is all that is needed to achieve denervation.

Finally, Dr. Dale has called attention to use of endoscopic thoracic sympathectomy. Recently, there has been a report on the use of radio-frequency percutaneous upper-thoracic sympathectomy using "C"-arm fluoroscopy for guidance of the electrode.[10] This technique may be performed on an outpatient basis, and perhaps is less costly than direct surgery. Further experience is needed to verify this new approach.

COMMENTARY REFERENCES

1 Gask GE, Ross JP: *The Surgery of the Sympathetic Nervous System.* William Ward, Baltimore, 1934.

2 Downs AR, Gaskell P, Morrow I, Munson CL: Assessment of arterial obstruction in vessels supplying the fingers by measurement of local blood pressures and the skin temperature response treat—correlation with angiographic evidence. *Surgery* 1975, 77:530–539.

3 Hirai M: Arterial insufficiency of the hand evaluated by digital blood pressure and arteriographic findings. *Circulation* 1978, 58:902–908.

4 Pearce WH, Ricco J-B, Yao JST: Upper extremity vascular diagnosis, in Zwiebel WJ (ed), *Introduction to Vascular Ultrasonography*. Grune & Stratton, New York, 1982, pp 215–227.

5 Lafferty K, de Trafford JC, Roberts VC, Cotton LT: Raynaud's phenomenon and thermal entrainment: An Objective Test. *Br Med J* 1983, 286:90–91.

6 Nielsen SL, Lassen NA: Measurement of digital blood pressure after local cooling. *J Appl Physiol* 1977, 43:907–910.

7 Porter JM: Raynaud's syndrome and associated vasospastic conditions of the extremities, in Rutherford RB (ed): *Vascular Surgery*. Saunders, Philadelphia, 1977, pp 597–604.

8 Hollier LH, Joyce JW, Oldenburg WA: Atheromatous embolization to the hand, in Bergan JJ, Yao JST (ed): *Evaluation and Treatment of Upper and Lower Extremity Circulatory Disorders*. Grune & Stratton, Orlando, Florida, 1984, pp 203–215.

9 Kieffer E: Arterial complications of thoracic outlet syndrome, in Bergen JJ, Yao JST (eds): *Evaluation and Treatment of Upper and Lower Extremity Circulatory Disorders*. Grune & Stratton, Orlando, Florida, 1984, pp 249–275.

10 Wilkinson HA: Radiofrequency percutaneous upper-thoracic sympathectomy: Technique and review of indications. *N Engl J Med* 1984, 311:34–36.

22 EXTRACRANIAL CEREBROVASCULAR DISEASE

Reconstructive operations upon the arteries which supply the brain not only are the most common of all vascular procedures but also, in some centers, outnumber hernia and gallbladder operations and approach the popularity of coronary artery bypasses. Indeed, the carotid operation has beeen irreverently termed by surgical residents "the hernia of vascular surgery"!

These procedures are all-or-none cases in the sense that most patients undergo a straightforward operation, recover promptly without complications, and are discharged within a few days. The low risk factor has even been used, although unjustifiably, as an indication for operation upon a minor asymptomatic lesion.

On the other hand, the patient who has an intraoperative thrombotic or embolic episode with a resultant neurologic deficit falls into a no-reward category with long-term disability, if not death—a tragic result for all concerned. Such patients, fortunately uncommon, nonetheless serve to warn the enthusiastic surgeon that tragedy may attend any patient who undergoes such a procedure. Fortunately, this risk is in the order of 2 or 3 percent, less in some hands.

HISTORICAL BACKGROUND

Eastcott, Pickering, and Rob in 1954 first reported reconstruction of the carotid artery by resection and anastomosis of an atherosclerotic carotid bifurcation using general anesthesia with hypothermia (Table 22-1).[1] Actually, similar procedures had been accomplished but not published in Buenos Aires[6] and in Houston[3] earlier (reminiscent of the controversy regarding the development of general anesthesia by Long and Morton 150 years ago). These reports triggered the explosive clinical development of extracranial cerebrovascular arterial surgery.

The three accompanying photographs (Figures 22-1 to 22-3) show my first carotid operation in 1956 using general anesthesia, hypothermia produced by brief immersion of the total body in a tub of ice, and further protection by an external shunt consisting of two no. 12 needles connected by tubing. A homologous arterial graft was used to replace the severely diseased carotid bifurcation. This physicist is still alive and well 29 years later.

STROKE STATISTICS

The physician, and especially the surgeon, bases his or her advice upon probabilities which are determined by clinical statistics. Many relating to strokes are published in journals not readily accessible to surgeons.[10] Some of the important figures are summarized in Table 22-2, but it must be remembered that statistics are always subject to interpretation and influenced by bias.*

*I received an early introduction to conflicting statistical data at the University of Rochester, where two different studies of breast malignancies were done at slightly different times. Neither group of authors were aware of the retrospective study being conducted by the other, with the result that different conclusions were made.

TABLE 22-1 IMPORTANT EVENTS LEADING TO CAROTID ARTERY RECONSTRUCTION

Year	Physician	Event
1856	Savory[2]	Autopsy association of stroke with carotid artery occlusion
1914	Hunt[3]	Clinical relation of carotid artery disease and stroke
1927	Moniz[4]	Angiography
1951	Fisher[5]	Suggested correction of segment carotid lesions causing cerebral symptoms
1951	Carrea team[6]	Carotid repair (not reported until 1955)
1953	DeBakey team[7]	Carotid repair (not reported until 1959)
1954	Eastcott, Pickering, Rob[1]	First published report of carotid artery reconstruction

FIGURE 22-1 Carotid repair in 1956 was conducted under general anesthesia with hypothermia. The brain was additionally protected by an external shunt, whose loop is shown in the *lower portion* of the photograph. Twelve-gauge needles were used for entry into the carotid artery. The clamp is shown underlying an intraluminal web.

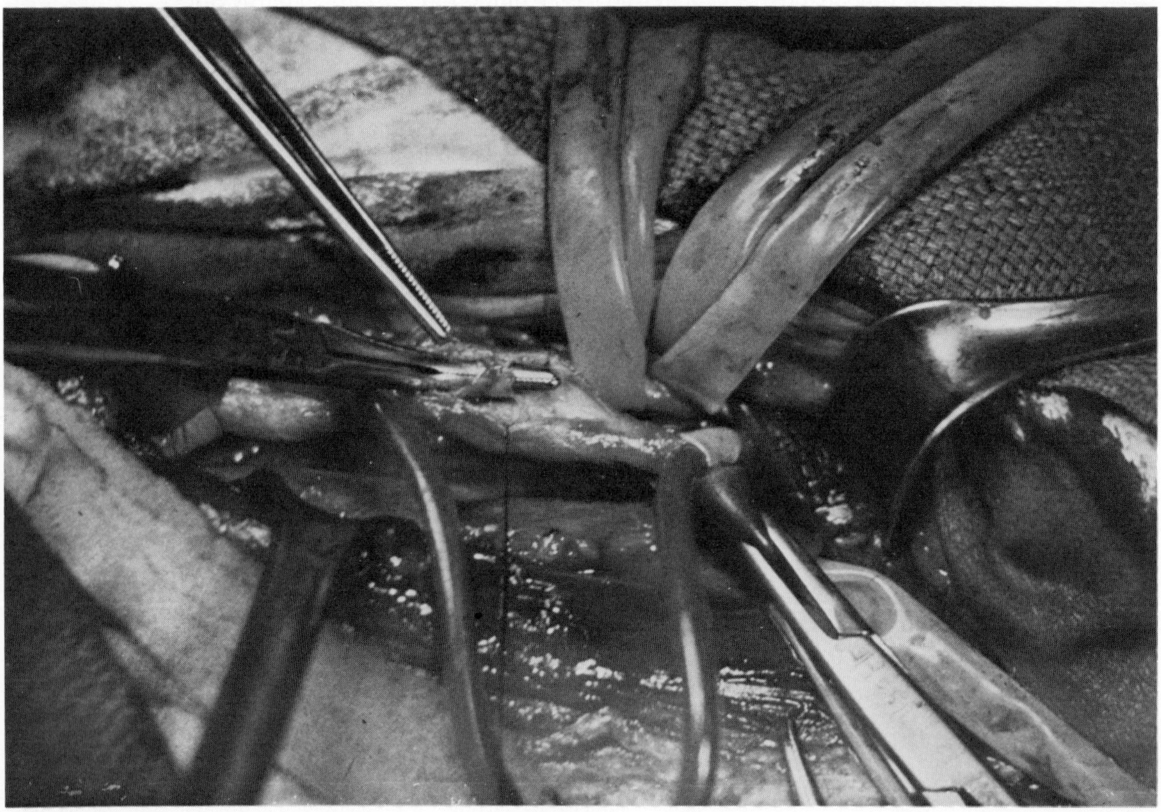

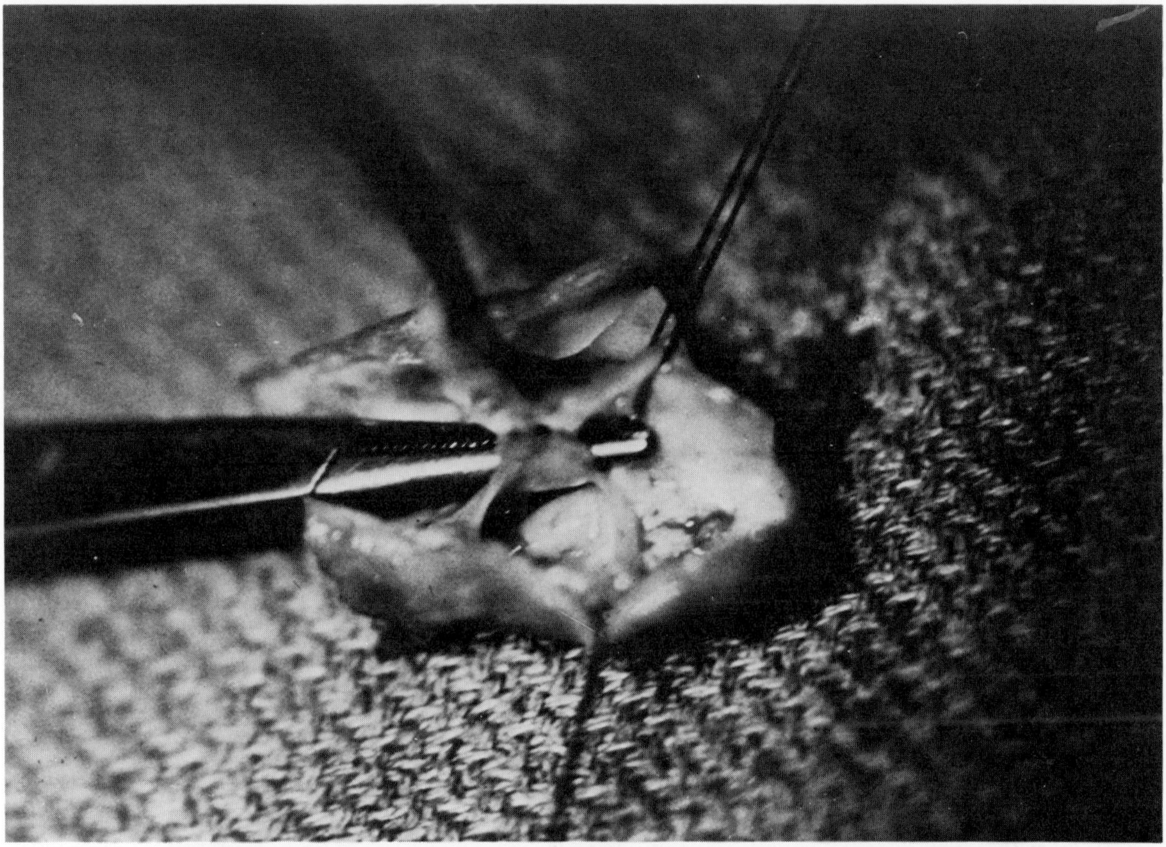

FIGURE 22-2 The deeply ulcerated internal carotid artery was resected and replaced by a homologous arterial graft.

DIAGNOSTIC STUDIES

Noninvasive Techniques

It is beyond the scope of this summary to discuss the controversies, the intricacies, and the techniques of the several methods of detecting abnormal flow in the arteries which supply the brain. Currently all these are screening and not critical diagnostic procedures.[14] Many have been oversold, not only to the public but also to physicians.

An accurate noninvasive test for the presence and extent of carotid disease is not yet available. As Ernst remarked editorially in 1983, "until studies are standardized and refined to be at least as accurate as arteriography, . . . results will be questioned." Arteriography remains the "gold standard" for carotid arterial diagnosis.[15]

Computerized Tomography (CT) Scan

The CT scan provides information about cerebral infarction as well as tumors, vascular malformations, and intracranial hematomas, any of which may mimic arteriosclerotic arterial lesions. The scan is not always necessary but in many instances provides additional information and is indicated on an individualized basis.

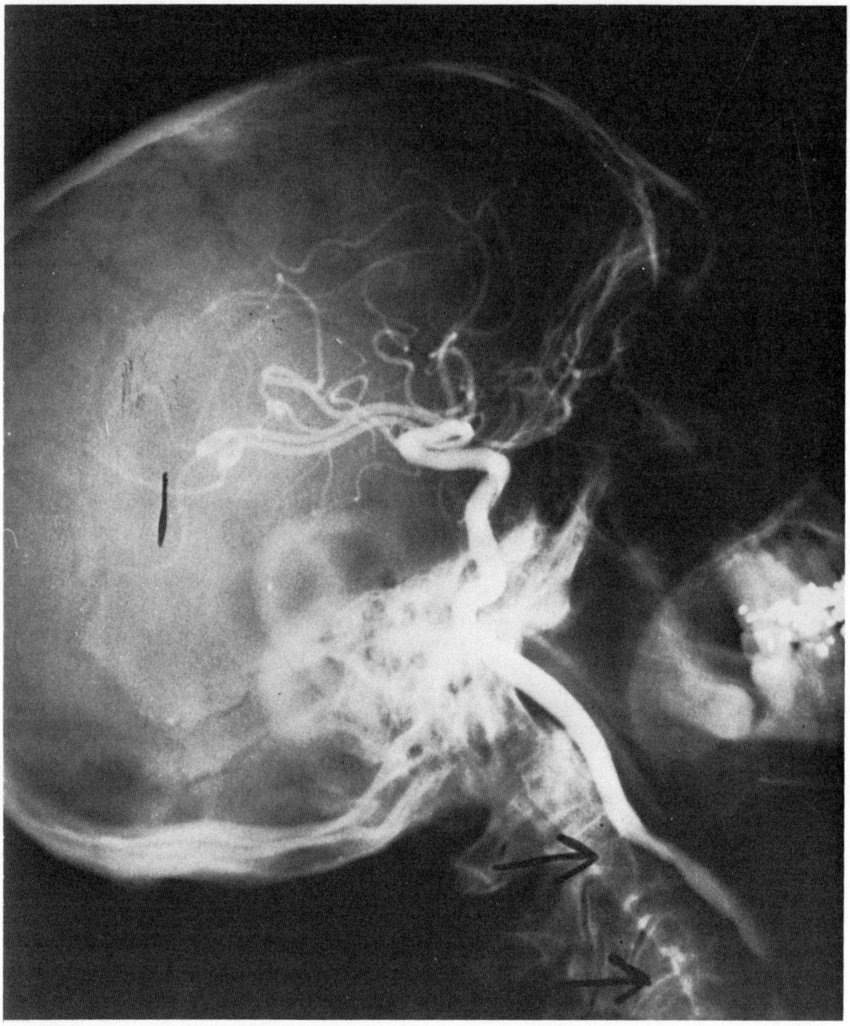

FIGURE 22-3 A postoperative arteriogram 6 months later showed patency of the grafted carotid artery, which has continued to date.

TABLE 22-2 SOME COLLECTED STROKE STATISTICS

There are 500,000 new strokes yearly in the United States. (40% die).[8]
There are 1 million stroke patients alive and disabled currently.[8]
The initial mortality from strokes is 20 to 30%.[9]
23% of TIA patients have strokes at 1 year, 37% at 3 years, and 45% at 5 years.[11]
10 to 15% of TIA patients eventually have strokes.[12]
12% of asymptomatic but hemodynamically positive patients had strokes within 2 years.[13]
33% of neck bruits are significant.[19]
There were 0.6 to 1.8% operative deaths, 0.7 to 2% permanent deficits, and 0.9 to 5.1% neurologic complaints in 8 series since 1979.[66]

Patients with a completed stroke and a fixed neurologic deficit should have a CT scan to demonstrate the infarct. If this is normal, a contrast-enhanced scan may locate an infarct in some of the patients, such as the 18 percent of "normal" CT scans in the experience of the Rosenthal group. A radionuclide scan is another alternative for patients who still have no demonstrable abnormality, to show whether the blood-brain barrier is intact and, if so, to suggest angiography at once.[16]

Angiography

Angiography may be conducted by any of several techniques. Whatever method is chosen should include adequate visualization of the aortic arch and its branches of the extracranial vessels. The major intracranial branches also require visualization at the same time. A good argument can be made for *arch aortography* through an indwelling catheter along with selected injections into the common carotid arteries as individually indicated. This has replaced direct arterial needle puncture ("four-vessel") techniques for most people. The *digital intravenous subtraction angiography* technique currently emerging will in some instances provide visualization adequate to allow operative planning. Presently it serves chiefly as a scouting or screening technique, and usually further angiographic study is required prior to an operative procedure. Whether it or noninvasive studies can replace conventional angiography in many patients remains to be seen.[17,18]

CLINICAL SYNDROMES AND THEIR MANAGEMENT

A brief focal episode of neurologic dysfunction that resolves within 24 hours is a *transient ischemic attack* (TIA). Repetition is characteristic. Whether TIAs are usually due to embolism or to flow variations through a stenotic artery is not certain, although embolization is increasingly indicted. A *completed stroke* consists of a fixed, nonprogressive neurologic deficit which lasts longer than 24 hours and is due to cerebral infarction. A third syndrome is the *reversible ischemic neurologic deficit* (RIND), which lasts longer than 24 hours but resolves completely within several weeks. It is believed to result from sustained ischemia not severe enough to produce an infarct.

Bruits

A *bruit** denotes turbulence in arterial flow as the sound of rapids denotes turbulence in a creek. If the artery is completely obstructed, there is no noise. Since tight stenosis may not and complete occlusion does not cause a bruit, and an ulcerated lesion may be silent, it is clear that significant lesions do occur in the absence of bruits.

It must at once also be recalled that not all noises in the neck originate in the carotid arteries. Reflection of cardiac murmurs often occurs, and there are other causes. Thus, Kartchner and McRae's analysis of 1287 cervical bruits indicated that less than one-third were hemodynamically significant. These noises are not clear-cut indications for an operation, but they do require evaluation.[19]

Carotid bruits also require evaluation. If neurologic findings are present, there is no need to waste time and money on noninvasive studies; angiography is needed. If there are no symptoms, the situation may be evaluated by noninvasive methods, reserving angiography for those who have a hemodynamic abnormality.

*We speak of the English *murmur* of the heart, while the French *bruit* occurs in the neck.

Asymptomatic Stenoses

The question of whether or not an asymptomatic stenosis should be operated upon seems settled in the minds of many vascular surgeons, yet this view is not completely certain, has many exceptions, and still provokes controversy among internists and neurologists as well as surgeons. Let us examine the evidence on both sides of this undetermined question.

Jesse Thompson has over the years advocated an aggressive operative approach for these carotid lesions. His group compared the results of nonoperative therapy with operation in selected groups of patients (Table 22-3), concluding that their surgical patients fared better over a period of years than did those managed nonoperatively. It is difficult to know whether the two groups were comparable—the series was retrospective. The mortality of both was nil. The later fatal stroke rate was the same.[20] The natural history of the small group of untreated patients was different from those in other reports. Kartchner also has supported prophylactic operations by citing a 12 percent stroke rate among 371 patients without antecedent symptoms who were serially evaluated by noninvasive studies.[19]

Advocates of prophylactic repair of asymptomatic stenoses sometimes cite the low risk (in the hands of an expert) as an indication. The Imparato no-death, no-deficit series[21] supported Thompson's zero mortality among 167 procedures for asymptomatic lesions.[22] Naturally, low risk is commendable but hardly an indication for an operation. However, a host of other vascular surgeons, the majority of our colleagues, today follow this aggressive advice for operation, generally with good results.

The fewer advocates of observation rather than immediate operation do present a rational argument. Humphries and the Cleveland Clinic group in 1976 discussed whether asymptomatic carotid stenosis greater than 50 percent required operation. Among 182 carotid arteries of 168 patients there was only 1 who went directly from a symptom-free state to a completed stroke. Most (81 percent) remained symptom-free up to 12 years, while 16 percent developed transient ischemic attacks which led to carotid endarterectomy. This analysis suggested observation of asymptomatic stenosis until TIAs developed.[23] Levin and Sondheimer operated upon one side and observed the other side on 60 patients with bilateral carotid artery lesions, finding similar evidence for a nonoperative approach until TIAs developed.[24]

Barnes's group in 1981 reviewed the situation and followed 44 patients with asymptomatic stenoses, concluding that since no one had "clearly documented the incidence of stroke without antecedent TIA," prophylactic carotid endarterectomy was not indicated and observation until TIAs occur was the better course.[25]

Mohr editorially commented that the risk of stroke without a warning TIA was so low that surgical management did not surpass nonsurgical treatment.[26] A year later, in 1983, he again

TABLE 22-3 RETROSPECTIVE COMPARISON OF ENDARTERECTOMY PATIENTS WITH THOSE WITHOUT OPERATIONS BY THOMPSON, PATMAN, AND TALKINGTON

	No operation	**Endarterectomy**
No. of patients	138	132
Time of follow-up	6 to 184 months (mean 55)	to 180 months (mean 45)
Operative deaths	0	0
Later strokes		
Fatal	2.2%	2.3%
Nonfatal	15.2%	2.3%
Later TIAs	26.8%	4.5%

Source: Thompson JE, Patman RD, Talkington CM: Asymptomatic carotid bruit: Long-term outcome of patients having endarterectomy compared with unoperated controls. *Ann Surg* 1978, 188:308.

reviewed the published evidence and concluded that "the risk of stroke without prior TIA is low enough that the best surgical statistics do not prove superior to medical management." The trend toward surgery was noted, however, along with another call for a prospective randomized study, even though the number needed for a correct statistical evaluation was estimated at 4000.[27]

The asymptomatic carotid bruit does mark the patient as being in an early stage in the clinical evolution of cerebrovascular disease. If a significant lesion is demonstrated by noninvasive techniques, angiography is performed. This often leads on to endarterectomy for those with significant stenoses or plaques. Stenoses of 50 percent require consideration. Those over 80 percent are considered to be serious, since that is the point where the stenosis-flow curve begins to diminish sharply (Figure 22-4).

Today's conventional wisdom teaches that stenoses of consequence include bilaterally tight ones, those with contralateral complete carotid occlusion, those in the artery supplying the dominant hemisphere, and those associated with present or past atherosclerotic lesions elsewhere. If an ulcerated plaque is associated, the stenosis is usually of less importance than the rough area likely to release emboli. These indications are so broad that the vascular surgeon easily finds an indication to perform a carotid operation when there is a noise in the neck!

Carotid endarterectomies are presently being done too often; critical prospective studies have

FIGURE 22-4 Tight stenosis of the internal carotid artery caused considerable reduction in pressure and a resultant gradient, which was corrected by endarterectomy with patch grafting.

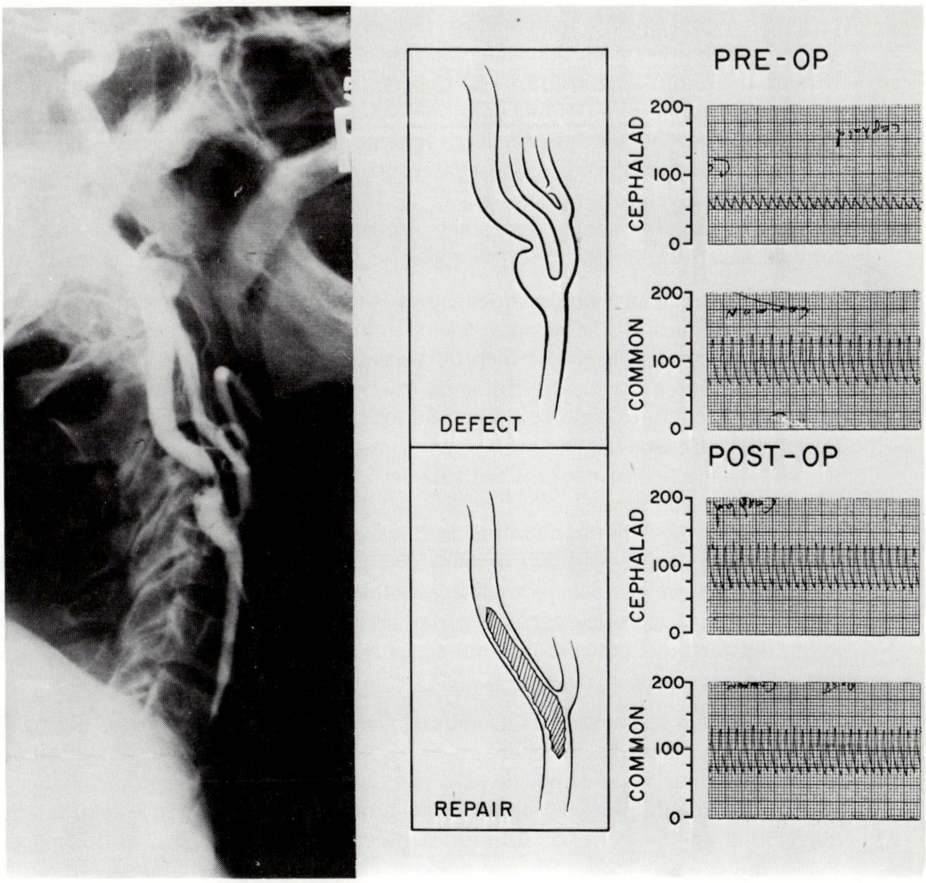

not yet determined the true risks of operative versus nonoperative treatment during a prolonged period of time. Medicare, yearly case load requirements, and the relatively low risk factor presently combine to produce an excessive number of carotid procedures to correct radiologic lesions.

Illustrative Case An 81-year-old male had two episodes of vertigo 3 years apart which responded well to meclizine hydrochloride (Antivert). Another bout led to a noninvasive study, which suggested carotid stenosis and led on to the arteriogram shown in Figure 22-5. There was a long stenosis of about 50 percent in the internal carotid artery, along with at least one and perhaps two ulcers.

The patient was discharged on antiplatelet medication.

Comment The angiogram along with a brief history was submitted to five nationally recognized vascular surgical authorities by letter. Two advised operation, two advised antiplatelet therapy, and one did not respond.

The patient has had no further difficulty so far (19 months later).

It does appear that the correct management of patients with asymptomatic stenoses is not yet certain. Fields's summary of the available facts in 1983 led to his conclusion that "the natural history of asymptomatic carotid stenosis is unknown," so a satisfactory answer awaits a well-conducted prospective randomized study.[28] To me it seems inappropriate to advise an operation which is expensive and has at least some danger, when its merits are unproven.

How Threatening Is a Tight Asymptomatic Stenosis? Occasionally a thin thread of radiopaque material shows a tight stenosis (90 percent or greater) of the internal carotid artery. The general wisdom has been that this is so threatening that an immediate operation must be done because there is a "significant risk of undergoing thrombosis within the next 12 hours following study."[9] Documentation of this opinion is uncertain. Perhaps if acute thrombosis occurs, it will cause a stroke. On the other hand, such complete occlusion merely reduces the blood flow another fraction, so it may not be significant. The Turnipseed, Vasko, and Lubow series had 10 patients in that category who progressed to complete occlusion after ateriography "asymptomatically and were discovered incidentally at operation."[29] The need for an emergency endarterectomy is unproven. An early elective repair seems more reasonable (Figure 22-6).

Management of Asymptomatic Stenoses Prior to Other Major Surgery For some time it was believed that carotid stenoses posed such a threat of stroke that they should be corrected prior to major elective surgery elsewhere.[20] It has gradually become recognized that this is more a bogey man than a real threat. Ropper's 1982 prospective study of 735 patients having elective surgery showed an overall incidence of stroke of 0.7 percent. There was no difference between those with bruits (0.9 percent of 104) and those without (0.6 percent of 631).[30] Many series have shown that the risk of stroke is not sufficient to indicate a carotid operation prior to whatever other procedure is needed.[13,25,31,32]

Completely asymptomatic bruits need not delay or contraindicate needed surgery. Noninvasive study is in order, with angiography reserved for a few. This may be delayed until after the needed procedure has been completed, so that angiography is performed in the postoperative period. Tight stenosis or a deep ulcer may require thought regarding a preliminary carotid operation, but for most patients it is not sensible to say "we must first perform a major vascular operation in your neck and later correct the problem that is troubling you."

Management of Combined Carotid and Coronary Arterial Stenoses Recognition of the sizable incidence of cardiac disease as a major risk among candidates for carotid endarterectomy (49 percent[33] and 50 percent[34] in two series) has raised the question of whether coronary revascularization should precede, follow, or be done concomitantly. Jones in 1983 discussed indications based upon experience at Emory University and the reports of others, concluding that a staged strategy was proper for symptomatic carotid disease combined with a stable cardiac sit-

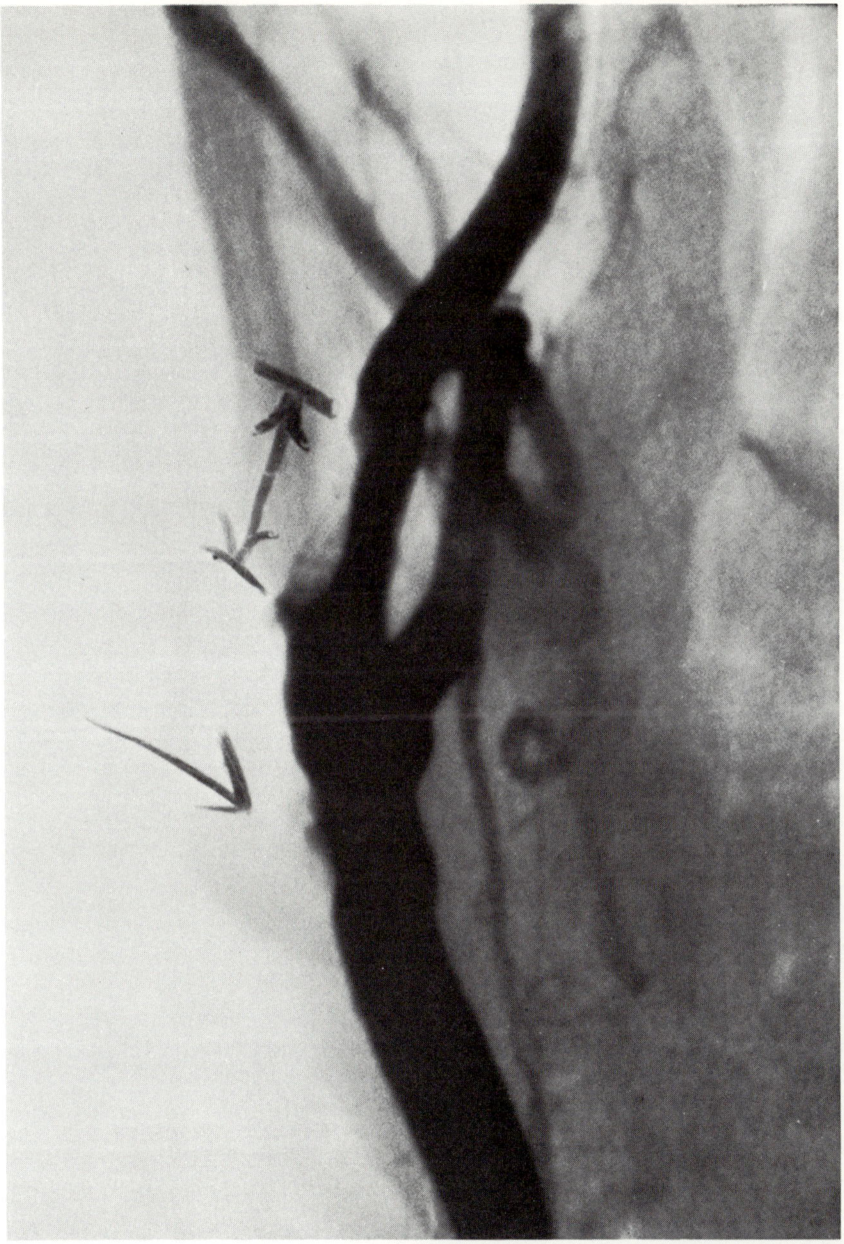

FIGURE 22–5 A long 50 percent stenosis *(brackets)* was associated with the appearance of ulcerated plaques in this 81-year-old male. He was discharged on antiplatelet therapy.

uation and that combined operations should be reserved for those with notable cardiac disease or left main coronary arterial obstruction.[14]

Other statistics were reported the same year. One group in Boston had a 5 percent death rate but no neurologic defects among 41 patients undergoing simultaneous carotid and coronary operations.[35] On the other hand, another Boston team preferred carotid endarterectomy with

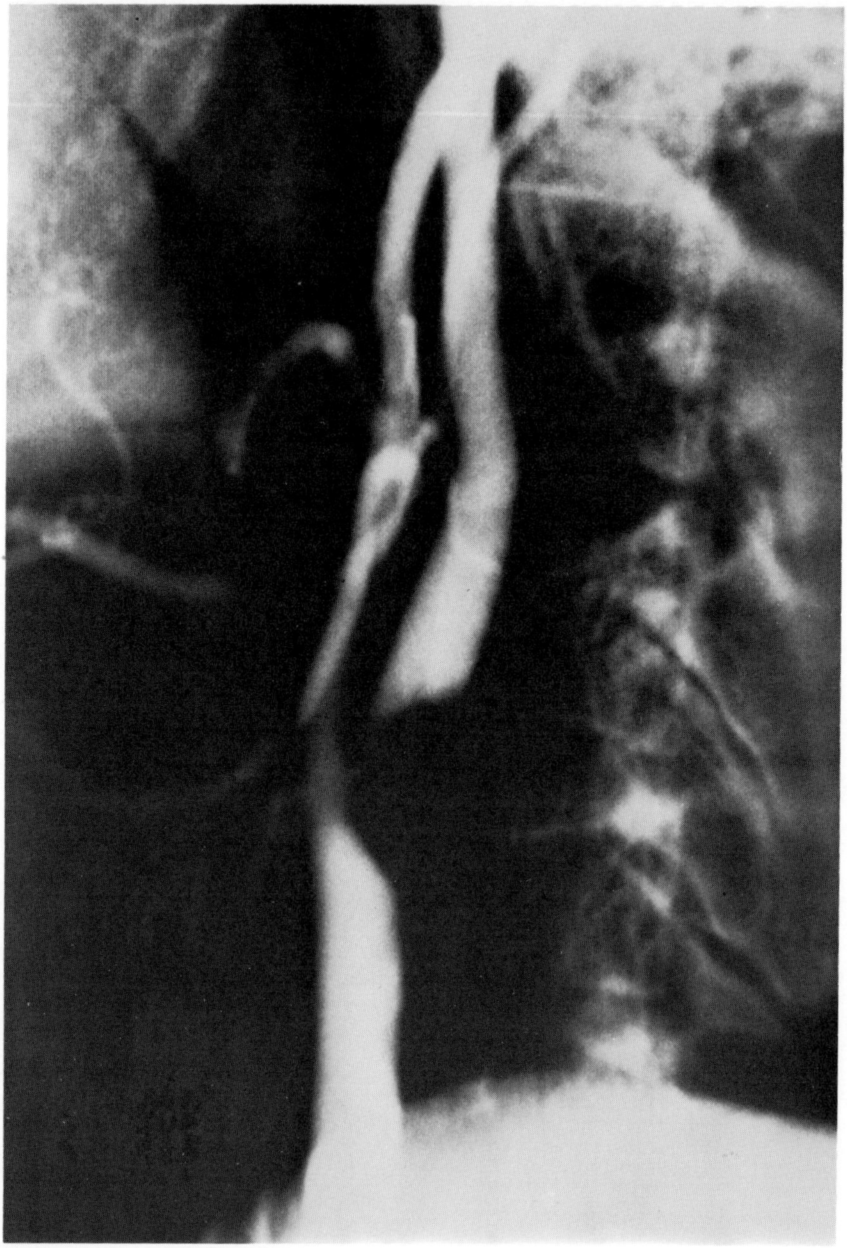

FIGURE 22-6 Tight stenosis was essentially complete and required early elective endarterectomy.

careful nonoperative cardiac management, citing 0.9 percent mortality among 364 patients.[36] Another 22 patients, who had concomitant procedures, had a 4.5 percent death rate. Thus the combined risks of the procedures are similar for both groups, but the low carotid risk of the latter series suggests the strategy of initial carotid operation, since the combined procedures are more dangerous.

Plaques and Ulcerations Long recognized as potential sources of TIAs, plaques and ulcerations are more dangerous than are stenoses alone. Successful management of TIAs by anticoagulant drugs suggests cessation of embolism. Surgically removed atheromas which are "clean" are often associated with a lack of recent symptoms, while those with continuing symptoms often harbor lesions covered with platelets and fibrin (Figure 22-7).[37] Particulate matter has been observed in the retinal arteries during transient monocular blindness.[38] However, whether such emboli arise from the carotid artery or are released from the heart or aorta is not clear.

Imparato's concept that a carotid plaque due to hemodynamic trauma develops hemorrhage with attendant conversion to ulceration covered by atherosclerotic debris and elements of blood clot[39] seems to explain the various pathologic lesions which are discovered in the carotid arterial system. Lusby and his California associates found recent hemorrhage in plaques in 93 percent of symptomatic patients but in only 27 percent of nonsymptomatic ones. They were able to simulate the local lesions in canine models.[40]

Further clinical analysis of ulcerative lesions by Dixon and associates at the University of California at Los Angeles correlated the angiographic appearance of ulcers in 153 asymptomatic patients with the likelihood of a stroke without an antecedent TIA. Some 3 percent with small type A, 21 percent with large type B, and 19 percent with compound type C ulcers developed such strokes, so they recommended carotid endarterectomy for large ulcerated lesions whether or not symptoms had occurred.[41]

FIGURE 22-7 Fresh thrombus covers a deep ulceration in this specimen of an atherosclerotic material removed from the internal carotid artery.

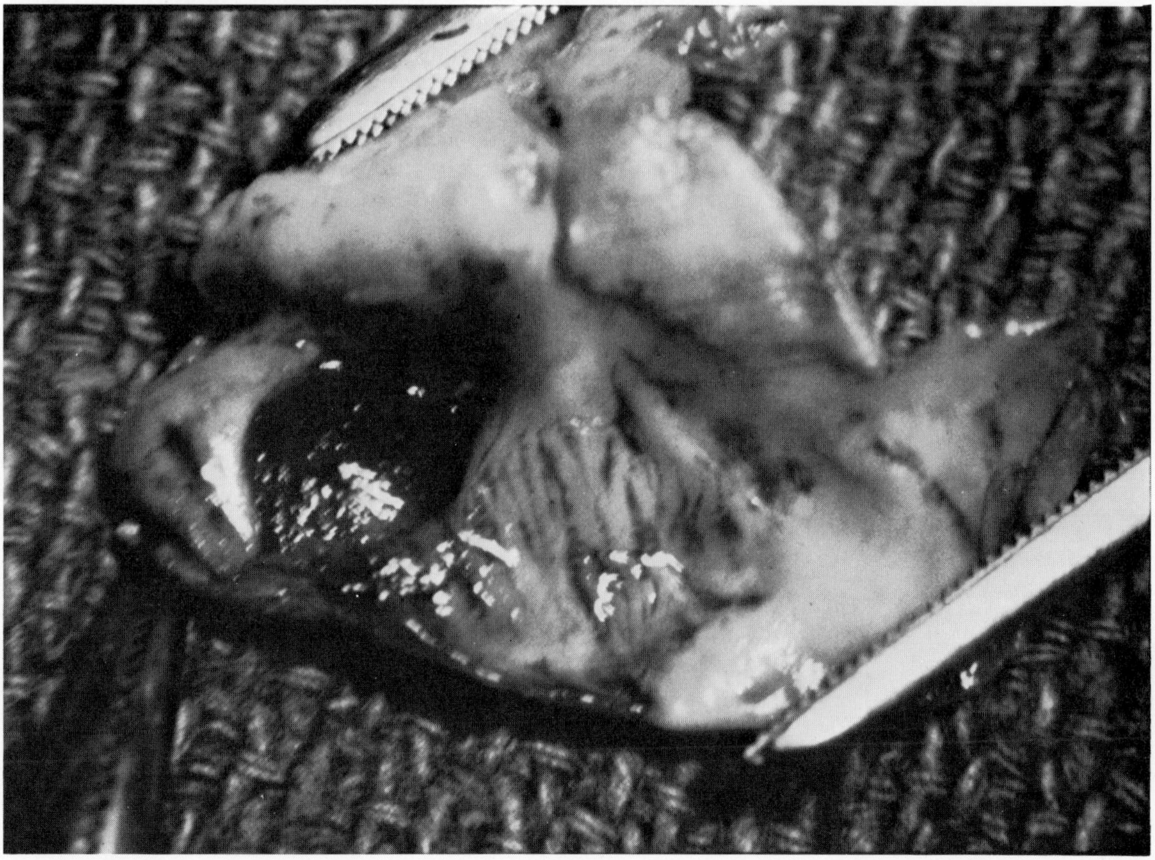

The threat of ulcerated plaques is serious, more so than stenosis alone, and suggests early surgical intervention.

Common Carotid Artery Occlusion Approximately 2 percent of patients evaluated for asymptomatic carotid artery disease have occlusion of a common carotid artery. Some are symptomatic to the extent that revascularization is needed. This has been generally deemed impossible.

In 1984 Riles, Imparato, Posner, and Eikelboom reviewed 24 such patients, and preoperative visualization by conventional angiography was obtained in only 4. It was possible, however, to reconstruct 15 of the 24 by either thromboendarterectomy or venous bypass from the subclavian to the external or internal carotid artery. More recently their experience with rapid sequential media-enhanced computerized tomographic scanning indicated that the internal carotid patency could sometimes be determined by that method.[42] A single personal experience with this technique demonstrated a false positive. The scan indicated internal carotid artery patency, while surgical exploration showed complete absence of the lumen. Further evaluation of this extended diagnostic technique is needed.

Complete Chronic Occlusion of the Internal Carotid Artery The clinical presentations of patients with complete occlusion of the internal carotid artery vary from those of asymptomatic patients whose chronic lesions are discovered incidentally (Figure 22-8) to those of patients with crescendo TIAs to those of patients with mild or severe fixed neurologic deficits.

The diagnostic problem is difficult, since the conventional radiographic technique usually does not penetrate the collateral arteries enough to opacify the upper reaches of the internal carotid artery. If careful evaluation of the intracranial cross-circulation demonstrates retrograde filling of the cavernous and petrous portions of the internal carotid artery, it may be possible to clean it by removal of soft clot with a Fogarty catheter.

Poor results in attempts to reopen chronically completely blocked internal carotid arteries have led to pessimism, since the success rate has been too low to justify the operation. Fields has termed it "an exercise in futility."[43] Thompson and Talkington's large experience led them also to advise a nonsurgical strategy for asymptomatic patients and a cautious approach to others.[44]

On the other hand, certain patients may be benefited. Kish and associates reported two such and recommended an attempt if the cavernous portion of the carotid was visualized arteriographically in a patient with symptoms referable to that side.[45] More recently Welling's group in Cincinnati performed early operation upon 24 complete occlusions, with 15 (63 percent) early successes. Indications included 3 strokes in evolution, 4 crescendo TIAs, and 8 fixed neurologic deficits. Since the neurologic deficit patients did not benefit despite technical success, the actual clinical success rate was 29 percent.[46]

An operative decision should be based upon the clinical situation as well as the angiographic findings.[29] There is certainly no reason to explore a totally occluded internal carotid artery in an aysmptomatic patient. Others with profound fixed deficits also fall into the nonoperative category, thereby leaving patients with TIAs and those with minor deficits as possible candidates for a procedure whose results are uncertain.

It should be recalled that patients who survive complete occlusion of the carotid artery have less risk of dying from another stroke than from heart disease. In the series collected by Hafner the subsequent stroke rate varied between 6 percent and 23 percent, while the cardiac risk was greater.[47]

Acute Thrombosis of the Internal Carotid Artery

Acute thrombosis is a different problem, particularly when it occurs in the hospital or postoperatively. Immediate operation offers hope of recovery for some of these patients, while delay for diagnostic or other procedures increases the failure rate for thrombectomy. Kwaan, Connolly,

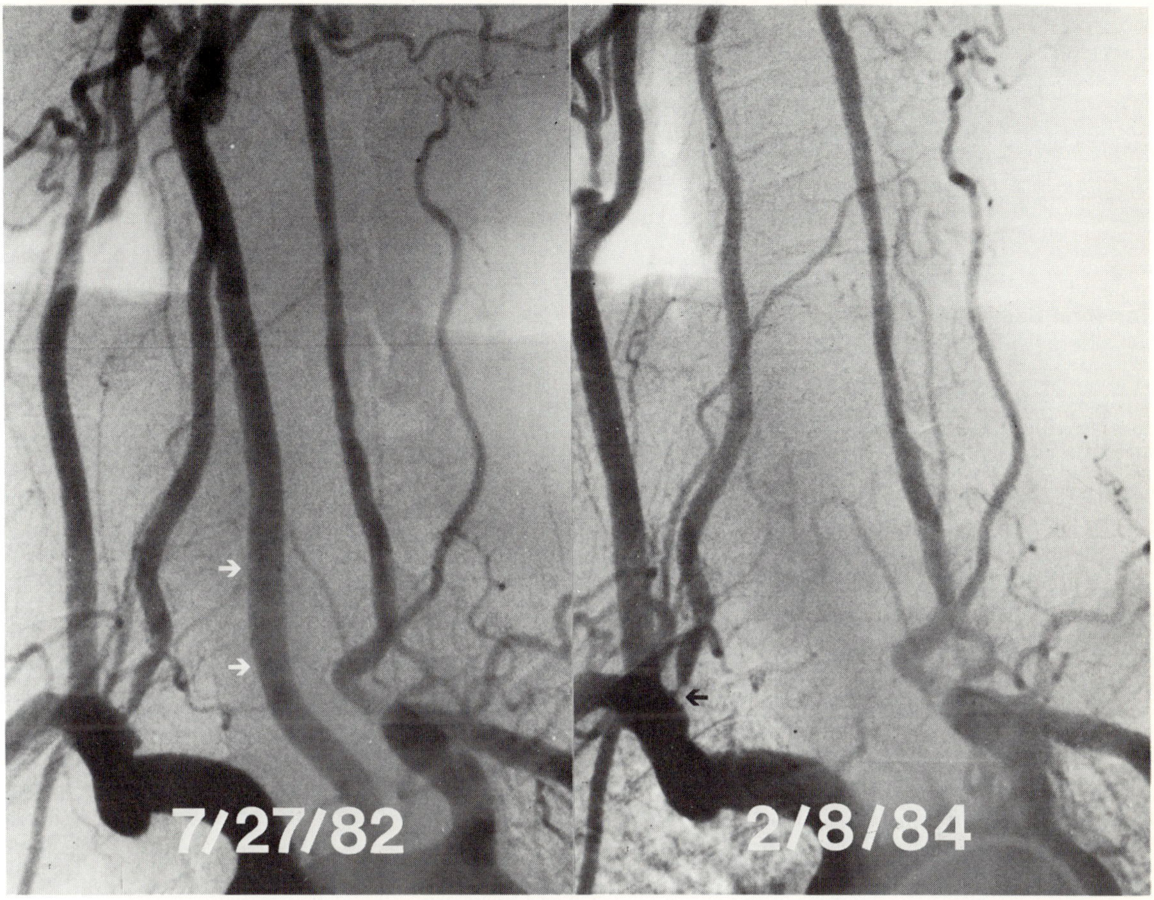

FIGURE 22-8 In July 1982 the left carotid artery acutely thrombosed in the immediate postoperative period after endarterectomy. Its early correction returned complete function. The *left* arteriogram, made just prior to discharge, showed the widely patent left carotid artery. Nineteen months later the *right* arteriogram showed complete absence of the left carotid arterial system, although the patient had no symptoms. Some progression of stenosis *(black arrow)* had occurred at the origin of the right vertebral artery. The patient has remained completely asymptomatic since then.

and Sharefkin documented the benefits of an immediate operation,[48] and Donaldson and Drezner recently reemphasized this with three recoveries among six such patients.[49]

The duration of thrombosis is often unclear, but revascularization results depend upon the time interval, so if an operation is to be done, it should not be delayed. In the 47-patient series of Hafner and Tew there was 100 percent postoperative patency among the 12 patients whose internal carotid arteries were revascularized within 7 days after thrombosis began, whereas the patency rate fell to 61 percent for surgery between 15 and 30 days after thrombosis and to 50 percent after a month.[47]

Prevention of Recurrent Stroke

The role of carotid surgery for the patient with a previous stroke and residual deficit is not clear. The analysis by Bardin and associates of the reports of others and of their own experience with 127 patients showed a higher risk of death and permanent neurologic deficits following operations in stroke patients than in patients without previous strokes. When the stroke rate after carotid surgery was compared with the estimated yearly stroke rate of 6 to 12 percent among patients not having operations, Bardin's group found "no significant improvement . . . by carotid surgery."[50] Thompson disagreed, on the basis of a different estimate of strokes among patients not having operations in his own practice.[51] Again, these reported series support the authors' biases and are not controlled prospective series. The indication for surgery is not clear. Common sense suggests caution in advising a prophylactic procedure upon a patient who has already had a stroke and is disabled. It resembles a revascularization operation on the side of a previous above-knee amputation.

Vertebral-Basilar Syndrome

The manifestations of ischemia in the vertebral-basilar arterial system are more difficult to recognize, including one or another of the following: vertigo, ataxia, limb weakness, general or local paresthesia, perioral paresthesia, visual disturbances, and palsy of cranial nerves.

The indications for surgical correction have similarly been vague. Fields has stated that "an isolated stenosis at the origin of one vertebral artery is virtually never an indication for operation," unless there is a problem with the contralateral vertebral artery (such as hypoplasia or vertebral arthritis impinging on it). It is usually better to improve the circulation through the circle of Willis by carotid arterial reconstruction.[43] Stanley Crawford agreed that "most patients who have vertebral-basilar symptoms have both vertebral and carotid artery . . . [lesions, which] are relieved by simple carotid artery operation."[52]

The occasional patient with bilateral vertebral stenoses or vertebral stenosis with contralateral vertebral absence or hypoplasia may need surgical relief. Another indication is persistence of symptoms after successful carotid endarterectomy (Figures 22-9 and 22-10). If operation is necessary, it can be done with little risk, as shown by the large series of Edwards and Mulherin.[53] Berguer and Feldman had no deaths and 84 percent relief of symptoms in their 34-patient series.[54] Ouriel and his Rochester associates in 1984 reported 107 cases with nonhemispheric symptoms, concluding that carotid operation was useful for many patients with vertebral lesions although the results were far from perfect 2 years later.[55]

Malone and associates have suggested that vertebral arterial transplantation to the carotid artery may be done at the time of carotid endarterectomy through an incision lengthened somewhat inferiorly.[56] This combined approach is useful on occasion.

Cerebral Cognitive Function

Whether carotid endarterectomy improves cognition and personality, as indicated by Doyle Haynes's study,[57] has not been absolutely confirmed, although it is obviously a desirable and hoped-for end result.

The National Cooperative Study of Extracranial Cerebral Vascular Disease raised considerable question about such conclusions regarding cerebral function.[58] Javid's group reported improved memory and learning in 31 patients studied before and 3 months after operation.[59] Jacobs's team found improvement in 12 patients with low-flow–endangered brains when compared with a control group.[60]

The verdict is not clear, but the optimistic attitude of both the patient and family after surviving a therapy perceived by them as dangerous and dramatic must be recognized.

Bilateral Operations

Correcting both sides at the same operation[61] is contraindicated because of the complications which may result from one side, not to mention both. The second procedure should be staged to

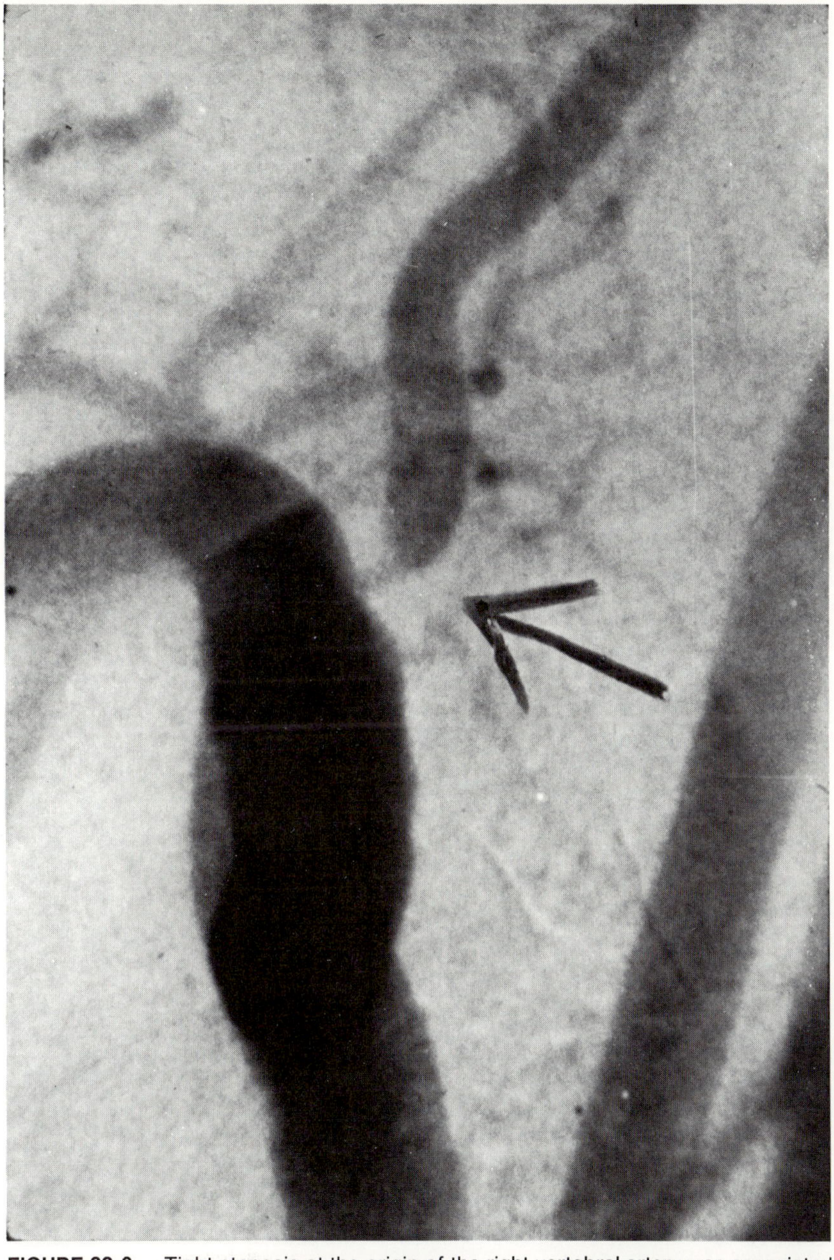

FIGURE 22-9 Tight stenosis at the origin of the right vertebral artery was associated with vertigo and ataxia.

occur 5, 7, or more days later. It is probably better to discharge the patient promptly (at 3 to 4 days) and allow stabilization prior to operating upon the contralateral artery 14 to 21 days later.

The delay allows examination of the various cranial nerves during the interim. Laryngoscopy to ascertain vocal cord function should be done to find vocal cord abnormalities which may be

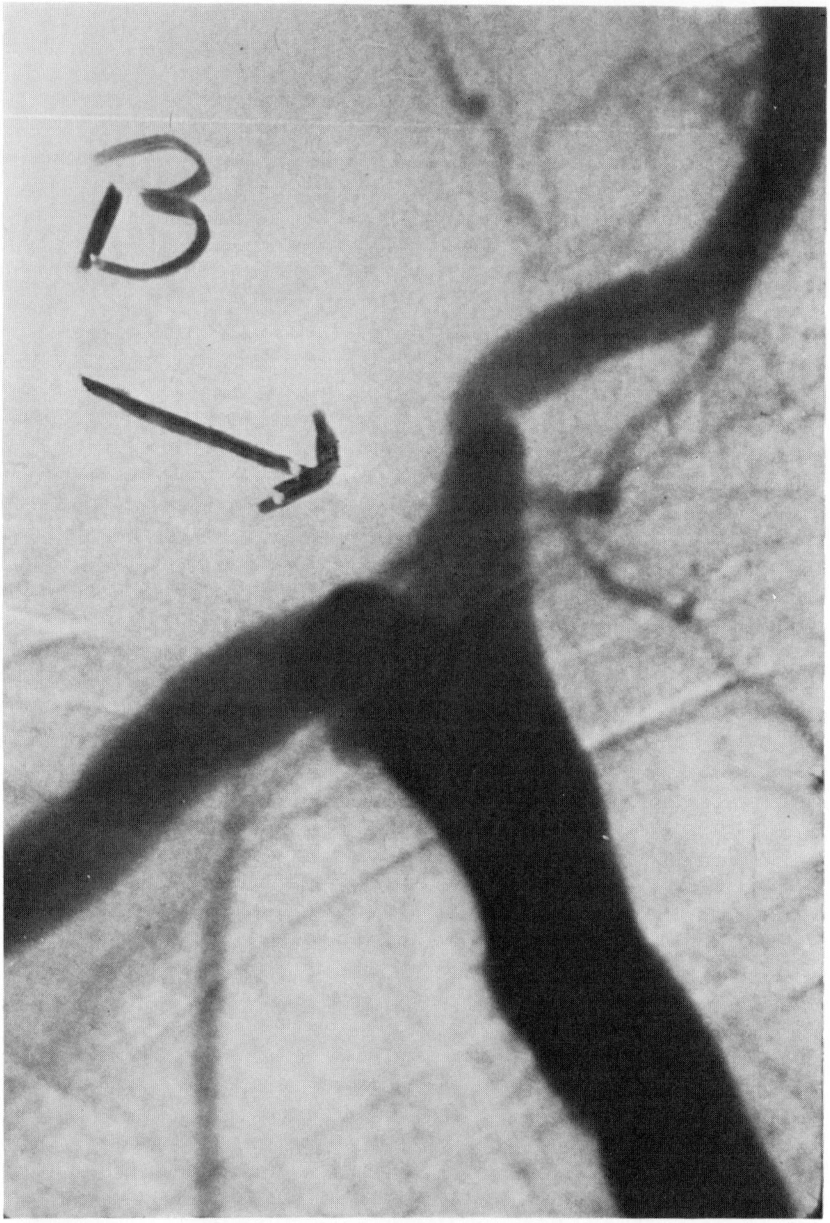

FIGURE 22-10 The postoperative arteriogram shows patency following venous patch grafting.

unrecognized clinically or which may be due to postanesthesia edema. Any form of nerve damage at once suggests further delay or even abandonment of the second side.

Fibromuscular Dysplasia

A nonatherosclerotic lesion of unknown cause, well-known in the renal arteries, fibromuscular dysplasia also occurs occasionally in the carotid artery as well as in peripheral arteries of large or medium size. The large series reported by Wylie's group in 1979 had 96 percent females among 68 patients with symptoms. Most were treated by dilation to 4 mm through a carotid arteriotomy. A few had an additional endarterectomy at the bifurcation. There were no deaths and only two transient neurologic deficits. A single arterial perforation occurred.[62] The experience of others[63] has been similar.

It is remarkable that no operation for this has yet been performed in our hospital, where a volume of carotid endarterectomies are done yearly (667 in 1983). Inquiry among colleagues indicates that their experience is similar to mine in that occasional instances of fibromuscular dysplasia of the carotid arteries have been seen but to date none have been judged to require operation.

Illustrative Case C.H., a 57-year-old female, had a history of weakness and stumbling. Noninvasive study suggested significant stenosis of the carotid arteries bilaterally. Angiography showed bilateral fibromuscular dysplasia of both internal carotid arteries (Figure 22-11). There were no neurologic signs. A Holter cardiac monitor over a 24-hour period showed several episodes of second-degree heart block (Figure 22-12). A cardiac pacemaker was implanted and gave relief.

Comment The carotid artery fibromuscular lesions were coincidental to the cardiac arrhyth-

FIGURE 22-11 Bilateral fibromuscular dysplasia of the carotid arteries was associated with recurrent brief episodes of unconsciousness.

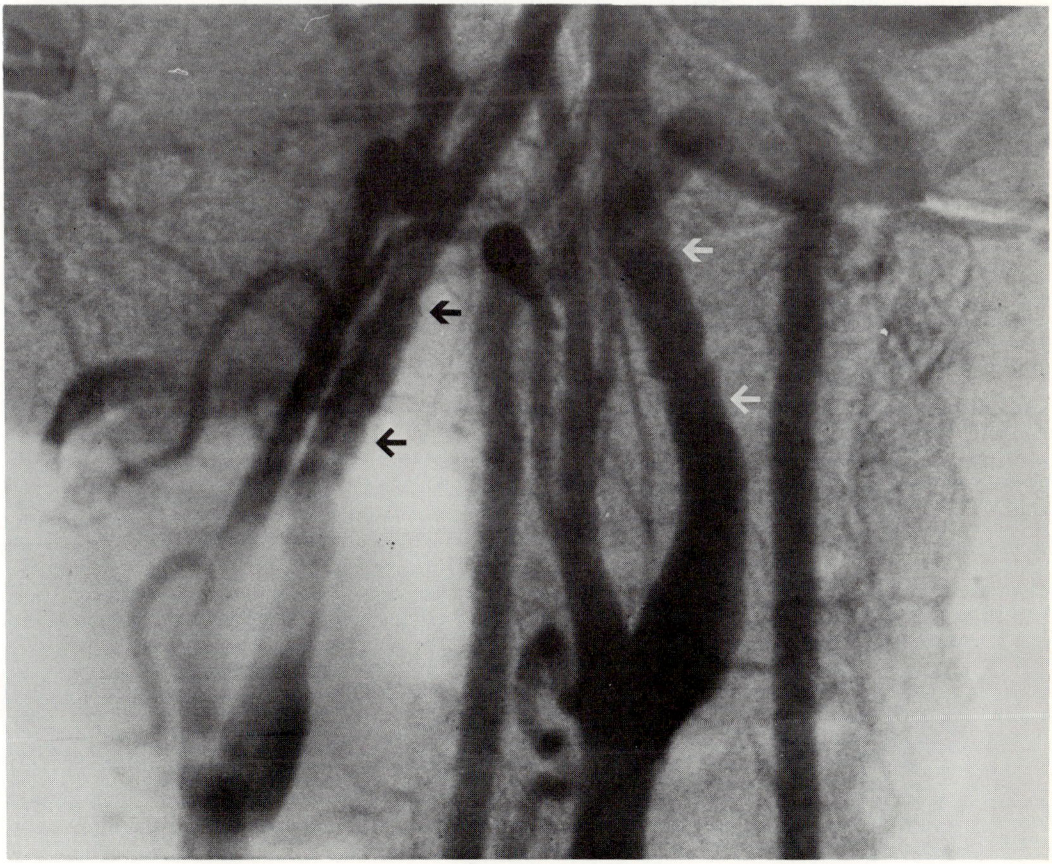

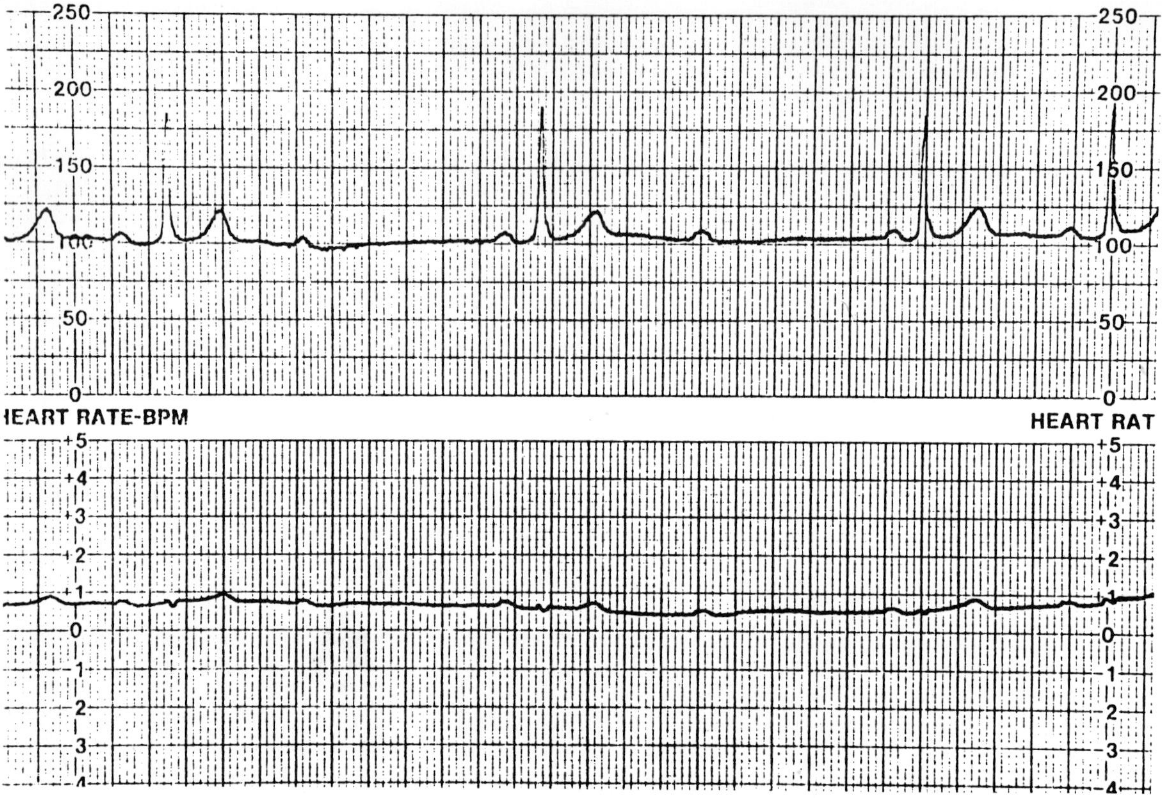

FIGURE 22-12 Electrocardiographic study with a Holter monitor showed the recurrent atrioventricular block, which was the cause of the recurrent episodes of unconsciousness. A permanent pacemaker was placed.

mia. There was no indication for surgical intervention in this unusual situation. There is no implication that these two lesions are commonly associated.

SUMMARY OF CLINICAL INDICATIONS

It is patently impossible to list absolute indications for carotid repairs. The following modification of the suggestions of W. S. Fields in 1979 seems reasonable.[43] The knowledgeable reader will recognize a few digressions and reversals of his opinions, based on later data and upon personal views. It should also be recognized, as Fields himself knew, that specific cases may be cited to refute any of these principles:

1 Complete carotid occlusion with severe neurologic deficit contraindicates operation, whose risk is large.

2 A stable deficit will not be altered by an operation, which is preventive and not therapeutic.

3 TIAs without deficit provide the best indication for operation if the stenosis is over 50 percent on the appropriate side or if there is an ulcerated plaque.

4 Bilateral stenosis with TIAs should have operation on the side appropriate to the symptoms. Time should pass before the other side is repaired, since that may not be needed.

5 Bilateral stenoses with nonlateralized symptoms should first have operation upon the worse stenosis.

6 Symptomatic unilateral occlusion and contralateral stenosis require operation only upon the stenosis.

7 With tandem lesions operative benefit may occur if the more severe lesion is in the extracranial but not in the endocranial portion of the artery.

8 Ulcerated carotid lesions are indications for surgery.

9 An asymptomatic stenosis is not an absolute indication but may be considered for endarterectomy if the surgical team has low morbidity and mortality rates.

ANESTHESIA

The local anesthesia used in the past to allow intraoperative monitoring of the state of consciousness when the carotid artery was clamped has with a few exceptions been replaced by general anesthesia, which usually offers better oxygenation through an endotracheal tube without the depressant drugs often necessary to control a patient struggling with pain in an uncomfortable position under local anesthesia.

There do remain a few staunch advocates of local anesthesia, including Imparato[39] and Connolly.[64] Peitzman and associates reported 13 percent nonneurologic complications with use of general anesthesia versus 3 percent with regional anesthesia.[65] Hafner in 1984 had only 1 death (0.2 percent) among 481 local anesthesia procedures, while there were 4 (5 percent) among 89 using general anesthesia.[66] Whether these statistics indict all general anesthesias or only those of the authors is unclear.

Certainly if local anesthesia is to be used, the surgeon must be an absolute expert and be supported by an anesthesiologist skilled in managing sedatives as well as agents for blood pressure control. At the same time an adequate source of oxygen must be provided into the nasopharynx. Most surgeons believe that the difficulties of using local anesthesia, along with emotional stress to both the patient and the surgical team, outweigh the possible advantages and that careful general anesthesia with tracheal intubation is the procedure of choice. It is not likely that local anesthesia has much future usefulness.

SHUNTS

Surgeons have always feared that even brief interruption of blood flow to the brain by occlusion of the carotid artery would cause an ischemic stroke. Past results of unilateral ligation of the common carotid artery for trauma and tumors have justified that fear. Thus some method of protection of the brain during carotid repair was considered even for the early cases in the 1950s.

The question of shunting during occlusion continues today without a generally accepted answer. Vascular surgeons have divided into three camps, namely, (1) those who always use a shunt, (2) those who never use a shunt, and (3) those who selectively use a shunt, based on one or another parameter. All groups currently present considerable documentation for their position. Let us first examine the concept of routine shunting.

Routine Shunting

There are several arguments for placement of an indwelling shunt in every patient. First is the development of experience so that the entire team is quite familiar with the procedure, thus avoiding the clumsy technique which may result if it is used only occasionally. Second, there is some advantage to having a shunt in place during closure of the internal carotid arteriotomy, to guarantee a widely patent lumen. Third is avoidance of the time and equipment needed to monitor pressure or brain waves, so the entire procedure is more efficient. Fourth, if residents are involved, they will be getting important experience using shunts. Finally, there is the knowledge that the well-perfused brain will tolerate careful removal of all shreds and fragments from the internal surface of the artery, as well as accurate placement of a suture line to prevent rolling up of a superior intimal flap in cases where complete "feathering" does not occur. With shunt protection the entire procedure may be done with care and delicacy.

The members of our vascular service all have concluded that routine shunting is advantageous and use it with rare exceptions. Technical difficulties are few. The tube can be moved about so that it does not interfere with the clean-out or the closure. Thrombosis is not a problem. Embolization is avoided by thoroughly flushing the vessel before placing the shunt and by flushing the shunt before placing the superior end. Placement and removal times are usually less than 2 minutes and always less than 3 minutes. Preference for any one of the several available shunts varies with the individual surgeon.

Selective Shunting

Some surgeons rely upon one or another indirect measurement which is believed to reflect dangerously low perfusion of the brain during clamping. The simplest and the oldest method is to clamp the carotid artery and observe the state of consciousness for several minutes with the patient under local anesthesia. On this basis the surgeon decides whether to proceed without a shunt or whether it is necessary to place one. This method of gross observation is not available to surgeons who use general anesthesia.

A 3- or even 5-minute period of carotid cross-clamping does not always show which patient will tolerate a longer period. Bland, Chapman, and Wylie reported that 11 patients who tolerated a brief test did develop a neurologic deficit after the operation.[67] Competent surgeons such as John Connolly, however, still believe that the "assessment of consciousness and motor ability are the only absolute guides to shunting."[64]

There next developed the measurement of internal carotid artery pressure as an indication of the need to shunt. The arterial pressure is measured before and after temporary occlusion of the common and external carotids so that it reflects the back pressure within the internal carotid artery. Various levels have been recommended as acceptable. Moore uses 25 mmHg as the critical level and also arbitrarily shunts anyone who has had a previous cerebral infarction on the side of operation.[68] Connolly, on the other hand, found pressure measurements to be unreliable. He based his decision upon the finding that 25 percent of 101 patients tolerated cross-clamping and subsequent shuntless endarterectomy despite stump pressures below 50 mmHg and 32 percent of those who lost consciousness had stump pressures over 50 mmHg.[64]

Electroencephalographic criteria indicating the need for shunting include flattening of waves or slowing during trial clamping of the artery.[69,70] Callow's experience with 274 carotid operations convinced him of the superiority of the electroencephalogram (EEG) over measurement of stump pressure to indicate selective shunting.[71] The Ricotta, Charlton, and DeWeese series of 100 patients without death or neurologic deficit also argues that the EEG selects those who need shunts (15 percent).[72] Rosenthal, Stanton, Zeichner, and Lamis warn of the importance of shunting all patients who have had previous strokes or reversible ischemic neurologic deficits lasting several days, since stump pressures and EEG monitoring may be unreliable in them.[73]

No Shunt

The nonshunter carries the considerable burden of providing low-risk performance without intraoperative neurologic complications or deaths. There are some such series, a fact which continues to trouble the routine shunters and the selectivists. Certainly, the operation is simpler and quicker without shunting. A controlled prospective study has not yet been done on this problem.

The Cleveland group who earlier did not shunt[74] had a "highly significant improvement in the incidence of postoperative stroke" after their policy was shifted to shunting.[75]

In 1980 Whitney and associates, on the basis of 1081 standard carotid endarterectomies and a review summarizing 12 other series done without shunts, presented a strong argument for shuntless operations.[76] Comparison of their figures with those of Thompson (using a shunt routinely) showed a mortality rate only 0.4 percent higher, a permanent stroke rate 0.65 percent higher, and a temporary stroke rate 0.44 percent higher, which they believed were not statistically significant numbers. The ensuing discussion only served to reinforce the previous arguments of shunter Thompson[77] and nonshunters Baker[78] and Harrison.[79]

Another low-risk series without shunts was reported by Cooley's group, who had a 0.6 percent mortality rate and a 1.3 percent permanent neurologic deficit rate, suggesting to them that emboli rather than cerebral ischemia caused the problem.[80] Rosenthal and associates' series also suggested that embolism or technical error rather than inadequate flow to the brain was the cause of neurologic deficits. Their results with shunts (1.6 percent with deficits among 318) and without (2.2 percent with deficits among 274) are quite similar.[73]

Baker, Dorner, and Barnes's 304 unshunted patients had 8 (2.7 percent) patients who awoke with a neurologic deficit. Later 8 more developed such, so the final figure was 3 percent with temporary and 1.6 percent with permanent neurologic lesions, along with 0.6 percent mortality.[81] Baker and associates in 1984 updated their no-shunt series to include 940 endarterectomies with 0.6 percent mortality, 2.6 percent permanent stroke, and 2.2 percent temporary neurologic symptom rates. Since those with a contralateral carotid occlusion plus a low stump pressure had an 11 percent incidence of neurologic deficit, they suggested that these should be shunted.[82] It would be simple to shunt all those with contralateral occlusion or tight stenosis and ignore pressure.

The controversy concerning shunting therefore continues and perhaps only reinforces individual prejudice in the absence of a prospective study. The nonshunters are in the minority, but there are strong arguments on that side; several large series support their view. Perhaps a no-shunt approach with exceptions, including severe contralateral disease, will finally emerge as the correct procedure.

The routine shunters also present good results and arguments. I am one of them. After one becomes experienced, the technique is only a minor inconvenience. The chief fear is that the tube may tear off embolic material, and if it is not really vital to perfusion, the procedure would be simpler without it.

The position of the selective shunters is less tenable, as often occurs with fence sitters. The acceptable stump pressure is debatable, the meaning of abnormal EEGs is not clear, and the small incidence of use of shunts precludes expertise. The recent account of a 7-minute placement time with later stroke attests to the difficulty which may occur when shunt placement is not a routine, even for an otherwise experienced surgeon (intentionally not referenced here).

Shunt Techniques

Currently available shunt devices range from a simple indwelling Silastic tube to others with expanded ends which allow retention by special clamps or encircling ligatures to expensive tubes with balloons on each end and side arms.

The Javid shunt has become quite popular, is useful for most patients, and is easily retained by special clamps which prevent its bulbous ends from becoming dislodged.[83] The body of the shunt lies outside the lumen and can be moved about to allow easy internal endarterectomy.

Simple straight Silastic tubes are available in a variety of sizes. A disadvantage to their use is that they lie entirely within the lumen, thereby increasing, to some extent, the difficulty of dissection. Even if not implemented routinely, however, they are useful for placing into an internal carotid vessel whose lumen is too small to accommodate a Javid shunt.

OPERATIVE TECHNIQUE

There is more standardization of surgical technique than of indications. There are variations, but all agree that an efficient procedure through a completely opened common and internal carotid artery is important, with feathering of the superior edge or suturing if needed.

I prefer general anesthesia with maintenance of normal temperature, blood pressure, and blood gas levels. Shunting is routine. All shreds of tissue are carefully removed. Meticulous monofilament suture closure is performed. Total time of shunting ranges from 15 to 30 minutes. I usually assist and direct the vascular fellow, which allows efficient management of the team, better exposure than the fellow can provide, preparatory directions for instruments and materials prior to their actual use, and more experienced tactical management. There is no doubt that the younger surgeon sews, ties, and cuts well.

The patch graft closure advocated routinely by some experts[21] is, in the experience of others, "only rarely necessary."[22] In most cases it simply adds time and complicates the closure. At worst it may be applied too loosely and lead to aneurysm or thrombosis.[84] It is rarely needed. Our vascular surgeons all practice the sound advice of Charles Hafner who says that "a very meticulous and accurate technical performance of the endarterectomy is probably the most important single factor in the outcome."[66]

Vertebral Arterial Reconstruction

Edwards and Mulherin reviewed their extensive experience with 132 operations upon the vertebral arteries. They preferred vertebral anastomosis to the side of the carotid artery rather than endarterectomy or bypass. They emphasized (1) a medial approach through the divided sternocleidomastoid muscle, (2) due care for the vagus and recurrent nerves, (3) ligation of the thoracic duct, (4) preservation of the internal mammary artery, and (5) end-to-side anastomosis of the vertebral to the carotid artery.[53]

Berguer and Feldman's 34-patient experience led them also to prefer reimplantation of the vertebral artery into the side of the common carotid, rather than a bypass. Three of their patients had simultaneous carotid endarterectomy and vertebral transplantation.[54]

There is no doubt that vertebral transplantations can be done safely, but the indications for such are still controversial. The operation is not often needed.

Completion Studies

Angiography to evaluate the operative procedure has hardly been accepted in the extremities, to say nothing of the carotid arteries, where the risks of injecting radiopaque material are still not completely understood. A series of 131 completion arteriograms led the Andersen group to conclude that there was a "delicately weighed balance between the beneficial and harmful effects," so they stopped routine arteriography in 1978.[85]

It is also argued that the results of carotid procedures are so good that little is to be gained by completion angiography, which might suggest meddlesome reentry into the artery. Nevertheless, it is now being said that "it is not acceptable to wait until the patient is awake to assess the result of surgery," implying that the 15- to 30-minute time difference may be important in terms of a neurologic deficit.

Zierler, Bandyk, and Thiele analyzed 150 completion carotid angiograms, finding 23 (15 percent) with abnormalities. Of the 23, 7 were located in the external branch and 16 in the internal. Only 8 defects (5 percent) were thought worthy of immediate repair,[86] considerably less than the 25 percent unacceptable results in another series reported 17 years previously,[87] but in the range of the 8 percent recently reported by others.[85]

Noninvasive techniques have been advocated as replacements of angiography, but none have yet become standard. Use of postoperative pressure studies have been abandoned as not useful in finding tags and flaps of intima.

As noted by Imparato, there are probably a number of patients who "experience no neurologic deficits . . . but who nevertheless have serious changes occurring at the operative site," not manifest because of the collateral circulation.[88] Later angiograms document this point in completely asymptomatic patients with complete occlusion of a carotid artery. It is likely that a noninvasive technique will soon emerge as the best solution of this problem.

COMPLICATIONS

Cerebral Embolism

Prevention is the order of the day. Intraluminal flushing, careful placement of the shunt so that it lies beyond the lesion in the internal carotid artery, and flushing of the shunt after placement in the proximal carotid artery first are important in preventing embolization.

The patient should remain in the operating room through the early period of postanesthesia recovery until extremity motion and other evidences of intact neurologic status are present. If the patient does not awaken promptly or has evidence of a neurologic deficit, it has been suggested that completion angiography and noninvasive studies should be immediately performed to determine the situation. A surer way is to reinstitute anesthesia, reopen the wound and the vessel, and thereby ascertain immediately whether there is embolus or clot lying within the repaired artery. This settles the issue at once without delay for studies and provides whatever relief is possible.

The patient who awakens and develops a neurologic deficit later in the recovery room may be evaluated by noninvasive means or angiography. Experience, however, again suggests that delay for these should be avoided and the patient should immediately be returned to the operating room for surgical exploration. This will salvage many immediately and provoke no particular harm if an intracerebral event has occurred. This policy follows the advice of Kwaan, Connolly, and Sharefkin, who in 1979 altered their approach by avoiding time delay for angiography or other studies and returning the patient to the operating room for immediate exploration, with complete salvage of all three patients.[48]

Illustrative Case T.B., a 54-year-old male, had a previous right carotid thromboendarterectomy 2 weeks prior to contralateral operation for arterial stenosis and an ulcerative plaque. He awoke promptly after the second operation and moved all extremities and talked while in the operating room.

An hour after he reached the recovery room, there occurred paralysis of the right arm and leg, aphasia, and loss of consciousness. He was returned immediately to the operating room, where the wound and artery were rapidly opened 20 minutes after the complication occurred. Soft red clot was removed from the internal carotid artery. There was a large calcific atherosclerotic plug, which had washed up from below and which had occluded the bifurcation. The artery was flushed and closed with a polytetrafluoroethylene (PTFE) patch graft.

Thirty minutes after restoration of blood flow and closure of the wound the patient moved his extremities; ninety minutes later there was bilaterally equal strength and he was oriented completely. Recovery was uneventful.

He returned to normal life. He was rehospitalized to study leg claudication 19 months later. The aortic arch was visualized during angiography. The left carotid arterial system was entirely missing (Figure 22-8). The patient was discharged without further treatment and during the ensuing 5 months continued to be asymptomatic.

Comment Immediate removal of the occluding material allowed early complete recovery to the extent that the patient's golf handicap remained unchanged. Avoidance of delay was achieved by the operating room supervisor's clearing a room for immediate use and by the surgeon's leaving another case in order to prevent any delay in exploration of the carotid artery.

There is no explanation for the complete lack of symptoms 2 years later, during which time that same carotid arterial system had become completely occluded.

Infections

Infections are rare following arterial operations in the neck. There were none in our previous study of antibiotic prophylaxis, so the group was dropped from that series.[89] During the 4 years which have elapsed since that publication, there has occurred in our hospital (with 667 carotid operations in 1983) only a single instance of infection in a cervical wound through which a carotid thromboendarterectomy was performed.

Bleeding and Hematoma

If absolute hemostasis is obtained by suture ligatures on large veins and ties on others, with electrocoagulation limited to control of small oozing points, the instance of postoperative hemorrhage is low. Nevertheless, the risk of a rapidly expanding hematoma in the neck in terms of compromise of the airway is so great that some type of drainage should be provided. Better than the old Penrose drain is a suction drain placed through a stab wound. Such should be placed in every cervical wound regardless of its apparent dryness at closure. This has proved critically important in two of my cases in the last several years, when bleeding suddenly occurred in the recovery room. In both cases the suction drain gave an immediate indication of bleeding (500 mL in 5 minutes in one case); it also temporarily decompressed the wound so that a respiratory problem did not occur.

Bleeding obviously requires immediate control. Sutures must be removed to allow egress of blood and to allow a gloved finger to be placed within as a digital tamponade while the patient is rapidly transferred to the surgical unit. Unless an endotracheal tube can be immediately placed, this is safer than attempting to transport a rapidly evolving bleeder through the hall to the operating room.

False Aneurysm

False aneurysm fortunately is unusual,[22] even though small bites are made with a single-layer continuous suture. The only personal experience with such occurred 3 weeks postoperatively, when the entire continuous suture line pulled out of one wall of the carotid artery. It was corrected by replacement with a secondary suture line. Considerable bleeding did occur during the surgical approach before both ends of the carotid could be controlled. A double suction unit and adequate blood replacement managed the problem.

Hypertension

Hypertension is common following the operation and requires temporary pharmacologic control. While this has been attributed to baroreceptors in the carotid sinus nerve supply,[90] the mechanism is uncertain. Surely other factors are involved. I always dissect and cut these nerves.

Trimethaphan (Arfonad) administered intravenously as 500 mg in 500 mL in 5 percent dextrose is rapidly effective. Sodium nitroprusside (Nipride), 50 mg in 500 mL in 5 percent dextrose, may also be used as an intravenous drip. It is uncommon for these to be needed beyond 12 to 24 hours postoperatively.

Cranial Nerve Injuries

Temporary or, less often, permanent injuries to the several cranial nerves which lie within the area of dissection are more common than ordinarily believed.[91] These are summarized in Table 22-4.

At best these complications are frequently overlooked, and at worst they are ignored, as long as the patient lives and does not have a stroke. The *morbidity of carotid surgery is higher than generally admitted* by vascular surgeons. The patient is grateful for his or her life without stroke, and the usual statistics often do not reflect these cranial nerve problems. The Cleveland Clinic group reported 38 nerve injuries in 30 patients among 240 operations. These included 14 recurrent laryngeal, 13 hypoglossal, 6 mandibular, and 5 superior laryngeal nerve injuries.[92] Baker, Dorner, and Barnes reported temporary nerve complications in 6 percent of patients.[81] The high incidence in the hands of experienced surgeons warns of the danger.

TABLE 22-4 CRANIAL NERVE INJURY

Nerve	Location	Result of injury
Greater auricular	At the upper incision inferior to the parotid, ascending on the sternomastoid muscle	Numbness over the earlobe and nearby skin
Marginal mandibular branch of facial	Inferior to the mandible lying on the deep fascia	Motor damage of the mouth and lower lip
Hypoglossal	Crossing inferior to the digastric muscle	Deviation of the tongue and difficulty chewing
Superior laryngeal	Crossing near the superior thyroid artery posterior to the carotids	Vocal cord weakness
Recurrent laryngeal	The inferior portion of the field	Vocal cord paralysis
Vagus	Occasionally anterior to the carotid artery	Includes vocal cord weakness
Glossopharyngeal	Superior and posterior	Dysphagia

Any of the peripheral cranial nerves which enter or cross the operative field may be damaged. Everyone pays considerable attention to preserving the hypoglossal nerve, to prevent deviation of the tongue and swallowing problems. A steel retractor should not be placed on the nerve, nor should the nerve be elevated by a hook or suture. If the ansa branch is divided a centimeter from the main nerve, its end may be gently elevated with a ligature without appreciable disturbance of the hypoglossal nerve. Such division of the ansa hypoglossi does not produce a clinically significant lesion.

The superior laryngeal nerve is temporarily or permanently injured more commonly than has been generally recognized. This lesion results in hoarseness of either temporary or permanent nature and can be detected by direct examination of the vocal cords. In the early postoperative period the hoarseness may be attributed to inflammation secondary to the endotracheal tube. If a bilateral carotid operation is required, direct examination of the cords should be done prior to operation on the second side. Vocal cord damage may be a considerable contraindication to entering the contralateral side, particularly if the lesion there is asymptomatic.

The vagus nerve ordinarily lies posterior to the carotid artery and is visualized there but occasionally lies anterior. Since a secondary carotid procedure is sometimes necessary, the operative report should carefully note the anatomic position of the vagus nerve if it lies away from its usual posterior course.

The glossopharyngeal nerve lies high in the field posterior to the internal carotid artery and is not usually in danger unless a quite high dissection is required. Dissection should be kept as close to the artery as possible to avoid such a problem.

The facial nerve's cervical branch may be injured in the superior part of the wound, particularly if dissection is carried superiorly.

Recurrent Carotid Stenosis

The incidence of symptomatic stenosis following carotid endarterectomy of 3 percent[93] to 4.5 percent[94] is probably minimal in view of the 10 percent[95–97] or even 19 percent[98] recurrence rates detected by noninvasive studies. Suggested risk factors include tobacco, hypertension, hyperlipidemia, abnormal platelets, and technical errors as well as other associations such as bilaterality and gender.

Fortunately, the reoperative risks are reasonable. Clagett's team had no deaths, 1 brief neurologic deficit, and 1 nerve injury among 29 reoperations. No patient died or suffered permanent damage.[99] Routine noninvasive studies have been suggested to detect recurrent stenoses.[97] Whether this is antistroke-effective or cost-effective for large numbers of patients has not yet been determined.

FIGURE 22-13 Tight stenosis of the right internal carotid artery was corrected by endarterectomy in June 1980. Minimal stenosis of the left carotid artery was not treated.

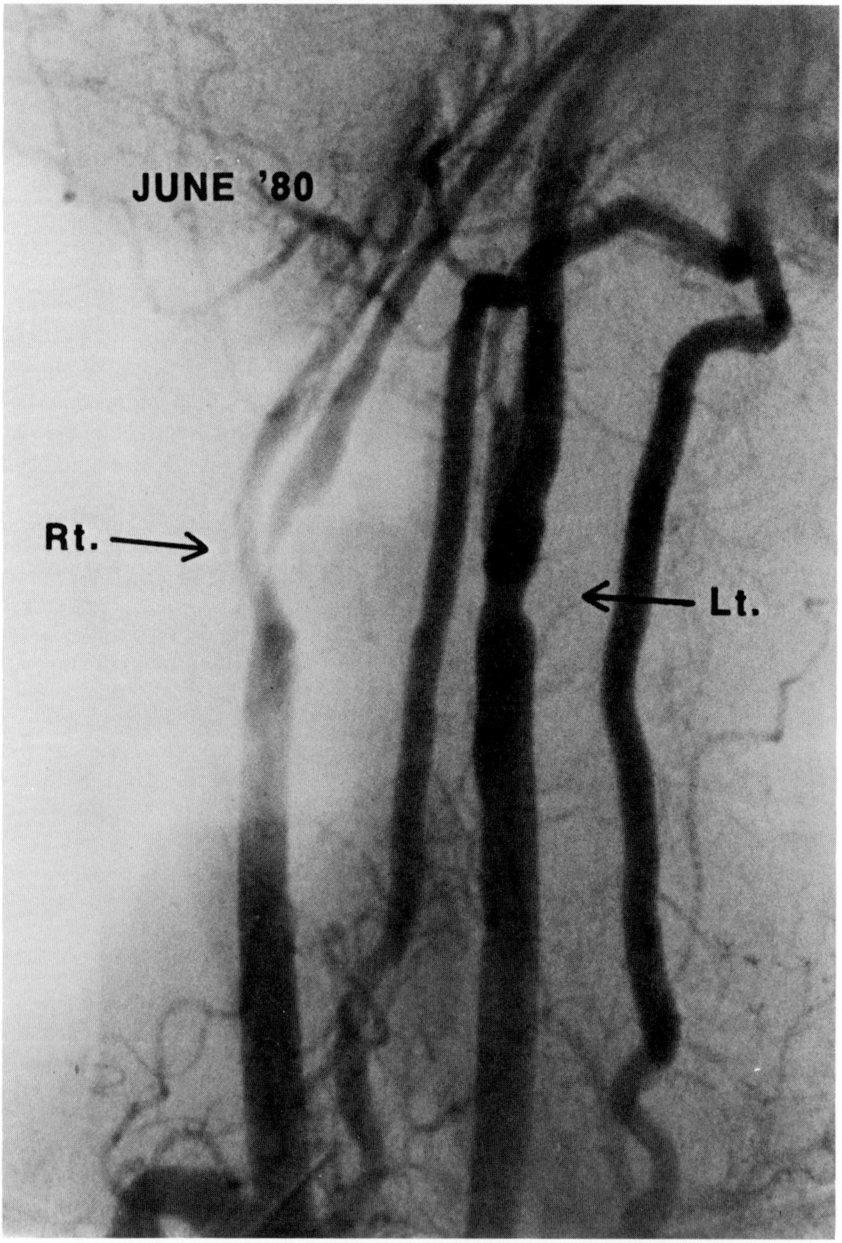

The Contralateral Artery after Endarterectomy

The question of how to manage the contralateral artery with more or less stenosis (but without referable symptoms) after successful endarterectomy of one side (Figures 22-13 to 22-15) fre-

FIGURE 22-14 Twenty-five months later the right carotid repair was patent, with slight narrowing at the site of a superior tacking suture line (shown at the *arrow*).

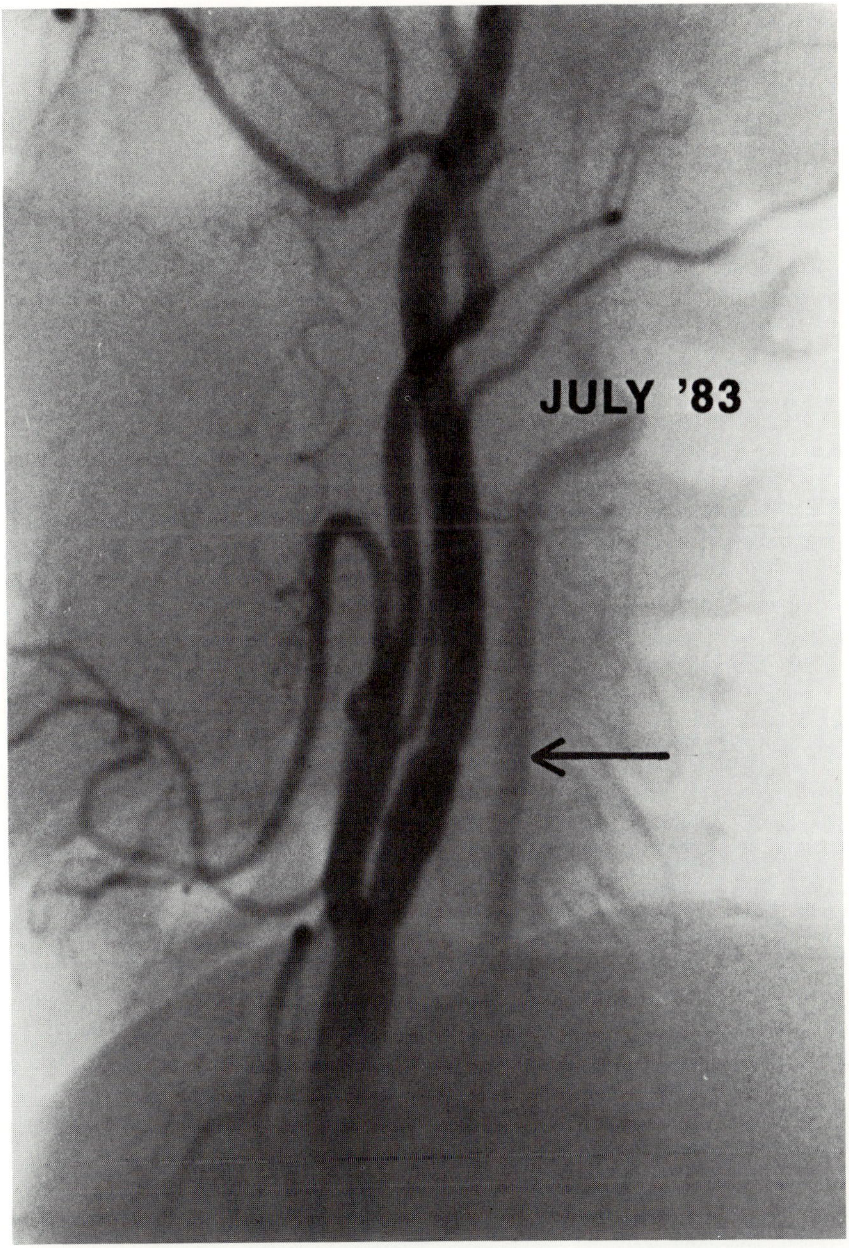

quently arises. Bergan's conservative advice was based on the fact that only 6 of 102 patients had referable symptoms. Several later developed TIAs and required operation.[100] More recently Roederer and his associates in Seattle reported a 134-patient series followed for 48 months. They found none of the 9 deaths to be stroke-related. Ten percent did develop TIAs. They also advocated conservatism until symptoms appear or a stenosis greater than 80 percent develops.[101]

FIGURE 22-15 Twenty-five months later the minimal left carotid lesion had progressed considerably. Endarterectomy was performed.

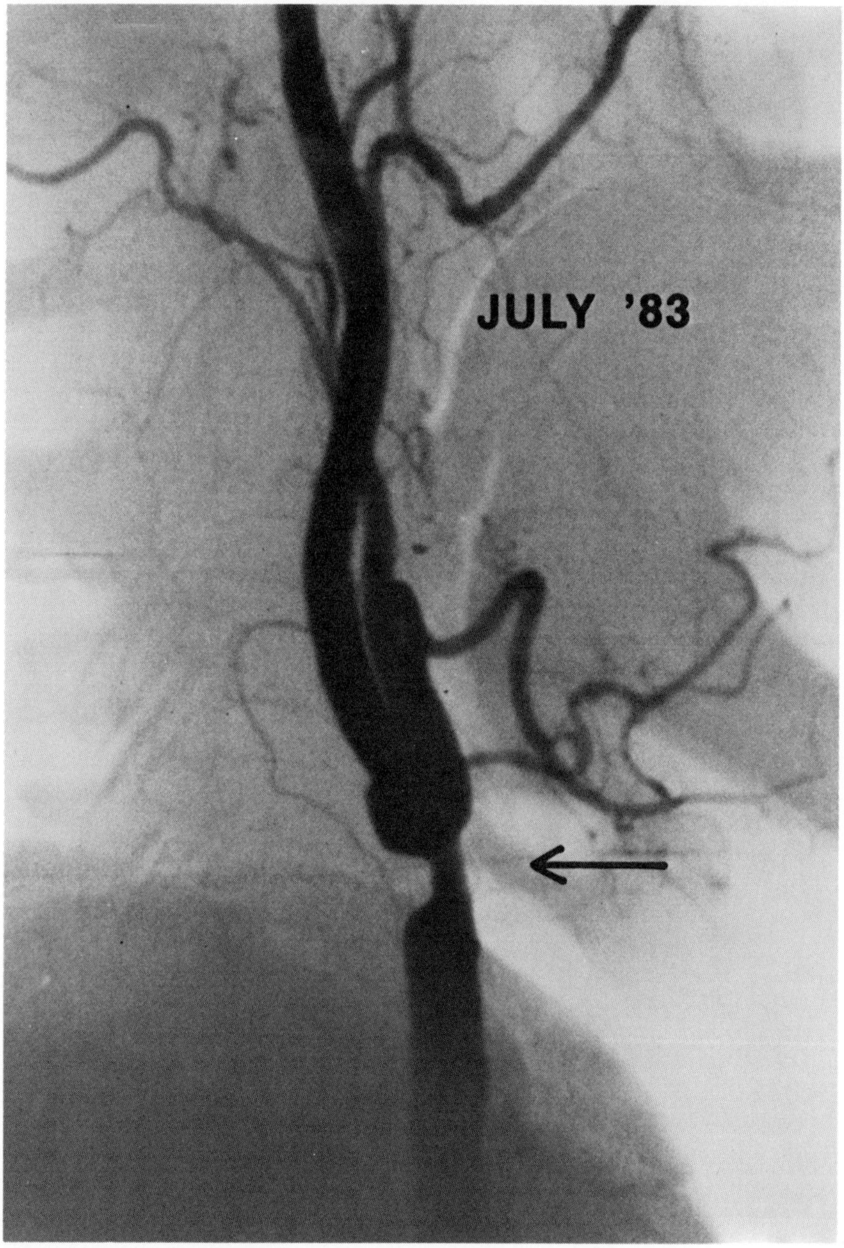

Lesions of Other Supraaortic Arteries

Atherosclerotic lesions of the supraaortic arteries previously were repaired by a variety of intrathoracic grafts and endarterectomies, which occasionally may still be required[102,103] (Figure 22-

FIGURE 22-16 The postoperative arteriogram demonstrates patent transfer of the subclavian artery to the side of the common carotid artery, carrying the patent vertebral artery along with it. The *lower arrow* demonstrates the remaining stump of the transected left subclavian artery.

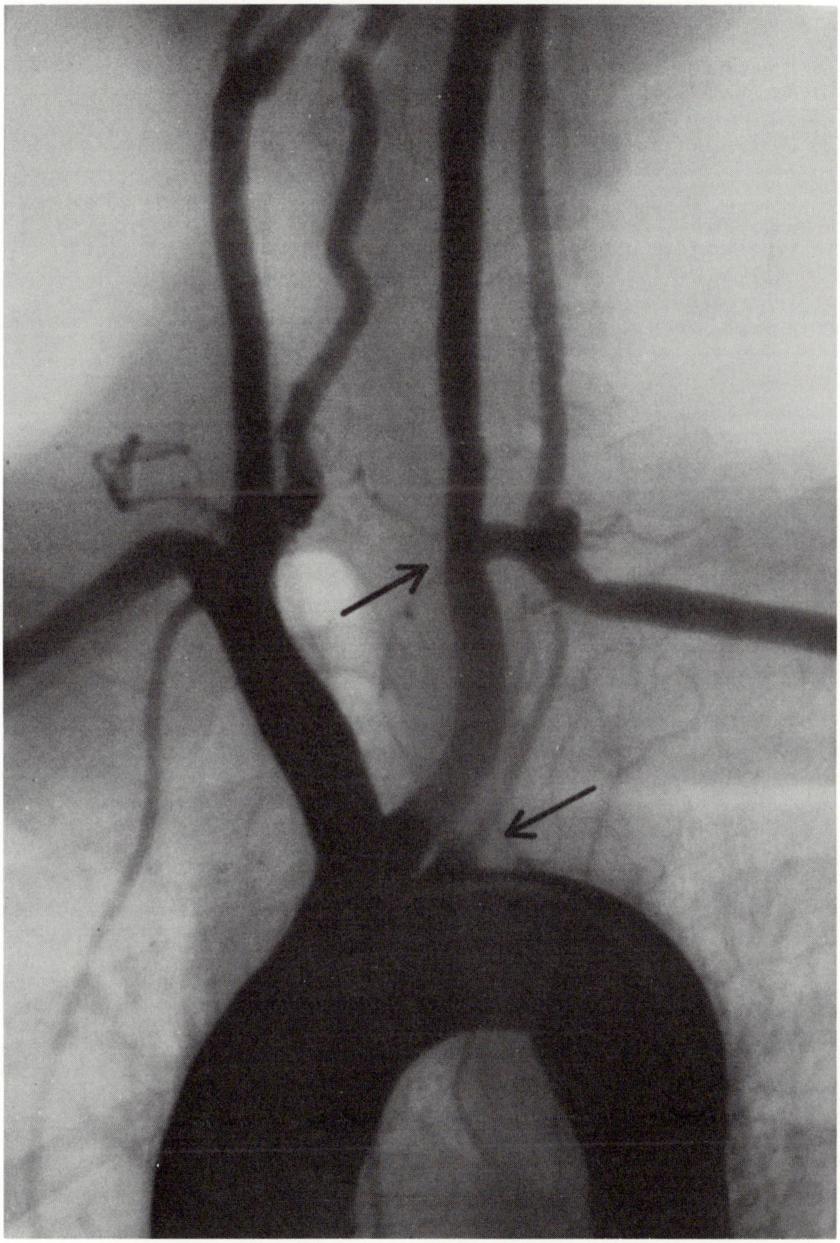

16). With increasing experience it has become apparent that extrathoracic bypasses are simpler, safer, and effective.

REFERENCES

1 Eastcott HH, Pickering GW, Rob CG: Reconstruction of internal carotid artery in a patient with intermittent attacks of hemiplegia. *Lancet* 1954, 267:994.
2 Savory WS: Case of a young woman in whom the main arteries of both upper extremities and of the left side of the neck were completely obliterated. *Med Chir Tr Lond* 1856, 39:205.
3 Hunt JR: The role of the carotid arteries in the causation of vascular lesions of the brain with certain remarks on certain special features of the symptomatology. *Am J Med Sci* 1914, 147:704.
4 Moniz E: L'encephalographique arterielle: Son importance dans la localization des tumeures cerebrales. *Rev Neurol* 2:172, 1927.
5 Fisher M: Occlusion of the internal carotid artery. *Arch Neurol Psychiatr* 1951, 65:346.
6 Carrea R, Molias M, Murphy G: Surgical treatment of spontaneous thrombosis of the internal carotid artery in the neck. *Acta Neurol Lat Am* 1951, 1:71.
7 DeBakey ME, Crawford ES, Cooley D, Morris G: Surgical consideration of occlusive disease of innominate, carotid, subclavian and vertebral arteries. *Ann Surg* 1959, 149:690.
8 Yatsu SM, Coull BM: Stroke, in Appel SH (ed): *Current Neurology* 1981, vol 3, p 159.
9 Moore WS, Quinones-Baldrich WJ: Extracranial cerebrovascular disease, in Moore WS (ed): *Vascular Surgery: A Comprehensive Review.* Grune & Stratton, New York, 1983, chap 18.
10 Robinson RW, Demirel M, LeBeau RJ: Natural history of cerebral thrombosis, 9 - 19 year follow-up. *J Chronic Dis* 1968, 21:221.
11 Whisnant JP, Matsumoto M, Elveback LR: The effects of anticoagulant therapy on the prognosis of patients with transient cerebral ischemic attacks in a community. *Mayo Clin Proc* 1973, 48:844.
12 Heyman A, Levinton A, Millikan CH, Sahs AL, Whisnant JP, Jefzger MD, Ostfeld AM, Stallones RA: Transient focal cerebral ischemia: Epidemological and clinical aspects. *Stroke* 1974, 5:277.
13 Kartchner, MM, McRae LP: Carotid occlusive disease as a risk factor in major cardiovascular surgery. *Arch Surg* 1982, 117:1086.
14 Jones EL, Craver HN, Michlak RA, Murphy DA, Guyton RA, Bone BK, Hatcher CR, Reichwald NA: Combined carotid and coronary surgery: When is it necessary? *J Thorac Cardiovasc Surg* 1984, 87:7.
15 Ernst, CB: Editorial comment. *Arch Surg* 1983, 118:1171.
16 Rosenthal D, Stanton PE Jr, Lamis PA: Carotid endarterectomy: The unreliability of intraoperative monitoring in patients having had stroke or reversible ischemic neurologic deficit. *Arch Surg* 1981, 116:1569.
17 Eikelboom BC, Ackerstaff RGA, Moll FL, DeVries AR: Accuracy and usefulness of combined duplex scanning and digital subtraction angiography, in Greenhalgh R, Rose FC (eds): *Progress in Stroke Research 2.* Pitman, Bath, 1983, p 178.
18 Ricotta, J, Holen J, Schenk E, Plassche W, Green R, Gramiak R, DeWeese J: Is routine angiography necessary prior to carotid endarterectomy? *J Vasc Surg* 1984, 1:96.
19 Kartchner MM, McRae LP: Noninvasive evaluation and management of the asymptomatic carotid bruit. *Surgery* 1977, 82:840.
20 Thompson JE, Patman RD, Talkington CM: Asymptomatic carotid bruit: Long-term outcome of patients having endarterectomy compared with unoperated controls. *Ann Surg* 1978, 188:308.
21 Imparato AM, Riles TS, Gorstein F: The carotid bifurcation plaque: Pathologic findings associated with cerebral ischemia. *Stroke* 1979, 10:238.
22 Thompson JE: Complications of endarterectomy and their prevention. *World J Surg* 1979, 3:155.
23 Humphries AW, Young JR, Santilli PH, Beven EG, deWolfe BG: Unoperated, asymptomatic significant internal carotid artery stenosis: A review of 182 instances. *Surgery* 1976, 80:695.
24 Levin SM, Sondheimer FK, Levin JM: The contralateral diseased bruit asymptomatic carotid artery: To operate or not? An update. *Am J Surg* 1980, 140:203.
25 Barnes RW, Liebman PR, Marszalek PB, Kirk CL, Goldman MH: The natural history of asymptomatic carotid disease in patients undergoing cardiovascular surgery. *Surgery* 1981, 90:1075.
26 Mohr JP: Asymptomatic carotid artery disease. *Stroke* 1982, 13:431.
27 Mohr JP: Asymptomatic carotid artery disease. *Symp Soc Clin Vasc Surg* March 1983, p 112.

28 Fields WS: Management of the patient with an asymptomatic carotid bruit. *Vasc Diag Treat* July–August 1983, p 39.

29 Turnipseed WD, Vasko JS, Lubow M: Surgical management of the totally occluded carotid artery. *Surgery* 1977, 82:689.

30 Ropper AH, Wechsler LR, Wilson LS: Carotid bruit and the risk of stroke in elective surgery. *N Engl J Med* 1982, 307:1388.

31 Treiman RL, Foran RF, Cohen JL, Levin PM, Cossman DV: Carotid bruit: A follow-up report on its significance in patients undergoing an abdominal aortic operation. *Arch Surg* 1979, 114:1138.

32 Evans WE, Cooperman N: The significance of asymptomatic unilateral carotid bruits in preoperative patients. *Surgery* 1978, 183:521.

33 Ennix CL, Lowrie GM, Morris GC, Crawford ES, Howell JF, Reardorn MJ, Weatherford SC: Improved results of carotid endarterectomy in patients with symptomatic coronary disease: An analysis of 1546 consecutive carotid operations. *Stroke* 1979, 10:122.

34 Hertzer NR, Feldman BJ, Beven EG, Tucker HM: A prospective study of the incidence of injury to cranial nerves during carotid endarterectomy. *Surg Gynecol Obstet* 1980, 151:781.

35 Emery R, Cohn L, Whittemore M, Mannick J, Couch N, Collins J: Co-existent carotid and coronary artery disease: Surgical management. *Arch Surg* 1983, 118:1035.

36 O'Donnell TF, Callow AD, Willet C, Payne D, Cleveland RJ: The impact of coronary artery disease on carotid endarterectomy. *Ann Surg* 1983, 198:705.

37 Gunning AJ, Pickering GW, Robb-Smith AHT, Russell RR: Mural thrombosis of the internal carotid artery and subsequent embolism. *Q J Med* 1964, 33:155.

38 Fisher CM: Observations of the fundus oculi in transient monocular blindness. *Neurology* 1959, 9:333.

39 Imparato AM: Discussion of Thompson JE: Complications of endarterectomy and their prevention. *World J Surg* 1979, 3:163.

40 Lusby RJ, Ferrell LD, Ehrenfeld WK, Stoney RT, Wylie EJ: Carotid plaque hemorrhage: its need in production of cerebral ischemic ulcers. *Arch Surg* 1982, 117:1479.

41 Dixon S, Pais SO, Raviola C, Gomes A, Machleder HI, Baker JD, Busuttil RW, Barker WF, Moore WS: Natural history of non-stenotic asymptomatic ulcerative lesions of the carotid artery. *Arch Surg* 1982, 117:1493.

42 Riles T, Imparato A, Posner M, Eikelboom B: Common carotid occlusion: Assessment of the distal vessels. *Ann Surg* 1984, 199:363.

43 Fields WS: Selection of patients with ischemic cerebrovascular disease for arterial surgery. *World J Surg* 1979, 1:147.

44 Thompson JE, Talkington CM: Carotid endarterectomy. *Ann Surg* 1976, 184:1.

45 Kish GF, Adkins AC, Slovin AJ: The totally occluded internal carotid artery: Indications for surgery. *Am J Surg* 1977, 134:288.

46 Welling R, Cranley J, Krause R, Hafner C, Arbaugh J, Roedersheimer L: Surgical therapy for recent total occlusion of the internal carotid artery. *J Vasc Surg* 1984, 1:57.

47 Hafner CD, Tew JM: Surgical management of the totally occluded internal carotid artery: A 10 year study. *Surgery* 1981, 89:710.

48 Kwaan JHM, Connolly JE, Sharefkin JB: Successful management of early stroke after carotid endarterectomy. *Ann Surg* 1979, 190:676.

49 Donaldson M, Drezner A: Surgery for acute carotid occlusion: Therapy in search of predictability. *Arch Surg* 1983, 118:1266.

50 Bardin J, Bernstein E, Humber P, Collins G, Dilley R, Devin J, Stuart S: Is carotid endarterectomy beneficial in prevention of recurrent stroke? *Arch Surg* 1982, 117:1401.

51 Thompson JE: Discussion of Malone JM, Moore WS, Hamilton R, Smith M: Combined carotid-vertebral vascular disease: A new surgical approach. *Arch Surg* 1982, 117:1401.

52 Crawford ES: Discussion of Thevenet J: Surgical management of atheroma of the aortic dome and origin of supra-aortic trunks. *World J Surg* 1979, 3:187.

53 Edwards WH, Mulherin JL: The surgical approach to significant stenosis of vertebral and subclavian arteries. *Surgery* 1980, 87:20.

54 Berguer R, Feldman AJ: Surgical reconstruction of the vertebral artery. *Surgery* 1983, 93:670.

55 Ouriel K, May AG, Ricotta JS, DeWeese JA, Green RM: Carotid endarterectomy for nonhemispheric symptoms: Predictions of success. *J Vasc Surg* 1984, 1:339.

56 Malone JM, Moore WS, Hamilton R, Smith M: Combined carotid-vertebral vascular disease: A new surgical approach. *Arch Surg* 1980, 115:783.

57 Haynes CD, Gideon DA, King GD, Dempsey RL: The improvement of cognition and personality after carotid endarterectomy. *Surgery* 1976, 80:699.

58 Blaisdell FW: Discussion of Haynes CD, Gideon DA, King GD, Dempsey RL: The improvement of cognition and personality after carotid endarterectomy. *Surgery* 1976, 80:704.

59 Javid H, Julian OC, Dye WS, Hunter JA, Najafi H, Goldon MD, Serry C, Delaria GA: Seventeen year experience with routine shunting in carotid artery surgery. *World J Surg* 1979, 3:167.

60 Jacobs LA, Ganji S, Shirley JG, Morrell RM, Brinkman SD: Cognitive improvement after extracranial reconstruction for the low flow–endangered brain. *Surgery* 1983, 93:683.

61 Satiani B, Liapis C, Pflug MS, Vasko JS, Evans WE: Role of staging in bilateral carotid endarterectomy. *Surgery* 1978, 84:784.

62 Effeney DJ, Ehrenfeld WK, Stoney RJ, Wylie EJ: Fibromuscular dysplasia of the internal carotid artery. *World J Surg* 1979, 3:179.

63 Perry MO: Discussion of Effeney DJ, Ehrenfeld WK, Stoney RJ, Wylie EJ: Fibromuscular dysplasia of the internal carotid artery. *World J Surg* 1979, 3:179.

64 Connolly J: Discussion of Rosenthal D, Stanton PE Jr, Lamais PA: Carotid endarterectomy: The unreliability of intraoperative monitoring in patients having had stroke or reversible ischemic neurologic deficit. *Arch Surg* 1981, 116:1573.

65 Peitzman AB, Webster MW, Loubeau JM, Grunday BL, Bahnson HT: Carotid endarterectomy under regional (conductive) anesthesia. *Ann Surg* 1982, 196:59.

66 Hafner CD: Minimizing the risks of carotid endarterectomy. *J Vasc Surg* 1984, 1:392.

67 Bland JE, Chapman RD, Wylie EJ: Neurological complications of carotid artery surgery. *Ann Surg* 1970, 171:459.

68 Moore WS: Use of internal carotid artery back pressure in evaluating the need for cerebral protection during carotid endarterectomy. Postgraduate Course #1, American College of Surgeons, April 1981, p 9.

69 String T: Discussion of Rosenthal D, Stanton PE Jr, Lamis PA: Carotid endarterectomy: The unreliability of intraoperative monitoring in patients having had stroke or reversible ischemic neurologic deficit. *Arch Surg* 1981, 116:1573.

70 Whittemore A, Kauffman J, Kohler T, Mannick J: Routine electroencephalographic (EEG) monitoring during carotid endarterectomy. *Ann Surg* 1983, 197:707.

71 Callow AD: Discussion of Rosenthal D, Stanton PE Jr, Lamis PA: Carotid endarterectomy: The unreliability of intraoperative monitoring in patients having had stroke or reversible ischemic neurologic deficit. *Arch Surg* 1981, 116:1569.

72 Ricotta J, Charlton M, DeWeese J: Determining criteria for shunt placement during carotid endarterectomy: EEG versus back pressure. *Ann Surg* 1983, 198:642.

73 Rosenthal D, Zeichner W, Lamis P, Stanton P: Neurologic deficit after carotid endarterectomy: Pathogenesis and management. *Surgery* 1983, 94:776.

74 Hertzer NR, Beven EG: A retrospective comparison of the use of shunts during carotid endarterectomy. *Surg Gynecol Obstet* 1980, 151:81.

75 Lees CD, Hertzer NR: Postoperative stroke and late neurologic complications after endarterectomy. *Arch Surg* 1981, 116:1561.

76 Whitney DG, Kahn EM, Estes JW, Jones CE: Carotid surgery without a temporary indwelling shunt: 1,917 consecutive procedures. *Arch Surg* 1980, 115:1393.

77 Thompson JE: Discussion of Whitney DG, Kahn EM, Estes JW, Jones CE: Carotid surgery without a temporary indwelling shunt: 1,917 consecutive procedures. *Arch Surg* 1980, 115:1393.

78 Baker WD: Discussion of Whitney DG, Kahn EM, Estes JW, Jones CE: Carotid surgery without a temporary indwelling shunt: 1,917 consecutive procedures. *Arch Surg* 1980, 115:1393.

79 Harrison JH: Discussion of Whitney DG, Kahn EM, Estes JW, Jones CE: Carotid surgery without a temporary indwelling shunt: 1,917 consecutive procedures. *Arch Surg* 1980, 115:1393.

80 Ott DA, Cooley DA, Chapa L, Cuelho A: Carotid endarterectomy without temporary intraluminal shunt: Study of 309 consecutive operations. *Ann Surg* 1980, 191:708.

81 Baker WM, Dorner DB, Barnes RW: Carotid endarterectomy: Is an indwelling shunt necessary? *Surgery* 1977, 82:321.

82 Baker W, Littooy F, Hayes A, Dorner D, Stubbs D: Carotid endarterectomy without a shunt: The control series. *J Vasc Surg* 1984, 1:50.

83 Javid H, Dye WS, Hunter JA: Surgical treatment of cerebral ischemia. *Surg Clin North Am* 1974, 54:239.

84 Dale WA, Lewis MR: Lateral vascular patch grafts. *Surgery* 1965, 57:37.

85 Andersen CA, Collins GJ, Rich NM: Routine operative arteriography during carotid endarterectomy: A reassessment. *Surgery* 1978, 83:67.

86 Zierler R, Bandyk D, Thiele B: Intraoperative assessment of carotid endarterectomy. *J Vasc Surg* 1984, 1:73.

87 Blaisdell FW, Linn R, Hall AD: Technical result of carotid endarterectomy: Arteriographic assessment. *Am J Surg* 1967, 114:239.

88 Imparato AM: Discussion of Zierler R, Bandyk D, Thiele B: Interoperative assessment of carotid endarterectomy. *J Vasc Surg* 1984, 1:81.

89 Kaiser WB, Clayson KR, Mulherin JL, Roach AB, Allen TR, Edwards WH, Dale WA: Antibiotic prophylaxis in vascular surgery. *Ann Surg* 1978, 188:283.

90 Cafferata HT, Merchant RF, Depalma RG: Avoidance of postcarotid endarterectomy hypertension. *Ann Surg* 1982, 196:465.

91 Verta MJ, Applebaum EL, McClusky DA, Yao JST, Bergan JJ: Cranial nerve injury during carotid endarterectomy. *Ann Surg* 1977, 185:192.

92 Hertzer NR, Lees CD: Fatal myocardial infarction following carotid endarterectomy: 335 patients followed 6–11 years after operation. *Ann Surg* 1981, 194:212.

93 Cossman D, Callow AD, Matsumoto G: Early restenosis after carotid endarterectomy. *Arch Surg* 1978, 113:275.

94 Cantelmo NL, Cutler BS, Wheeler HB, Herrmann JB, Cardullo PA: Noninvasive detection of carotid stenosis following endarterectomy. *Arch Surg* 1981, 116:1005.

95 Baker WH, Hayes AC, Mahler D, Littooy FN: Durability of carotid endarterectomy. *Surgery* 1983, 94:112.

96 Turnipseed WD, Berkoff HA, Crummy A: Postoperative occlusion after carotid endarterectomy. *Arch Surg* 1980, 115:573.

97 Kremen JE, Gee W, Kaupp HA, McDonald KM: Restenosis or occlusion after carotid endarterectomy. *Arch Surg* 1979, 114:608.

98 Zierler R, Bandyk D, Thiele B, Strandness E: Carotid artery stenosis following endarterectomy. *Arch Surg* 1982, 117:1408.

99 Clagett G, Rich N, McDonald P, Salander J, Youkey J, Olson D, Hutton J: Etiologic factors for recurrent carotid artery stenosis. *Surgery* 1983, 93:313.

100 Bergan JJ: Carotid endarterctomy: A follow-up study of the contralateral non-operated carotid artery. *Ann Surg* 1978, 188:748.

101 Roederer GO, Langlois YE, Lusiani L, Jager KA, Primozich JF, Lawrence RJ, Phillips DJ, Strandness DE: Natural history of carotid artery disease on the side contralateral to endarterectomy. *J Vasc Surg* 1984, 1:62.

102 Thevenet J: Surgical management of atheroma of the aortic dome and origin of supra-aortic trunks. *World J Surg* 1979, 3:187.

103 Crawford E, Stowe C, Powers R: Occlusion of the innominate, common carotid and subclavian arteries: Long term results of surgical treatment. *Surgery* 1983, 94:781.

Invited Commentary

Allan D. Callow, M.D.
Boston, Massachusetts

Thanks to the author's extensive experience and with his vantage point of participating in the evolution of carotid surgery, a complex topic with many controversial aspects has been presented in a deceptively simple but reliable and authoritative fashion.

Several points deserve comment and emphasis. Preoperative and intraoperative arteriography may not continue as the "gold standard" of carotid artery disease. Improvements in B-mode real-time duplex imaging may yield more detailed preoperative information as well as immediate operative evaluation in the operating room. Although stenoses of 80 percent or more are described as serious in patients with asymptomatic carotid bruits, they should not be considered the only indication for prophylactic surgery. Embolization may occur from areas of stenosis substantially less than 80 percent. TIAs and strokes in the territory of the cervical carotid artery are rarely due to low flow. Emergency endarterectomy may be considered for frequent transient ischemic attacks with waxing and waning of neurologic deficits, appropriate to the side of the lesion, and also for the carotid artery undergoing acute thrombosis with or without occlusion.

A continuing problem is our inability to identify the transition of a smooth, stable lesion to an unstable and potentially ulcerated plaque. Although it is true, as the author states, that the threat of ulcerated plaques is serious and more so than stenosis alone, there is no reliable test available which will detect conversion of the nonulcerated to the ulcerated plaque or the onset of an intraplaque subsurface hemorrhage.

Recommendations concerning the use of a shunt on a selective or routine basis, or not at all, are of little help to the beginning vascular surgeon. What may be of some assistance is the observation that cerebral perfusion must be reduced during carotid cross-clamping, because the collateral circulation is reduced in patients with (1) a history of a remote or recent stroke, (2) an infarct present on CT scan, (3) the presence of a contralateral occluded carotid, and (4) the combination of vertebral-basilar insufficiency and carotid territory signs and symptoms. These patients are at high risk of underperfusion during endarterectomy. The incidence of perioperative stroke should be reduced by the use of routine shunting.

Although there may be a rare case where sutures at the superior end of the plaque are necessary, their routine use suggests an incomplete endarterectomy. As stated, "a very meticulous and accurate technical performance of the endarterectomy is probably the most important single factor in the outcome."

Hypertension must be controlled following operation. In our experience, the overwhelming majority of cardiac and subsequent neurologic deficits were significantly correlated with postoperative hypertension.

Although it is true that extrathoracic bypass is a simpler, safer, and effective procedure for lesions of the brachiocephalic arteries, there is an occasional need for median stemotomy and a single-, double-, or triple-armed bypass graft from the arch of the aorta. The indication is in the individual with bilateral internal carotid occlusion plus reduced or even absent vertebral artery flow and in whom an extraintracranial bypass may be necessary.

23 CAROTID BODY TUMOR

Paralleling the development of vascular surgery, technical advances in the surgical management of the nonchromaffin paragangliomas known as chemodectomas or carotid body tumors have placed the risks of the excision of these tumors at an acceptable level.

Paragangliomas are tumors of the extraadrenal paraganglion system which occur in diverse locations, including the jugulotympanic region, lung, bladder, intestines, and the carotid body.[1]

The tumor is usually unilateral, but among the occasional familial cases there is some bilaterality.[2]

Chemoreceptors of the carotid body, from which these tumors rise, affect blood pressure, pulse, and respiration by sensing through the glossopharyngeal nerve the O_2, CO_2, and pH levels in the blood. Carotid body tumors are commonly nonfunctional,[3] but occasional patients with symptoms like those of pheochromocytoma have been reported.[4]

Most of these tumors are benign, although malignant lesions with distant metastases sometimes occur.[5] Rush in 1962 found that 5 percent of 104 reported cases had developed distant metastases and that 12 percent had local recurrences[7].

While these chemodectomas may affect the nearby nerves, including the vagus, recurrent laryngeal, glossopharyngeal, and hypoglossal nerve and the stellate ganglion, the usual presenting complaint is a mass with more or less discomfort.[7] The differential diagnosis includes carotid aneurysm, branchiogenic cyst, and metastatic node lesions.

ILLUSTRATIVE CASE

A 57-year-old female originally had surgical removal of a carotid body tumor in 1974. It thereafter slowly recurred, so by October 1982 it had become a 4 × 4 cm, slightly tender mass in the right midneck with an accompanying bruit. An arteriogram showed divergence of the internal and external carotids and patency of the entire system. The tumor itself was heavily outlined by the radiopaque material (Figure 23-1).

Operation was conducted through the usual oblique skin incision anterior to the sternocleidomastoid muscle. The internal jugular vein was separated laterally by division of all its crossing tributaries. Proximal control of the common carotid artery was easily obtained. Dissection was carried posterolaterally to expose the vagus nerve and then superior to locate the internal and external carotid arteries (Figure 23-2). The glossopharyngeal and the hypoglossal nerves were visualized and protected.

The main mass of the tumor was carefully dissected away from the vessels by splitting it anteriorly, beginning at the inferior aspect. Meticulous dissection in the plane of the adventitia was carried out until the tumor lay attached only to the proximal portion of the internal carotid artery, where it was tightly bound by old scar tissue which defied removal. A 2-cm section of

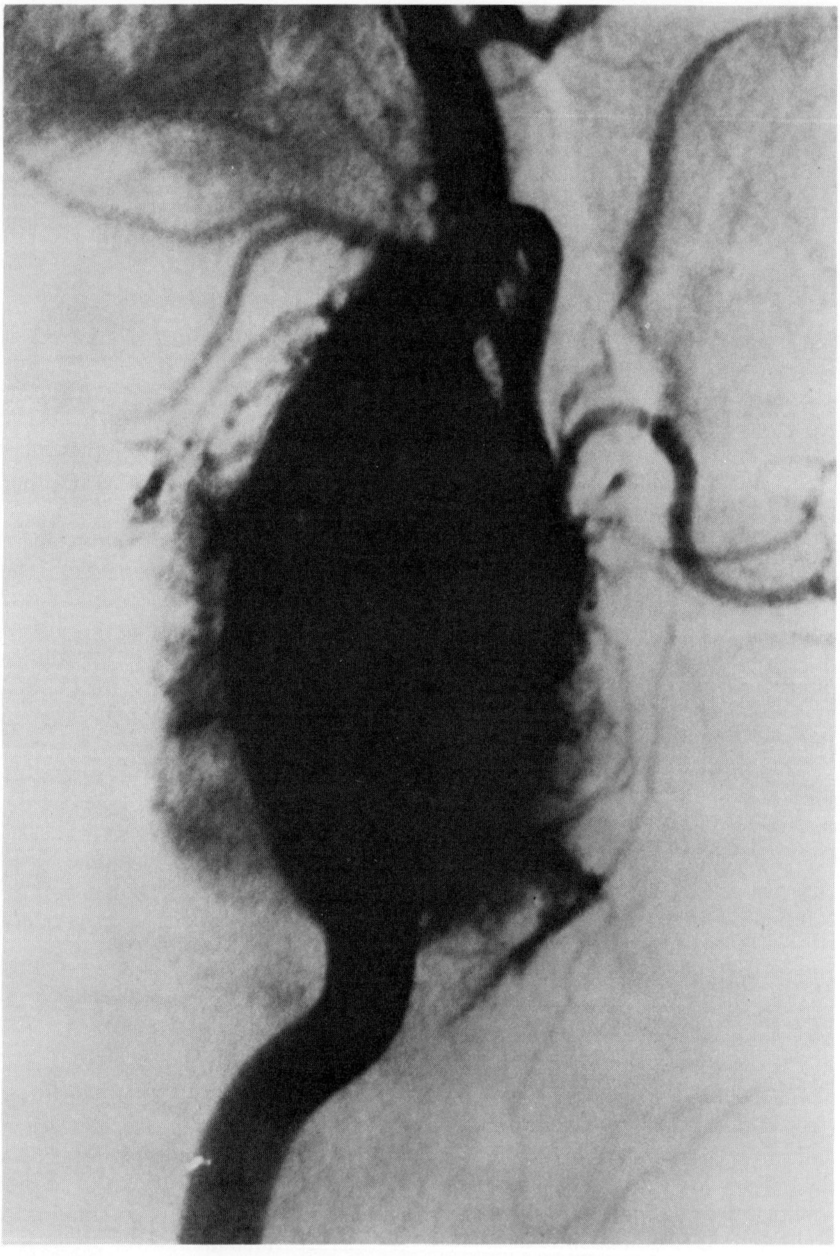

FIGURE 23-1 The arteriogram showed divergence of the internal and external carotids with patency. The tumor was heavily outlined by the radiopaque material.

internal carotid artery was therefore removed with the mass (Figure 23-3). A Javid shunt was placed within the artery, and an ovoid anastomosis was constructed between the superior end of the carotid artery and this original aperture on the side of the common carotid artery, using continuous 6-0 polypropylene. The total shunting time was 17 minutes.

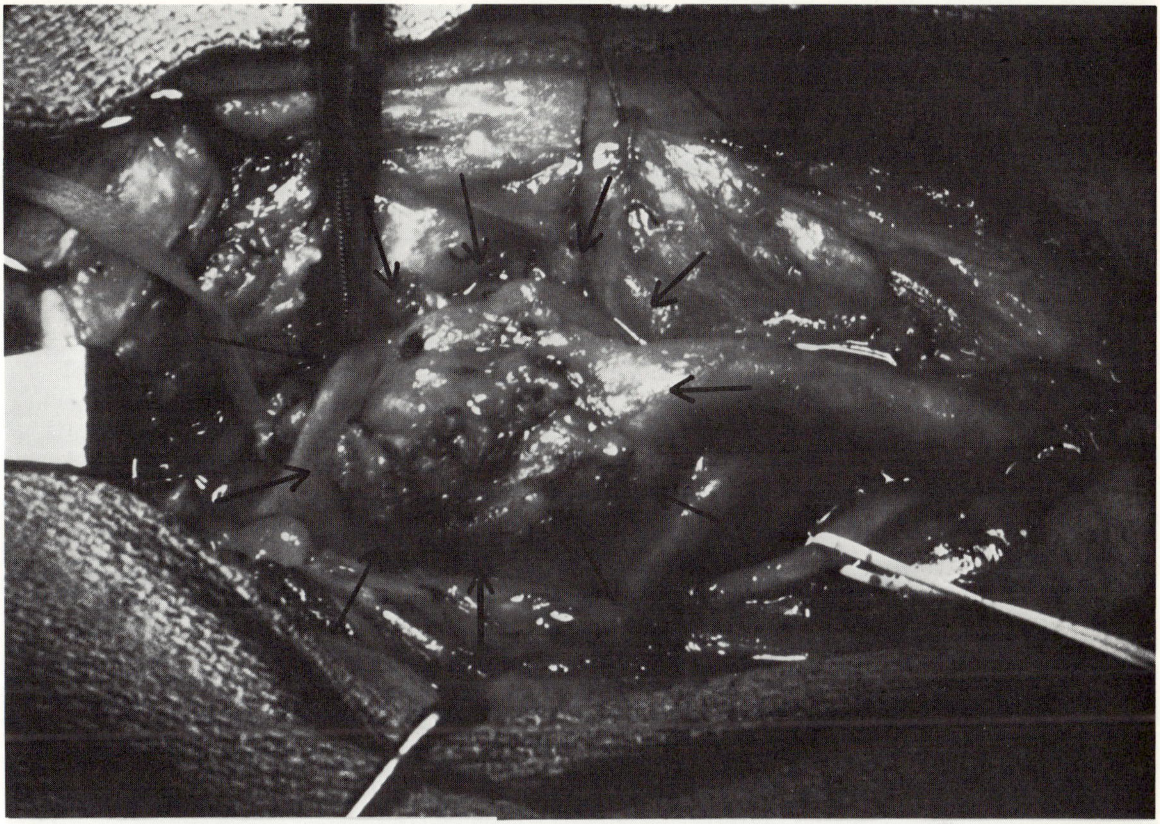

FIGURE 23-2 The tumor lay in the bifurcation of the carotid artery and surrounded both the internal and external branches. This operative view looks through the lateral exposure, with the tumor mass still in situ. The white loop at the *lower right* retracts the vagus nerve, which runs to the left up under the already dissected internal jugular vein. The vessel loop at the *left* encloses the superior portion of the internal carotid artery. The hemostat points toward the crossing hypoglossal nerve. The *arrows* outline the tumor mass.

At conclusion the field was dry; in the postoperative period there was no particular amount of drainage through the suction drain, which was left in place for 48 hours. There was no evidence of neurologic damage or other complication, and the patient was discharged on the fifth postoperative day.

DISCUSSION

Diagnostic Procedures

Angiography not only allows definitive diagnosis but also discloses carotid arterial stenosis or occlusion, uncommon as it is.[8] It should invariably be performed. Ultrasound and computerized tomography (CT) scanning may be useful but do not replace angiography and are therefore usually superfluous.

Operation versus Observation

The availability of modern arterial reconstructive techniques has lowered the risk of operation to the extent that excision by an experienced vascular surgeon should be offered for these lesions

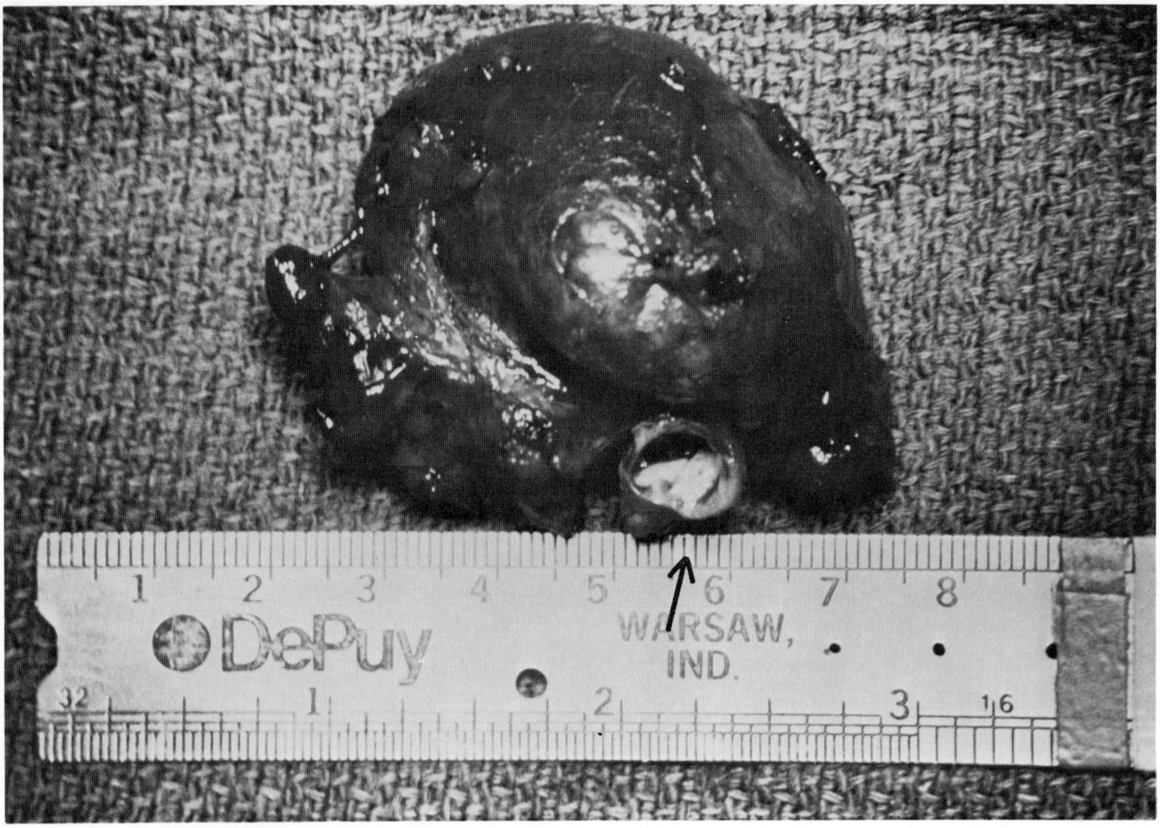

FIGURE 23-3 The recurrent tumor could not be separated from the internal carotid artery near the bifurcation, so a portion of that was resected along with the specimen. The *arrow* indicates the opening in the resected internal carotid artery.

with few exceptions.[9,10] However, growth is usually slow and malignancy is unusual, so contraindications such as advanced physiologic age, decompensation of an important functional system, or any condition which limits life expectation may suggest a nonoperative strategy.

The chief problem of surgical removal of the tumors has been their intimate association with the carotid arteries and the hazard of artery ligation or resection. The 25 percent mortality and 30 percent hemiplegia rates among survivors of carotid artery interruption in earlier experience led to the concept that operation should be limited to relatively young patients with small tumors, those with severe symptoms, and those in whom rapid growth suggested malignancy.[3]

Modern experience with the management of large arteries, particularly the carotids, and the several kinds of indwelling shunts now available as well as saphenous vein graft replacements, has now reduced the risk of surgical resection to a reasonable level, so operation is indicated for carotid body tumors in most patients. The 4 percent mortality (1 patient died of later myocardial infarction) among the 24 patients of Javid and associates;[11] the 38 patients without death reported by Chambers and Mahoney;[12] and the 19 without mortality reported by Krupski, Effeney, Ehrenfeld, and Stoney[4]* document the reasonable risk factor when modern methods are used.

*The report of Krupski and associates is an exceptionally comprehensive yet concise review.

Planning the Dissection

Proximal control of the common carotid artery should be obtained promptly. Isolation of internal and external carotid arteries superior to the mass is an early aim but may require delay to allow exposure laterally, followed by an approach from the side to the important structures high in the neck, which include the hypoglossal and glossopharyngeal nerves. During this portion of the dissection the vagus nerve should become apparent. (Recall that occasionally it lies anterior to the carotid artery.) Instances of postoperative nerve dysfunction are well-documented (Table 23-1), suggesting care in dissection of these nerves, which usually lie on the perimeter of the tumor.

Inability to obtain distal control of the carotid arteries because of high extension of the tumor may occasionally cause abandonment of the procedure before uncontrollable hemorrhage occurs.

Sometimes the internal jugular vein must be sacrificed; ordinarily it can be separated, with division of its crossing contributory veins as they are encountered.

Considerable discussion has been devoted to conducting meticulous dissection in the subadventitial plane of the carotid artery. Actually, this is the adventitial plane directly outside the media, where every cut and snip produces bleeding. This strongly suggests that all these tissues should be meticulously divided between clamps and tied to control blood loss. By inserting the tip of a clamp or the point of the scissors under the tumor and just outside the artery, a plane can usually be developed to allow clamping and division so that the arteries can be gradually dissected out of the tumor. Only a small minority of arteries require resection if the proper plane is achieved. If complete removal of the tumor becomes necessary, the surgeon should not hesitate to resect and repair the artery rather than leave tumor tissue in place.[13]

Management of the Carotid Arteries

Since the chief hazard of removal of a chemodectoma is disturbance of the carotid arterial supply to the brain, it behooves the surgeon to protect this throughout the procedure. Simple ligation of either carotid artery is outmoded because of its danger and the availability of methods for reconstructing the artery.

Any procedure upon such tumors should be begun only by a surgeon whose skill and team

TABLE 23-1 MORBIDITY AND MORTALITY OF OPERATIONS UPON CAROTID BODY TUMORS

Author	Institution	No. of operations	Vascular reconstructions	Strokes	Nerve injuries	Deaths
Rosen[10]	U. Toronto	24	8	0	8	1
Lees[9]	Cleveland Clinic	15	2	1	4	0
You-xian[15]	Shanghai, China	60	14	2	20	1
Chambers[12]	Washington and Baltimore, 1946–1968	38	5	0	*	0
Shamblin[16]	Mayo Clinic	70	NA†	16	NA†	3
Javid[11]	Rush-Pres-St. Luke's Med Ctr, Chicago	24	8	0	7	1
Dent[14]	U. Michigan	16	5	0	0	0
Van Asperen de Boer[8]	U. Leyden	34	NA†	1	10	0
Farr[17]	Memorial, New York	62	6	4	1	1‡

*Unstated.
†Not available.
‡Since 1945.

provide the ability to reconstruct the carotid artery if that proves necessary. A donor vein (preferably the saphenous) site should be prepared and draped for possible use.

Only rarely has the carotid already become occluded, so no collateral circulation is to be expected; an intraarterial shunt should be included in the plans for the procedure. The shunt can be temporarily placed through an anastomosis or a vein graft while the anastomoses are being constructed.

Alcott and associates in 1981 proposed that if a preoperative balloon occulsion caused unconsciousness or if the cephalad occluded carotid pressure was below 50 mmHg that the carotid should not be resected, or if it were, required an internal shunt.[13] Whether this is a valid indication is no more clear than are studies during carotid endarterectomies. Since use of the shunt is simple and results with it are excellent at present it seems rational to use it regardless of pressure and to resect the artery if it is necessary to complete tumor removal.

Hemostasis

The importance of meticulous hemostasis and careful dissection has been recognized for a long time. In this case approximately 500 ligatures and suture-ligatures were placed, and electrocautery was used. No metal clips were placed for fear that these might later be dislodged. Despite the continuous attention to hemostasis during the entire 4-hour procedure, it was necessary to transfuse 3000 mL of blood. There was no time during the procedure when it appeared that the situation was becoming uncontrolled, but a recurrent tumor such as this forces the realization that another in the future might require staging or be virtually impossible to operate upon safely. An excellent team, proper exposure, and sufficient patience are requisites for success.

REFERENCES

1 Dial P, Marks C, Bolton J: Current management of paragangliomas. *Surg Gynecol Obstet* 1982, 155:187.
2 Rush BH: Familial bilateral carotid body tumors, *Surgery* 1963, 157:633.
3 Thompson JE: Disorders of the arterial system: Carotid body tumors, in Sabiston DC (ed): *Davis-Christopher Textbook of Surgery,* vol 1. Saunders, Philadelphia, 1981, p 1903.
4 Krupski WC, Effeney DJ, Ehrenfeld WK, Stoney RJ: Cervical chemodectoma: Technical considerations and management options. *Am J Surg* 1982, 244:215.
5 Levitt SA, Sheps SG, Espinoza RE, Remine WH, Harrison EG: Catecholamine-secreting paraganglioma of glomus–jugular region resembling pheochromocytoma. *N Engl J Med* 1969, 281:805.
6 Staats EF, Brown RL, Smith RR: Carotid body tumors, benign and malignant. *Laryngoscope* 1966, 76:907.
7 Rush, BF: Current concepts in the treatment of carotid body tumors. *Surgery* 1962, 52:679.
8 Van Asperen de Boer FRS, Terpstra JL, Vinic M: Diagnosis, treatment and operative complications of carotid body tumors. *Br J Surg* 1981, 68:433.
9 Lees, CD, Levine HL, Bevin EG, Tucker HM: Tumors of the carotid body: Experience with 42 operative cases. *Am J Surg* 1981, 141:362.
10 Rosen IB, Palmer JA, Golberg M, Mustard RA: Vascular problems associated with carotid body tumors. *Am J Surg* 1981, 142:45.
11 Javid H, Chawla SK, Dye WS, Hunter JA, Najafi H, Goldin MD, Sperry C: Carotid body tumor: Resection or reflection. *Arch Surg* 1976, 11:344.
12 Chambers RG, Mahoney WD: Carotid body tumors. *Am J Surg* 1968, 116:554.
13 Olcott C IV, Fee WE, Enzmann DR, Mehigan JT: Planned approach to the management of malignant invasion of the carotid artery. *Am J Surg* 1981, 142:123.
14 Dent TL, Thompson NW, Fry WF: Carotid body tumors. *Surgery* 1976, 80:365.
15 You-xian F, Qun S: Surgical treatment of carotid body tumors: Review of 63 cases. *Chin Med J* 1982, 95, 417.
16 Shamblin WR, ReMine WH, Sheps SG, Harrison EG Jr: Carotid body tumor (chemodectoma): Clinicopathologic analysis of ninety cases. *Am J Surg* 1971, 122:732.
17 Farr HW: Carotid body tumors: A 40 year study. *CA* 1980, 30:260.

Invited Commentary

Jesse E. Thompson, M.D.
Dallas, Texas

Carotid body tumors are uncommon lesions whose removal is hazardous because of their location in the neck, adjacent to numerous essential structures. As stated, they should be managed by an experienced surgeon capable of handling problems with the carotid artery should they arise.

While most carotid body tumors are benign, the incidence of malignancy reported in the literature varies from 5 to 50 percent. The criteria of malignancy are controversial. Biological behavior cannot be predicted from the histologic appearance. The tumors may invade locally (e.g., into the carotid artery), give rise to regional lymphatic node metastases, or produce distant hematogenous metastases. They may also be considered malignant because of their location adjacent to vital structures in the neck. They do not regress spontaneously but grow slowly and progressively; an occasional tumor is aggressive and grows very rapidly. It is obvious that the best treatment is complete excision once the diagnosis is made.

A painless mass in the region of the carotid bifurcation should arouse suspicion of a carotid body tumor. While radionuclide scanning, sonography, and computerized tomographic scanning are useful diagnostic adjuncts, arteriography is mandatory for definitive diagnosis and proper planning of the operative procedure. Biopsy, both needle and open, should be avoided because of the hazards of bleeding and of complicating the subsequent operation.

As mentioned in the text, with innovations in vascular surgical techniques during the past 30 years, indications for operative removal of carotid body tumors have been liberalized, so the vast majority of patients should be offered operation. Only those patients with limited life expectancy, for whatever reason, or the rare neglected case that is inoperable because of local conditions in the neck remain for nonoperative management.

Technical aspects of the operation are of critical importance, and dissection must be meticulous, since complications may arise from injury to cranial nerves, from injury to the carotid artery itself, or from cerebral ischemia giving rise to strokes. Dissection in the subadventitial plane allows most carotid body tumors to be removed while the carotid artery is left intact. Occasionally, the internal carotid artery must be resected, as in the illustrative case, because of previous surgery, tumor invasion, or prior irradiation. The use of temporary carotid shunts followed by appropriate graft replacement makes carotid artery resection a safe and acceptable procedure in complicated cases. Since the blood supply to these tumors arises almost entirely from the external carotid artery, John Connell of Melbourne, Australia, has described a simplified technique of tumor removal. In selected cases, he first divides the external carotid artery and then resects a portion of it along with the tumor, employing an internal shunt from common carotid to internal carotid. This provides cerebral protection, allows easy identification of the internal carotid during subadventitial dissection, and markedly reduces operative blood loss.

As emphasized in the text, with modern methods of diagnosis and operation, most carotid body tumors can now be resected successfully with low morbidity and mortality rates (Table 23-1). In fact, several recent series have been published showing no surgical mortality or serious neurologic complications.

24 INFECTIONS

The incidence of infection following vascular surgical procedures is low, but the results of infection for the individual patient are terrible. Indeed, infected grafts are the bête noire of the vascular surgeon to the extent that today a high rate of infection would force curtailment of grafting operations.

Infection rates have declined in the past decade. In the largest study to that date Szilagyi in 1972 reported a 5.2 percent infection rate among 3347 vascular reconstructions (1.9 percent for synthetic grafts).[1] A later study of 400 patients showed an overall infection rate of 1.5 percent. Only 1 of these had a graft infection.[2]

In 1983 Bunt collected and summarized 575 reported vascular infections.[3,4]* Obviously, many have been unreported. It is generally believed that infection rates now range between 1.5 percent and 3 percent.[5,6]

As Caesar divided Gaul, so Szilagyi divided wound infections into three classes: superficial (class 1), subcutaneous (class 2), and graft (class 3).[1] Class 1 and 2 infections can usually be managed by prompt drainage and antibiotic therapy, without long-term ill effects. However, until such infections are eradicated, they have the potential of penetrating deeper and involving the artery and/or the graft. Thus, early, vigorous, and continued therapy is mandatory.

Class 3 infections involving the artery and/or graft are at once limb- and life-threatening. Mortality rates of 29 percent,[7] 41 percent,[8] and 75 percent[9] and amputation rates of 30 percent or more attest to their great hazard.

The vascular wound infection rates in our hospital are shown in Table 24-1. These low rates reflect the continuing effort of every member of the vascular surgical service—nurses, residents, and surgeons—to achieve a zero rate of infection by paying attention to every detail of prophylaxis and prevention.

It is also interesting to note that costs rise somewhat for class 1 and 2 infections but increase markedly for class 3, reflecting the considerably longer hospital time and care needed (Figure 24-1).

Organisms

Staphylococcus aureus outranks all other varieties of organisms which may occur, causing about 50 percent of the infections, with *Escherichia coli* a distant second at 10 to 20 percent.[8] Table 24-2 summarizes our previously reported experience with pathogenic organisms during 1976–1977.[10]

*Bunt's two articles in 1982 and 1983 provide an overall view of infections, along with a large list of pertinent references.

TABLE 24-1 VASCULAR SURGERY SERVICE INFECTIONS IN 1983 AT ST. THOMAS HOSPITAL, NASHVILLE

Month	No. of vascular operations*	No. of infections: Superficial	Deep	Total	Percent infected
January	120	4	0	4	3.3
February	109	3	1	4	3.7
March	118	0	1	1	0.8
April	109	1	2	3	2.8
May	114	2	0	2	1.8
June	136	3	0	3	2.2
July	118	1	1	2	1.6
August	138	1	1	2	1.4
September	124	1	2	3	2.4
October	115	5	1	6	4.3
November	107	4	0	4	3.8
December	58	0	1	1	1.7
Total	1366	25 (1.8%)	10 (0.7%)	35	2.6

*Varicose vein operations and sympathectomies are omitted.

FIGURE 24-1 Costs rise with the increasing severity of wound infections.

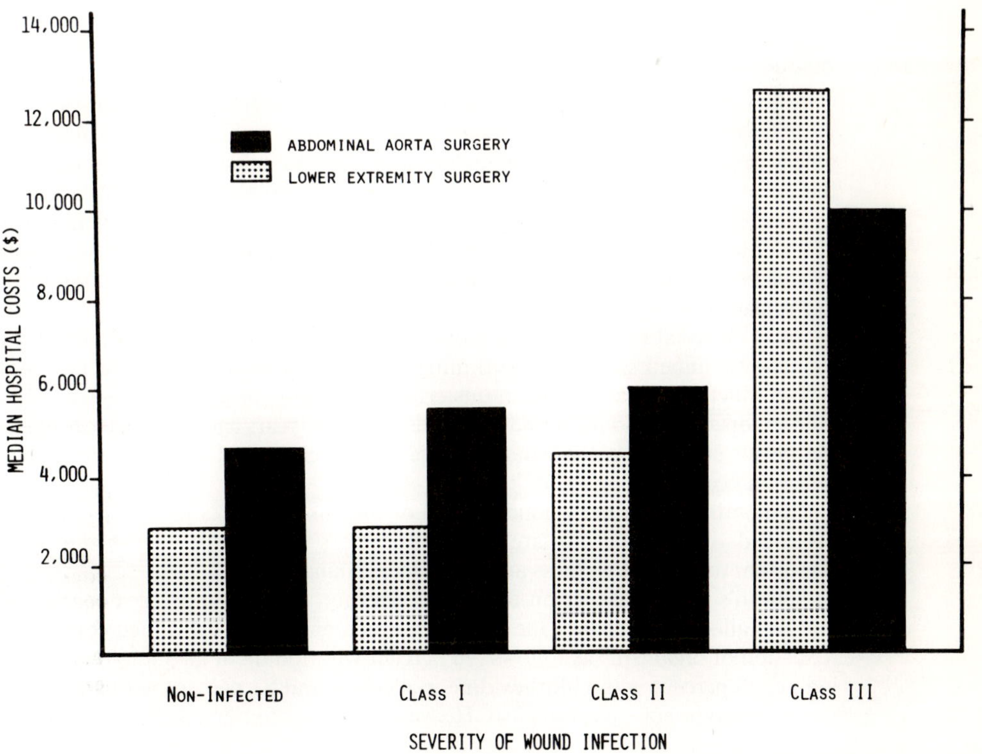

TABLE 24-2 BACTERIAL PATHOGENS ISOLATED FROM WOUND INFECTIONS, 1976–1977

Pathogen	Number of pathogens by category of infection 1	2	3	Total number of pathogens
Staphylococcus aureus (coagulase-positive)	3	5	1	9
Mixed staphylococci and gram-negative bacilli	0	1	1	2
Gram-negative enteric bacilli	0	2	2*	4
Mixed enteric bacilli and gram-positive cocci	0	2	0	2
(No culture)	1	0	0	0
Total	4	10	4	18

*One patient developed a urinary tract infection and sepsis due to cefazolin-sensitive *E. coli* 48 hours after graft implantation; graft dehiscence occurred 13 days postoperatively; cultures obtained on the seropurulent fluid at the time of reexploration while the patient was on antimicrobials were sterile.

PREVENTION

Despite all efforts it is unlikely that any open wound can be maintained more than briefly without bacterial contamination. It therefore behooves the surgeon (1) to minimize this inoculation, (2) to guard the body's defensive mechanisms, and (3) to destroy contaminating organisms as far as possible.

Preventing Inoculation of the Wound

Considerable attention to wound contamination by bacteria from the air itself has centered about joint replacements, since the implanted foreign body must be kept sterile. From Charnley and others in England came recommendations that clean outside air be rapidly circulated through the operating room and that the team members be isolated with hoods and impervious gowns to prevent bacterial entry into the wound.[11] Later information, however, denied this "salutary effect of laminar air flow on the incidence of wound infections."[12] Cruse also objected to these expensive installations and used simple ways to achieve minimal infection rates (0.7 percent in hip replacements).[13] Following study of the expected benefits versus costs, when the new St. Thomas Hospital in Nashville was constructed, it was concluded that such elaborate operating rooms were unnecessary; our continuing experience attests to the correctness of this decision.

Introduction of bacteria from unsterile instruments or grafts is an error which is rare in the modern operating room. In one of my cases several years ago one unsterile graft did get as far as the towels adjacent to the wound before it was recognized as being unsterile. Fortunately, no infection occurred.

Contamination of the wound by skin organisms continues to be a problem. The usual acidic pH and dryness of the skin are important factors which limit microbial growth. It is therefore important to prevent wetness and other local changes.

Selwyn's recent discussion of skin preparation not only provides considerable information but also allows insight into the variables which encourage continued controversy. He reported reduction of organisms as follows: 96 percent with iodine in alcohol, 89 percent with povidone-iodine, 88 percent with chlorhexidine in alcohol, and 82 percent with aqueous chlorhexidine—variations to be sure, but not great. He went on to recommend a chlorhexidine-detergent-alcohol rinse for scrubbing the hands for 2 minutes, avoiding a brush (except for the nails), since that damages the skin and encourages subsequent bacterial colonization.[14]

The surgeon's gloves are so frequently punctured, especially as the duration of the procedure increases, that I have worn two gloves on the left hand for many years, since that is where the hard wear from forceps occurs. Double gloves do not significantly decrease the tactile sense.

It is the conventional wisdom that the skin and its edges should not be touched by the hands, instruments, or grafts. Adherent plastic drapes are useful. There are, however, a minority who disagree. Cruse, for example, cited a clean-wound infection rate of 1.5 percent with use of only cotton drapes versus 2.3 percent with adhesive plastic.[15] It is also notable that two experienced vascular surgical colleagues have never bothered to avoid skin contamination, without creating any problem with postoperative infections. The matter requires further study.

Preoperative skin preparation by povidone-iodine and showering cleanses the skin and provides a residual film. Cruse and Foord's prospective study of 23,649 surgical wounds in Calgary, Alberta, Canada showed a reduction of infections in clean wounds from 2.3 to 1.3 percent in patients who had preoperative antiseptic (hexachlorophene) showers.[16]

Shaving is postponed until a few minutes before the surgical incision is made, to minimize the time in which organisms can multiply in the tiny nicks and abrasions which the razor produces. Seropian and Reynolds reduced wound infections from 5.6 to 0.6 percent by using depilatory cream.[17] The skin irritation produced by chemical depilation may be severe enough to preclude its general use. Perhaps close clipping rather than either shaving or depilation will prove to be the optimal method.

Wound Management

There is general agreement that careful wound-management techniques are mandatory to produce a minimal rate of infection. Increasingly, experience has shown the importance of even more careful hemostasis, debridement of devitalized tissue, avoidance of opening tissue planes unnecessarily, and use of appropriate sutures in proper positions.

Open rubber dam drains have given way to closed suction drainage, the latter being freely used for 24 to 48 hours in large wounds, in obese individuals, and after secondary procedures in which oozing is difficult to stop completely. A closed suction drain is less dangerous than is a collection of serum or blood within the wound.

Because of its overuse, electrocautery is probably the most dangerous of the several available hemostatic methods. While "charcoal doesn't bleed," neither does it heal, and the tissues must absorb the burn products prior to final healing. The study of Cruse and Foord indicated doubling of the infection rate in all wound categories when the electrosurgical unit was used extensively.[16] Metal clips and fine ligatures are preferable to extensive use of electrocautery (although tissue toleration of these burns is surprising).

It has been stated that "wounds become infected in the operating room and the surgeon is primarily responsible,"[15] and it is, of course, common but unpublished knowledge that some surgeons have better results than others. This silence will end and known infection rates will come to mark openly surgeons and their results. They will reflect wound management.

An Irish report of a 25 percent infection rate among 53 groin wounds without antibiotic prophylaxis is contrasted with 2 percent infection among 152 groin wounds managed with antibiotics. The contrast attests to the importance of the antimicrobial agents but suggests that these drugs may "cover" poor technique, particularly since the same group reduced infections after varicose vein operations from 7 percent to zero by using antibiotics.[18] The same varicose vein procedure done in 1000 patients here without antibiotics had a 0.3 percent infection rate.

Williams, on the other hand, had no infections among 460 groin incisions, which he "ascribed . . . to wound care."[19]

Antibiotic Prophylaxis

The efficacy of perioperative antimicrobial prophylaxis of wound infection in peripheral vascular surgery has been widely debated. Controlled studies have been rare, in part because the low wound infection rate associated with peripheral vascular surgery would require a series of a very large size to achieve statistically significant results. In the absence of such controlled studies, proponents of pre-, peri-, and postoperative antimicrobial prophylaxis have emphasized the high morbidity and mortality associated with graft infections, the success of prophylaxis in uncontrolled reports, and the reproducible efficacy of antimicrobials in experimental studies. Opponents of unrestricted prophylaxis have pointed out that the relatively low infection rate in peripheral vascular surgery does not justify the needless exposure of the vast majority of patients to potentially toxic antimicrobials. Additionally, results from occasional clinical studies have suggested that prophylactic antimicrobials may not be useful in peripheral vascular surgery. Thus, Simmons and Stoley commented that the prophylactic use of antibiotics should undergo the greatest scrutiny, since their common use, especially in surgery, is supported by very few appropriately designed, randomized, controlled clinical trials.[20]

In an effort to solve this problem we conducted a randomized blind propsective study to contrast cefazolin with placebo saline among 565 patients.[10] All patients undergoing elective aortic or peripheral vascular surgery were eligible for the study, provided there was no area of wet gangrene or cellulitis and no history of severe penicillin allergy. Informed consent was obtained. Only 2 patients declined entry into the program after its explanation; 1 was excluded because of history of severe penicillin reaction, and 18 were omitted inadvertently.

The efficacy of cephalosporins against staphylococci and the relatively low incidence of toxic and allergic reactions associated with their use prompted selection of this class of antimicrobial. Cefazolin was chosen from among the cephalosporins because of its high sustained serum levels, lack of renal toxicity, low cost, and ease of administration.

The Placef (placebo-cefazolin) study was administered by the pharmacist, who supplied the floor nurse with the solution, to be given with on-call medications prior to operation; another similar dose was given intravenously every 6 hours for four more doses. The Placef solution contained either 1 g of cefazolin in 100 mL of saline or 100 mL of saline alone. The two were indistinguishable, and the code was broken only after the wound follow-up was completed.

Wounds were inspected daily, and if infections occurred, they were classified as superficial (class 1), subcutaneous (class 2), or graft (class 3). Patients were also inspected daily for evidence of antibiotic sensitivity.

Since no infections occurred among 103 consecutive patients undergoing carotid or brachiocephalic arterial surgery, such were thereafter excluded from the study.

The results of 462 patients undergoing abdominal aorta and/or lower-extremity vascular repairs are shown in Table 24-3.

The differences in infection rates of the wound itself (class 1 and class 2) were statistically significant ($p < 0.0002$). There were only four infections of the graft; this difference was not statistically significant. However, all occurred in placebo patients, of whom two died and the other two lost limbs.

It appears from our study that the primary effect of cefazolin prophylaxis was to prevent all potential infections due to staphylococci. Side effects of the prophylactic antibiotic were compared with those of the saline. When the study was concluded and the code was broken, it was learned that skin rash (two instances) and arm vein phlebitis (two instances) had occurred only in patients receiving placebo. No patient had a cefazolin-induced complication. Moreover, it was apparent that resistant bacterial flora had not been induced by the cefazolin prophylaxis, since there was no increase in the incidence of cefazolin-resistant strains in the treated patients as compared with the controls. The site of occurrence of infections is shown in Table 24-4 and Figure 24-2.

TABLE 24-3 WOUND INFECTION AMONG 462 CLEAN VASCULAR PATIENTS

Prophylaxis	No. of patients	No. of infections: Superficial (class 1)	Subcutaneous (class 2)	Graft (class 3)	Percent infected
Placebo	237	4	8	4	6.8
Cefazolin	225	0	2	0	0.9

TABLE 24-4 RATIO OF PATIENTS WITH INFECTION TO PATIENTS WITHOUT INFECTION, BY SITE OF INCISION AND PROPHYLACTIC REGIMEN

Site	Prophylactic regimen: Cefazolin	Placebo	Total
Abdomen	1/86 = 1.2%	8/98 = 8.2%	9/184 = 4.9%
Groin	0/179 = 0%	2/179 = 1.1%	2/358 = 0.6%
Leg	1/117 = 0.9%	6/111 = 5.4%	7/228 = 3.1%

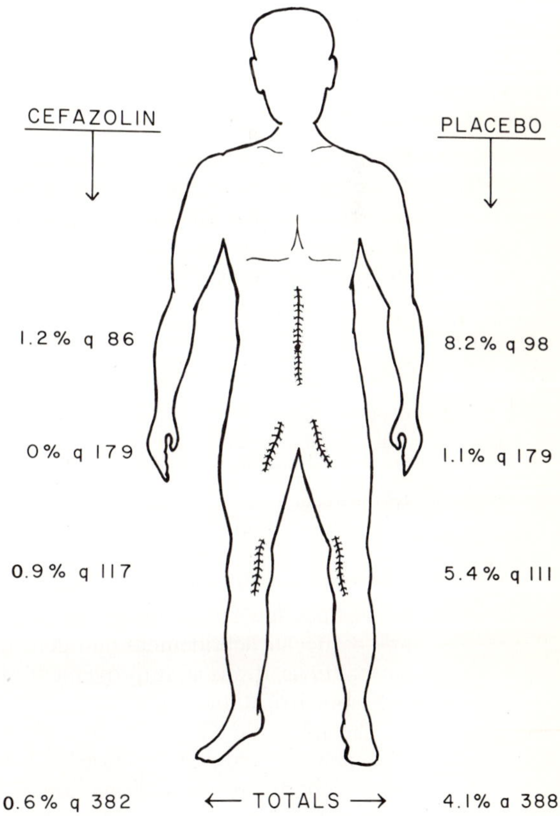

FIGURE 24-2 The incidence of infections at different operative sites. In the prospective double-blind study this was less in each area when antibiotic pretreatment was used.[10]

Analysis of the infection rates by site of incision is of interest, since the groin incisions (0.6 percent infected) fared better than did either those in the abdominal wall (4.9 percent) or those in the lower thigh and leg. Perhaps this reflects our great concern for groin incision, which elsewhere, and also earlier in our experience, has caused more problems than the others. We now exercise extreme care in the management of groin incisions.

It is important to recognize that the number of grafts which became infected in our study was too small to allow statistical proof of the virtue of the prophylactic cefazolin in preventing class 3 infections. However, all of the four such patients (Table 24-3) received placebo saline rather than antibiotics. Additionally, there were significantly more class 1 and 2 infections among saline recipients. Further accumulation of data was stopped at that time in the belief that no more patients should be subjected to the risk involved when they received no antibiotics.

It was concluded that cefazolin was effective in the prophylaxis of infections, and its use therefore continues as 1 g cefazolin administered intravenously prior to operation and 1-g doses following at 6-hour intervals for four doses.

More recently, Stone and associates reemphasized the importance of antibiotic dosage prior to incision and reported that the continuation of antibiotics after the patient left the recovery room did not alter the incidence of wound infection or of postoperative intraabdominal infections.[21]

Antibiotic-Bonded Synthetic Grafts

These grafts are attractive in terms of a high local concentration of the antimicrobial during and immediately after the grafting procedure. Laboratory studies suggest increased resistance over a 6- to 12-week period to organisms implanted at the original operation.[22] The later characteristics are unknown.[23] These grafts have not been evaluated clinically, nor are they yet available for use.

Irrigation of Wounds

Surgeons have traditionally washed wounds with saline prior to closure, sometimes with additives, on the basis that wound debris were removed and that bacterial contamination was decreased mechanically if not otherwise. Two general classes of additives have been advocated: first, one of a variety of antiseptics, the current favorite being povidone-iodine; and second, one or a mixture of the antibiotics.

Antiseptics

The original use of carbolic acid in wounds by Joseph Lister occurred prior to any program of asepsis. Although now recognized as a great victory over infection, at the time it was controversial and was widely accepted on the Continent before it was in the United States or in Great Britain, where the concept originated. The use of this toxic antiseptic faded as asepsis became recognized.

During World War I, Alexis Carrel along with Dakin developed an antiseptic sodium hypochlorite solution, which they used for the constant irrigation of war wounds which were closed about indwelling tubes.[24] This technique became known as the Carrel-Dakin system. The regimen comes down to the present as Dakin's solution. Although the idea of closing wounds without any particular debridement and depending on antiseptic irrigation to encourage healing seems strange to us, it was an improvement over the previous practice of the same closure without any antiseptic irrigation.

The antiseptic era essentially ended about the middle of the present century as principles of wide debridement and drainage for heavily contaminated wounds became well-recognized and were supported by the systemic use of antimicrobial drugs. Along with this there developed the concept that antiseptics killed tissue cells as well as surface bacteria, while hardly affecting bacteria already in the tissues. A return to antiseptic irrigation is therefore a retrogression rather than a forward step.

The development of iodophors such as povidone-iodine predictably has attracted surgical interest because the solution looks like an antiseptic and smells like one. Whether or not it prevents infection or in fact does nothing more than harm the wound is uncertain. The English surgeon Gilmore reviewed the evidence in 1980 and concluded that "there is no doubt that, allied to good surgical technique, topical povidone-iodine will reduce wound infection."[25] Further evidence casts doubt upon that opinion. Rodeheaver and his associates tested povidone-iodine against *Staphylococcus* injected into guinea pig wounds and found "no therapeutic benefit when compared with control wounds treated with saline solution." In fact, if detergents were added to the iodophor, the effect was deleterious and wounds exposed to that combination had significantly higher infection rates than untreated controls. They recommended that aqueous iodine solutions and iodophor surgical scrub solution not be used in open wounds.[26] Nichols discussed that report and summarized his experience with iodophor peritoneal irrigation in animals with fecal peritonitis and concluded that it was dangerous as well as ineffective.[27] Rogers, Blouin, and O'Leary contrasted povidone-iodine with saline in 187 surgical patients in a veterans hospital here and found "no significant difference . . . between those patients whose wounds were irrigated with normal saline and . . . with povidone-iodine."[28] Zamora's editorial comments in 1984 regarding wound irrigation with providone-iodine were succinct. He noted the variation in experimental models and their reports, strongly suggested no higher concentration than 1%, and concluded that "it only appears worthwhile to use it in contaminated and dirty cases."[29]

No antiseptic or antimicrobial drugs are used for irrigation of wounds on our vascular service; the irrigant consists only of sterile isotonic saline.

MANAGEMENT OF INFECTIONS

Superficial Infections

Infections of the skin (class 1) and subcutaneous tissues (class 2) overlying vascular grafts are certainly more threatening than similar ones in nonvascular patients. If a groin incision for node biopsy or an abdominal wound for gastrectomy becomes infected, it can be opened widely with the expectation of resolution of infection, the development of granulations, and slow but sure healing. Antibiotics may be used, but once wide drainage is established, they are not critical.

The management of skin and subcutaneous infection of the abdominal wall after aortic grafting is no different, since the graft lies at a distance and is far separated from the infection. Open drainage solves the problem. Attempts to resolve the matter by removing one or two sutures and inserting a drain are often fruitless—the infection requires removal of enough of the skin sutures to guarantee complete unroofing so that no pockets of pus remain. Failure to provide wide drainage may occur because the surgeon is reluctant to recognize the complication or because there is faulty understanding of the management of an infected wound.* Some infections subside after a small drain is placed, but the practice is risky and often leads to even further delay in healing.

Infections in groin and lower-limb incisions are different because of the proximity of the underlying graft, whose involvement is at once threatened by any type of skin or subcutaneous infection. Early recognition is important in preventing spread of the superficial infection to the underlying graft. If there is a real question of infection in a groin or limb wound, it should be explored in the operating room rather than observed expectantly. Exploration may be ended in the fat if the infection does not extend deeply, with the expectation of prompt granulation and healing of the superficial layers. On the other hand, if the process is found to extend deeply, involving the graft and/or the anastomosis, cultures aid in selecting the appropriate antibiotic

*It is ironic that those surgeons who least understand the management of infections are so often called upon to treat them.

therapy while local procedures are directed toward removal of conditions which encourage bacterial proliferation.

Infected Grafts

One of the advantages of an *autogenous graft* such as the saphenous vein is its resistance to infection. If the complication is recognized early and the wound is widely opened to provide prompt and complete drainage, the appearance of the pulsating vein graft lying at the bottom is frightening, but it may be expected to remain patent or to thrombose without any great danger of hemorrhage. Over the years we have managed several such infections by widely opening the wound, packing it with saline-soaked gauze (avoiding iodoform- or iodophor-soaked sponges), changing the dressings with mask-and-glove precautions, and awaiting granulation and secondary closure of the wound. If the graft thombroses, the wound should be allowed to close firmly prior to a secondary revascularization.

In the past it was general experience that infection would persist or recur until a synthetic graft was removed. Szilagyi expressed this concept by saying that "success in salvaging an infected arterial prosthesis is a very rare exception to the rule."[30] Nevertheless, the numerous reports of such success without removal of a patent graft suggest the alternative plan of sterilization, by either antibiotic or antiseptic drugs, and retention of the graft in the extremity. If that program is undertaken, the risk of serious, life-threatening hemorrhage from an infected anastomosis must be recognized and accepted.

Successful salvage of femoral grafts in groin wounds has occurred repeatedly since Carter, Cohen, and Whelan reported their seven cases treated by antibiotic instillation[31] and Shumacker and Mandelbaum reported their two in 1963.[32] Smith, Lowry, and Perdue rescued eight of nine infected limb grafts by this technique as long ago as 1967.[33] In 1977 Liekweg and Greenfield reported 81 percent recovery among 17 patients with infected groin grafts who were treated by irrigation with antibiotics.[8] A system of continuous irrigation of antibiotic solution through an indwelling catheter for 7 to 10 days was also described by Popovsky and Singer, whose three patients healed groin infections with synthetic grafts in place.[34] Ghosn, Rabbat, and Trudel healed three infected aortobifemoral grafts without removal of the graft. After surgical drainage and debridement of the groin an antibiotic irrigation system via indwelling tubes was maintained for 1 to 4 months. The mortality rate of 23 percent, with amputations in 8 percent of the survivors, was better than some reported results, but because of the long hospitalization periods required this procedure is not recommended if similar results can be obtained more quickly.[35]

Personal experience with a few infected groin grafts indicates that early exploration with debridement and wound closure protected by antibiotics often succeeds. Operative removal of any hematoma, along with excision of necrotic fat, at once rids the wound of excellent culture media. The wound may then be treated by irrigation with an appropriate antiseptic or antibiotic or closed with frequent instillation of antibiotics through indwelling catheters. After the wound is debrided, it is closed snugly about the graft with two or three layers of deeply placed continuous 3-0 Dexon sutures. The skin is closed with interrupted 4-0 Dacron mattress sutures. As Figures 24-3 and 24-4 show, two no. 18 polyethylene tubes are led from the depths of the wound, through each of which 2 mL of antibiotic solution is injected every 2 hours for 5 days.

An alternative is to leave the wound open and irrigate with a solution such as dilute povidone-iodine, as demonstrated by Kwaan and Connolly.[36] A bag fitted about the wound confines the solution as well as wound excretions and allows run-off into a bedside container. This program may result in granulation and healing, or some form of flap closure may be needed to close the wound over the graft.

In some patients an infected femoral graft must be removed because it has thrombosed or because the anastomosis has bled or is bleeding. Some of these grafts may not require immediate revascularization. Delay until the wound is solidly healed is in order.

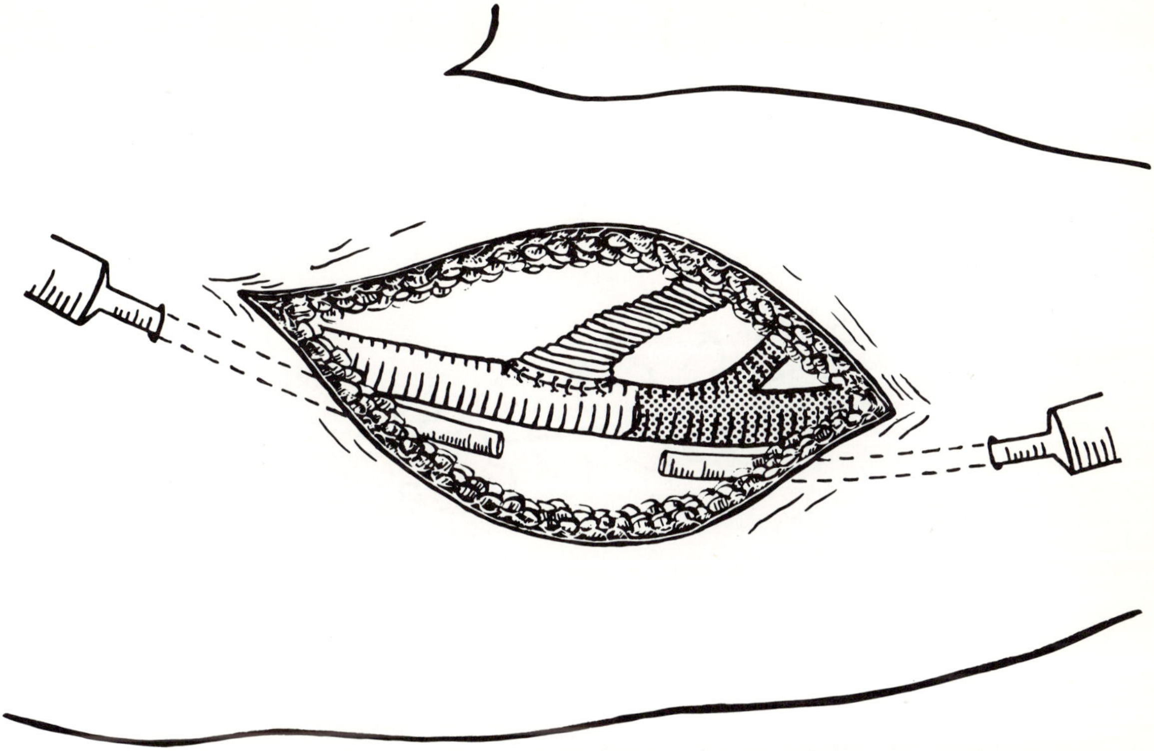

FIGURE 24-3 An early infection of a graft in the groin may sometimes be successfully treated by immediate debridement of the wound and secondary closure. Small polyethylene catheters are led out through stab wounds prior to multilayer closure over the still-patent graft.

If immediate revascularization is required, an extraanatomic pathway is needed to avoid the infected field.[37] The obturator foramen pathway was described by Shaw and Baue in 1962 for extraanatomic bypass.[38] If the obturator foraminal route is chosen, the surgeon should note the precautions against vascular injury suggested by Guida and Moore. The membrane across the foramen should be opened posterior to the neurovascular bundle.[39] Difficulties with intraoperative hemorrhage from the obturator artery recounted by VanDet and Brands further emphasize this hazard.[40] A good route to the foramen is via an extraperitoneal approach in which a hand is placed within the pelvis to guide a long clamp, which is passed proximally from a midthigh route posterior to the adductor magnus muscle.

Simpler routes are available through the tissues of the lateral abdomen or medially via the suprapubic area or the perineal tissues, so the obturator pathway is not used frequently.

Aortic Graft Infection

Infection of an aortic graft at once threatens not only one or both lower limbs but life as well. Comprehensive diagnostic measures and drastic surgical treatment are needed at once. The twofold problem consists not only of removal of the infected synthetic material but also of revascularization, since only occasional patients will tolerate ligation of the aorta without losing one or both lower extremities.

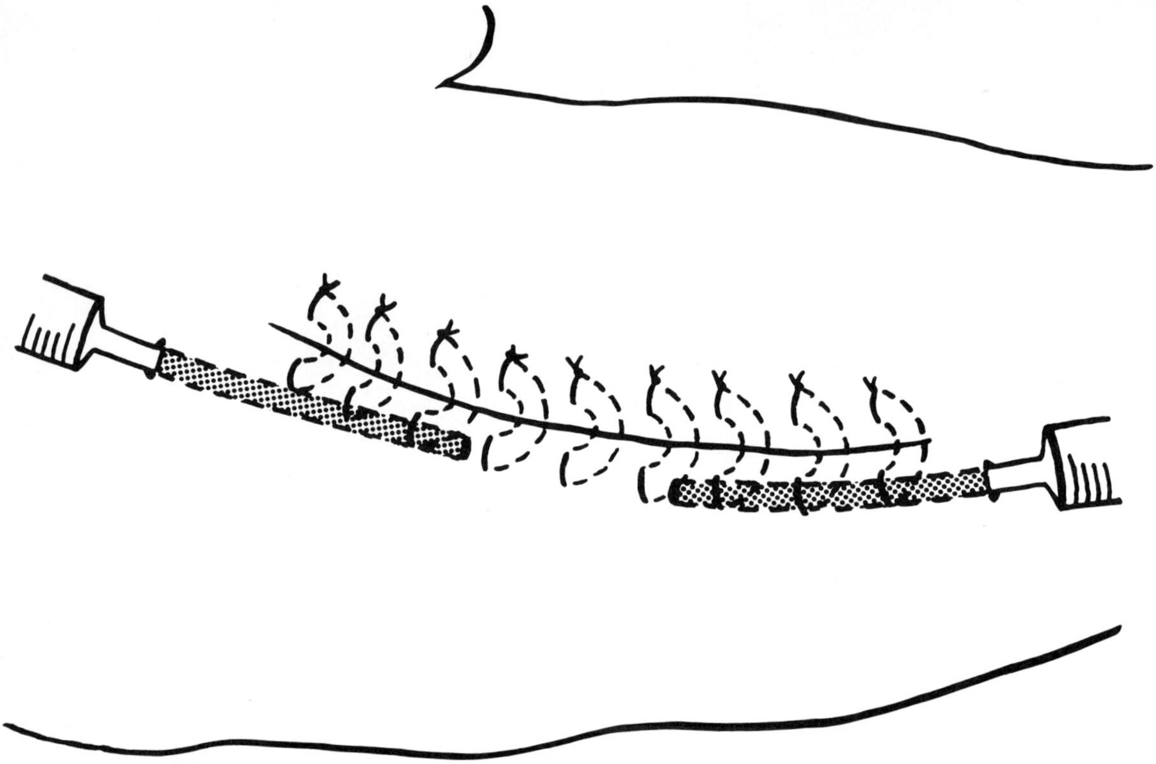

FIGURE 24-4 Local instillation of 2 mL of antibiotic solution into each indwelling polyethylene catheter is done every 2 hours for 5 days.

Diagnosis Chronic infection of an aortic prosthesis without distal extension to the femoral anastomosis may be difficult to detect. Back or abdominal pain, fever, and systemic signs may suggest the diagnosis. If a graft limb has been anastomosed in the groin area, the initial indication may be formation of an abscess or a chronic sinus there.

Special studies include injection of a sinus with radiopaque material to determine its extent and proximity to the graft. Needle aspiration for culture material may be repeated. Computed tomography (CT) scans with contrast enhancement may show whether gas or fluid has accumulated about a deeply placed graft. Ultrasound may also be useful. Gastrointestinal endoscopy is indicated if there is any question of an aortoenteric fistula. Finally, surgical exploration may be necessary to establish the diagnosis.

Sometimes the infection is localized to one groin while the aortic portion and contralateral limb of the graft remain uninfected. Again, sinograms, ultrasound, and CT scans are helpful in determining whether a proximal extension of the infection has occurred.

If the infection is limited to the groin anastomosis, the proximal portion of the graft may be salvaged by detaching it through a noninfected area. The extraperitoneal space is entered through a high extraperitoneal incision to expose the clean iliac limb of the graft distal to the bifurcation. The graft is divided and its ends oversewn. A culture is made to determine whether infection exists at the point of division. Soft tissues in the area are then sutured between the divided ends to seal off the proximal portion of the graft, which is to be retained.

While it has been suggested that as much as 2 weeks is necessary to allow sealing of the tissues placed between the divided ends of the graft, this is usually too long. As soon as cultures have proved to be sterile, after the lapse of 3 or 4 days the distal infected portion of the graft may be removed. In one quite surprising instance it became apparent that local measures were cleaning up the groin wound; the distal nonpatent graft was simply allowed to remain in place.

Illustrative Case A 74-year-old male in January 1975 had an aortobifemoral Dacron graft, which by June of 1975 had formed a false aneurysm in the right groin. It was replaced with a new segment of Dacron. A week later the groin wound and graft had become infected with *Staphylococcus aureus.*

Infection persisted despite antibiotics, wide opening of the wound, and local treatment. Twelve days later through an extraperitoneal approach the proximal limb of the Dacron graft was divided, the proximal end was oversewn, and the soft tissue was sutured between the ends, the plan being to remove the distal portion of the graft through the open wound in the groin several days later. The limb remained viable, and the wound granulated over the thrombosed distal portion of the graft and eventually completely healed with that foreign body in place. In the 9 years which have elapsed since then, the patient has not been seen personally, but oral communication has indicated no further wound problem. He continues to walk.

Comment Infection of the graft was explained by the positive culture obtained from the wound at the time of the second operation. There is no explanation for the complete healing of the wound, which still retains the Dacron graft. Happily, collateral circulation prevented loss of the limb or even severe symptoms. Such a favorable result cannot be expected to occur often.

Management If infection has extended to involve the proximal portion of the graft, both limbs, or the entire graft, then it must be removed completely. Closure of the proximal aortic stump is fraught with the danger of continued infection leading to necrosis and hemorrhage. The standard closure has been to place monofilament synthetic mattress sutures plus a distal over-and-over suture.

The high incidence of rupture of the closed proximal aortic stump (30 percent in Kiernan's series from the Mayo Clinic[41] and 4 of the 6 deaths among the 21 patients in the Buchbinder series[42]) has prompted a search for a better method to close the aorta after removal of an infected graft. Shah and the Karmody group in 1983 reported clinical success using a pedicled seromuscular jejunal patch placed over the sutured end of the proximal aorta. One patient did well for a subsequent year. Two others died too soon to determine long-term results, but their aortas were intact at 4 days and 6 weeks respectively.[43]

It has also been suggested that the renal arterial origins be repositioned (to the splenic on the left and the hepatic on the right) so that suture closure of the proximal aorta can be made in healthy tissue just distal to the superior mesenteric artery. That is a needlessly complicated technique which does not allow escape from the already infected field of operation.

Revascularization to prevent limb loss is usually necessary after removal of an aortic graft. Observation at the operating table or in the recovery room is unreliable and dangerous.[44] A recent proposal that revascularization be delayed was based upon a retrospective study of only 20 patients, among whom there was extremely high mortality following immediate revascularization. This was judged to be due to the longer procedure and the need for more blood.[45] The argument is not convincing either to me or to others.[46] Revascularization should be established prior to or at the time of removal of an aortic graft.

Often the infection is a chronic smoldering lesion; in such cases there is time to establish an extraanatomic bypass a few days prior to removal of the graft.[47] Alternatively, the bypass may be completed just prior to removal of the infected graft.

If the infected field is entered before the extraanatomic bypass is performed, the graft may be removed and all wounds closed prior to repreparing, redraping, and performing of a clean extraanatomic procedure. The operator should place the distal limbs of the axillobifemoral graft to the superficial femoral artery in its midportion, thus avoiding passing the graft through an infected field.

An alternative method of revascularization is one-stage removal of the infected aortic graft along with endarterectomy of the aorta and the iliac and femoral vessels. This provides removal of the infected synthetic material and uses autogenous vessels to carry blood through the infected field. Ehrenfeld and his San Francisco associates in 1979 reported a 13 percent death rate and 6 percent amputation rate among 24 patients on whom this technique was used. The series was updated in 1983 to 14 percent mortality and 25 percent limb loss. The series had a lower risk with use of autogenous reconstruction (14 percent of 56) than with extraanatomic bypass (41 percent of 29).[47] Seeger and his Norfolk team lost only 1 of 11 such patients (9 percent mortality). Their procedure was an eversion thromboendarterectomy of the aortoiliac segment with attached saphenous or arm veins.[48] It is clear that autogenous tissue revascularization should be considered for these repairs, although the incidence of late infections is not yet known.[49]

In view of the high mortality and amputation rates associated with graft removal and extraanatomic bypass, several voices have suggested that the infected aortic graft need not always be removed. Knight, Farnell, and Hollier irrigated a Dacron aortic graft infected with *Fusobacterium necrophorum* with 2500 ml of 0.5% povidone-iodine daily for 18 days, which resulted in sterilization of the graft with no recurrence of infection at the 25-month follow-up.[50] On the other hand, Liekweg and Greenfield reported a 69 percent mortality rate when this nonoperative management was used.[8] Current standard therapy requires removal of an infected aortic graft.

REFERENCES

1 Szilagyi DE, Smith RF, Elliott JP, Vrandecic MP: Infection and arterial reconstruction with synthetic grafts. *Ann Surg* 1972, 176:321.

2 May ARL, Darling RC, Brewster DC, Darling CS: A comparison of the use of cephalothin and oxacillin in vascular surgery. *Arch Surg* 1980, 115:56.

3 Bunt TJ: Synthetic vascular graft infections: I. Graft infections. *Surgery* 1982, 93:733.

4 Bunt TJ: Synthetic vascular graft infections: II. Graft-enteric erosions and graft-enteric fistulas. *Surgery* 1983, 94:1.

5 Bernhard VM, Towne JB: Complications in vascular surgery, in Moore WS (ed): *Vascular Surgery: A Comprehensive Review.* Grune & Stratton, New York, 1983, p 765.

6 Moore WS: Infection of vascular grafts: Incidence, bacteriology and pathogenesis, in Bernhard VM, Towne JB (eds): *Complications in Vascular Surgery,* Grune & Stratton, New York, 1980, pp 483–489.

7 Bouhoutsos J, Chauatazas D, Martin P, Morris T: Infected synthetic arterial grafts. *Br J Surg* 1974, 61:108.

8 Liekweg WG, Greenfield LJ: Vascular prosthetic infections: Collected experience and results of treatment. *Surgery* 1977, 81:335.

9 Fry WJ, Lindenauer SM: Infection complicating the use of plastic arterial implants. *Arch Surg* 1967, 94:600.

10 Dale WA, Kaiser AB: Prevention of infection in vascular surgery, in Karran S (ed): *Controversies in Surgical Sepsis.* Praeger, New York, 1980, pp 277–284.

11 Charnley J: Theater design, in Karran S (ed): *Controversies in Surgical Sepsis.* Praeger, New York, 1980, pp 1–13.

12 Laufman H: Operating room air. *J Surg Practice* 1979, 8:12.

13 Cruse P: Prevention of sepsis. Discussion in Karran S (ed): *Controversies in Surgical Sepsis.* Praeger, New York, 1980, p 68.

14 Selwyn S: Skin preparation, the surgical scrub and related rituals, in Karran S (ed): *Controversies in Surgical Sepsis.* Praeger, New York, 1980, p 23.

15 Cruse P: Surgical infection surveillance, in Karran S (ed): *Controversies in Surgical Sepsis.* Praeger, New York, 1980, p 327.

16 Cruse P, Foord R: A five-year prospective study of 23,649 wounds. *Arch Surg* 1973, 107:206.

17 Seropian R, Reynolds BM: Wound infections after preoperative dipilatory versus razor preparation. *Am J Surg* 1971, 121:251.

18 Pitt HA, Postier R, MacGowan W, Frank L, Surmak A, Sitzman J, Bouchier-Hayes D: Prophylactic antibiotics in vascular surgery. *Ann Surg* 1980, 192:356.

19 Williams RD: Discussion of Pitt HA, Postier R, MacGowan W, Frank L, Surmak A, Sitzman J, Bouchier-Hayes D: Prophylactic antibiotics in vascular surgery. *Ann Surg* 1980, 192:356.

20 Simmons HE, Stoley PD: This is medical progress? Trends and consequences of antibiotic use in the United States. *JAMA* 1974, 27:1023.

21 Stone HH, Haney BB, Kolb LD, Geheber CE, Hopper CA: Prophylactic and preventive antibiotic therapy. *Ann Surg* 1979, 189:691.

22 Greco RS, Harvey RA, Smilow PC, Tesoriero JV: Prevention of vascular prosthetic infection by a benzalkonium-oxacillin bonded polytetrafluoroethylene graft. *Surg Gynecol Obstet* 1982, 155:28.

23 Moore WS, Chvapil M, Sieffert G, Keown K: Development of an infection resistant vascular prosthesis. *Arch Surg* 1981, 116:1403.

24 Dale WA: The beginnings of vascular surgery. *Surgery* 1974, 76:849.

25 Gilmore OJA: The use of antiseptics, in Karran S (ed): *Controversies in Surgical Sepsis.* Praeger, New York, 1980, p 53.

26 Rodeheaver G, Bellamy W, Kody M, Spatafora G, Fitton L, Leyden K, Edlich R: Bactericidal activity and toxicity of iodine-containing solutions in wounds. *Arch Surg* 1982, 117:181.

27 Nichols RL: Discussion of Rodeheaver G, Bellamy W, Kody M, Spatafora G, Fitton L, Leyden K, Edlich R: Bactericidal activity and toxicity of iodine-containing solutions in wounds. *Arch Surg* 1982, 117:186.

28 Rogers D, Blouin G, O'Leary J: Povidone-iodine wound irrigation and wound sepsis. *Surg Gynecol Obstet* 1983, 157:426.

29 Zamora J: Povidone-iodine and wound infection. *Surgery* 1984, 95:121.

30 Szilagyi DE: Editorial comment on Popovsky J, Singer S: Infected prosthetic grafts: Local therapy with graft preservation. *Arch Surg* 1980, 115:203.

31 Carter SC, Cohen A, Whelan TJ: Clinical experience with management of the infected Dacron graft. *Ann Surg* 1963, 158:249.

32 Shumacker HB, Mandelbaum I: Continuous antibiotic irrigation in the treatment of infection. *Arch Surg* 1963, 86:384.

33 Smith RB, Lowry K, Perdue GD: Management of the infected arterial prosthesis in the lower extremity. *Am Surg* 1967, 33:711.

34 Popovsky J, Singer S: Infected prosthetic grafts: Local therapy with graft preservation. *Arch Surg* 1980, 115:203.

35 Ghosn PB, Rabbat AG, Trudel J: Why remove an infected aortofemoral graft? *Can J Surg* 1983, 26:330.

36 Kwaan JHM, Connolly JE: Successful management of prosthetic graft infection with continuous povidone-iodine irrigation. *Arch Surg* 1981, 116:716.

37 Tilson M, Sweeney T, Gusberg R, Stansel H: Obturator canal bypass grafts for septic lesions of the femoral artery. *Arch Surg* 1979, 114:1031.

38 Shaw RS, Baue AE: Management of sepsis complication in arterial reconstructive surgery. *Surgery* 1962, 53:75.

39 Guida PM, Moore WS: Obturator bypass technique. *Surg Gynecol Obstet* 1969, 128:1307.

40 VanDet RJ, Brands LC: The obturator foramen bypass: An alternative procedure in ileofemoral artery revascularization. *Surgery* 1981, 89:543.

41 Kiernan PD, Pairolero PC, Huber JP, Mucha P, Wallace RB: Aortic graft–enteric fistula. *Mayo Clin Proc* 1981, 55:731.

42 Buchbinder D, Leather RP, Shah DM, Karmody AM: Pathologic interactions between prosthetic aortic grafts and the gastrointestinal tract. *Am J Surg* 1980, 140:192.

43 Shah DM, Buchbinder D, Leather RP, Corson J, Karmody AM: Clinical use of the seromuscular jejunal patch for protection of the infected aortic stump. *Am J Surg* 1983, 146:198.

44 Ehrenfeld WK, Wilbur BG, Olcott CN, Stoney RJ: Autogenous tissue reconstruction in the management of infected prosthetic grafts. *Surgery* 1979, 85:82.

45 Turnipseed WD, Berkoff HA, Detmer DE, Acher CW, Belzer FO: Arterial graft infections. *Arch Surg* 1983, 118:410.

46 Read R: Discussion of Turnipseed WD, Berkoff HA, Detmer DE, Acher CW, Belzer FO: Arterial graft infections. *Arch Surg* 1983, 118:410.

47 Reilly LM, Altman H, Lusby RJ, Kersh RA, Ehrenfeld WK, Stoney RJ: Late results following surgical management of vascular graft infection. *J Vasc Surg* 1984, 1:36.

48 Seeger JM, Wheeler JR, Gregory RT, Snyder SO, Gayle RG: Autogenous graft replacement of infected prosthetic grafts in the femoral position. *Surgery* 1983, 93:39.

49 Goldstone J: Discussion of Reilly LM, Altman H, Lusby RJ, Kersh RA, Ehrenfeld WK, Stoney RJ: Late results following surgical management of vascular graft infection. *J Vasc Surg* 1984, 1:43.
50 Knight CD Jr, Farnell MB, Hollier LH: Treatment of aortic graft infection with povidone-iodine irrigation. *Mayo Clin Proc* 1983, 58:472.

Invited Commentary

Wesley S. Moore, M.D.
Los Angeles, California

The opening discussion correctly points out the high morbidity and mortality associated with vascular graft infection. The author reviews the important literature, which documents a low incidence of this complication and then attempts to compare the incidence of infection in his own hospital in the course of 1 year. He reports that there were 1366 vascular operations in 1983, only 10 of which (0.7 percent) resulted in deep wound infections. (The author does not state what percentage of the total operations employed vascular grafts and how many deep wound infections actually became graft infections later.) One other problem associated with looking at a single year's institutional experience is that not all graft infections are manifested by an initial acute wound infection. The majority of graft infections do not present until months or years after initial implantation. In review of our own experience over a 10-year interval, we found that the median time of presentation for graft sepsis was 3.5 months following implantation, with many cases presenting after 1 year. Therefore, looking at the most recent 1-year experience is likely to understate the actual incidence of graft sepsis.

There is appropriate emphasis upon prevention. The author also summarizes his own important randomized clinical study documenting the efficacy of antibiotic prophylaxis in preventing wound infection and its probable efficacy in reducing the incidence of graft sepsis. He emphasizes the importance of meticulous groin wound management as an important aspect in preventing graft sepsis. To this discussion I can only add the importance of skin closure technique. In my own experience, the use of transcutaneous skin sutures increases the incidence of wound complications in the groin. The use of subcuticular suture, Steri-strips, or, more recently, skin clips has materially contributed to improved rates of primary healing.

It is difficult to make the diagnosis of occult graft sepsis. Abdominal CT scanning and perigraft aspiration are helpful ways to establish the diagnosis prior to operation. It should also be pointed out that indium 111 oxime labeling of white blood cells has been extremely useful in identifying graft sepsis prior to exploration. I have had personal experience with this test in two cases of occult graft sepsis in the aortic position. Both cases were correctly identified by this technique prior to exploration.

Finally, the problem of late graft infection needs mention. Infected grafts that present months to years after placement may represent dormancy of organisms introduced at the time of graft placement or they may represent late infection from transient bacteremia. There is now ample experimental evidence combined with anecdotal clinical experience to suggest that grafts, like prosthetic or diseased heart valves, are susceptible to infection of bacteremic origin. For this reason, I make a point of cautioning my patients and their physicians to employ antibiotic prophylaxis when they are likely to be exposed to transient bacteremia, such as may occur during dental procedures, urologic procedures, endoscopy, etc.

25 REVASCULARIZATION OR AMPUTATION

The main effort of vascular surgeons today is directed toward reconstruction to prevent loss of an extremity by amputation. Nevertheless, not all legs can be saved and patients may still be rehabilitated by an amputation which heals promptly, conserves as much function as possible, and allows early use of a prosthesis. The total program for a patient whose leg is threatened should be correlated to ensure that revascularization is done if possible or, if not, to decide when and at what level amputation should occur. Prosthesis fitting and training must follow closely.

Revascularization procedures and amputations are not really alternative strategies for most patients; the indications usually point clearly to one or the other. A few patients present difficult decisions, but most are clearly candidates for revascularization or, if that appears unlikely of success, for amputation.

The experienced vascular surgeon revascularizes when possible but also skillfully performs the necessary amputation when advanced ischemia, severe tissue necrosis, and/or severe infection necessitate it, and thereafter supervises the prosthetist and physical therapist through the rehabilitation process.

THE AGGRESSIVE APPROACH FOR LIMB SALVAGE

Twenty years ago successful distal calf arterial reconstructions were performed,[1] and in 1967 the aggressive approach to revascularization of the threatened limb was further documented, including the salvage of the limbs of 58 percent of 100 consecutive patients who had either toe or foot gangrene or pain at rest requiring opiates for control. Of these 58 successes 52 were the end results of revascularizations, 5 others followed sympathectomy, and 1 was spontaneous.[2]

This aggressive approach to limb salvage has continued (Figure 25-1). Patients facing amputation are studied for the possibility of revascularization, and that is offered to most. This policy is attested by a recent retrospective analysis of 55 amputations, which showed that 87 percent had some form of revascularization procedure attempted or completed prior to the amputation. Occasionally patients or their families elect amputation, but most choose an attempt at salvage even in the face of a frank statement of the approximate chances of success.

This aggressive plan for limb salvage has since been widely accepted, with some notable exceptions discussed below. Recent reports affirm the principle. Gardner and Ochsner in 1983 recorded 121 bypasses to the distal calf vessels with 4 percent mortality and loss of only 10 of 86 threatened limbs (2 of these were 2 years later), producing an immediate salvage rate of 91 percent.[3]

Perdue's group documented the successful salvage of 90 percent of 40 legs by grafting to tibial arteries (along with 92 percent overall success among 308 limbs). Further, the 5-year salvage rate was 49 percent for the femorotibial group.[4]

Veith and his 12 associates in 1981 salvaged 584 of 755 patients (77 percent) who presented with a limb threatened by ischemia. Of the 551 who had surgical revascularizations, there was a 66 percent 6-year cumulative salvage rate.[5] In 1982 Veith reported 26 bypasses to distal calf arteries, with 83 percent 1-year and 74 percent 2-year limb salvage. He preferred vein grafts (12 cases) but concluded also that polytetrafluoroethylene (PTFE) was an acceptable "conduit" (14 cases),[6] a statement which may not receive general agreement.

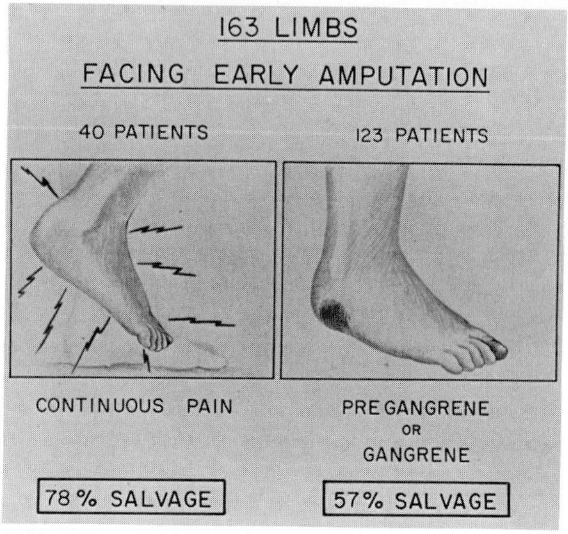

FIGURE 25-1 A consecutive series of 163 limbs threatened with loss because of continuous ischemic pain requiring opiates or unhealing ischemic lesions.

COMPARISON OF RISKS

Callow recently discussed costs of amputation (57 days and $24,000) versus below-knee salvage procedures (27 days and $18,000).[7] It is accepted that revascularization costs less than amputation: it is submitted that the hospital times for both are excessive. The femoropopliteal graft patient should go home about the seventh or eighth postoperative day and the amputee on the tenth day. The hospital times and costs in that series were excessive.

Verta, Moreno, and Viello concluded that revascularization not only preserved function but also was safer and less expensive than amputation, based upon their results summarized in Table 25-1.[8] These patients were not matched for extent of disease, but the significantly different results further document the advantages of salvage procedures. Reichle's group in 1979 analyzed 98 femorotibial grafts. There was 7.1 percent mortality and 43 percent had limb salvage for 5 years or until death.[9] Sproull's 100 salvage cases had 85 percent early success and "none of the failures resulted in amputation."[10]

Eickhoff commented upon the risks of amputation versus revascularization among 1393 patients in Denmark, noting the thrice greater risk of amputation, probably because of more-advanced disease and a higher incidence of diabetes. The amputation-to-revascularization mortality ratio decreased from 6:1 below 60 years of age to 1:1 beyond age 80.[11] The risk of revascularization procedures (5.2 percent among 750) was considerably less than the risk of amputation (21 percent of 134) in an English report by Thomas in 1983.[12] These reports indicate that surgeons experienced in performing distal revascularizations achieve high salvage rates with a risk less than that of amputation.

TABLE 25-1 TIBIAL BYPASS VERSUS AMPUTATION

	Bypass graft	Amputation
No. of patients	27	25
Mortality	4%	12%
Hospital days	32	52
Hospital cost	$12,602	$14,903
Patients walking	93%	28%
Patients maintaining original function level	74%	28%

Source: Verta MJ, Moreno N, Viello J: Salvage by-pass or primary amputation in the patient of seventy: is there really a choice? *J Cardiovas Surg* (Torino), 1983, 4:401.

DOES FAILURE OF REVASCULARIZATION COMPROMISE A LATER BELOW-KNEE AMPUTATION?

It has been feared that if a distal tibial revascularization failed, it would compromise healing of a later below-knee amputation, causing loss of the knee and an above-knee amputation. Interruption of collateral pathways, propagation of clot, infection, and other wound complications singly or together are recognized as possible causes of this.

Veith's group analyzed 61 primary amputations, half above- and half below-knee, of which 81 followed failure of a revascularization operation, and concluded that "the risk of jeopardizing the knee joint should not be considered a major contraindication to limb salvage procedures."[13] On the other hand, Stoney in 1982 discussed the question of whether to attempt revascularization or to perform a primary below-knee amputation, favoring the latter and reflecting a strategy which he and Wylie have espoused for some time, citing only 24 percent survival with a functioning graft 1 year after vein graft reconstruction for foot gangrene.[14] Their argument requires consideration, although documentation of how the distal graft failure caused loss of the knee is doubtful.

Some other reports suggest that failed below-knee procedures increase the likelihood of loss of the knee. Couch and associates retrospectively studied limb survival after femoropopliteal reconstruction and believed that half their above-knee amputations were necessitated by failure of limb salvage procedures.[15] Schlenker and Walkoff believed all 10 of their above-knee amputations could have been avoided.[16] Kazmers, Satiani, and Evans analyzed their amputations on the basis of popliteal artery pressure.[17] The hazards to below-knee amputation of failed distal revascularization were shown for patients with high popliteal pressures (above 60 mmHg) by the 81 percent of 45 without a preceding vascular operation who healed, while only 52 percent of 45 with a prior operation healed.[18] Szilagyi concluded that an unsuccessful graft operation for limb salvage had approximately a 60 percent chance of raising the level of amputation to a point above the knee, while a below-knee amputation would probably have been successful if done primarily instead of a graft.[19]

Dardik's analysis of the 15 percent failures of later below-knee amputation among 552 leg revascularizations led to the conclusion (which I do not believe is demonstrated) that revascularizations "increased morbidity associated with a failed vascular by-pass by converting a potential [below-knee] amputation to an [above-knee] level."[20]

Thus, a number of experienced vascular surgeons warn that a below-knee revascularization may be hazardous in terms of not only failing to prevent loss of limb but also causing loss of the knee and an above-knee amputation. Others strongly support an aggressive surgical approach to limb salvage and argue that when this philosophy is properly applied, it saves limbs and does not needlessly jeopardize a later amputation if that proves necessary. On the one hand it is suggested that inexperience with distal bypass leads to problems, while on the other it is implied that higher amputations are not recognized as due to failure of revascularization.

An overview of the matter suggests that further experience is needed to determine finally what policy is better for most patients. It seems likely that improvements in predicting the results of distal bypasses and of amputations will occur as diagnostic techniques continue to develop accuracy, while at the same time the skilled surgical techniques for small distal bypasses become more widespread. My own strategy has always aimed toward limb preservation by revascularization, and there has been the clinical impression that, even if that failed, a later below-knee amputation was not compromised.

Illustrative Case

A 51-year-old male in 1974 developed acute ischemia of the left calf and foot. An attempt was made to place a vein graft to the posterior tibial artery at the ankle, but the procedure was abandoned without completion because of the tiny distal vessel. Two months later below-knee amputation was performed with excellent healing (Figure 25-2). Some 2 years later the prosthesis was rubbing on the anterior portion of the stump, and when healing could not be obtained, the 2-year-old below-knee amputation was revised to an above-knee amputation which healed.

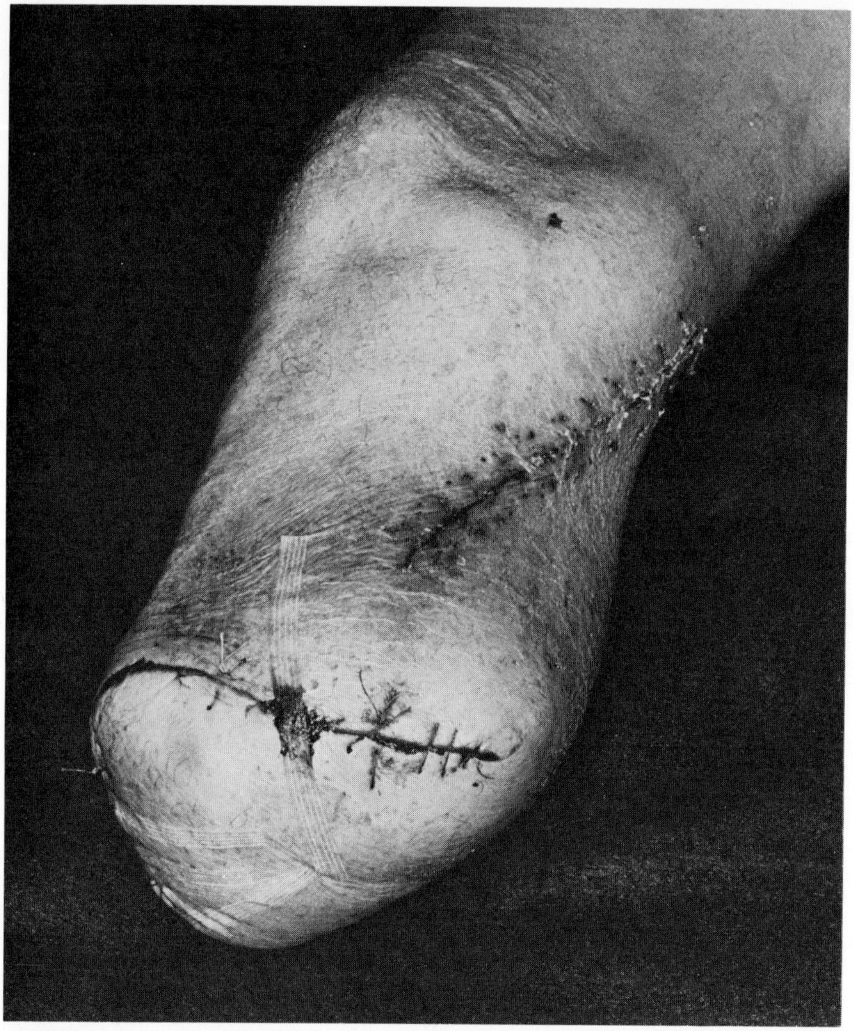

FIGURE 25-2 The healing wound of a popliteal bypass which failed twice. The below-knee amputation wound was not compromised.

Five years later, in 1979, when the patient was 59, because of severe ischemia of the contralateral right leg a femoropopliteal vein graft was placed. After 2-year patency it failed, and in April 1981 composite arm veins were used to replace it. This graft failed immediately and was replaced 3 days later with a PTFE graft, which also failed. Because of the proximal extent of severe ischemia an above-knee amputation was performed 2 days later. This initially appeared to heal, but 4 months later, in August 1981, the suture line had broken down, so a midthigh amputation was performed which thereafter healed successfully.

Comment This case illustrates the complex problem of limb ischemia and its relief. On the left side the attempt at peripheral revascularization did not interfere with healing at the below-knee level, although 2 years later the skin was not sufficiently resistant to withstand the friction of the prosthesis, which led to an above-knee amputation.

The other limb was revascularized successfully for 2 years, but secondary revascularization then was unsuccessful. The extent of ischemia proximally was severe and eventuated first in an above-knee amputation, which was revised to a midthigh amputation. It would be difficult to blame this high amputation upon the previous revascularization or upon failure of the secondary procedure, since the latter simply did not alleviate the ischemia which was already preventing a below-knee success.

Patients in that situation have been advised of the estimated chance of success, based on personal (not literature) statistics, prior to an attempt at tibial or peroneal revascularization. As the estimate has approached a low figure, the advice has usually been for primary amputation. A few patients, however, with fully informed consent, insist upon a last-ditch effort.

It has been my impression that knees were not being lost as a result of the aggressive approach to salvage of the leg and foot. In order to document this, I studied a recent group of 55 consecutive personally performed amputations (Table 25-2). It was found that 87 percent of the amputees had a previous attempt at or completion of operative revascularization, reflecting the policy of attempting salvage. The two below-knee amputations which were later revised to the above-knee level did not per se indicate whether or not the vascular procedure caused loss of the knee, but rather that there was a 93 percent rate of below-knee healing. The 51:49 ratio of above- to below-knee procedures was surprising, since the below-knee level was always considered the choice, if it would heal. The ratio therefore indicated that half the patients were not judged able to heal at the below-knee level. The question then occurred as to whether a previous reconstructive procedure had caused something which would change the choice from below- to above-knee. That question could only be answered by individually scanning each record and making a judgment call. Admittedly this decision may have been biased, but it did not appear that revascularizations had changed the amputation level.

The study of these records did suggest that perhaps the provision of a blood supply by a graft so that the foot remained viable also prevented the development of a collateral circulation, so if the graft failed after several years, there was no secondary supply to the leg below the knee to allow a below-knee amputation to be viable. That line of reasoning is a bit questionable. If correct, it means that a patent graft saves the foot and allows walking for months or years, but when it fails, the undesirable above-knee amputation is likely.

TABLE 25-2 55 RECENT CONSECUTIVE AMPUTATIONS

Age of patient	No.	Healed	Proximal revision	Mortality	Previous revascularization
		28 above-knee amputations (51% of total)			
50 to 60	8				
61 to 70	5				
71 to 80	10				
81 to 90	5				
Total	28	25 (89%)	3	6 (21%)	26 (93%)
		27 below-knee amputations (49% of total)			
40 to 50	3				
51 to 60	1				
61 to 70	6				
71 to 80	11				
81 to 90	6				
Total	27	25 (93%)	2*	2 (7%)	22 (82%)

*Patients later had an above-knee amputation.

INDICATIONS FOR REVASCULARIZATION

In the absence of an immediate need for amputation a reconstructive procedure should be considered. The fact that one or more toes or rays or even all of these will be lost does not rule out a repair to save the heel and allow walking. Areas of local gangrene on the heel are common, but they will heal if a blood supply is provided.

Clinical Evaluation

Revascularization for claudication is an elective procedure for patients with disabling symptoms and will not be discussed here.

Progression of the atherosclerotic process beyond a single occlusion which produces claudication to the multiple stenoses and occlusions associated with rest pain is uncertain, but when it occurs, the symptoms become drastically changed. The constant pain of severe ischemia usually begins as night pain because of lessened peripheral perfusion as the cardiac output and blood pressure diminish with rest and sleep. Walking may relieve the pain. Eventually the severe symptoms become constant, usually with an obviously ischemic foot. Areas of brown or purple discoloration of the toes and/or heel signal impending dry gangrene. Minor injuries (some iatrogenic) fail to heal. The syndrome calls for early relief, certainly prior to exhaustion from pain or the development of extensive tissue necrosis and infection.

Complicating Factors

The presence of severe pulmonary, cardiac, cerebral, hepatic, or other disease or combinations may point toward amputation rather than reconstruction. However, if the complicating disease process is stable or is reversible, a vascular repair under spinal anesthesia is often less difficult for the patient to survive than is amputation with its resultant invalidism. A history of myocardial infarction, of angina, of a previous cerebral vascular accident, of pulmonary emphysema, or of similar processes need not prevent salvage in most cases. Even the presence of inoperable or recurrent malignant tumors does not always indicate amputation rather than limb salvage, for the obvious reason that the patient obtains considerably better palliation from salvage of the extremity than from its loss! The presence of such serious lesions elsewhere may, however, act as a relative contraindication to arterial repair, particularly in instances where the outlook for success appears to be limited.

Chronologic Age Age is not itself as important as irreversible degeneration of the physiologic processes. Figure 25-3 indicates that while the limb salvage rate declines with advancing age, there are still successes in patients over 80. An 83-year-old male (Figure 25-4) whose leg was saved by placement of a vein graft from the femoral

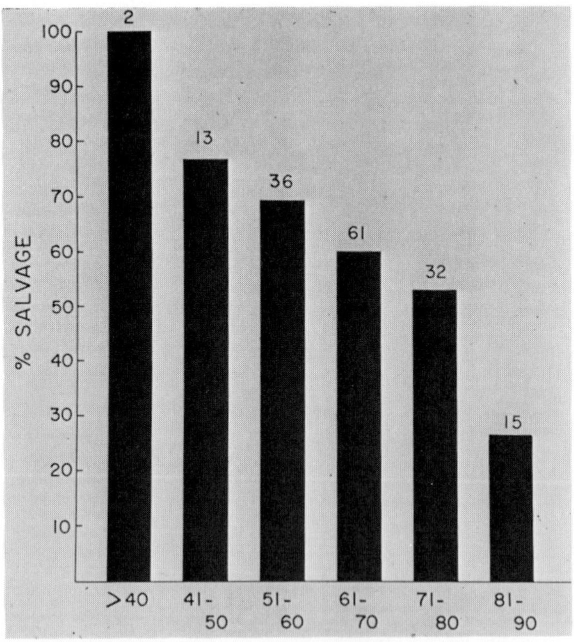

FIGURE 25-3 Limb salvage rates by age in 159 consecutive operations on extremities.

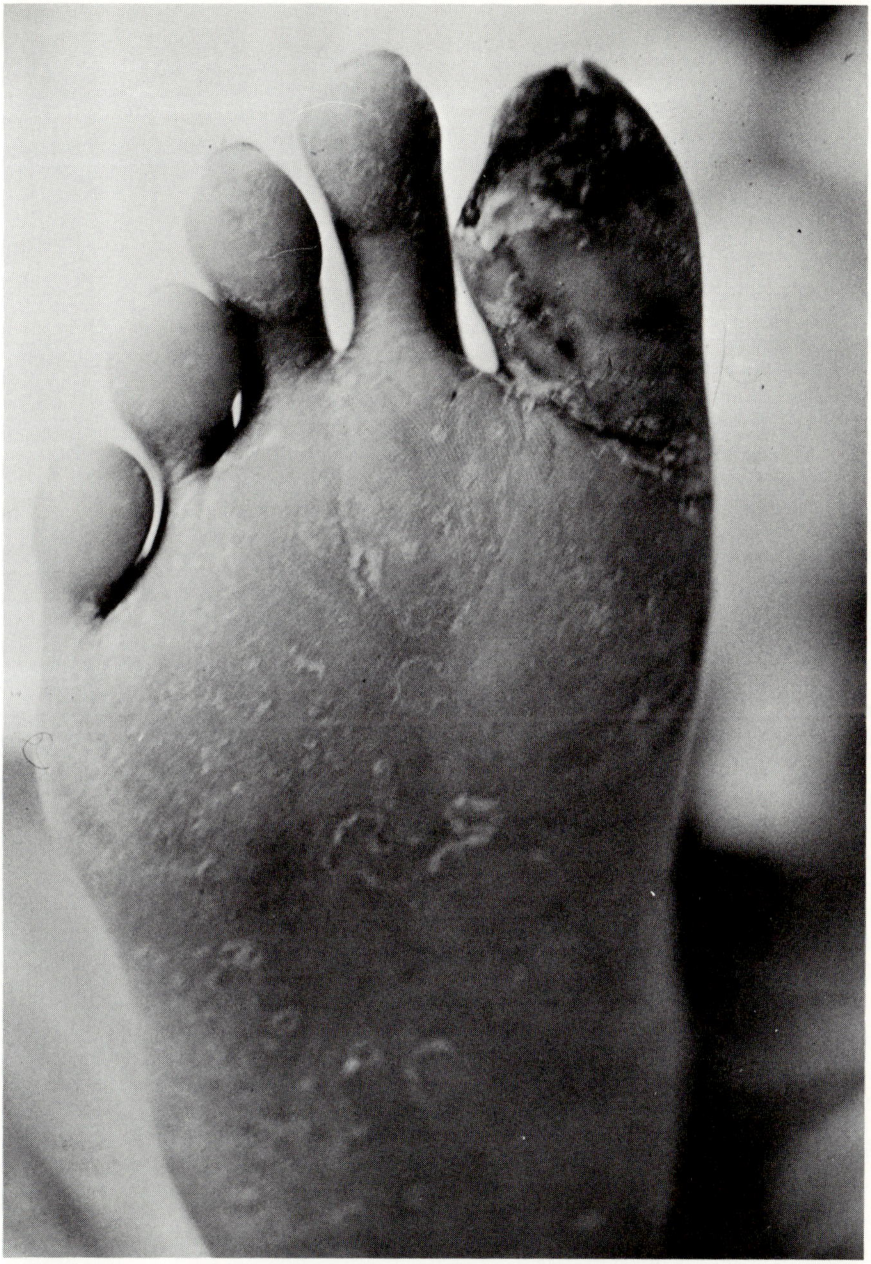

FIGURE 25-4 Ischemic necrosis of the great toe of an 83-year-old male.

to the anterior tibial artery below the knee (Figure 25-5) and later amputation of the gangrenous toe and metatarsal head, which were beyond salvage, is shown in Figure 25-6.

Diabetes Two generally held opinions regarding diabetic patients are at least controversial and perhaps completely untrue, namely, their supposed difficulty in wound healing and the propensity of the diabetic to develop more arterial disease as well as lesions which occur in smaller rather than larger arteries.

There is a persistent legend that wounds of diabetic patients heal poorly. This may be true in the presence of uncorrected metabolic lesions of several kinds, but *controlled diabetic patients heal wounds as well as do any others.*

Personal experience leads to two recommendations for diabetics. First, the same indications for revascularization procedures should be used for diabetics as for nondiabetics. Second, a more conservative approach to amputation may be adopted in diabetics than in nondiabetics if tissue loss is inevitable. An open-toe–metatarsal head amputation appears more likely to heal in the diabetic with toe gangrene than in the nondiabetic.

Angiography

An aggressive approach to salvage of the limb is warranted by the documented evidence that well over half of threatened limbs may be saved. Angiography is the key to salvage and is indicated for all threatened limbs.

The actual technique of angiographic visualization may be variable. The essential needs are to see clearly (1) the inflow of the aortoiliac system, (2) the profunda femoris and its branches, and (3) the distal calf and foot vessels, including the pedal arch. A sufficient volume of contrast material and delayed exposures are often needed to visualize adequately the calf and foot, since the material must bypass occlusions via small collateral arteries. If the distal vessels are not seen, there may be the necessity to repeat the examination to be certain, rather than to amputate at once. This must be done in the radiologic unit or the operating room. Most patients have a patent distal artery somewhere (Figure 25-7).

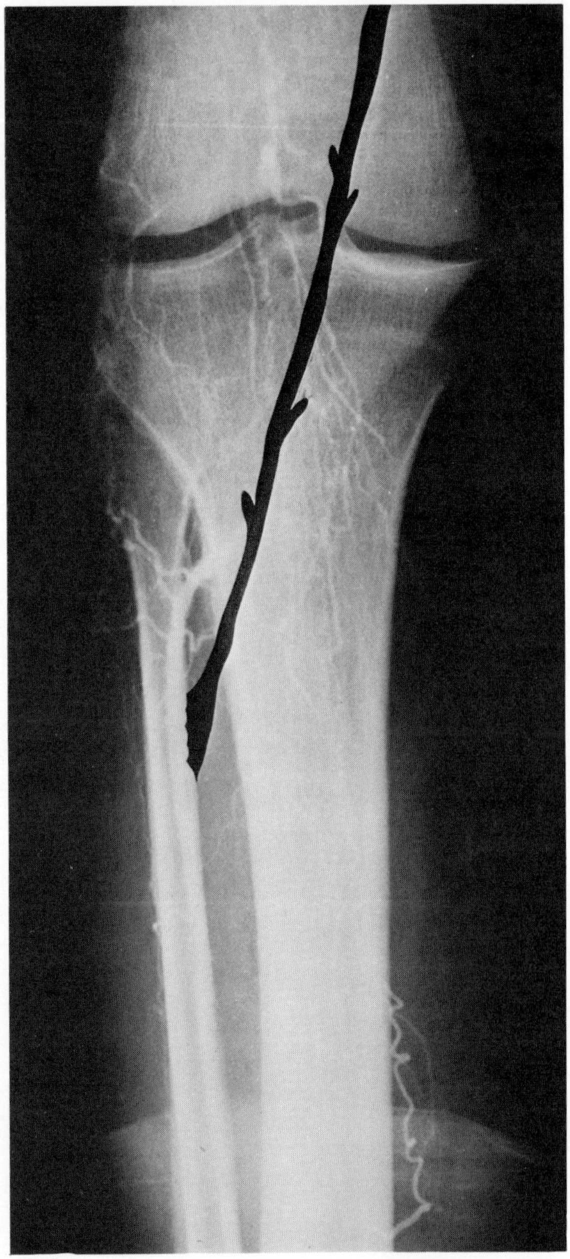

FIGURE 25-5 Revascularization by reversed autogenous vein graft to the remnant of anterior tibial artery provided a viable foot with a toe beyond salvage.

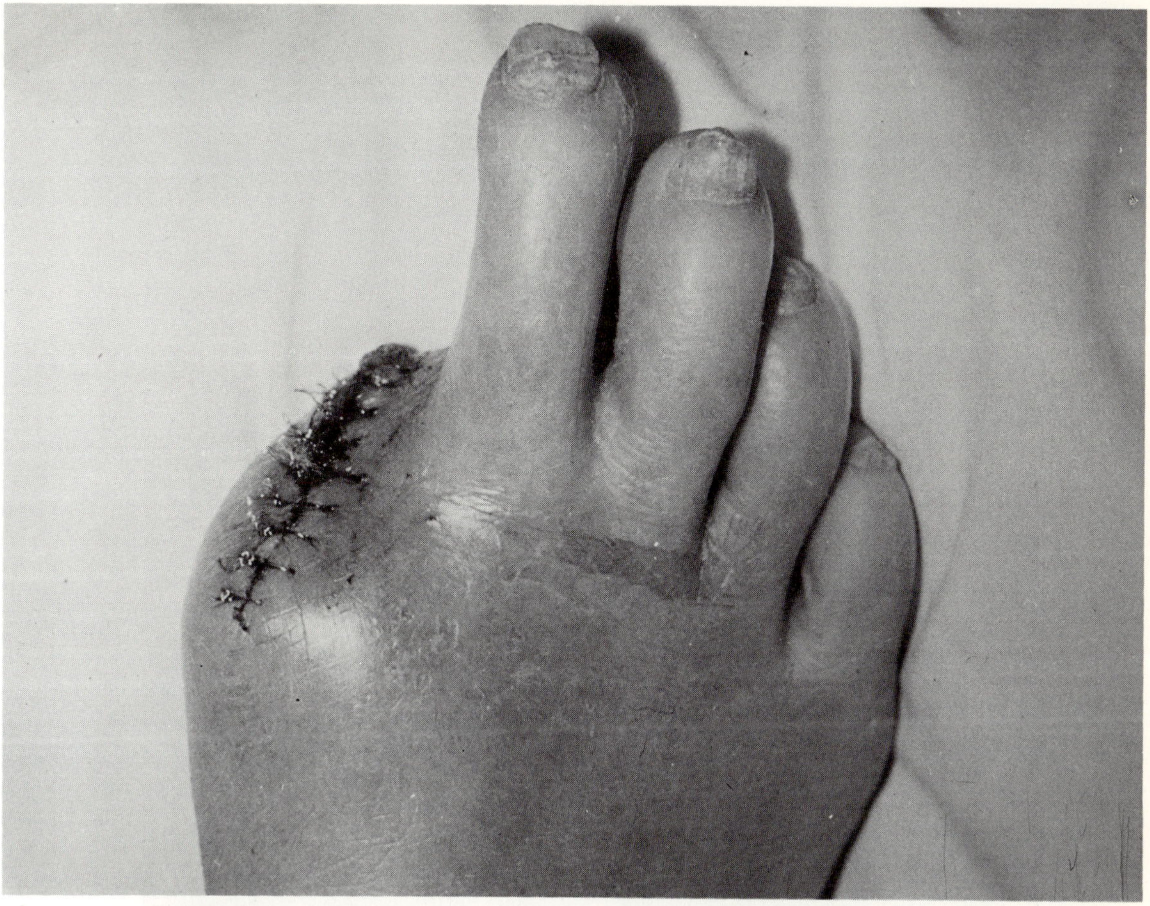

FIGURE 25-6 The first toe and adjacent metatarsal head were amputated on the fifth day after the successful revascularization.

Illustrative Case A 64-year-old male in 1975 had a femorofemoral PTFE graft plus bilateral PTFE grafts for incapacitating claudication and early ischemia in the right foot. In 1980, 5 years later, these grafts failed and were replaced by a new PTFE graft between the femoral arteries, with extensions to both popliteal arteries. Eight months later the right limb failed, and a tertiary PTFE femoropopliteal bypass was placed to the popliteal artery below the knee. This failed and 4 weeks later a below-knee amputation was carried out. The distal edges of the flap were somewhat ischemic and the skin suture line broke down. Four weeks later the below-knee amputation was revised to a point $1\frac{1}{2}$ inches higher on the bone, and the wound healed slowly. Walking with a prosthesis was delayed for 4 months. The left limb has remained asymptomatic.

Comment Despite a series of vascular reconstructions the patient was still using the left leg 9 years later and at the same time walking on a below-knee prosthesis on the right. There was difficulty in healing at that level, but with attentive care it did occur and save the knee. The several vascular operations salvaged function on one side and did not cause loss of the knee on the other.

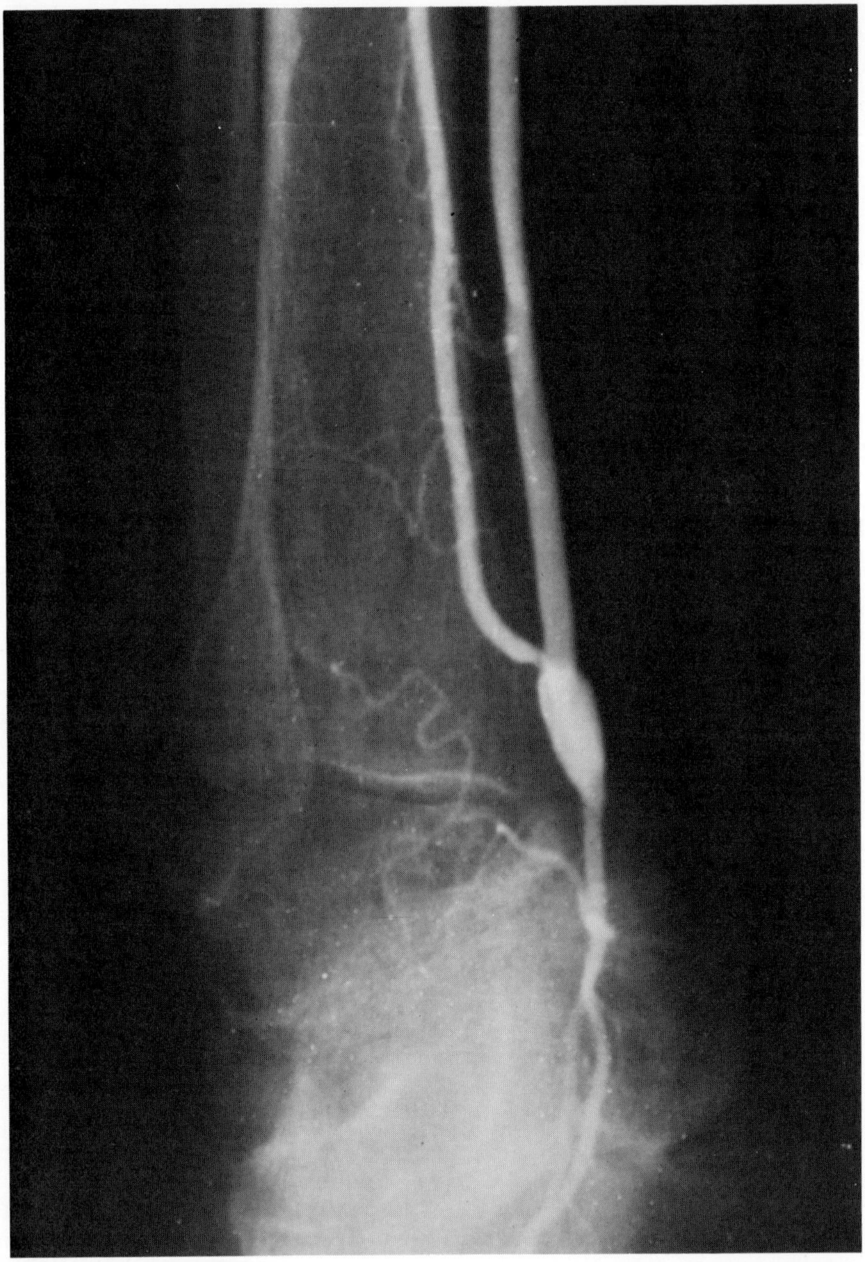

FIGURE 25-7 The reversed autogenous vein graft is the material of choice for revascularization of the posterior tibial artery at the level of the ankle.

INDICATIONS FOR PRIMARY AMPUTATION

The extent of tissue necrosis or gangrene in the toes and foot is an important indicator of whether an immediate below-knee amputation should be done. If the heel cannot be saved in a form which will allow walking, there is little reason to consider a complicated and risky revascularization procedure. Immediate below-knee amputation and early prosthesis fitting should be done. Attempts to cut necrotic tissue away from the posterior foot and form complicated covering flaps usually fail in an ischemic foot (although the young patient with traumatic loss may very well heal the same). It is for this reason that proximal forefoot amputations are usually only preliminary to higher ones and are therefore contraindicated.

The extent of infection sometimes forces an early amputation. Life-threatening gas gangrene certainly demands emergency amputation at a high level. Extensive involvement of the foot and ankle, with lymphangitis and cellulitis spreading proximally, may be better managed by a distal "chop" removal of tissue than by an attempt at drainage and later revascularization. Lesser degrees of infection often respond well to wide drainage and systemic antibiotics, allowing time for angiography and revascularization.

Some limbs have such extensive loss of arterial supply, along with only small residual distal vessels, loss of the pedal vascular arch, and other angiographic features, that the chance of a successful graft is small (Figure 25-8). As the likelihood of long-term patency diminishes, the indications for an early amputation increase. The factors which may affect the decision are discussed below.

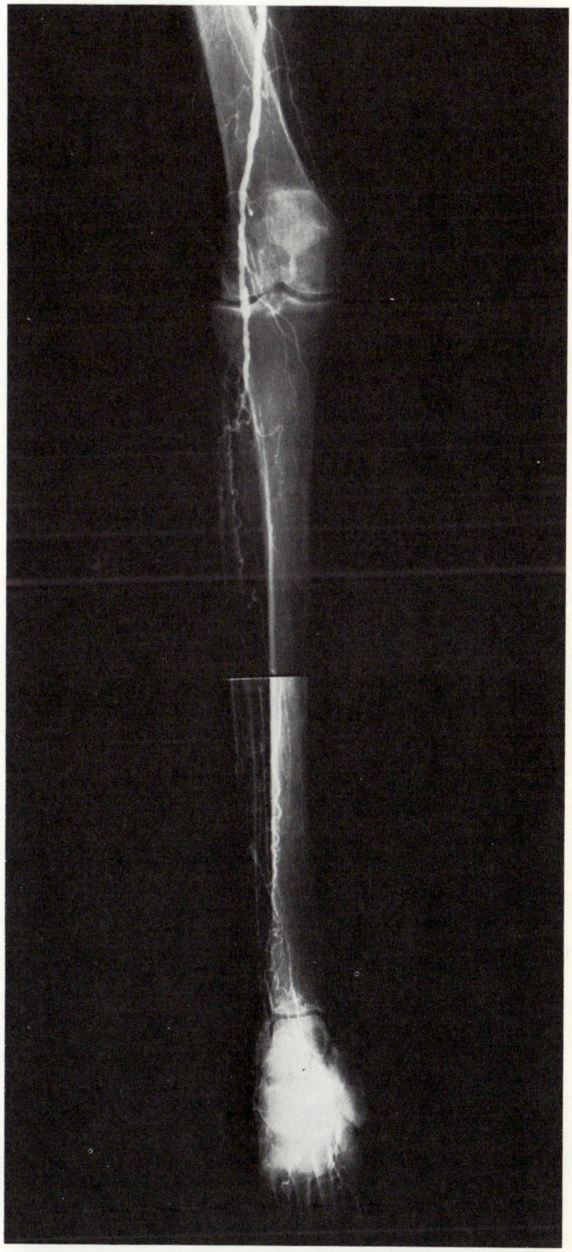

FIGURE 25-8 The femoropopliteal segment of vessel in this patient was irregular but patent, while the distal vessels were stenosed and occluded to the extent that below-knee amputation was recommended instead of an attempt at revascularization.

Illustrative Case

An 85-year-old male had acute ischemia with discoloration of the right foot for 4 days. Because of blindness, cardiac disease, and his bedridden condition there was no consideration of revascularization or of below-knee amputation, so an above-knee amputation was performed with excellent healing. Six weeks later, because of femoral and popliteal embolism contralaterally, an embolectomy and bypass femoropopliteal graft were successfully carried out on the left side.

Comment The later contralateral embolectomy was done to prevent loss of the second limb. The graft was placed because at the time of operation it was not certain that the popliteal artery would remain patent unless a large blood flow was brought to it by a graft.

DECISION FOR REPAIR OR AMPUTATION

In the final analysis today different experiences lead to opinions which vary, so a standard approach has not yet been achieved. It is typical of a field whose development is incomplete and whose problems are not yet solved. The distal revascularization question today is reminiscent of our discussions of aneurysms 20 years ago. Individualization must be the order of the day, since standardization is not yet possible.

In an attempt to recognize and weigh the effects of all the factors involved in the decision to perform a vascular reconstruction or an amputation, Table 25-3 was constructed.

The extent of ischemia may be so severe that a reconstructive vascular procedure would be pointless, since it would still be necessary to amputate above the heel level. Several times we have misjudged this factor and surgically produced a situation where there was a patent graft but an amputation was necessary because the gangrene involved the heel and could not be reversed. If the heel cannot be saved, amputation is indicated. It is doubtful that a major vascular procedure should be done to save the knee.

The distal arteries which are available for repair have a great bearing upon the decision. It is still not completely determined whether distal calf anastomoses (Figure 25-5) will remain open long enough to make them attractive or whether they and anastomoses to isolated popliteal segments have too little hope of long-term success to be indicated. I believe they are worthwhile.

The operator can estimate preoperatively the availability of suitable grafts in some patients by examining their legs and thighs for veins by looking for arm veins, or by using some other alternative method if these should not be suitable. The long-term results of prosthetics placed to ankle-level arteries are so poor that early amputation is usually preferable.

Failure of a previous vascular repair must to some extent discourage secondary and tertiary reconstructions, yet at times a modification or addition will salvage the extremity. More than once a later sympathectomy has remarkably improved toe changes which a patent femoropopliteal graft failed to correct. New occlusions of course require reconstruction.

If the patient is bedridden or about to die from cancer, it is usually not justifiable to advise a major vascular pro-

TABLE 25-3 FACTORS AFFECTING THE DECISION FOR REVASCULARIZATION OR AMPUTATION

Patient	Family / Surgeon / Environment
1 Extent of ischemia Toes, heel, foot, etc. Clinical syndrome Pain Gangrene Infection **2** Availability of arteries for run-off Number and quality Location Distal disease **3** Availability of graft **4** Previous vascular operations Cardiac Carotid **5** Other diseases Diabetes Tumor Miscellaneous (lung, rectal, etc.) **6** Physiologic age Overall risk Life expectancy **7** Psychologic factors Desire for rehabilitation Courage **8** Economic factors Work or retirement Finances	**Family** **1** Availability **2** Cooperation **Surgeon** **1** Training and experience Attention to details Surgical judgment **2** Personal philosophy **Environment** **1** Equipment For angiography Instruments Blood Assistants **2** Anesthesia **3** Consultants For complications For physical therapy

cedure, but there are undoubtedly exceptions to this. One such patient was extremely grateful for salvage of his extremity even though he died of carcinoma of the pancreas 6 months later. Certain forms of heart disease may be a contraindication to vascular repair, but many successfully treated patients are already victims of cardiac disease. Furthermore, there is less cardiac strain for the revascularized patient than for the amputee wearing a prosthesis.

The overall chance of success of reconstruction is not affected by the chronologic age of the patient, but the physiologic age is of more significance. The 86-year-old patient needs his or her limb just as much as the 65-year-old and if questioned will defend his or her right to walk even when compared with a 25-year-old! The post-70 patient has proved superior physical status by survival, and it is incorrect for a younger physician to deny him or her a chance for salvage merely on the basis of chronologic age.

From discussions with patients and observation of their courses I have the opinion that salvage for less than 6 months is not worthwhile but that a year or longer is, so perhaps insistence upon 2-year patency to justify a revascularization procedure is too strict.

The patient's desire for help and his or her courage are difficult to describe yet are obvious to all who work in this field. To be considered here is the possibility of failure of an initial reconstructive procedure (or even of multiple reconstructive procedures) and the necessity for later amputation. The patient may wish to have an amputation to avoid the chance of multiple operations.

Increasingly, one must consider economic factors as affecting surgical indications. While it has been customary to assume that money plays no part in surgical indications, this is untrue and it must be recognized that the total cost of rehabilitation by revascularization may be less than that of rehabilitation by amputation and prosthesis, as shown in Table 25-1. It should, however, be recalled that failure with subsequent complications may lead to a long hospitalization and multiple procedures.

The availability of family and friends and their willingness to cooperate in the rehabilitation effort may influence the surgical decision to some extent, since the individual patient is certainly not an isolated entity.

The previous training and experience of the surgeon was emphasized by Edwin J. Wylie in his presidential address to the Internatiomal Cardiovascular Society when he pointed out that there was a considerable difference between the success rate of revascularization carried out by the experienced vascular surgeon and the rate involving the occasional operator.[21] There are many surgical procedures which are so standardized that they are probably done as well by 1 individual as by 100 others. Vascular operations are more demanding and less tolerant of error, and their results depend to a considerable degree upon the skill of the individual operator. A gastroenterostomy probably functions about the same regardless of its author, but a small intestinal anastomosis in a premature infant requires unusual skill. Many vascular repairs are analogous to the latter, particularly when smaller vessels become involved. There are "blood and sweat" inherent in revascularization procedures; unfortunately, there are also "tears and toil."

The personal philosophy of the surgeon involves intangibles which we recognize yet hardly dare label. The boundary between courage and foolhardiness is thin and often dimly perceived. The pressure to avoid sins of commission may obscure even deadlier sins of omission. Surgical virtuosity is not an adequate substitute for sound judgment. At some point science must allow humanity to enter.

Finally to be considered is the environment surrounding the patient. Angiography is a basic necessity if salvage is to be attempted. Proper instruments, blood, and other tools must be available. Anesthesia services have tremendous variation from place to place and even from hospital to hospital. The availability of safe regional block or low spinal anesthesia allows considerably more latitude in the performance of peripheral arterial operations than is the case if general anesthesia is invariably necessary.

The aggressive approach to leg salvage leads toward vascular reconstruction to prevent loss of the extremity. Nevertheless, not all legs can be saved, and patients may still be rehabilitated by an amputation which heals promptly, conserves function, and allows early use of a prosthesis. The total program for a patient whose leg is threatened should be correlated to ensure revascularization if possible or, if not, to decide when and at what level amputation should occur. Prosthesis fitting and training must thereafter follow closely. It is harmful for efforts to be separated. In plain words, patients fare better if the surgeon who performs the vascular repair is also responsible for an amputation, should that become necessary; at least, the surgeon should remain an active consultant in determining timing, site, and other aspects of amputation. There is no contest between repair and amputation but rather a continuing effort to maintain ambulation by the best available means.

REFERENCES

1 Dale WA: Grafting small arteries: Experiences with shunts below the knee. *Arch Surg* 1963, 86:22.

2 Dale WA: Salvage of the arteriosclerotic leg by vascular repair. *Ann Surg* 1967, 165:844.

3 Gardner PA, Ochsner JL: Operations for lower extremity salvage. *J Cardiovasc Surg* (Torino) 1983, 4:401.

4 Perdue GD, Smith RB, Vesey CR, Ansley JD: Revascularization for severe limb ischemia. *Arch Surg* 1980, 115:168.

5 Veith FJ, Gupta SK, Samson RH, Scher LA, Fell SC, Weiss P, Janko G, Flores SW, Rifkin H, Bernstein G, Haimovici H, Gliedman M, Sprayregen S: Progress in limb salvage by reconstructive arterial surgery combined with new or improved adjunctive procedures. *Ann Surg* 1981, 194:386.

6 Sampson RH, Gupta SK, Scher LA, Veith FJ: Treatment of limb threatening ischemia despite a palpable popliteal pulse. *J Surg Res* 1982, 32:535.

7 Callow AD: Discussion of Veith FJ, Gupta SK, Samson RH, Scher LA, Fell SC, Weiss P, Janko G, Flores SW, Rifkin H, Bernstein G, Haimovici H, Gliedman M, Sprayregen S: Progress in limb salvage by reconstructive arterial surgery combined with new or improved adjunctive procedures. *Ann Surg* 1981, 194:400.

8 Verta MJ, Moreno N, Viello J: Salvage by-pass or primary amputation in the patient of seventy: Is there really a choice? *J Cardiovasc Surg* (Torino) 1983, 4:401.

9 Reichle FA, Rankin KP, Tyson RR, Firestone AJ, Shuman C: Long term results of 474 arterial reconstructions for severely ischemic limbs: A 14 year follow-up. *Surgery* 1979, 85:93.

10 Sproull GJ: Discussion of Reichle FA, Rankin KP, Tyson RR, Firestone AJ, Shuman C: Long term results of 474 arterial reconstructions for severely ischemic limbs: A 14 year follow-up. *Surgery* 1979, 85:100.

11 Eickhoff JH: Revascularization of the lower limb. *Lancet* 1980, 2:262.

12 Thomas WEG, Byfield DM, Ring NP, Sheard SC, Stephenson RN, Baird RN: Vascular surgical audit—arterial reconstructions and amputations for lower limb ischemia. *Acta Chir Scand* 1983, 149:127.

13 Sampson RS, Gupta SK, Scher LA, Veith FJ: Level of amputation after failure of limb salvage procedures. *Surg Gynecol Obstet* 1982, 154:56.

14 Stoney RJ, James OR, Wylie EJ: Surgery for femoral popliteal atherosclerosis. *Arch Surg* 1971, 103:8.

15 Couch NP, Wheeler HB, Hyatt DF, Crane C, Edwards EA, Warren R: Factors influencing limb survival after femoropopliteal reconstruction. *Arch Surg* 1967, 95:163.

16 Schlenker JO, Walkoff JS: Major amputations after femoropopliteal by-pass procedures. *Am J Surg* 1975, 129:495.

17 Dean RH, Yao JST, Thompson RG, Bergan JJ: Predictive value of ultrasonically derived arterial pressure in determination of amputation level. *Am Surg* 1975, 4:731.

18 Kazmers M, Satiana B, Evans WE: Amputation level following unsuccessful distal limb salvage operations. *Surgery* 1980, 87:683.

19 Szilagyi DE, Hageman JH, Smith RF, Elliott JP, Brown F, Dietz P: Autogenous vein grafting in femoral popliteal atherosclerosis: The limits of effectiveness. *Surgery* 1979, 86:9.

20 Dardik H, Kahn M, Dardik I, Sussman B, Ibrahim IM: Influence of failed vascular by-pass procedures on conversion of BK to AK amputation levels. *Surgery* 1982, 91:64.

21 Wylie EJ: Vascular surgery—reflections on the past three decades. *Surgery* 1980, 88:743.

Invited Commentary

Ronald J. Stoney, M.D.
San Francisco, California

This is a controversial subject, namely, the optimal management of the patient with an extremity threatened by infrainguinal atherosclerosis. The author's preference is aggressive attempted leg salvage by revascularization, which is usually accomplished by an extremity bypass to the popliteal or suitable distal artery.

Nevertheless, he points out that many limbs (and I would hasten to add *patients*) are not candidates for salvage bypass and should be primarily amputated. Most legs heal at the below-knee level, allowing the realization of the ultimate objective, the resumption of bipedal gait, through effective prosthetic rehabilitation.

The overall assessment of the patient usually favors either revascularization or primary amputation. The ambulatory status of the patients, their potential for rehabilitation, the degree and extent of ischemia, the arteriographic status of the vessels, and the availability of a suitable graft all impact on the decision regarding optimal treatment. I agree that there is no contest between revascularization and amputation as therapeutic considerations. However, most surgeons consider amputation a personal defeat and accept the challenge of a revascularization, often with little likelihood of success, sometimes to the detriment of the patient's welfare.

The author emphasizes that most patients are offered a revascularization and reviews his own series of 55 amputees, of whom 87 percent had prior limb revascularizations attempted or completed. The preponderance of above-knee amputations in this group does raise the concern that the previous revascularization attempts did, in fact, impair healing at the below-knee level, as others have pointed out. Since the loss of the knee halves the rehabilitation potential of dysvascular amputees, one can only speculate how many of this group were denied the opportunity for successful rehabilitation to an ambulatory status?

Concern for the knee joint in patients facing amputation can, in selected instances, become an indication for revascularization. Usually this means that, if adequate perfusion through the profunda femoris artery can be provided, below-knee healing will occur and a functional limb will result. Above-knee amputations can be reserved for nonambulatory patients or those with advanced gangrene of the lower leg or patients who cannot be rehabilitated because of general debility, paralysis, or severe cardiopulmonary dysfunction.

The vascular surgeon should undertake responsibility for total care of a patient with advanced lower-extremity ischemia. The goal should be to achieve an ambulatory status for most patients by either successful revascularization of a functional limb or primary amputation and rehabilitation. If a revascularization is feasible, what is the probability of success or failure? Will success ensure healing of a functional limb? Will failure compromise the knee joint and subsequent rehabilitation? If an amputation is the alternate method selected, what is the probability for preservation of the knee? Will the patient be able to resume an ambulatory status with a prosthesis that will allow him or her to maintain the qualities present prior to amputation? Answers to these questions are important in order to understand the central theme of this chapter, namely, the optimal treatment for patients with limb-threatening ischemia.

26 AMPUTATIONS

Amputation for gangrene was described 5 centuries before Christ, but most people in ancient times did not live long enough for it to be necessary. The main indications until recently were trauma, particularly compound fractures, bone and joint infections, and tumors. At the New York Hospital in the decade ending in 1848, there were 91 major lower-extremity amputations with a mortality rate of 29 percent, but none were done because of ischemic gangrene.[1] Similar statistics were reported elsewhere in the United States[2] and Europe.[3]

Before anesthesia was available, a surgeon's reputation largely depended upon speed (often measured in seconds) rather than upon prevention of death (which was frequent) or of complications (which were expected). "Laudable" pus was welcomed because it signaled localization of the inevitable postoperative infection rather than its life-threatening spread.

The highly skilled technique which allowed Baron Larrey to perform 200 amputations in the 24-hour period following Napoleon's battle at Borodino in the Russian campaign of 1812 also allowed him to perform hip disarticulation in 14 to 15 seconds after primary ligation of the femoral vessels. The slightly inexact time was said to be due to some inaccuracy of the then available chronometers!

The discovery of anesthesia in the midnineteenth century removed the heavy pressure of operative speed from the surgeon's shoulders. Lister's doctrine of antisepsis soon attracted attention, spread, and evolved shortly into the aseptic method of surgery. By the late 1800s postamputation infections were no longer inevitable and the risk had sharply decreased. Sudden proximal spread of infection in ischemic tissues of the toes or foot, however, remained a threat to life that often required immediate high amputation until the development of antibiotic drugs in the 1940s. The arterial reconstructive techniques which began in the 1950s have proved to be widely useful and now allow salvage of many limbs which would previously have been lost. These developments now allow attention to be shifted away from severe postoperative infections and death to prevention of amputation as well as to wound healing and conservation of the function of the remainder of the limb.

INDICATIONS

The only indications for an immediate major amputation are life-threatening infections and continued pain in an extremity whose revascularization is not possible, along with occasional instances of trauma.

Infection may force an immediate ablation. One such incidence was the discovery of gas in the ankle and foot tissues of a patient about to undergo angiography to determine the feasibility of revascularization. He was transferred directly to the operating room for above-knee amputation. Most infections, however, are not so threatening and do well with drainage (sometimes accomplished by toe or foot amputation), antibiotics, and early revascularization. Restoration of arterial blood flow is better than penicillin!

If the loss of tissue is distal so that the heel is maintained, the walking function is preserved. A flesh-and-blood heel is better than a prosthetic one. If the heel cannot be salvaged in any event, there is usually not much reason to perform a vascular procedure proximally. Occasionally a bypass to preserve the knee and allow below- rather than above-knee amputation may be in order.

Continuous pain does require relief, and if blood flow cannot be restored amputation is necessary. In either event the situation demands early treatment one way or the other.

SITE OF AMPUTATION

Selection of the proper level for amputation is important, on the one hand, to proper healing without complications or the necessity for revision and, on the other, to the later function of the limb remnant and the total rehabilitation of the patient (Figure 26-1).

Walking after any major loss of the lower limb requires the expenditure of more energy than does the use of both natural legs and feet. Malone and Goldstone estimated the increases in expended energy shown in Table 26-1, where the advantage of below-knee over an above-knee prosthesis or crutch walking is immediately apparent.[4] It is also evident why a patient handicapped by cardiac or pulmonary disease may not be able to deliver the additional energy needed to get about after a major amputation.

An interesting report of the trends of amputation surgery indicated a significant increase in the percentage of below-knee amputations performed in the past decade at a veterans hospital (28 percent in 1969–1970 to 71 percent in 1979–1980), while there was no change at a nearby private hospital (50 percent versus 52 percent over the same time period). On the other hand, the percentage of revascularization procedures attempted prior to amputation was the same in the veterans unit, but in the private hospital the percentage increased resulting in more salvage of limbs.[5]

The risk of above-knee amputation is considerably greater than at the below-knee level. The high risk associated with above-knee amputation was emphasized in 1980 by the 10 series with mortality rates of 15 to 37 percent listed by Huston and associates.[6] Our earlier series showed a mortality rate of 20 percent among 284 in Rochester in 1959[7] and the same rate of 20 percent among 479 in Nashville in 1962.[8] The risk is, of course, due to more-advanced disease rather than to the operation itself. Indeed, the above-knee procedure is easier and quicker than operation at the below-knee level. For example a Canadian group of 141 patients had 31 percent above-knee mortality rate and 7 percent at the below-knee level.[9]

There is no single criterion to allow selection of the most distal site where primary healing will occur. Factors to be considered include the physical findings, the location of the most distal pulse, the angiogram, and evaluation by noninvasive tests and other newer studies.

Physical Signs

The color and temperature of the skin actually reveal little of the capacity of the tissues to heal at a given level. Further, the presence of an immediately proximal pulse is not necessary, although it is comforting. Warren and Kihn reported the primary healing rates at the below-knee level to be the same whether the popliteal pulse was present (52 percent) or absent (47 percent).[10] Eraklis and Wheeler noted that 13 of 16 below-knee amputations healed in the absence of a popliteal pulse.[11]

Amputations done two levels below a palpable pulse (below-knee amputation with the most distal pulse at the femoral artery) also often heal well, reflecting the importance of the profunda femoris blood supply. Block and Whitehouse reported that 42 of 43 diabetics healed below-knee

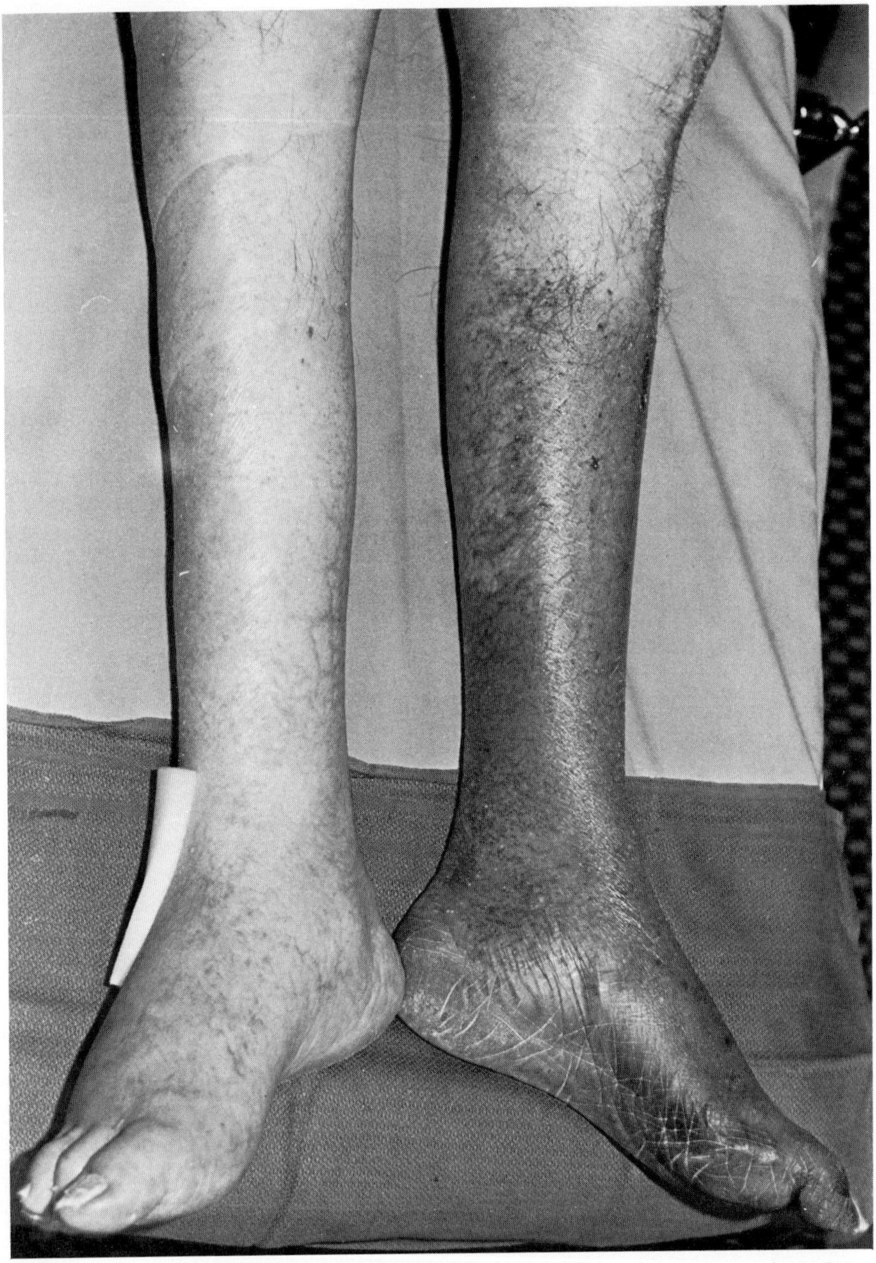

FIGURE 26-1 Late-stage acute thrombosis of the superficial and deep femoral arteries with violaceous skin changes high in the calf necessitated above-knee amputation.

amputations despite the fact that only 33 percent had palpable popliteal pulses.[12] Lempke's group had somewhat less success two levels below a palpable femoral pulse, finding 66 percent healing at the below-knee level versus 94 percent for the above-knee site.[13]

An amputation done three levels beyond a palpable pulse is even riskier, as noted by Wheelock, who reported that only 57 percent of transmetatarsal amputations healed if the femoral was the most distal palpable pulse.[14] This essentially contraindicates the procedure.

The pulse examination thus is a relative rather than a strict indication of the lowest site for amputation.

TABLE 26-1 ADDITIONAL ENERGY EXPENDITURE FOR AMBULATION

Below-knee amputation	10 to 40%
Above-knee amputation	50 to 70%
Crutch walking without prosthesis	60%
Wheelchair	9%

Source: Malone JM, Goldstone J: Lower extremity amputation (Chapter 31), in Moore WS (ed): *Vascular Surgery: A Comprehensive Review.* Grune & Stratton, New York, 1983, p 916.

Angiography

Demonstrated occlusion of the popliteal artery confirms absence of the pulse. Again, it does not necessarily predict failure of healing at the below-knee level. Lim and associates reported that 68 percent of below-knee amputations healed with the popliteal artery occluded, while 83 percent healed when it was patent.[15] Complete absence of run-off does suggest a higher risk of below-knee healing, while a patent distal vessel or vessels should suggest the possibility of a reconstructive graft.

Other Laboratory Predictive Studies

It is, of course, desirable to have a test, preferably noninvasive, which is more accurate than clinical judgment. A number of these have been devised, recommended by one or more investigators, and revised or rejected by others as experience accumulated.

Malone and Goldstone summarized these tests recently and concluded that "elective lower extremity amputation should not be performed without some form of preoperative testing."[4] They did not, however, document any readily available single test or group of tests which accurately predicted below-knee healing without giving false negatives, which lead to some unnecessary above-knee amputations. Their favorite, the xenon skin clearance test, by their own admission cannot be reproduced by others, so "its practicability and reliability remains to be determined."[4] Similar criticisms of the other available tests are in order.

Stockel's group recently suggested that a photoelectric technique of determining capillary blood flow[16] is simpler and less painful while just as accurate (89 percent of 45 amputations) as the isotope washout test in predicting healing.[17]

Nicholas and associates also have discussed the role of laboratory studies among 140 patients in predicting the correct level for amputation. They concluded that Doppler studies were useful to predict healing but would not always detect failures, and they recommended that the "vast majority . . . should have an effort to preserve the knee."[18]

Cheng's 1982 review of the various available tests for determination of the level of healing will be of interest to any surgeon who performs amputations. After summarizing the data on isotope washouts, skin perfusion pressures, and several techniques of Doppler sound studies, he concluded that skin capillary blood flow would yield the strongest correlation with healing. Moore's Xenon 133 intradermal injection[19] method is intricate; Kostuik's variation may be more practical.[20] In any event, Cheng finally concluded that "clinical judgment must still remain the major determinant of amputation."[21]

Actually, the situation appears similar to the need for preoperative tests to determine the outcome of lumbar sympathectomy for peripheral ischemia. In the 1950s, spurred by the reports of several noninvasive laboratory tests, we studied 300 patients by the recommended techniques without critical success and concluded that an experienced clinician could make as good a prediction as could the then available skin temperature and venous plethysmography studies, that is, about 85 percent. Testing was abandoned at Rochester as well as elsewhere, and no more accurate criteria have been developed since then.

This pessimism regarding currently available tests is not a suggestion that investigations cease—critical studies are needed—but that reality presently suggests a clinical decision. The knee should be saved whenever possible. Below-knee amputation should be the usual procedure, with a deviation to the above-knee level when necessary.

The above-knee is necessary if there are ischemic skin changes in the calf where the flaps will be made or if there is (heaven forbid!) an infected incision there. Absence of a femoral pulse and inability to revascularize the profunda also suggest that above-knee amputation (sometimes at the midthigh or high-thigh level) is needed. Finally, if the muscle tissue (as the below-knee procedure begins) appears nonviable by color, lack of bleeding, or response to pinching, the amputation site should at once be shifted to the above-knee level. For this reason the operative permit for all below-knee amputations should include the words *or above the knee, if necessary,* and the appropriate information should be provided to the patient and family preoperatively.

PREOPERATIVE CARE

Attention to uncontrolled disease and decompensated functional systems should be particularly directed toward diabetes and cardiac lesions, because of their high incidence in patients requiring major amputations.

There is a persistent legend that wounds of diabetic patients heal poorly. This may be true in the presence of uncorrected metabolic lesions of several kinds, but *controlled diabetic patients heal wounds as well as do any others.* Our statistics on final amputation healing in 479 amputations during a 5-year period in Nashville show slightly better percentages at both the above- and below-knee level of diabetics than for nondiabetics.[8]

The experience of others has been similar. Warren and Kihn studied 453 amputations in 14 Veterans Administration hospitals and stated that "primary healing occurred as frequently at all levels in the 162 diabetics as in the 251 non-diabetic patients."[10] Block and Whitehouse reviewed 43 amputations in diabetics and concluded that "below knee amputations are more likely to heal when performed for gangrene of the foot developing in the patient with diabetes mellitus than in the patient with occlusive arterial disease without diabetes mellitus."[12] Cranley, Krause, Strasser, and Hafner's 101 below-knee amputations had a success rate of 98 percent in diabetics and 68 percent in others.[22] Lempke and associates could find no unfavorable effect of diabetes upon the healing rate at any level.[13] Otteman and Staghlgren reviewed 523 amputations at the Philadelphia General Hospital and stated that "the rate of wound healing was not influenced by the presence of diabetes."[23] Harris, Schwartz, and DeWeese similarly showed no difference in the healing rates of below-knee amputations between 24 diabetics (77 percent) and 15 nondiabetics (71 percent).[24]

It may therefore be accepted that treated diabetics do heal amputation wounds as well as nondiabetics. Diabetes requires recognition so that it may be treated but should not influence the surgical decision so far as healing is concerned.

Anemia requires correction, and its association with hypovolemia in chronically ill patients should be recalled and treated if present.

The high incidence of wound difficulties demands every possible preoperative attention to prevent them. Twice-daily scrubs of the skin with chlorhexidine (Hibiclens), special attention to previous wounds and their sutures (with early removal and replacement by plastic strips), use of preoperative antibiotics for infections, and judicious incision and drainage of pocketed pus about the foot or toes are important.

It is frequently observed that patients who are toxic, febrile, and even uremic due to a gangrenous extremity fail to improve until amputation is carried out. Prompt removal of the offending part is in order. While there have been advocates of staged closure of the amputation wound to prevent infection, under these circumstances I have ordinarily made a culture from the amputation wound, closed the wound primarily, and followed it carefully in order to reopen it at once should infection occur. Such primary closure is usually tolerated satisfactorily if the amputation is performed in viable tissue well above the site of localized foot or toe infection. While guillotine or "chop" open amputations may be indicated in military field surgery, they have little or no place in civilian hospitals, where individual management is possible.

Physiologic Amputation by Refrigeration

The toxic effects of an infected foot or leg may be removed quickly by placement of an extremely tight tourniquet proximal to the infected area and quick lowering of the tissue temperature of the distal part (including the tourniquet site). Ordinary ice may be used, but dry ice is easier to manage. Still, Wray and Moretz described their experiences with this method in 130 extremities and reported approximately the same death and infection rates for iced and noniced amputations, although the iced ones were presumably poorer risks at the outset.[25]

My own experience with the technique ended 30 years ago. The development of a refined spinal anesthesia technique, recognition of the need for immediate drainage (with excision of necrotic tissue), and the use of antibiotics have outmoded the refrigeration of tissue.

Proximal Arterial Repair to Allow Below-Knee Amputation

Emphasis upon preservation of the knee has led some surgeons to revascularize the deep femoral artery by proximal graft or thromboendarterectomy to lower an amputation from the above- to the below-knee level.[15] It does not, however, seem good surgical judgment to perform a major vascular repair at the aortoiliac level in an attempt to shift the amputation lower to save a knee without an attached foot. If the heel can be saved, the indication for vascular repair is clear.

Preoperative Lumbar Sympathectomy

At one time it was suggested that preamputation lumbar sympathectomy would either permit a more distal amputation site to heal or benefit healing at any site.[24] This hypothesis cannot be documented and appears doubtful. In the Veterans Hospital study of Warren and Kihn it was found that there was no better healing rate in extremities following sympathectomy that in non-sympathectomized ones.[10] Lempke and associates found no statistically significant effect on the failure rate at any or all of the amputation sites.[13] Preliminary sympathectomy is not useful to aid healing of an amputation stump.

PRINCIPLES OF AMPUTATION SURGERY

Antibiotics have permitted most amputations to be closed primarily, since partial reopening with drug coverage usually controls an infection should it develop. If it is thought mandatory to leave the wound open, it is still possible to hold the central portions of the flaps together with two or three Dexon sutures so that later formal closure is not necessary. No guillotine amputation with the wound left completely open has been done in my series of thigh and leg amputations. The single above-knee amputation done as an emergency because of gas gangrene of the foot healed promptly with the central portion of the flaps sutured while each side was left open.

Important principles of operative management may be summarized as follows: (1) the amputation level should pass through vascularized tissue, with immediate change to a higher level if nonviable tissues are found, (2) there must be sufficient skin and soft tissue length in relation to bone length to allow closure without suture line tension, (3) undue tissue damage must be avoided, (4) the stump wound must be drained to remove the serosanguineous fluid which inevitably occurs despite meticulous hemostasis, and (5) post-operative dressings must avoid localized pressure on the stump. A sharp dissection technique from the anterior aspect of the extremity directly through to the posterior aspect has gradually evolved as the simplest and most efficient way of performing an amputation.*

Rough sponging, inclusion of large bits of muscle or fat in ligatures, excessively tight sutures, and excess foreign bodies (which include hematoma and serum collections) are well-known criteria of poor technique. To be similarly frowned upon are scraping periosteum from the bone end, chemical injections into the nerve, use of large plugs of bone wax, and multiple small scalpel cuts rather than tissue severance with a long amputation knife. Many operative descriptions include "loose closure of the skin," which allows fat to protrude and encrustations to form. Careful edge-to-edge closure is preferable to this.

Myodesis operations, whereby the distal ends of muscles are fixed to the bone end through drill holes,[27] should be avoided as likely to reduce the chance of primary healing if additional trauma, dissection, and suturing are done in a stump whose viability may already be in doubt. Tourniquet control of bleeding is contraindicated for fear of damage to the brittle arteriosclerotic vessels.

Every detail of operation should be directed toward an absolutely A-1 performance because of the known difficulty with healing of amputation wounds.

TECHNIQUES OF AMPUTATIONS

"Quite often the procedure is delegated to a junior member of the surgical staff who has had little experience and even less guidance in the actual technique of the operation."[28] This recent expression of a British surgeon unfortunately reflects the general attitude of many American surgeons as well, which indeed has changed little since, as a resident thirty-odd years ago, I recognized that my seniors' knowledge was on a par with their disinterest in amputations. For this reason some details of technique and care follow.

The surgeon should perform amputations, like other procedures, as simply as possible, avoiding unnecessary dissection of tissue planes, ensuring proper flap-to-bone length, emphasizing secure fascial closure, and providing for tube drainage of the subcutaneous tissue for 48 to 72 hours. The procedure can be done without much loss of blood in about 30 to 45 minutes, should not require dressing until about the fifth day, and should allow most patients to go home or to a nursing unit 7 to 10 days postoperatively. The 21- to 30-day or longer postoperative period reported in some articles is simply not tolerable at present-day cost levels. Amputees should visit the physical therapy department as outpatients.

Toe Amputation

Amputation of a toe without prior revascularization carries the danger of progression to gangrenous necrosis of the wound because the arteries may be unable to deliver enough blood to meet the increased metabolic need of a healing wound. Toe amputation is therefore hazardous in the ischemic foot and should be delayed until after revascularization. Once the blood supply is improved, there is no particular reason to delay toe amputation. It usually is wise to perform this 5 to 8 days after the vascular reconstruction.

An abscess in the toes or feet must be drained promptly, but toe gangrene alone is not an immediate indication for a major calf or thigh amputation. It does show the degree of ischemia which has occurred and is an indication for early angiography to determine the feasibility of revascularization. Vascular reconstruction should precede toe amputation, unless pus requires drainage. It is not optimally done along with the repair, because if the graft should fail, the best management of the toe usually is to leave it in situ rather than to risk an open wound whose ischemic edges are unlikely to heal. Thus, if the artery cannot be repaired or if the reconstruction

*Details of this technique, along with those of three other surgeons, are described and illustrated in another publication, to which the interested reader may refer.[26]

fails and infection does not force amputation, the toe should be left to slough spontaneously rather than be amputated with the risk of ascending gangrene and/or infection that threatens the entire limb.

Gangrenous toes which are necrotic beyond salvage require amputation even though the remaining portion of the extremity has been revascularized by arterial repair. It is usually wise to retract the skin flaps and remove the head of the adjoining metatarsal at the same time, although occasionally simple disarticulation of the toe and closure of the tissue over the cartilaginous end of the metatarsal may be done if it is certain that the soft tissues are well-arterialized. Removal of the metatarsal head allows the soft tissues to contact the vascular medullary portion of the bone and leads to better healing. At the same time, the shape of the foot is improved because the bulbous head of the metatarsal is gone (Figure 26-2). If the soft tissues are viable and without invasive infection, primary healing occurs following immediate closure of the wound. If there is doubt about vascularity, and particularly if infection is present, it may be advisable to leave the wound open to provide immediate drainage.

Transmetatarsal Site

The excellent results of transmetatarsal amputation reported by McKittrick in 1949, in the pre-revascularization era, indicated that it would be possible with the protection of antibiotics to avoid an immediate major amputation in many patients. Among 215 patients there were 2 deaths, and 82 percent were discharged without a high amputation.[29] This method was thereafter applied to similar patients by a variety of surgeons. Warren, Crawford, and McKittrick reported that 73 percent of their 43 healed,[30] and Wheelock stated that 63 percent of 428 remained healed for periods of 2 years or more.[31]

The transmetatarsal amputation is still useful in a few patients but has largely been replaced by vascular reconstruction plus toe amputation. If sufficient vascularization is not present or cannot be restored to allow surgical healing at the metatarsal head level, then there is considerable risk of failure at the transmetatarsal level.

Amputations proximal to the transmetatarsal site produce deformities of the remnant foot because of muscle imbalance. They should not be attempted unless some form of arthrodesis is done. This is contraindicated in arteriosclerotic patients.

Occasionally there is gangrene of multiple toes while the remainder of the foot is sufficiently well-vascularized to permit healing at the transmetatarsal level (Figure 26-3). A site is selected 3 cm distal to the base of the metatarsals, and a straight transverse incision is made through the skin, subcutaneous tissue, and fascia and carried around the medial and lateral sides of the foot to a level with the plantar surface of the first and fifth metatarsal (Figure 26-4). The incision is extended distally parallel to these bones to form a long plantar flap. This must be considerably longer than would appear necessary, in order to completely cover the ends of the severed metatarsals. More rather than less of the plantar flap should be saved if there is doubt about where the incision should be made.

With the distal end of the foot firmly controlled by the hand, a saw is used to cut across the metatarsals beginning anteriorly. As soon as this is completed, the scalpel is used to remove these from the plantar flap of tissue. Debridement is then carried out by the cutting away of tendons so that well-vascularized tissue forms the entire flap.

The plantar flap is pulled up over the end of the severed metatarsals, and the fascia sutured. No sutures are placed in the fat. A 4-0 synthetic suture closure of the skin follows. A through-and-through $\frac{1}{4}$-in Penrose drain is placed, and a nonbinding dressing is applied (Figure 26-5).

Malleolar Site

Syme's amputation at the malleolar level is not well-known. Occasional patients with foot gangrene extending too far proximal to allow a transmetatarsal level may be considered for this,

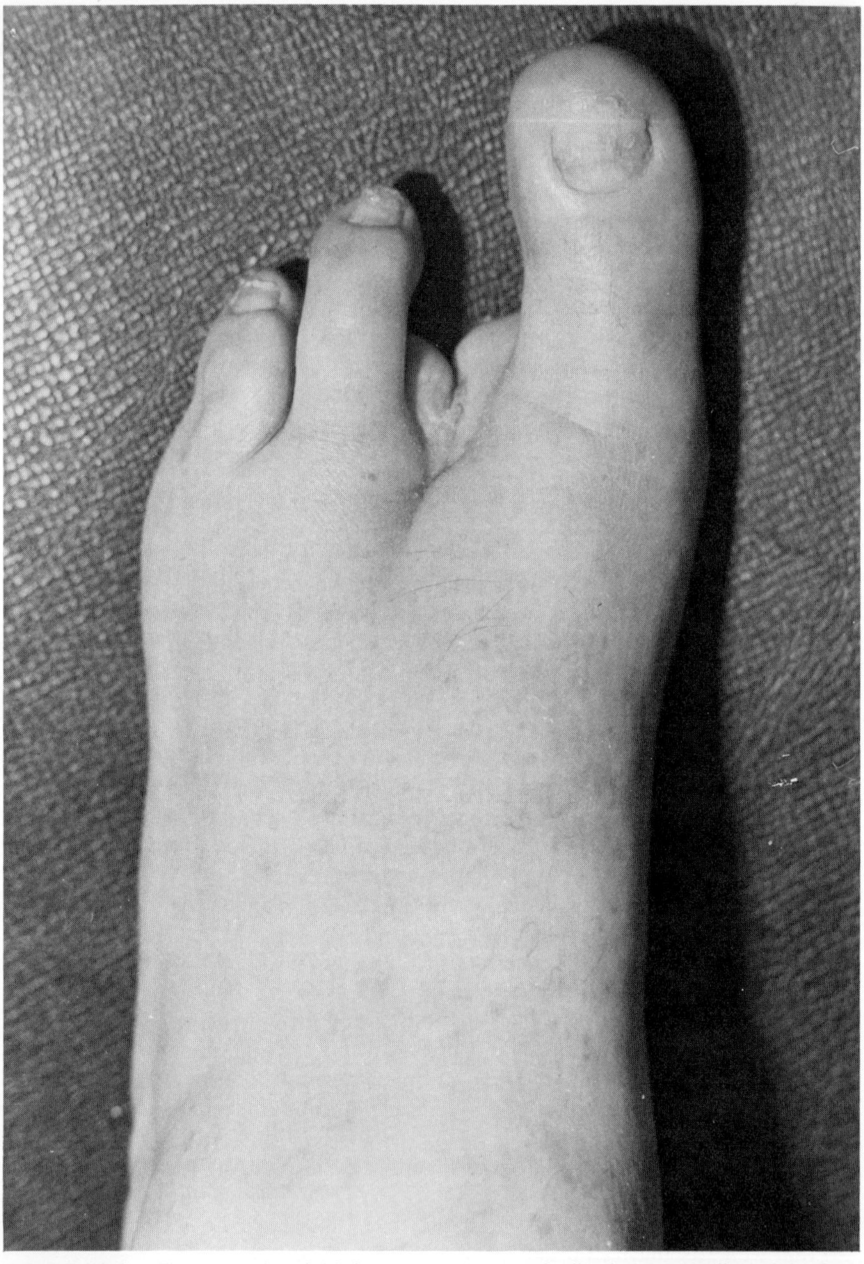

FIGURE 26-2 The second and third rays were removed, allowing remodeling of the foot.

although the prosthesis is awkward. It places the skin and fat of the heel over the cut end of the tibia and fibula and uses tissue which has been accustomed to weight bearing for that purpose. It is a good amputation for some because it allows some stumping about (to the bathroom or swimming) without crutches or prosthesis but may be unsuitable for others because of the bulkiness of the prosthesis.

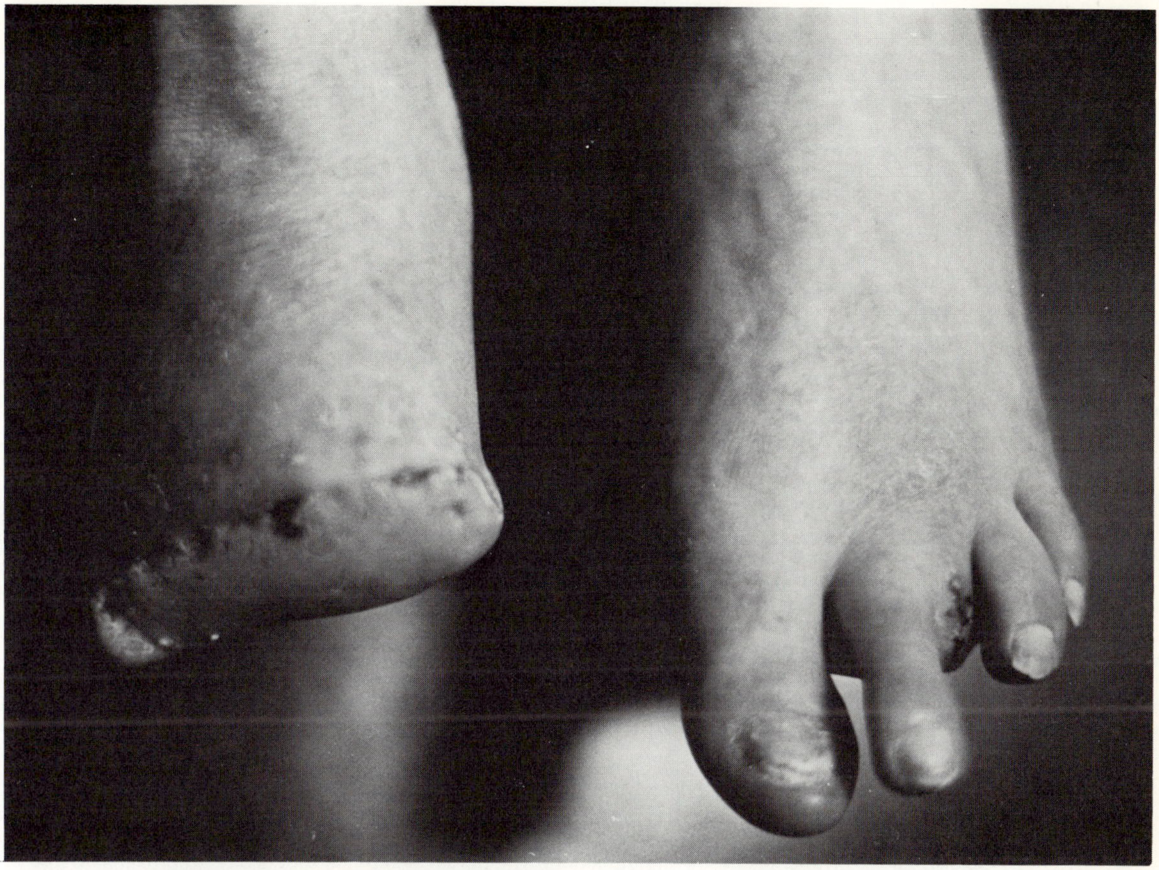

FIGURE 26-3 Healing bilateral local amputations allow the patient to walk.

Because of the absolute necessity for good arterialization of the heel flap, this amputation is not often chosen for a patient with ischemic gangrene.[32]

The chief operative danger during the Syme amputation is that of devascularizing the heel flap, whose arterial supply is chiefly derived from the posterior tibial artery on the medial side. The ankle should therefore be disarticulated through the anterior part of the incision, and the os calcis should be enucleated subperiosteally from within outward in order to protect the blood supply of the skin flap (Figure 26-6).

The anterior skin incision is made over the anterior line of the ankle joint and then is carried a bit diagonally in a posterior direction on both sides of the foot so that it passes 1 cm anterior to the tip of each malleolus on the sides of the ankle. The incision is carried across the plantar surface of the heel 1 cm posterior to the inner tubercle of the plantar surface of the os calcis. The incision is deepened to the periosteum of the bone.

With the foot in forceful plantar flexion the anterior tendons are cut at the level of the distal end of the anterior skin flap. The anterior joint capsule is incised transversely at the lower margin of the tibia. The medial and lateral ligaments supporting the ankle are next severed from inside outward, and the astragalus is completely dislocated by continued forceful plantar flexion so that the attachment of the Achilles tendon to the posterior tubercle of the os calcis is exposed. A sharp periosteal elevator is then used from the inside of the ankle joint to remove the periosteum,

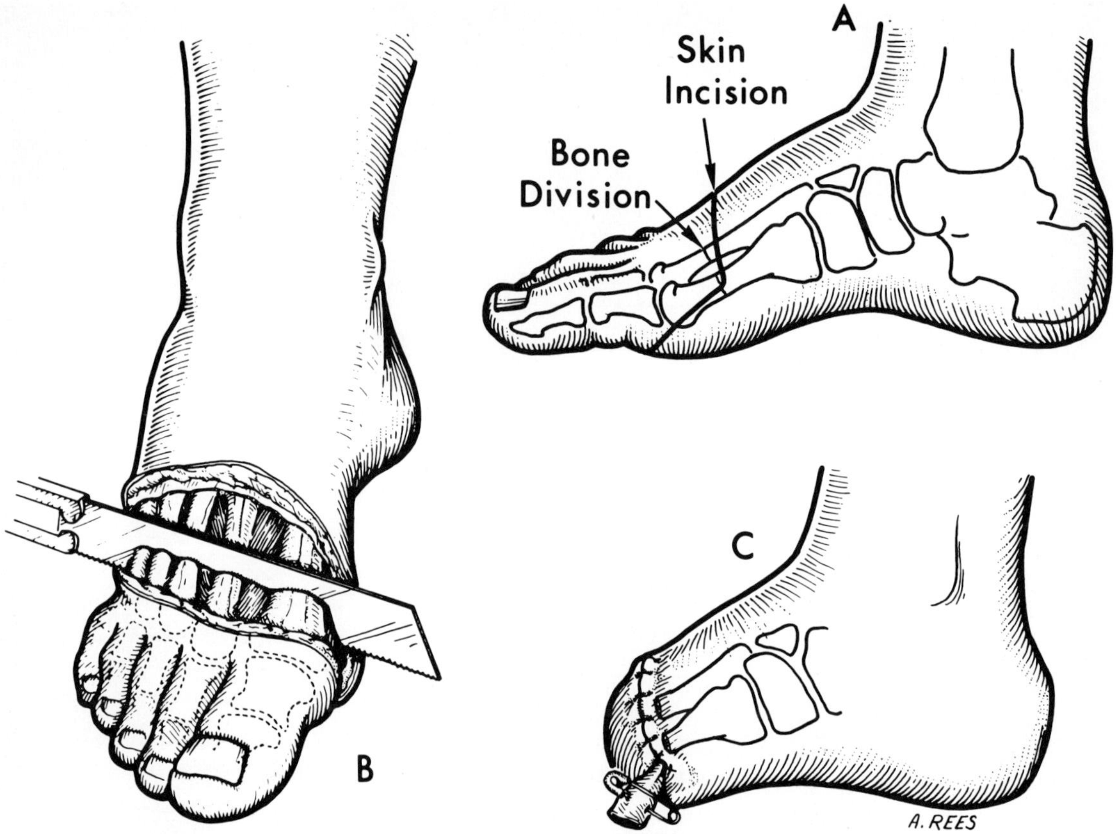

FIGURE 26-4 Transmetatarsal amputation. (*a*) The dorsal skin of the foot is incised proximal to the metatarsal heads; the plantar incision is carried distally to form a flap to cover the metatarsal ends. (*b*) Metatarsal shafts are cut in line with the skin. The plantar flap is fileted. (*c*) After closure of the fascia with interrupted sutures the skin is similarly closed, with a drain led out the corner.

starting at the attachment of the Achilles tendon, and this dissection is carried out subperiosteally to the point where the periosteum was originally incised through the skin incision. The distal foot is discarded. Stumps of visible tendons now may be pulled down, cut across sharply, and allowed to retract.

The anterior skin flap and the side flaps are then gently retracted so that the distal end of the tibia and fibula may be cut across with the saw just proximal to the joint surface. It is important to place this line distal to the inferior tibiofibular ligament, to prevent diastasis of these bones. This inevitably leaves a flare at the ankle, but removal of more bone results in an unsatisfactory stump due to spreading of the bones no longer bound together by ligaments. Careful placement of the posterior flap across the cut end of the bone and suture of the fat and skin is then performed. The "dog-ears" of skin and fat must be left medially and laterally and *not trimmed.* They ensure a broadly based blood supply and later atrophy, and they cause no difficulty. Additional fixation of the distal flap over the bone end is secured by placement of two crossed strips of sterile cloth held with dermatome glue, and a careful external dressing is placed. Maintenance of the distal flap for several weeks is important to prevent its dislocation.

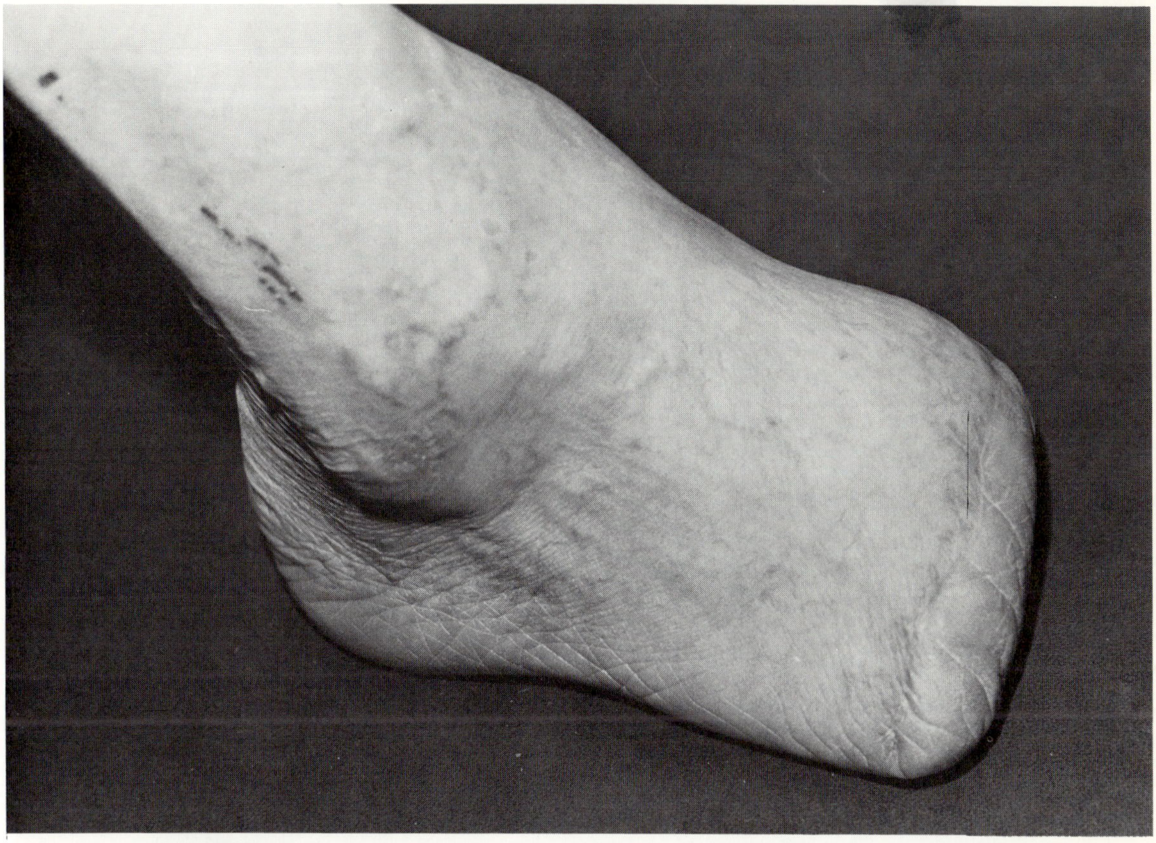

FIGURE 26-5 A painless foot and scar result from a well-healed transmetatarsal amputation.

Below-Knee Amputation

The ideal bone length of approximately 15 cm of tibia (varying with the patient's height) is marked by placing a needle through the skin into the periosteum of the tibia (Figure 26-7). The posterior skin and subcutaneous tissue flap are cut longer than the anterior flap so that the suture line will lie anterior to the bone end. With a simple anterior-to-posterior technique Gigli's saw is passed around, cutting the tibia and fibula individually. The fibula is recessed 2 cm on the lateral aspect of the leg by retraction of the soft tissues before it is cut. The anterior edge of the tibia is beveled and rounded with a file. Excess muscle is then removed from the posterior flap, and the fascia is closed without tension. A suction drain is led out through a stab wound laterally. A splint is placed to prevent contracture of the knee during the postoperative period and also to prevent painful motion during this time. It can be eliminated when the patient can move the knee without pain, 4 to 6 weeks later. (Details of technique for both the below- and above-knee amputations and their variations as described by four surgeons, including the author, may be compared.[26])

Below-Knee Amputation with Immediate Plaster Prosthesis

European surgeons Berlemont of France[33] and Weiss of Poland first practiced placing the below-knee prosthesis in the operating room.[34] Eugene Burgess of Seattle introduced this to North

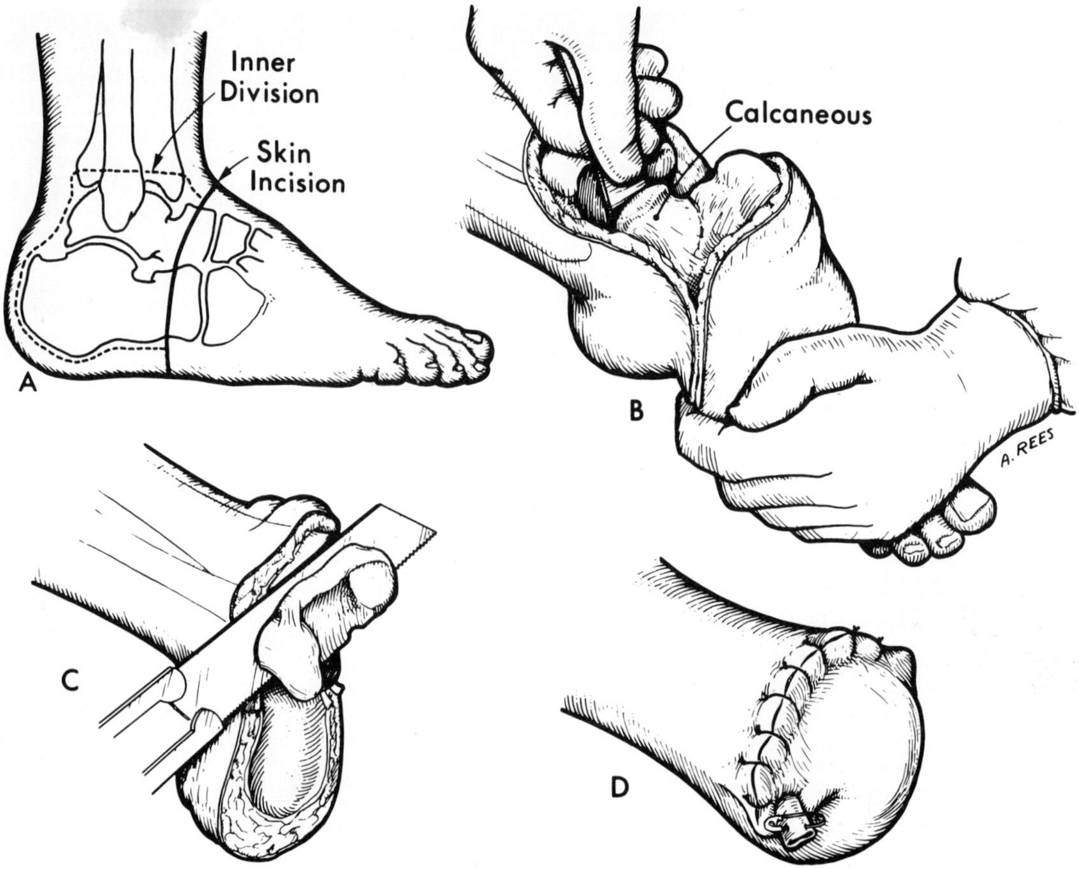

FIGURE 26-6 Syme's transmalleolar amputation. (*a*) A skin incision is made proximally, following which (*b*) the calcaneus is peeled out from within the heel flap. (*c*) With the heal flap retracted, the malleoli are removed. (*d*) The heel flap is sutured over the bone end and carefully stabilized by dressings.

America and has consistently advocated the technique.[35] Its advocates believe that (1) wound healing is not retarded, (2) edema is significantly reduced, (3) pain is lessened, and (4) early walking becomes possible, so muscular atrophy does not occur. Whether attachment of muscles to the bone end through drill holes aids development of collateral circulation seems doubtful, at best useless, and at worst harmful for an ischemic stump.

The immediate postoperative plaster prosthesis is applied after the skin is closed. A removable foot is incorporated into this immediately in the operating room (Figure 26-8). The patient is then encouraged to begin to walk on the prosthesis at once (Figure 26-9). The cast is changed 10 days and again 20 days after operation.

This method was used for 37 of my cases during the mid-1970s with the cooperation of a prosthetist, who applied the initial cast in the operating room as well as the secondary ones 10 and 20 days later. Most of the wounds did well, but a minority showed pressure effects upon one or the other skin flap (Figure 26-10). This ischemic effect did not seem to be due to the operation, since it sometimes occurred after the first or second cast change. It was due to a tight dressing pressing upon skin with poor circulation. These results convinced me that while the technique

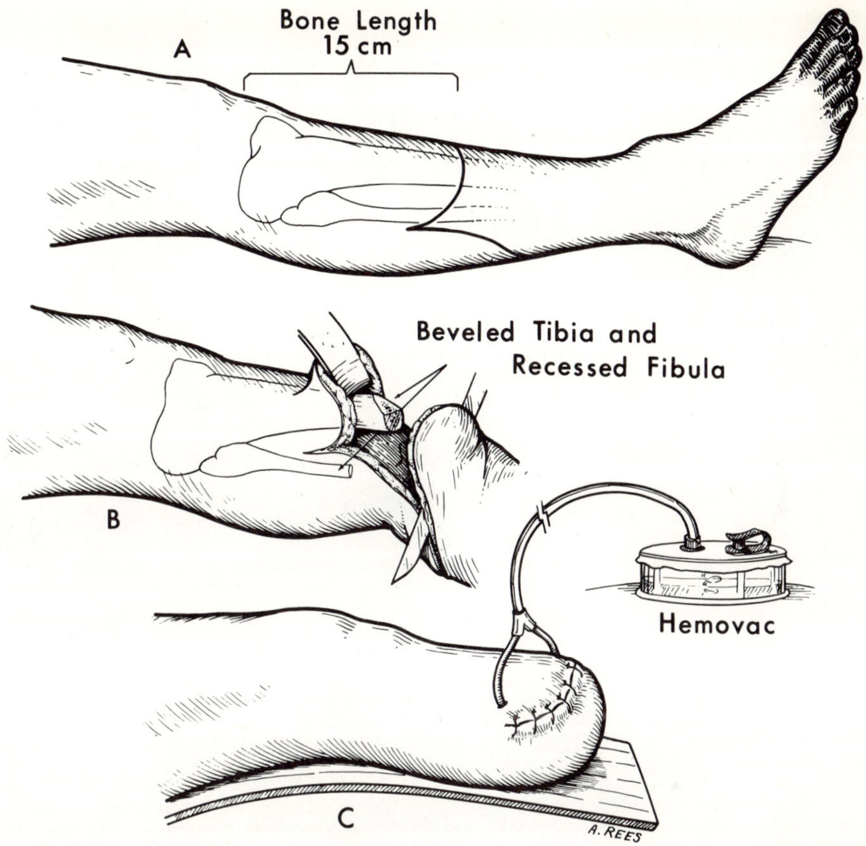

FIGURE 26-7 Below-knee amputation. (*a*) The short anterior and longer posterior flaps are cut through the skin, fat, and fascia to provide an optimum bone length of 15 cm for the average person. (*b*) The tibia is beveled 45° and the fibula recessed 2 cm. The posterior soft tissues are severed with the amputation knife. (*c*) The fascia and skin are closed with interrupted sutures. A suction drain is led out through a stab wound.

may be useful for young patients, the older atherosclerotic limb is better managed without a pressure dressing—a principle that long ago led to using noncompressive loose dressings for above-knee as well as other amputations. Further, the tight fascia and skin closure is a heresy in this field, where sufficiently long flap length has become a generally accepted principle. Immediate-fit prostheses have therefore been abandoned for elderly patients.

Above-Knee Amputation

Complicated tendinoplastic or patella-shifting procedures are technically more difficult, often have complications, and are not recommended. The femur should be cut approximately 10 cm proximal to the knee to allow room for a joint in the prosthesis. The skin-fat-fascia flaps should close easily over the bone end. No sutures should be placed in the fat, since they may cause inflammation and may devitalize the tissue.

A longer anterior and a shorter posterior flap then for a below-knee procedure are outlined by a firm cut through skin, fat, and fascia. The distal end of the anterior flap is cut over the middle

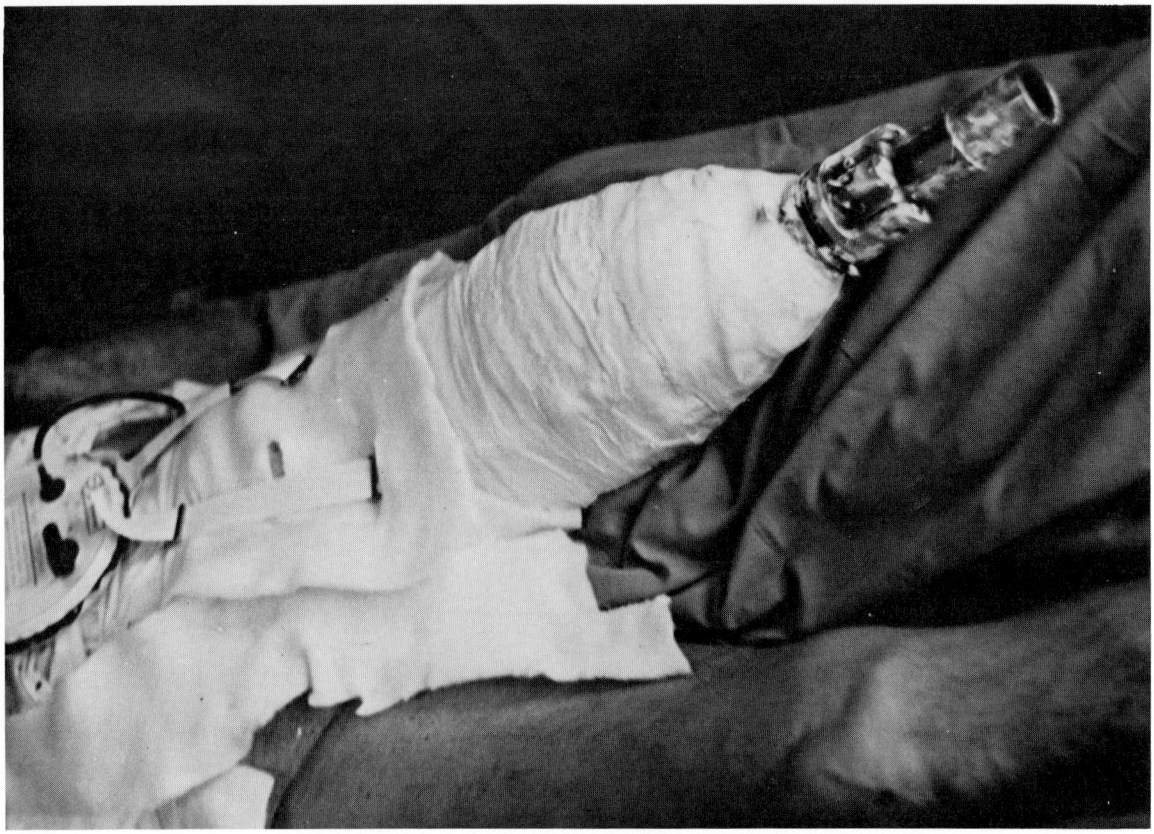

FIGURE 26-8 An immediately fitted elasticized-plaster prosthesis is placed just after below-knee amputation. The foot portion of the removable socket is placed later.

of the patella. The posterior flap does not extend as far distally (Figure 26-11). The fascia is cut. Allis clamps then elevate the anterior fascia, allowing access to the femur. A curved clamp is passed posterior to the bone to pull through the Gigli saw used to cut the bone.

A long amputation knife is used to sever the remaining posterior soft tissues. The amputated extremity is removed, and a few 3-0 Dexon ties are placed to control bleeding.

The operator may at this point easily stabilize the stump in a thigh-flexed position by passing a folded sheet around its posterior aspect and securing this to the table over the patient's shoulders. This provides excellent exposure for hemostasis and wound closure.

The previously severed vascular bundle is dissected so that the artery and vein may be individually doubly ligated with 0-0 silk. A single absorbable tie is placed about the nerve as high as possible, to control bleeding. The distal portion of the nerve is cut away. If bleeding continues to occur from the bone end, it is controlled with Gelfoam and pressure. The periosteum is not scraped away. Interrupted 0-0 Dexon sutures close the fascia. No sutures are placed in the fat. A few interrupted 4-0 Dacron sutures are placed in mattress fashion to support the flaps, and a meticulous continuous closure of the edges of the skin is done with continuous 5-0 Dexon, which sloughs away 2 to 3 weeks later (Figure 26-12).

Amputation wounds have a relatively large surface area and, like burns and abrasions, exude fluid despite the most meticulous hemostasis. Suction-drainage via a small stab wound is provided for 4 to 5 days.

Hip Disarticulation

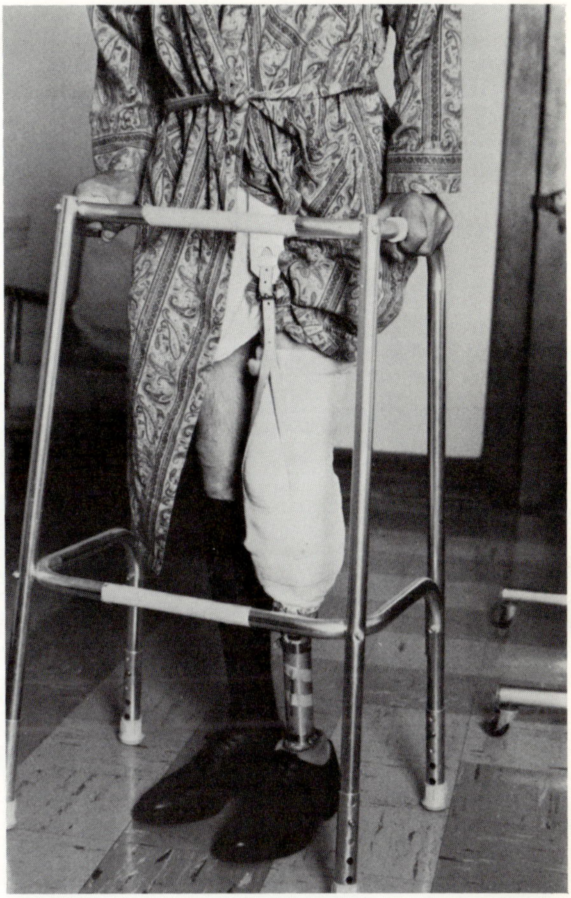

FIGURE 26-9 A below-knee amputee bearing weight on the immediately fitted prosthesis with attached foot 5 days postoperatively.

Removal of the entire lower extremity at the hip-joint level is difficult because of blood loss and operative trauma. It leads to the use of a cumbersome prosthesis (or none at all). Amputation at a lower level, in the midthigh or even the high thigh, is therefore preferred. The chief reason for hip disarticulation is widespread necrosis of the thigh muscles secondary to occlusion of the iliac vessels or of both the superficial and deep femoral arteries. This may follow high iliac occlusion, unsuccessful bypass grafting to the femoral artery with complete ascending thrombosis of vessels, or extensive bleeding into the thigh from a ruptured femoral aneurysm. It may be necessary after proximal iliac ligation to allow an infected synthetic graft to be removed.

The patient is placed supine on the operating table, and the hip is elevated 30° to aid exposure. Drapes are applied so that the lower part of the abdomen is exposed while the genitalia are covered.

The surgeon can perform preliminary vascular ligation by exposing the external iliac vessels retroperitoneally (deepening the usual herniorrhaphy incision through the transversalis fascia and pushing the peritoneal sac medially). This ensures ligature of the vessels outside the field of amputation and is desirable if there is any question of development of infection within the amputation site, which might lead to secondary hemorrhage. Alternatively, the femoral vessels may be initially ligated through the amputation exposure (Figure 26-13).

Medial and lateral flaps are placed so that they join over the area of the femoral vessels, and the resulting wound lies somewhat lateral and away from the perineum. Flaps are outlined from a point 6 cm above Poupart's ligament to a point 8 cm below it, with each end of the incision curving medially and laterally and then sweeping around the posterior aspect of the thigh 5 cm below the gluteal fold. After individual ligation the femoral artery and vein are divided. Other anterior structures, including the femoral nerve, the sartorius muscle, the rectus femoris muscle, and the tensor fasciae latae muscle are severed. With the extremity in adduction, the gluteus muscles attached to the greater trochanter are severed through their tendinous expansions. The iliopsoas muscle is next exposed by retraction of the severed muscles and is cut transversely to expose the anterior capsule of the hip joint. This capsule is entered around the margin of the acetabulum. The hip is flexed, adducted, and externally rotated so that the head of the femur may be dislocated. A bone holder is placed on the femoral neck, and the remaining portion of the posterior hip capsule is cut. The posterior musculature structures are then severed from

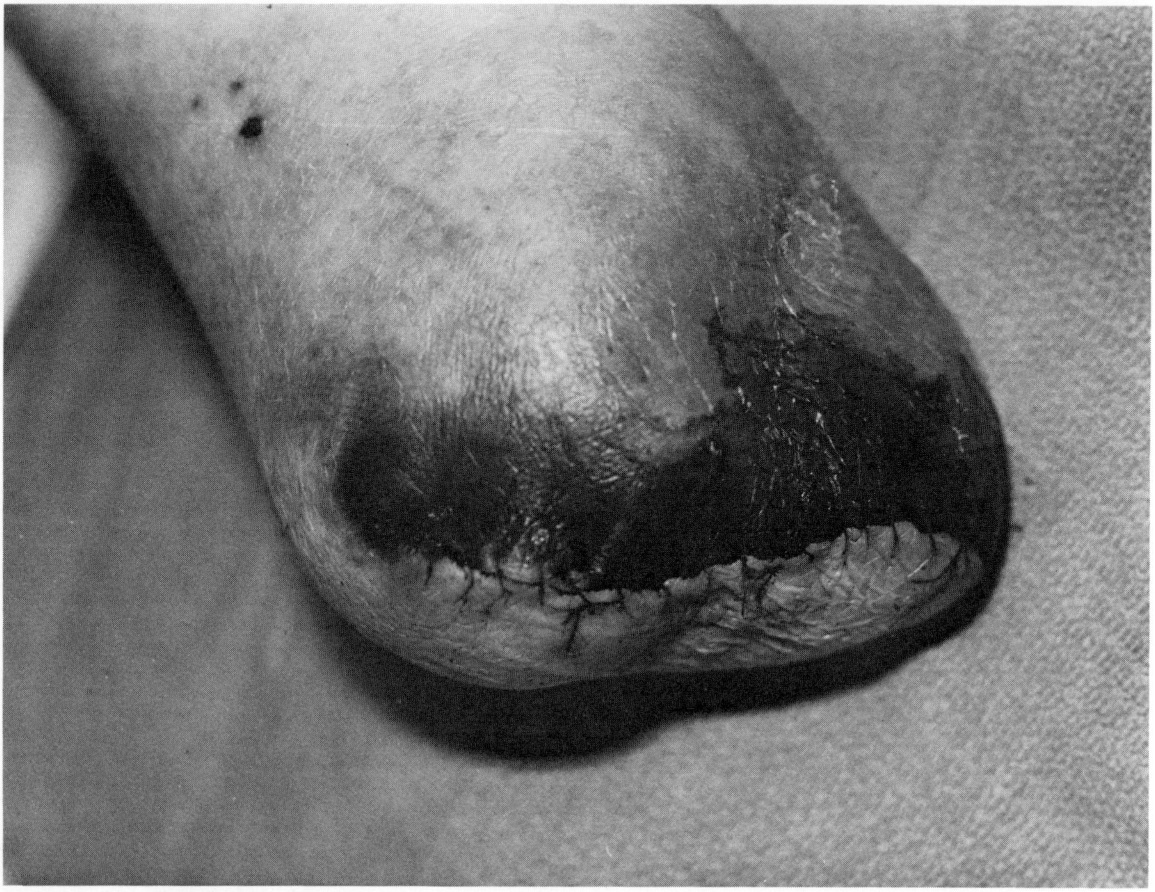

FIGURE 26-10 Anterior flap necrosis was apparent at the second dressing on the twentieth day after this below-knee amputation. Since the wound had been healing normally when the dressing was changed on the tenth day, it appeared that excessive pressure following the dressing change had caused this ischemic necrosis, which necessitated revision of the amputation.

within outward. The adductor muscle lining the medial flap is severed and tapered from above downward, and the extremity is removed. Fascia and skin closure are done in the usual layers, and suction drains are left in the hollow of the acetabulum. A firm dressing is applied to hold the flaps snugly together.

POSTOPERATIVE MANAGEMENT

Antibiotics Antibiotics are used prophylactically. An intravenous dose is given just before the anesthesia, followed by four others at 6-hour intervals.

Drain and Dressing Management These require individualization. Removal of the suction tubes is done after 2 to 5 days, depending upon the volume of drainage. On the fifth day the wound is inspected, and any excessively tight sutures are removed. Most of the sutures are left in place for 14 to 21 days. Throughout this period a loose dressing of carefully wrapped nonelastic but soft bandages is held in place with longitudinal strips of tape so that it does not slip down

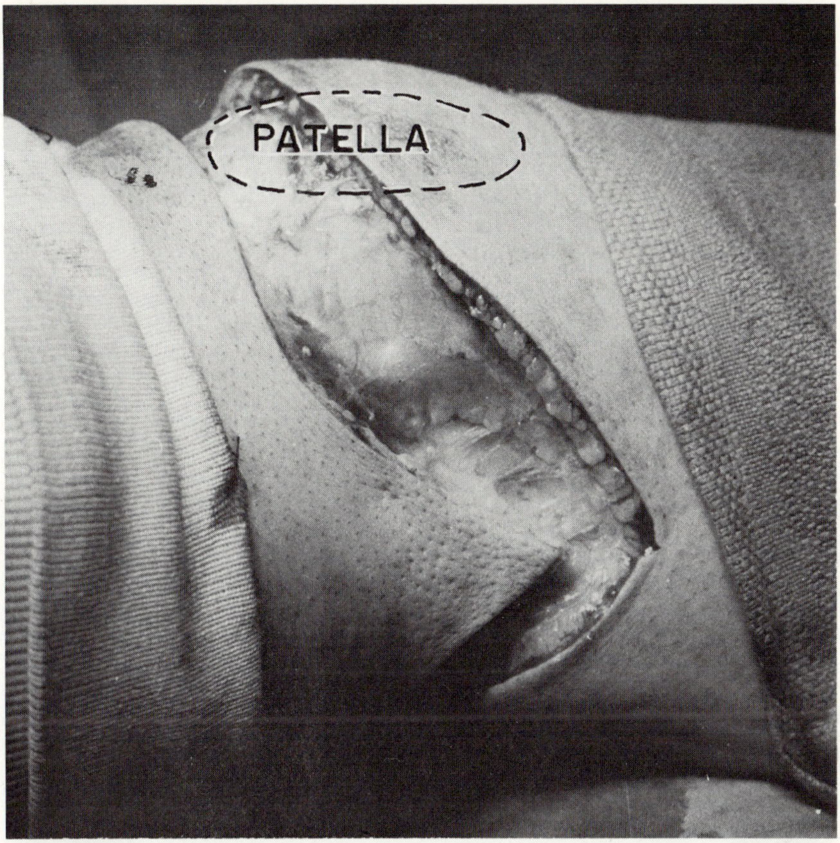

FIGURE 26-11 Above-knee amputation is begun by incising the skin, fat, and fascia for a somewhat longer anterior and shorter posterior fish-mouth flap. The lower margin of the anterior flap lies over the midpatella region.

around the end of the stump. Circumferential elastic bandaging has been abandoned as likely to cause undue pressure and resultant necrosis of the skin of the stump.

Above-knee amputation patients after 72 hours lie on the abdomen for 5 to 10 minutes twice daily to prevent flexion contracture of the hip. They also begin to travel in a wheelchair. After below-knee amputation a splint is used to prevent contracture. When the patient uses crutches or a walker in the early postoperative period, he or she is observed by an attendant to be certain that a fall does not occur. An overhead bed trapeze is useful during this period, to enable the patient to move about in bed and to maintain muscle tone in the upper extremities and shoulder girdles.

Physical Therapy Physical therapy is an essential part of rehabilitation. When possible, the patient is introduced to the therapist and the techniques prior to amputation.

On the second postoperative day the below-knee amputee begins active rehabilitation. An air bladder temporary prosthesis is placed about the limb, which is still encased in a dressing (Figure 26-14). Either the Jobst device or the Bonner airleg may be used.[36] Both provide side pressure rather than end pressure on the wound. The patient stands, using a walker, and swings the limb and touches it down but does not put weight on it. This occurs in twice-daily sessions. There are

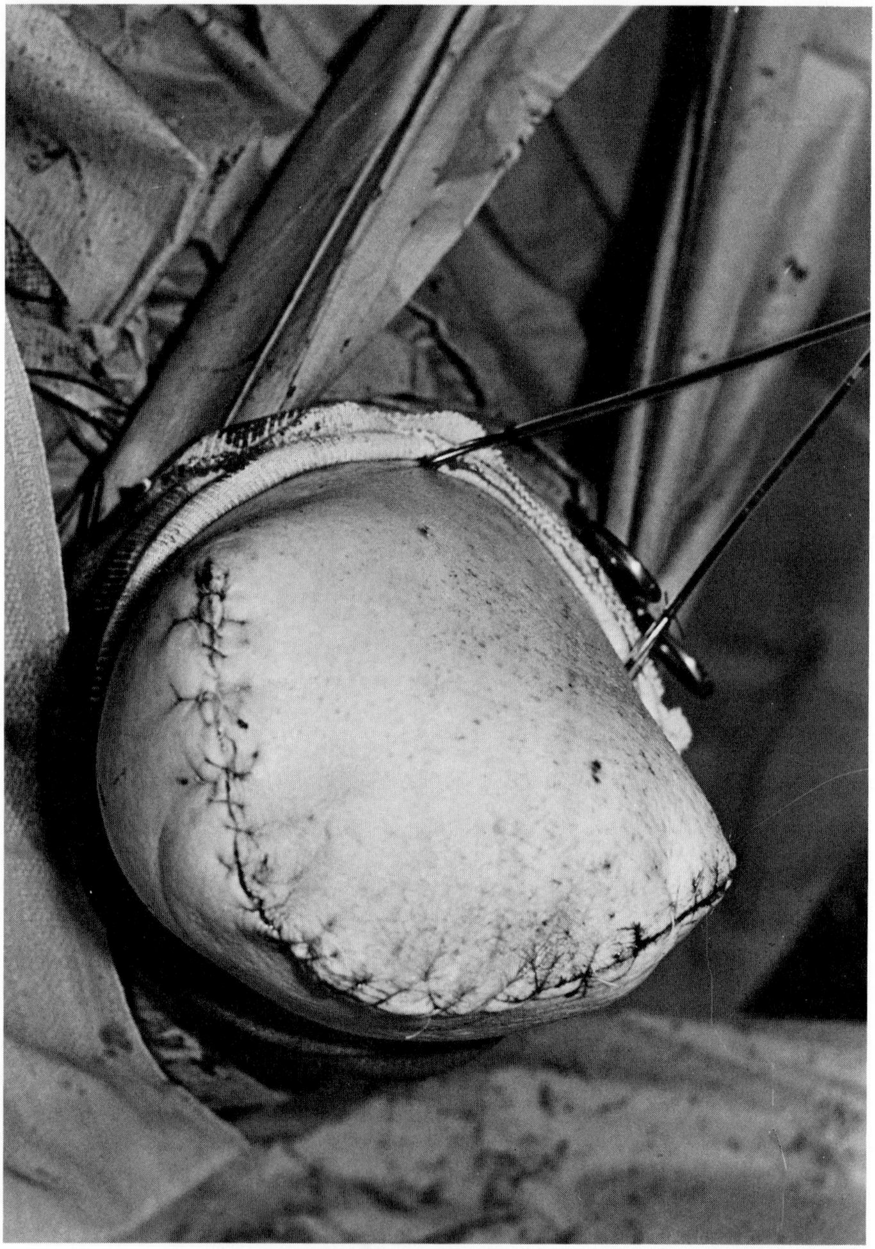

FIGURE 26-12 Above-knee amputation is concluded by closure of the fascia with interrupted sutures, drainage of the subcutaneous tissue with suction tubes, and closure of the skin appropriately.

hourly pulls on an overhead trapeze, and other therapy sessions in a wheelchair occur regularly. On the fifth day the wound is inspected, and if healing is normal, the patient begins to bear weight on the stump and pylon. A temporary plaster prosthesis is fitted on the seventh to ninth day (Figure 26-15), with the expectation of discharge 10 days after the amputation.

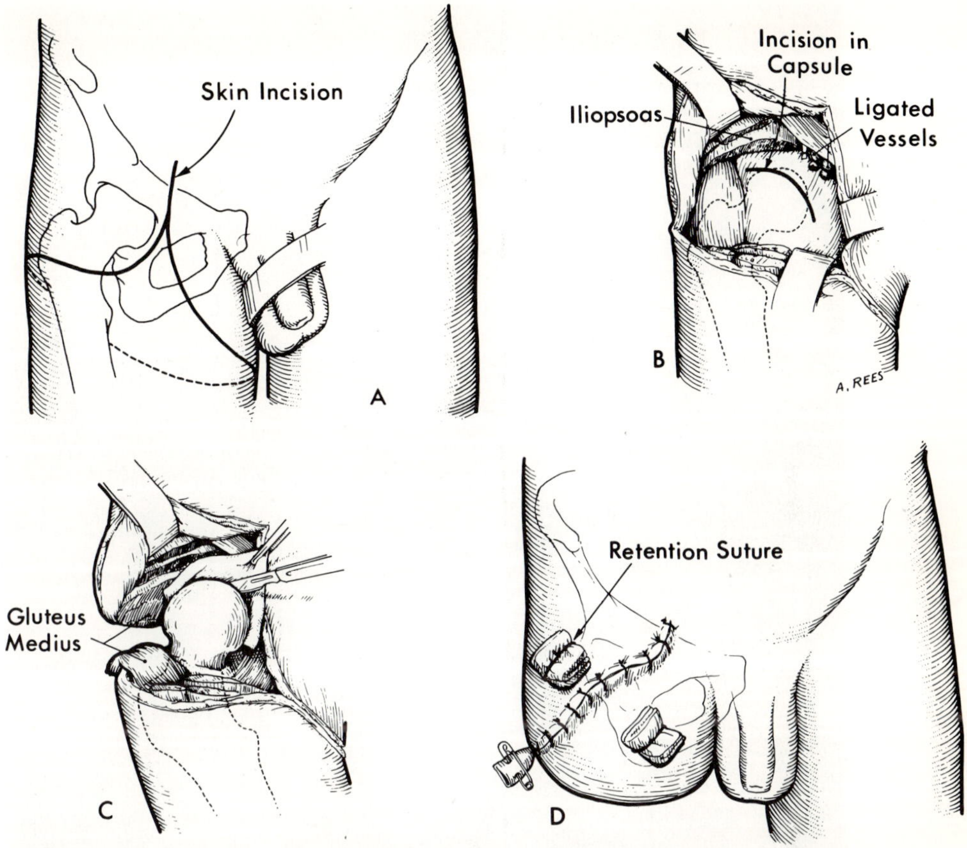

FIGURE 26-13 Hip disarticulation begins with (*a*) an incision through the skin and fat overlying the femoral triangle, through which the femoral vessels are individually suture-ligated and divided. (*b*) Dissection of the anterior and lateral soft tissues allows exposure of the capsule of the hip joint, which is opened. (*c*) Division of the posterior tissues and disarticulation of the joint complete the ablation. (*d*) Retention sutures are useful in supporting the heavy flaps. The cigarette drain shown has been replaced by tube suction drainage.

If the fifth-day inspection of the wound reveals any abnormality of the flaps, weight bearing is delayed for whatever time is necessary to allow proper healing.

After discharge there are daily visits to physical therapy. Ideally, the final prosthesis is fitted 6 to 8 weeks later, when the wound is solidly healed and only minimally painful.

Prosthesis Fitting Many surgeons know little (and care less) about the management of prostheses and tend to discard the patient once a necessary amputation has occurred. Rehabilitation is far from complete at that point and requires a cooperative effort between the surgeon, the prosthetist, and the physical therapist. This begins with planning of the amputation and continues through the period of fitting and training in the use of the artificial extremity. Arrangements should be made for the patient to be seen regularly by both the prosthetist and the surgeon (Figure 26-16), and communication should be maintained to prevent the patient from falling into limbo somewhere between them. The surgeon who listens to an experienced prosthetist learns many practical details of amputation, which are important in obtaining good functional results. The surgeon must also at times insist on the patient's behalf to the prosthetist that some

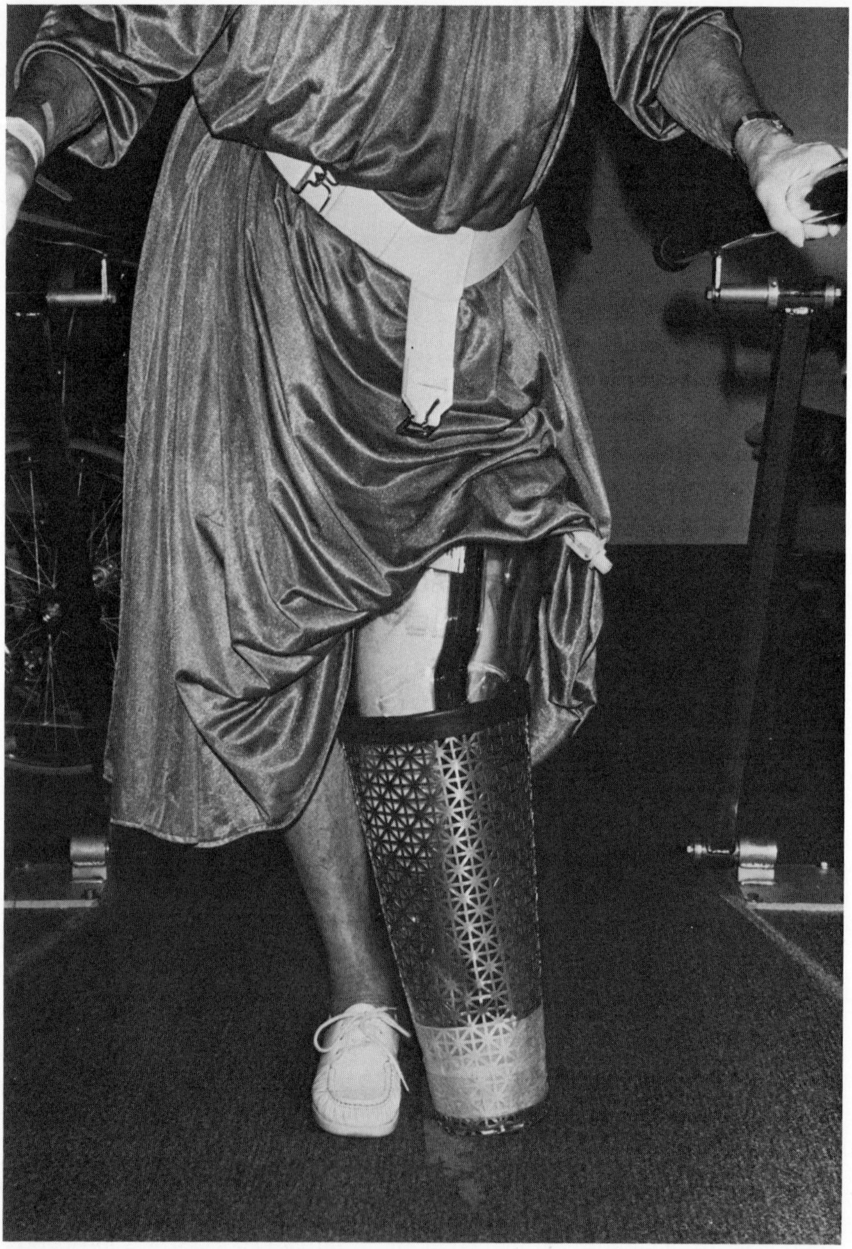

FIGURE 26-14 Five days postoperatively this below-knee amputee is beginning to walk on the temporary air bladder prosthetic device.

change in the artificial limb is required. I have little respect for the elitist surgeon who abandons the patient to the orthopedist and prosthetist for amputation and care after his or her vascular reconstruction fails.

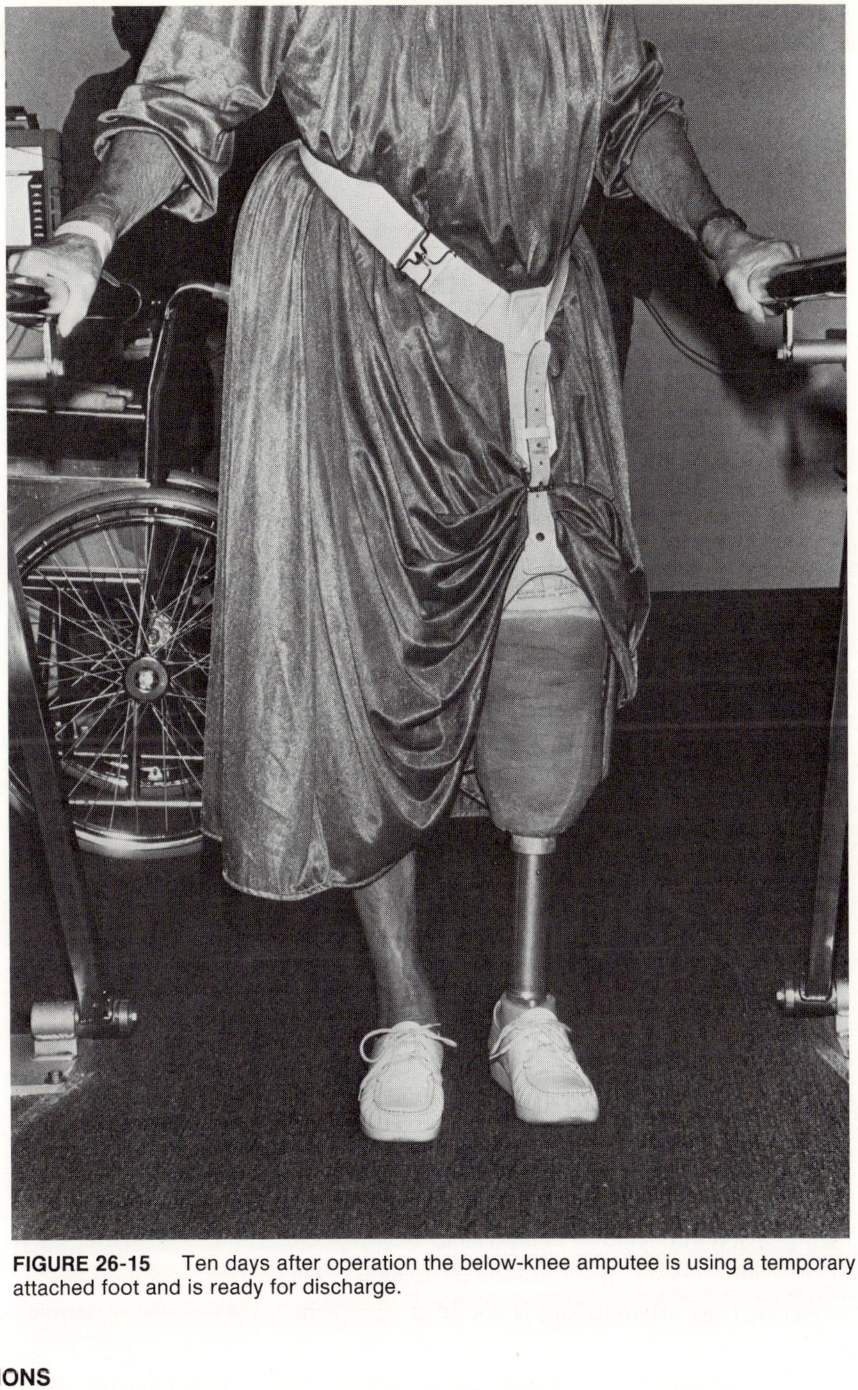

FIGURE 26-15 Ten days after operation the below-knee amputee is using a temporary pylon with attached foot and is ready for discharge.

COMPLICATIONS

Delayed Healing and Infection Delayed healing and secondary wound infections plague surgeons because the vascular supply, to say the least, is usually less than optimal. The desire to save as much as possible of the extremity further adds to the problem, since healing is progressively less certain as more distal sites are chosen. The surgeon should therefore be prepared to shift the amputation site to a more proximal one if nonbleeding muscle is found at the time of amputation or if there develops serious doubt about the healing capability of the subcutaneous tissue and skin.

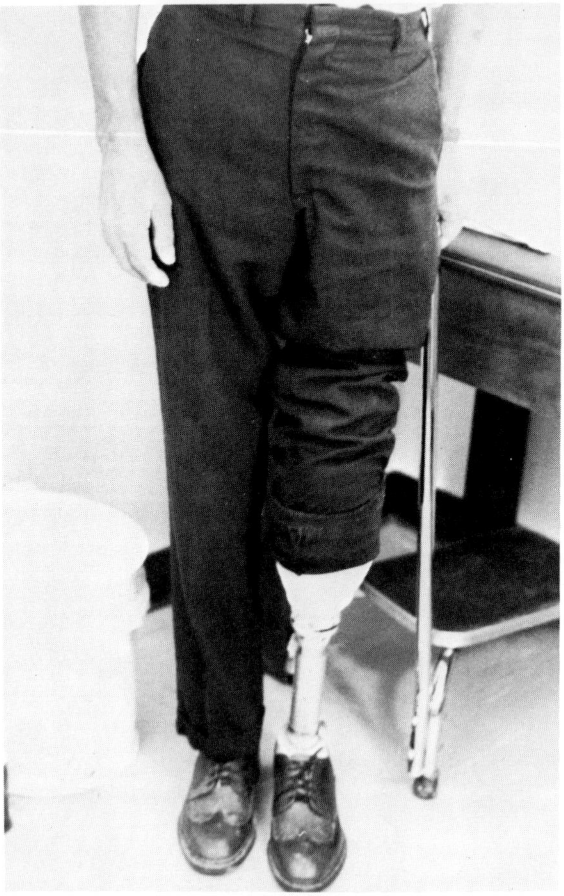

FIGURE 26-16 Four weeks following operation a below-knee amputee walks into the office.

Hematomas Hematoma and serum formation within wounds predispose them to infection more than any other thing, since this places an excellent culture medium within a poorly vascularized area. Prevention is undertaken by whatever means is available for a particular wound. In amputations, I tried earlier to prevent this by placing a through-and-through drain and then wrapping the stump firmly with elastic bandages. After several patients developed areas of skin necrosis due to excessively tight wrapping, this was changed. Now suction drainage is provided through a plastic tube placed through a proximal stab wound. No particular external pressure is attempted, and an absorbent but loose dressing is placed. This results in more comfort for the patient and satisfactorily removes serosanguineous drainage fluid.

Should infection occur, drainage must be promptly instituted by removal of corner sutures to allow escape of pocketed fluid or pus. Placement of a drain may be done through the end of the wound. Every effort should be made to secure open drainage without removal of the central sutures and thus exposure of the bone end. A broad-spectrum antibiotic should be begun and bacterial cultural procedures done.

Necrosis of Skin Flaps Necrosis may be treated expectantly if the area is small, since slough, granulation, and epithelialization occur in time. Large areas of necrosis indicate the need for early revision with removal of nonviable tissue (including more bone if necessary) and resuturing of vascularized tissues to allow primary healing (Figure 26-10).

Hemorrhage Hemorrhage is not often a problem, since the atherosclerotic vessels are usually occluded.

Phantom Limb This occurs to some extent after all amputations, but there are few serious problems. An explanation of the sensation is made to the patient without any dwelling upon the possibility of its continuation. The patient is encouraged by the knowledge that it ordinarily disappears spontaneously with progression of time.

Venous Thromboembolism Thromboembolism is an important unsolved problem. The incidence of phlebitis without pulmonary embolization is unknown. The minimal incidence of pulmonary embolism was 7 percent in the Rochester series of amputations[7] and 3 percent in the Nashville series.[8]

Frequently there is a loose thrombus lying within the popliteal vein when it is cut across. It appears reasonable to remove this by suction with a Fogarty catheter. Later embolism originating from recurrence of the same clot, from the contralateral leg, or from the pelvis explains why this removal cannot be expected absolutely to prevent thromboembolism.

Veal in 1943 reported 36 ligations of the common femoral vein at the time of amputation, without subsequent emboli,[37] but Perlow[38] and Papaioannoa[39] reported postligation embolism. In 1959 we reported the results of superficial femoral vein ligation at the time of amputation in 27 patients. Fifteen percent had pulmonary embolism despite the ligation. Since the procedure was ineffective because of embolization from a source outside the stump, it was abandoned.

Anticoagulation therapy using heparin appears to be too likely to cause hazardous bleeding. Long-acting anticoagulants such as warfarin are less effective and also are productive of complications. Thompson, Delblanco, and McAllister reported 24 patients thus treated without detectable embolization, but 3 anticoagulant complications occurred.[40]

The prophylactic merits of repeated intravenous doses of dextran have been cited. There were no instances of pulmonary embolism in 49 randomized patients with pelvic, hip, and femoral fracture who received dextran, while 8 of 77 patients receiving only saline had pulmonary embolization.[41] Dextran, however, remains unproven despite its popularity in some quarters.

Cerebral Vascular Accidents and Serious Cardiac Lesions These are the chief causes of death in patients who require amputations. Eighty-three percent of the deaths in the Nashville series were due to cardiovascular causes.[8] Their prevention is uncertain.

All of us finally must pay our debt to nature.

REFERENCES

1 Buel HW: Statistics of amputation in the New York Hospital, from Jan. 1, 1839 to Jan. 1, 1848. *Am J Med Sci* 1848, 16:33.

2 Hayward G: Statistics of the amputations of large limbs that have been performed at the Massachusetts General Hospital, from the establishment to Jan. 1, 1850. *Boston Med Surg J* 1850, 43:9.

3 Graham H: *Surgeons All.* New York Philosophical Library, New York, 1957.

4 Malone JM, Goldstone J: Lower extremity amputation, in Moore WS (ed): *Vascular Surgery: A Comprehensive Review,* Grune & Stratton, New York, 1983, p 916.

5 Rosenthal AM, Reddy NK: Revascularization surgery: Impact on lower extremity amputations. *Arch Phys Med Rehab* 1983, 64:125.

6 Huston CC, Bivins BA, Ernst CB, Griffen WO Jr: Morbid implications of above-knee amputations. *Arch Surg* 1980, 115:165.

7 Dale WA, Capps W: Major leg and thigh amputations. *Surgery* 1959, 46:333.

8 Dale WA, Jacobs JK: Lower extremity amputation: Results in Nashville, 1956–60. *Ann Surg* 1962, 155:1011.

9 Barber CG, McPhail NU, Scobie TK, Brennan MDC, Ellis CC: A prospective study of lower limb amputations. *Can J Surg* 1983, 26:339.

10 Warren R, Kihn RB: A survey of lower extremity amputations for ischemia. *Surgery* 1968, 63:107.

11 Eraklis A, Wheeler HB: Below-knee amputations in patients with severe arterial insufficiency. *N Engl J Med* 1963, 269:938.

12 Block MA, Whitehouse FW: Below knee amputation in patients with diabetes mellitus. *Arch Surg* 1963, 87:682.

13 Lempke RE, King RD, Kaiser GC, Judd D, Nahrwold D: Amputations for arteriosclerosis obliterans. *Arch Surg* 1963, 86:406.

14 Wheelock F: Transmetatarsal amputation and arterial surgery in diabetic patients. *N Engl J Med* 1961, 264:316.

15 Lim RC, Blaisdell FW, Hall AD, Moore WS, Thomas AN: Below-knee amputation for ischemic gangrene. *Surg Gynecol Obstet* 1967, 125:493.

16 Stockel M, Ovesen J, Brochner-Mortensen J, Emneus J: Standardized photoelectric technique as routine method for selection of amputation level. *Acta Orthop Scand* 1982, 53:875.

17 Holstein P: Level selection in leg amputation for arterial occlusive disease. *Acta Orthop Scand* 1982, 53:821.

18 Nicholas GG, Myers JL, Demuth WE: The role of vascular laboratory criteria in the selection of patients for lower extremity amputation. *Ann Surg* 1982, 195:469.

19 Moore WS: Determination of amputation level: Measurement of skin flow with Xenon, Xe 113. *Arch Surg* 1973, 107:798.

20 Kostuik JP, Wood D, Hornby R, Feingold S, Matthews V: Measurement of skin blood flow in peripheral vascular disease by epicutaneous application of Xenon 133. *J Bone Joint Surg* 1976, 58:833.

21 Cheng EY: Lower extremity amputation level: Selection using noninvasive hemodynamic methods of evaluation. *Arch Phys Med Rehab* 1982, 63:475.

22 Cranley JJ, Krause KJ, Strasser ES, Hafner CD: Below-the-knee amputation for arteriosclerosis obliterans. *Arch Surg* 1969, 98:77.

23 Otteman MG, Stahlgren LH: Evaluation of factors which influence mortality and morbidity following major lower extremity amputations for arteriosclerosis. *Surg Gynecol Obstet* 1965, 120:1217.

24 Harris PD, Schwartz SI, DeWeese JA: Midcalf amputation for peripheral vascular disease. *Arch Surg* 1961, 82:381.

25 Still JM, Wray CJ, Moretz WH: Selective physiologic amputation: A valuable adjunct in preparation for surgical operation. *Ann Surg* 1970, 272:143.

26 Dale WA, Wheelock FC, Jamieson CW, Burgess EM, Little JM: *Amputation of the Lower Extremity,* Little, Brown, Boston, 1978.

27 Dedrick R: Technique of myoplastic operations, *Ann R Coll Surg* 1967, 40:222.

28 Datta PK: The last resort. *Nurs Mirror* 1982, 41:154.

29 McKittrick LS, McKittrick JB, Risley TS: Transmetatarsal amputation for infection or gangrene in patients with diabetes mellitus. *Ann Surg* 1949, 130:826.

30 Warren R, Crawford ES, Hardy IB, McKittrick JB: The transmetatarsal amputation in arterial deficiency of the lower extremity. *Surgery* 1952, 31:1932.

31 Wheelock F: Transmetatarsal amputation and arterial surgery in diabetic patients. *N Engl J Med* 1961, 264:316.

32 Reeves MM, Quattlebaum FW: The lateral flap technique in supracondylar amputations. *Surg Gynecol Obstet* 1956, 102:751.

33 Berlemont M, Weber R, Willott JP: Ten years of experience with the immediate application of prosthetic devices to amputees of the lower extremities on the operating table. *Prosthetic Int* 1969, 3:8.

34 Weiss M: The prosthesis on the operating table from a neurophysical point of view. Report of a workshop panel on lower extremity prosthetic fitting, Committee on Prosthetics Research Development, National Academy of Sciences, February 1966.

35 Burgess EM, Romano RL, Zettl JH: *The Management of Lower Extremity Amputations.* U.S. Government Printing Office, Washington, 1969.

36 Bonner FJ, Green RF: Pneumatic airleg prosthesis: Report of 200 cases. *Arch Phys Med Rehab* 1982, 63:383.

37 Veal JR: Prevention of pulmonary complications following thigh amputation by high ligation of femoral veins. *JAMA* 1943, 121:240.

38 Perlow S: Amputation for gangrene because of occlusive arterial disease. *Am J Surg* 1962, 103:569.

39 Papaiouannou AN: A study of thromboembolism in patients with major amputations. *Ohio Med J* 1962, 581:903.

40 Thompson RC, Delblanco TL, McAllister FF: Complications following lower extremity amputation. *Surg Gynecol Obstet* 1965, 120:301.

41 Atik M, Harkess JW, Wichman H: Prevention of fatal pulmonary embolism. *Surg Gynecol Obstet* 1970, 130:403.

Invited Commentary

Jerry Goldstone, M.D.
San Francisco, California

This chapter is an excellent overview not only of the fundamental principles that guide the surgeon's decision to perform an amputation and selection of the appropriate level but also of technical details of the procedures themselves. There is appropriate emphasis on the care with which amputation must be approached—preoperatively, intraoperatively, and postoperatively—if one is to achieve the objective of satisfactory primary healing at the most distal possible level to attain full rehabilitation.

The various methods that have been employed to determine the proper level for amputation have been well reviewed in this chapter. Not mentioned was the presence of dependent rubor at the site of proposed amputation. Skin that develops dependent rubor is clearly ischemic and is a contraindication to amputation at that level.

The more sophisticated objective tests recently introduced all have inherent limitations. They represent a cumulative effort to identify preoperatively the approximately 20 percent of patients who have insufficient circulation to heal a below-knee amputation. We continue to use skin clearance of radioactive Xenon 133, which predicts amputation healing at all levels in greater than 90 percent of patients. Nevertheless, we agree with Dr. Dale's concerns regarding the difficulties in establishing this procedure as a practical clinical tool in most medical centers.

Recently, encouraging results have been reported of the use of transcutaneous Po_2 determinations combined with 100 percent oxygen inhalation. The oxygen inhalation increases the positive predictive value for below-knee amputations to 100 percent. Measurement of transcutaneous Po_2 is simple and avoids the problems inherent in measuring skin blood flow with radioactive xenon.

Severe infection complicating dry gangrene, especially in a diabetic patient, represents a limb- and life-threatening emergency. Although control of sepsis may sometimes be achieved with antibiotic therapy plus limited debridement and drainage, when the gangrenous infection involves a major portion of the foot and contaminates tendon and tissue spaces, a radical debridement (drainage) should be performed. This is most easily accomplished by open guillotine amputation of the foot at the level of the malleoli. This immediately eliminates the septic focus and allows drainage of contaminated lymphatics and tissue spaces in the lower leg. The presence of cellulitis and lymphangitis at the level of guillotine amputation is not a contraindication for this type of debridement. With this approach, we have had a decreased incidence of subsequent infection in the definitive amputation stump. In this respect I disagree with Dr. Dale's assertion that guillotine amputations have little or no place in civilian hospitals.

The importance of attention to technical details has also been appropriately emphasized in this chapter. Since healing of the skin is the major determinant of success or failure, particular care must be paid to handling it atraumatically, i.e., without the use of forceps, and to attaining close apposition of the skin edges. The use of a long posterior skin flap for below-knee amputations is another important feature that is well-founded both theoretically and clinically.

A technical complication of any kind can be disastrous to the healing of a distal amputation. This is especially true of wound hematomas. Nevertheless, we have rarely found it necessary to use drains of any kind in the dysvascular amputee. Drains may be useful in the traumatic amputation, where wound hemostasis has been difficult and tissue destruction extensive.

We continue to be enthusiastic about the use of the immediate postoperative prosthetic management technique for below-knee amputations. There are advantages to the use of a rigid dressing beyond those of early ambulation and rehabilitation, including limitation of stump edema and wound protection. The successful use of such an approach, however, requires the presence in the operating room of a skilled and dedicated prosthetist.

In addition to enumerating the principles and details of amputation, Dr. Dale demonstrates the sincere commitment to the care of patients requiring amputation that extends throughout the perioperative period and until maximum rehabilitation potential is achieved. This is a critical attitudinal factor encompassed by the philosophy that amputation should be looked at as a reconstructive rather than a destructive procedure. Amputation is not necessarily the ultimate failure, but rather the first step in a patient's rehabilitation.

27 TRANSLUMINAL ANGIOPLASTY

One of the important developments in vascular surgery during the last 20 years is the transluminal dilation of stenotic and even occluded arteries. The further modification of this technique, whereby a percutaneous approach avoids an open operation, is of even greater interest.

Charles Dotter in 1964 demonstrated that a firm but flexible series of bougies could be pushed distally through a tight or occluded segment of an artery and thereafter removed and that the opened vessel would retain patency for long periods, thus making unnecessary the considerably larger operation of either endarterectomy or a bypass graft (Figure 27-1).[1] By 1971 he had done 220 such procedures with "lasting success in 75–80 percent of cases."[2]

A decade later, in Zurich, Gruntzig described a better method of angioplasty, by which a polyvinyl chloride balloon (and later a polyethylene one) was suddenly and forcibly inflated (to 4 to 6 atmospheres) within the artery, achieving the angioplasty through the intact skin, if the small skin puncture for introduction be discounted (Figure 27-2).[3] The technique of percutaneous transluminal angioplasty (PTA) has since been used to the extent that thousands of such procedures are available for analysis, although the longest follow-up time is limited by its relatively recent origin.

The recent development by Fogarty of a linear extension balloon catheter[4] aimed particularly at intraoperative dilation of an artery by a surgeon without the need for complicated radiologic viewing devices has not yet been finally assessed (Figure 27-3). His success rate of 94 percent for the first 24 clinical uses suggests its virtues,[5] but further experience is needed for realistic evaluation.

MECHANISM OF ACTION

Originally, Dotter taught that the dilator "compacted" intraluminal thrombotic material as well as the thickened intima, thus restoring the lumen without rupturing the artery or forcing the material distally.

The Gruntzig balloon dilator, on the other hand, acutely ruptures or cracks the internal portion of the arterial wall without producing enough leakage of blood to cause a complicating hematoma (Figures 27-4 and 27-5).[6] Careful estimation of the correct size of the balloon is critical to success, since a diameter too small will not open the lumen sufficiently and one too large might cause widespread rupture and tearing of the vessel. Further, the balloon must expand circumferentially with enough force to crack the wall, yet it must not push out proximally and distally and thereby lose part of its expansive effect. Finally, the balloon must expand to a precise size, but not beyond the predetermined dimension.

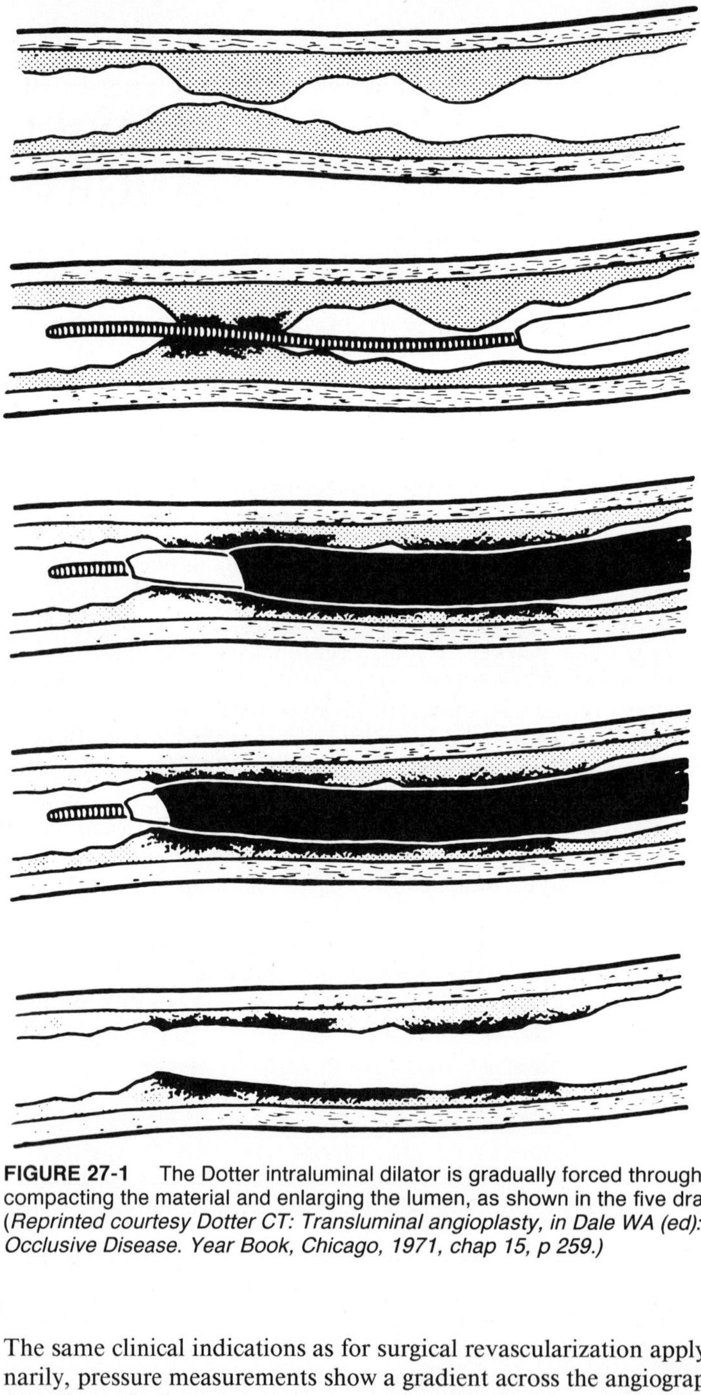

FIGURE 27-1 The Dotter intraluminal dilator is gradually forced through the stenotic area, thereby compacting the material and enlarging the lumen, as shown in the five drawings above downward. (*Reprinted courtesy Dotter CT: Transluminal angioplasty, in Dale WA (ed): Management of Arterial Occlusive Disease. Year Book, Chicago, 1971, chap 15, p 259.)*

INDICATIONS

The same clinical indications as for surgical revascularization apply to PTA (Table 27-1). Ordinarily, pressure measurements show a gradient across the angiographically demonstrated stenosis (Figure 27-6), but those without a gradient may be dilated before or during surgery either distal or proximal to the lesion.

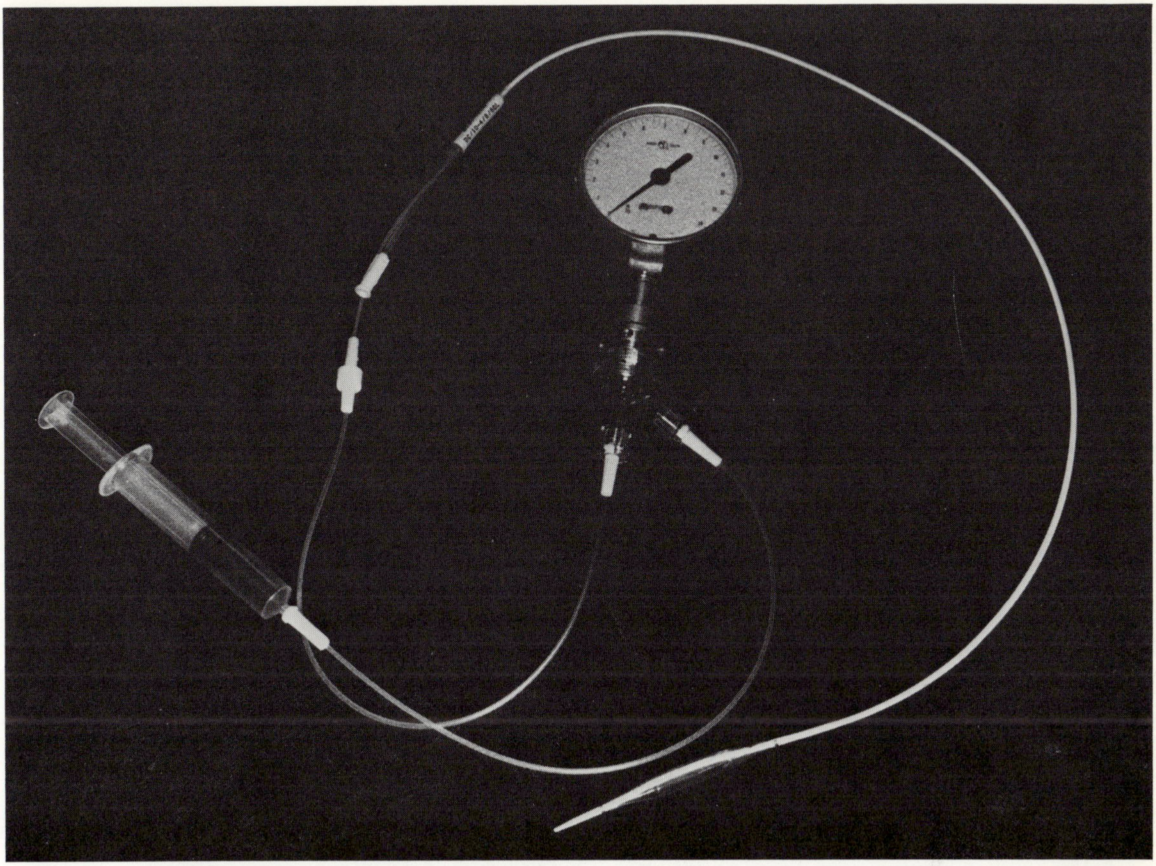

FIGURE 27-2 A Gruntzig balloon dilator.

It has become apparent that lesions which are short, of brief duration, and not calcified are better candidates, particularly in large vessels rather than small ones (Figure 27-7). Since complications including peripheral embolization occur in a small number, the results of this in a particular arterial bed must be carefully weighed before PTA is performed. Thus, the severe results of embolism to the brain generally contraindicate PTA of the carotid artery.

Failure of angioplasty usually does not preclude a later operative repair, nor does it make the patient worse, so it should often be considered prior to an operation, especially in patients who are poor risks for anesthesia and a complicated operation. The Toronto series of 384 showed clinical worsening in 4 percent of iliac and 14 percent of femoropopliteal PTAs, but these did not cause limb loss per se.[7]

COMPLICATIONS

The expected reduction in complications as materials improved and experience accumulated was documented by Zeitler's group. Among 2942 angioplasties for iliac and femoral lesions their complication rate over a 13-year period decreased from 14 to 4 percent while those requiring surgery after angioplasty diminished from 2.3 to 0.5 percent.[8] Their use of antiplatelet drugs prior to and after the procedure is therefore of interest.[9]

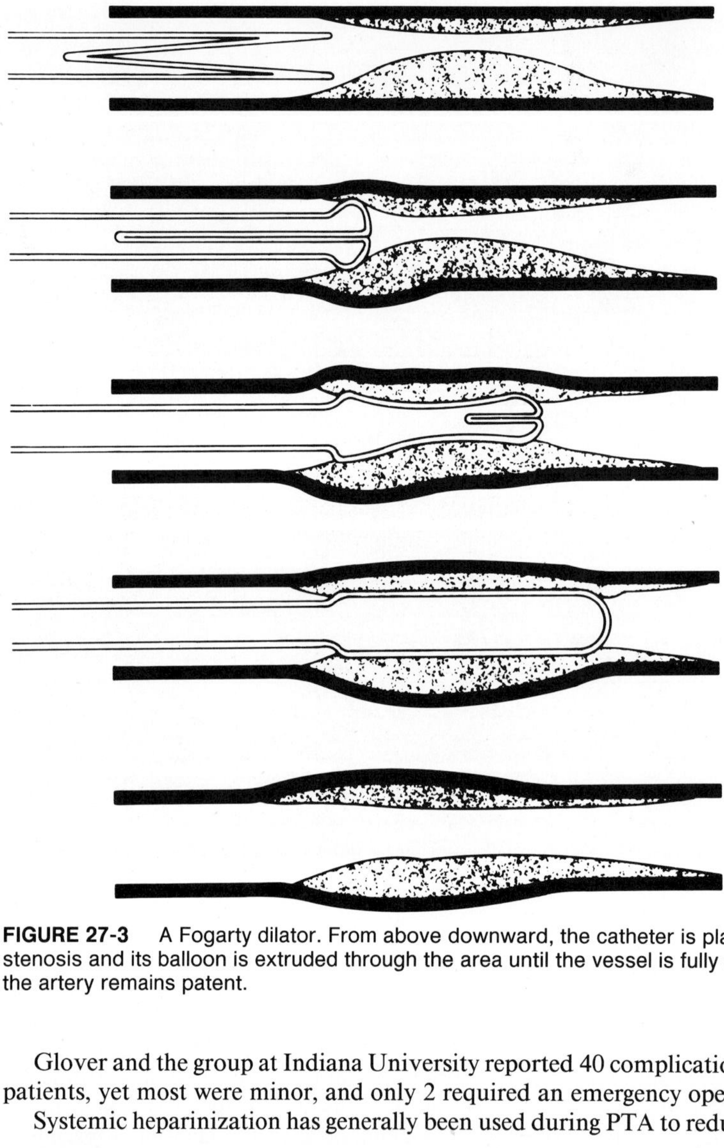

FIGURE 27-3 A Fogarty dilator. From above downward, the catheter is placed just at the end of the stenosis and its balloon is extruded through the area until the vessel is fully expanded. After withdrawal the artery remains patent.

Glover and the group at Indiana University reported 40 complications among 83 limb salvage patients, yet most were minor, and only 2 required an emergency operation.[10]

Systemic heparinization has generally been used during PTA to reduce clotting complications.

Hematomas Hematomas are not unexpected at the puncture site in the artery, particularly since systemic heparinization is usual. The rate of significant hematomas was 2.3 percent of 384 patients in the Toronto group.[7]

The risk is greater in hypertensives and when a proximal puncture site which overlies the retroperitoneal space, rather than one which is distal to the inguinal ligament, is used. The attention and devotion of the person holding pressure on the artery after removal of the catheter also affects this statistic. Our radiologists personally provide the pressure and the dressing to each patient.

Hemorrhage Sprayregen cited hemorrhage figures of 1.4 to 7.9 percent and false aneurysms of 0.5 to 2 percent in collected series.[11] The Roberts and Ring experience with 600 dilations

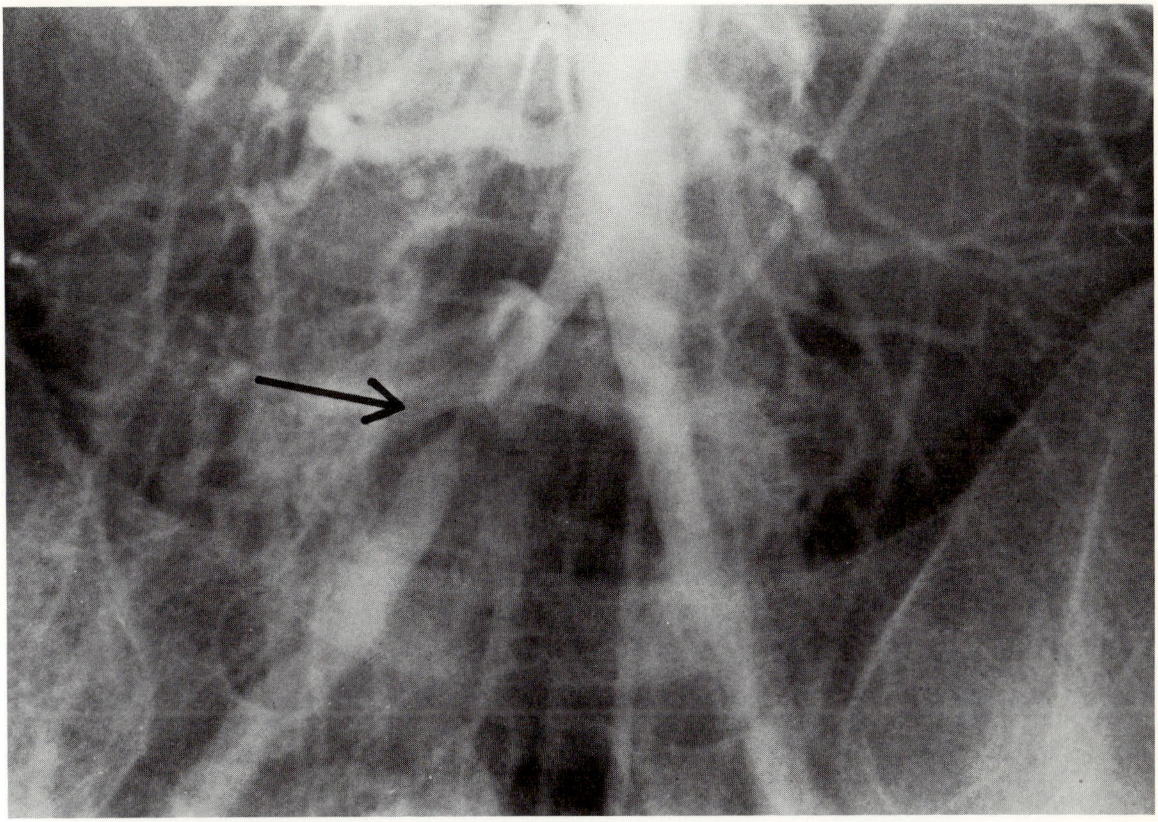

FIGURE 27-4 A short stenosis of the common iliac artery is the best indication for percutaneous transluminal dilation.

showed 3.5 percent overall complications, of which 1.2 percent were hemorrhage. There were no false aneurysms.[12] Ameli and associates had only 8 percent complications among 104 angioplasties done without heparin or antiplatelet drugs. If the three vessel perforations and one false aneurysm be deleted so that only four complications (two thromboses and two hematomas) are left, the revised complication rate becomes 4 percent, a figure comparable to the best for heparin use.[13]

Thrombosis and Embolism These are constant threats during and after PTA, varying considerably in several series and with the experience of the operator. Significant distal embolism was surprisingly seldom encountered in one series (1 percent).[14] It is generally supposed that 3 to 5 percent is usual.[9,15] The diagnosis is often doubtful and surgical correction is not always needed.

Perforation Perforation of the arterial wall sometimes occurs, usually without resultant difficulty. Whether this should at once indicate cessation of the attempt is unclear. Apparently most operators withdraw the catheter and try again.

Since any patient may require immediate surgical correction for these complications as well as for complete rupture of the artery,[15] the responsible vascular surgeon should be aware of planned angioplasties and be on call for whatever necessity may occur.

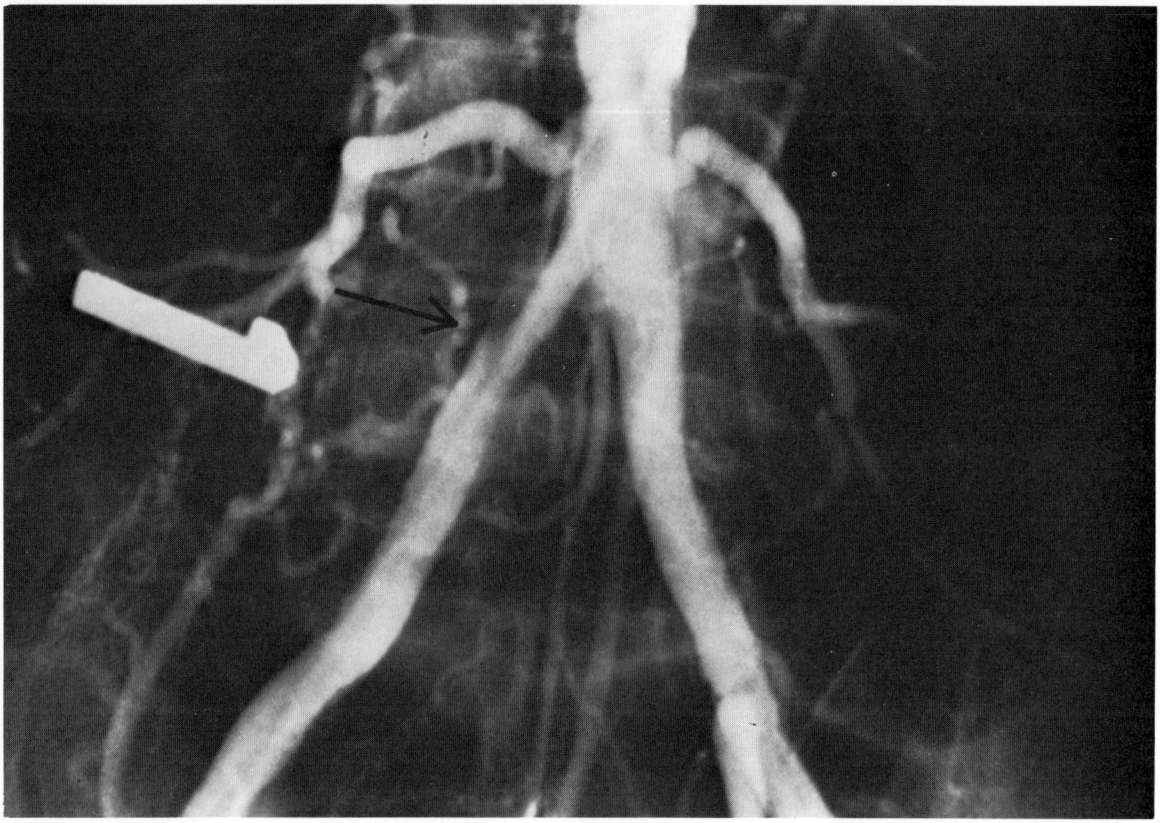

FIGURE 27-5 The 36-year-old male in Figure 27-4 had successful dilation with transient extravasation, shown by this immediately postoperative angiogram. His clinical relief has continued for 15 months.

WHO SHOULD PERFORM THE ANGIOPLASTY

The pat answer here obviously is someone who has learned the technique well, who performs enough to maintain experience, and who updates training and experience by continuing pursuit of new developments. In most institutions this will be one or more of the radiologists.

For at least three reasons the vascular surgeon should be generally familiar with the techniques and its results. First, the surgeon must be aware of the indications, hazards, and results in order to select proper lesions and patients for treatment. Angiography and surgical repair are better

TABLE 27-1 CURRENT INDICATIONS FOR PERCUTANEOUS TRANSLUMINAL ANGIOPLASTY

Stenosis in one of the following large arteries
Aorta
Iliac
Subclavian (beyond the vertebral origin)
Axillary
Stenosis in one of the following medium-size arteries
Superficial femoral or popliteal
Brachial
Carotid (in fibromuscular dysplasia)
Stenosis in one of the following small arteries
Renal (in a nonostial site)
Coronary
Limited length stenosis rather than occlusion
Recent origin
Absence of calcification

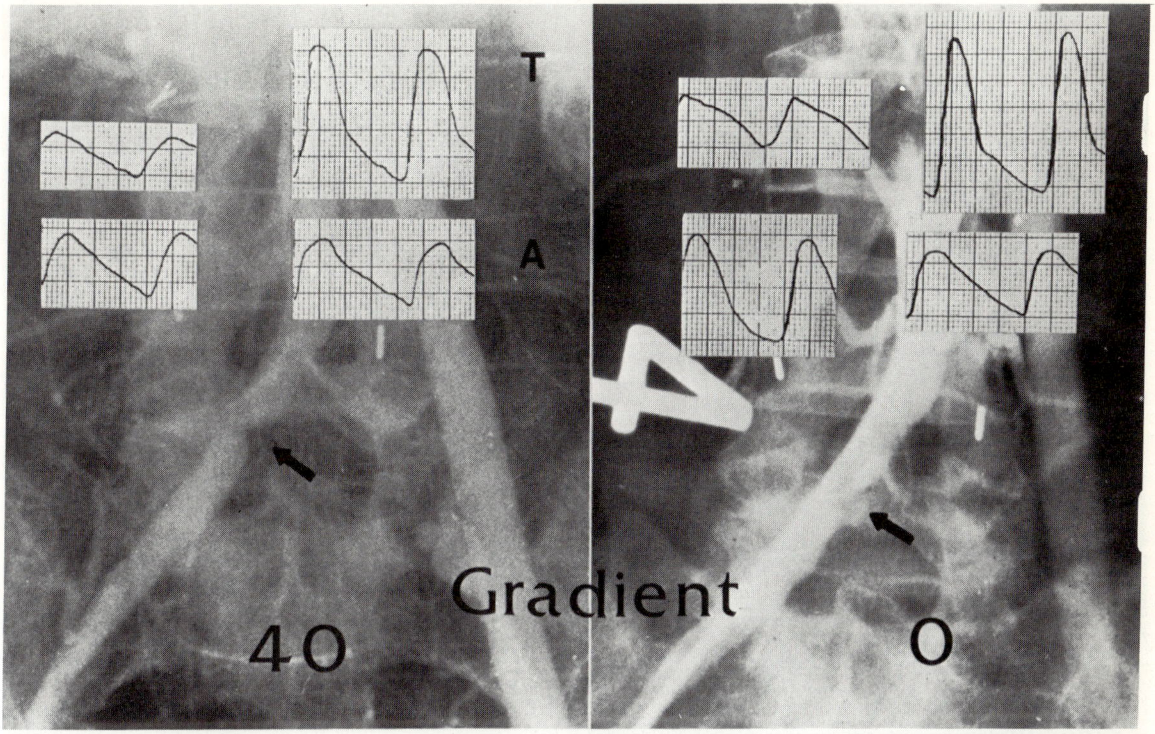

FIGURE 27-6 *Left,* a short stenosis of the right common iliac artery produced a 40-mmHg pressure gradient just prior to dilation, which was completely relieved, *right,* by the procedure. The pulse volume amplitudes at the thigh and ankle levels showed a 33 percent increase in the thigh measurement and a 50 percent increase in the ankle measurement on the right following the angioplasty.

viewed as complementary rather than as competitive, requiring the combined judgment of both subspecialists.

Second is the necessity to perform some dilations in the operating room during the course of surgical revascularization. The cooperative efforts of the radiologist and surgeon produce a better end result than from either one acting alone.

Finally, there are the occasional complications which require immediate operative help. This problem of cooperative management may be extended to a policy of referral of the patient for angioplasty either by or with the active consultation of a vascular surgeon. To put it bluntly, direct referral from a nonsurgeon to the radiologist has in certain hospitals and cities already created difficult administrative problems as well as patient tragedies. The judgment and skill of both the vascular surgeon and the radiologist are needed.

RESULTS OF ANGIOPLASTY

Neither angiography nor noninvasive tests are entirely predictive of clinical success after successful dilation. Thus, Samson's group noted no hemodynamic improvement in 33 percent of 37 angiographically successful iliac dilations, of which 9 had continued clinical success and limb viability. Twenty-six percent of 46 femoral PTAs were similar.[16] Reported statistics must therefore be evaluated cautiously.

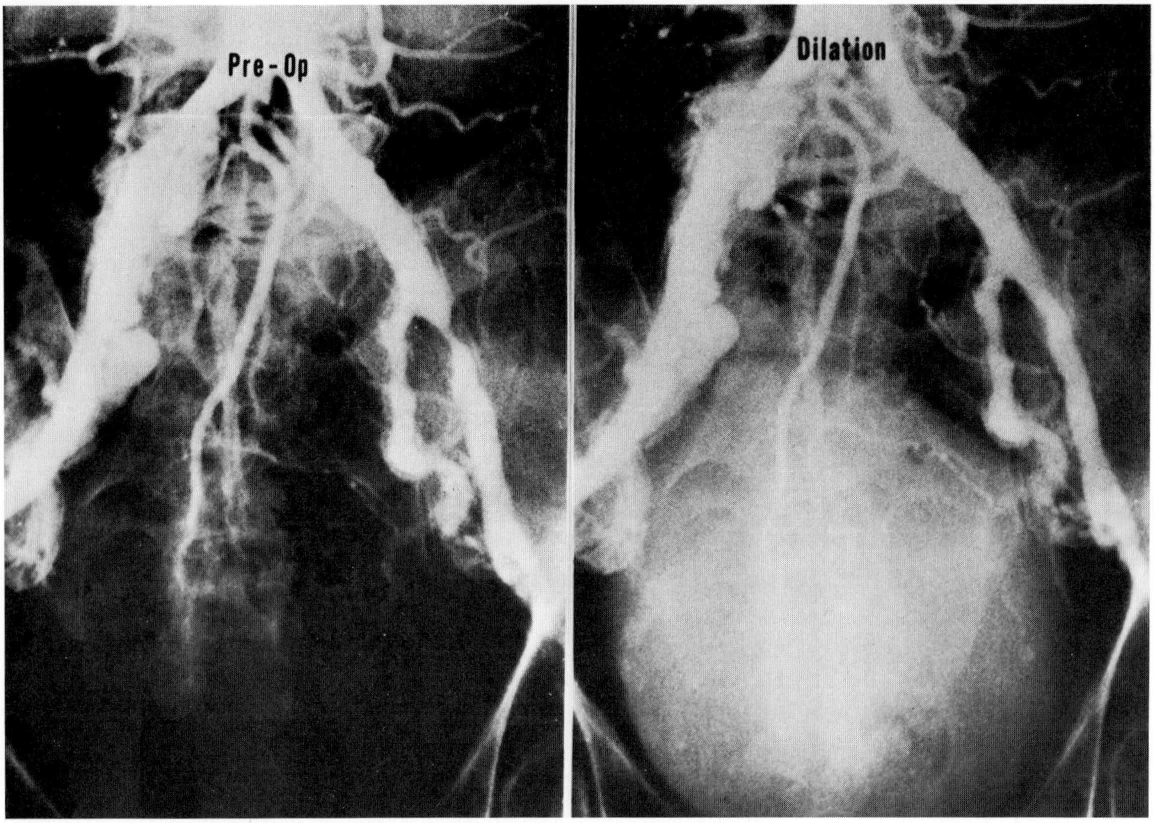

FIGURE 27-7 *Left,* the short stenosis of the left external iliac artery was easily dilated; *right,* with relief of symptoms.

The results of an attempt to produce a table of published results are not included here because they are confusing. The follow-up times are variable. Patency percentages are often calculated as the number of 2-year patencies divided by the total initially successful dilations. The patency rates would therefore be lower if figured against a denominator of all comers. The importance of objective documentation of results cannot be overemphasized. "Symptomatic relief alone is not sufficient to validate results."[17]

The short period of follow-up of most series is also noteworthy. Longer times may show different results. Schuler, for example, commented in 1984 that "we have been disillusioned with the long term results of PTA as three to five year results became available."[18] On the other hand, Katzen in 1984 suggested 96 percent initial success and 5-year patency of 85 to 95 percent for iliac angioplasties, and femoral results of 50 to 70 percent at 2 years.[19]

The group at Montefiore in New York made several useful comments based upon 206 attempted PTAs. First, they did not attempt to reopen long-occluded or totally occluded arteries, a variant from the indications used by some others. Second, the mortality rate was low (1 percent), but numerous nonlethal or nonthreatening complications occurred (25 percent). Third, repeated attempts at PTA were usually unsuccessful if the first failed. Fourth, recurrences were so common in the femoral arteries that they suggested surgical treatment rather than repetitive PTA.[16]

SPECIFIC LESIONS

Aortic Stenosis

Large-bore balloon catheters have not been available until recently, so few aortas have been dilated. Heeney and associates dilated six aortas with 10- to 15-mm balloons, as well as with two 6-mm balloons lying adjacent. There were no complications and five were successful.[20] Occasional other successes[21] suggest that improvement in catheters and increasing experience will lead to further indications for treatment of localized aortic lesions.[22]

Iliac Stenosis

This is the best single indication for PTA. Its results are good, particularly for a short lesion (Figures 27-8 and 27-9). Total occlusion of the common iliac artery is an exception, with greater risk and poorer results.[12] The 112 aorto-iliac angioplasties from Johns Hopkins University in 1983 had an initial success rate of 96 percent and a 24- to 36-month cumulative patency rate of 89 percent with a significant complication rate of 3.6 percent. Two of the patients with complications required surgery.[23]

Angioplasty is a practical answer for the patient who needs femoropopliteal revascularization but who also has an iliac inflow stenosis. If the inflow is left diminished the femoral graft may fail, yet operative correction of the iliac lesion may not be needed and no currently available tests allow a truly accurate determination. Percutaneous angioplasty via the contralateral femoral artery can usually be done without much difficulty. Several days later, with assurance of a proper inflow, the femoropopliteal revascularization can be done. These lesions may also be treated at the time of the operation.

PTA may be used to open a contralateral iliac stenosis just prior to placement of a femorofemoral graft. Occasionally the PTA has allowed enough collateral flow to relieve the necessity for the crossover graft.[24]

Femoral and Popliteal Lesions

These are less likely to have long-term success than are iliac stenoses,[17] yet failure does not prevent a later bypass (Figures 27-10 and 27-11). Short lesions fare better than longer ones. Roberts and Ring particularly recommended PTA for short stenoses of femoropopliteal grafts, citing 90 percent success in 30.[12] Sometimes it is worthwhile to dilate a distal femoral lesion through the groin incision when an aortofemoral graft is being placed. Preparation for that should be made when that combination is found.

Zarins' group in Chicago reported that restenosis occurred in 52 percent of 97 limbs of femoropopliteal PTAs in 78 patients but that toe and foot lesions had often healed by that time so that a further procedure was unnecessary.[25] This parallels experience with operative surgical revascularization.[26] Glover's group also noted the tendency to restenosis, to the extent that "only six of 19 lesions . . . maintained improved flow after one year."[10]

Carotid Lesions

The currently low risk of an operative procedure and the fear of cerebral embolism due to PTA have resulted in general avoidance of PTA for carotid lesions. Fibromuscular dysplasia, with its tendency to occur quite superior, is a lesion for which dilation via operative exposure is appropriate. Allowing the artery to back-bleed during the procedure should lessen the danger of embolism.[12] As noted in Chapter 22, the dysplastic lesion has been found infrequently in our hospital, and no one has operated upon one or dilated one to date.

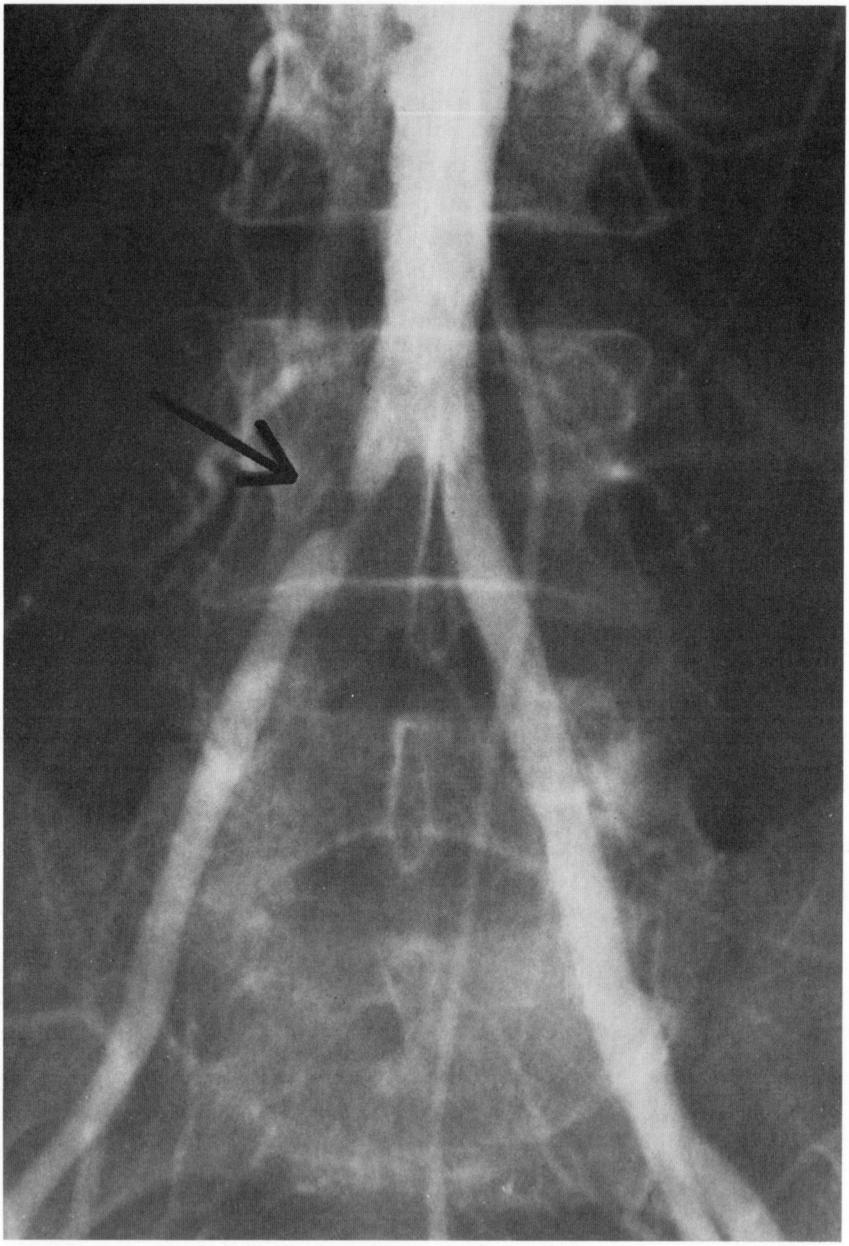

FIGURE 27-8 Tight stenosis of the right common iliac artery in a 53-year-old male.

Renal Lesions

Better results have been obtained with arteries affected by fibromuscular dysplasia than with those affected by arteriosclerosis. Also, treatment of a lesion within a renal vessel rather than at its ostium produces better results, probably because of difficulty in positioning the balloon accurately at the renal ostium.

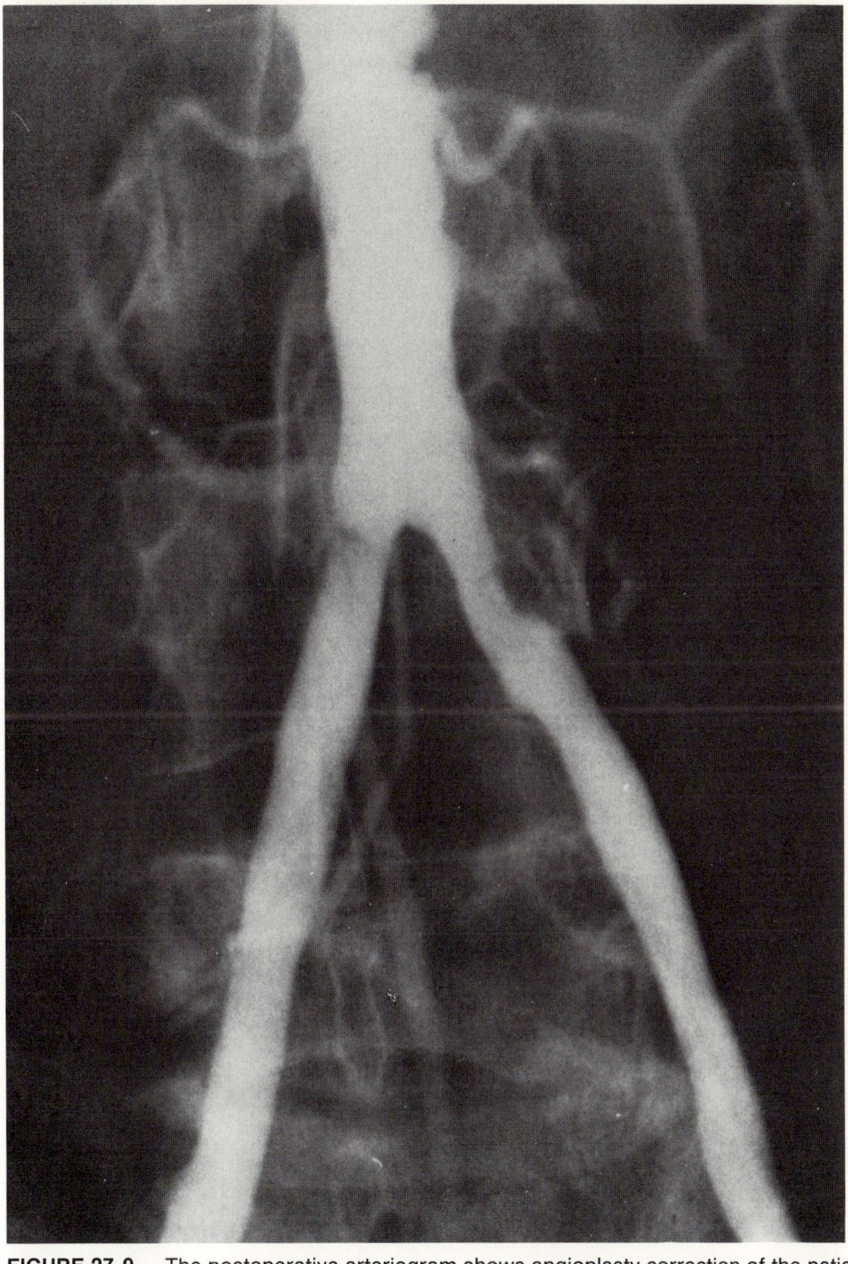

FIGURE 27-9 The postoperative arteriogram shows angioplasty correction of the patient shown in Figure 27-8.

Sos and associates' results are illustrative. They reported early technical success in 87 percent of patients with fibromuscular stenoses, in 57 percent of those who had unilateral arteriosclerotic lesions, but in only 10 percent with bilateral lesions. They had 20 percent success with arteriosclerotic ostial lesions but 75 percent if the lesion was nonostial. At an average time of 16 months later, hypertension was cured or improved in most patients in whom technical success had been

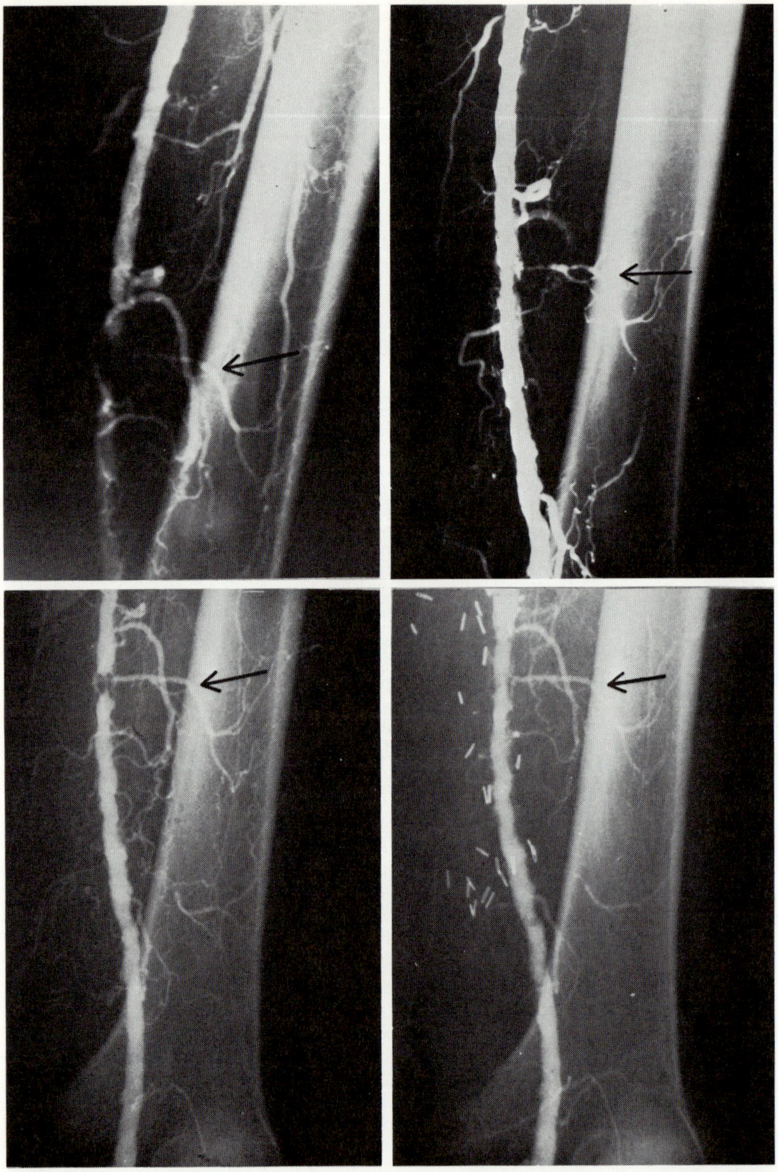

FIGURE 27-10 The *upper left,* a complete occlusion of the superficial femoral artery at Hunter's canal, was treated by PTA, resulting in the patency shown at the *upper right.* The *lower left* shows a recurrent lesion 3 months later. The *lower right* shows operative relief by direct open thromboendarterectomy.

achieved (93 percent for fibromuscular dysplasia and 82 percent for unilateral arteriosclerosis). Thus, if patients were properly selected, there was an excellent chance of long-term success.[27] Tegtmeyer's group reported 79 to 95 percent early successes in six series and a later patency rate of 70 to 90 percent. They believe that "the results of renal angioplasty compare favorably with surgical results."[28]

Levin, after reviewing the situation of 1984, concluded that PTA was better than surgery for

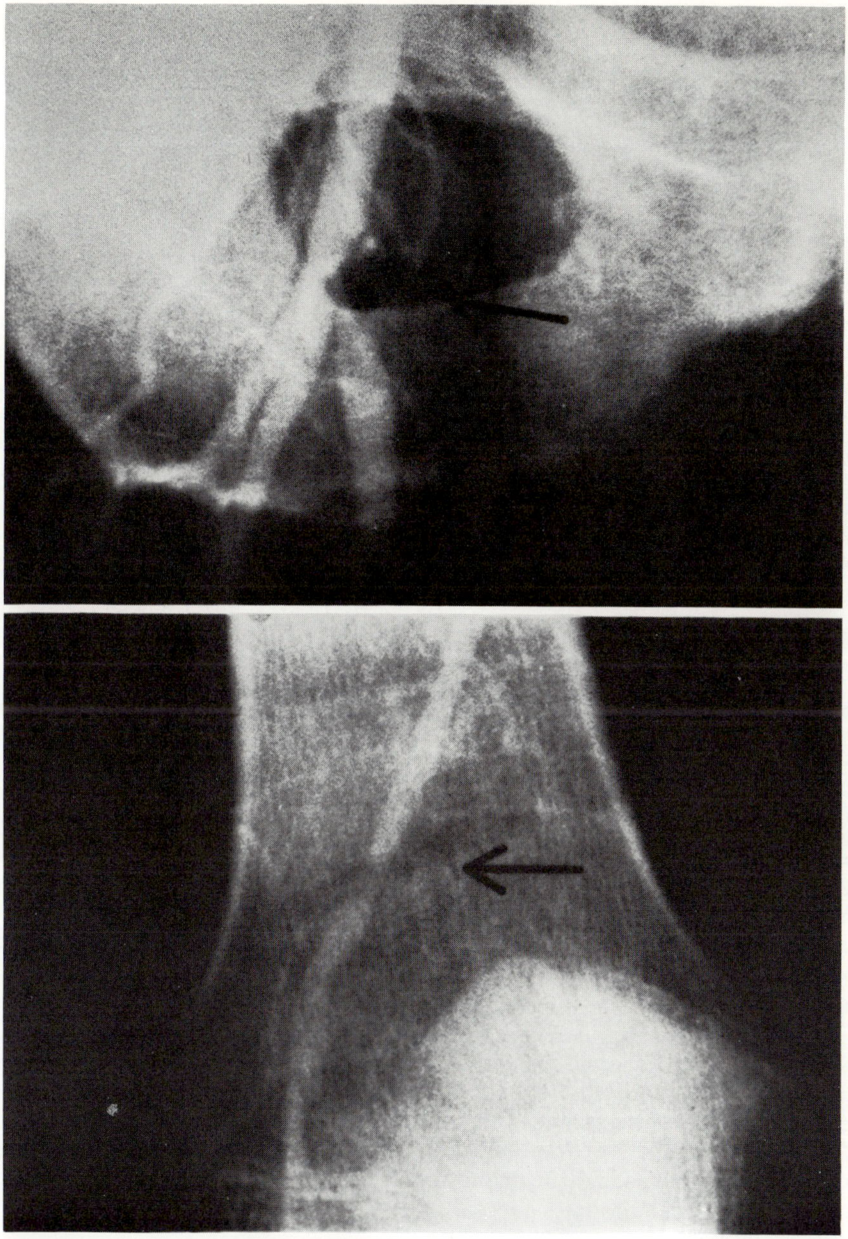

FIGURE 27-11 The *upper arrow* shows stenosis of the common femoral artery just at its bifurcation. This was corrected by open thromboendarterectomy. The *lower arrow* shows the tight popliteal stenosis which was dilated by passage of a Gruntzig catheter down from the femoral arteriotomy.

patients with lateralizing renal vein renins, that results in patients with fibromuscular dysplagia were superior to those in arteriosclerotics, and that lesions distal to the ostium were better candidates for PTA.[29]

Dean has warned that the high recurrence rate among atherosclerotic lesions treated by PTA

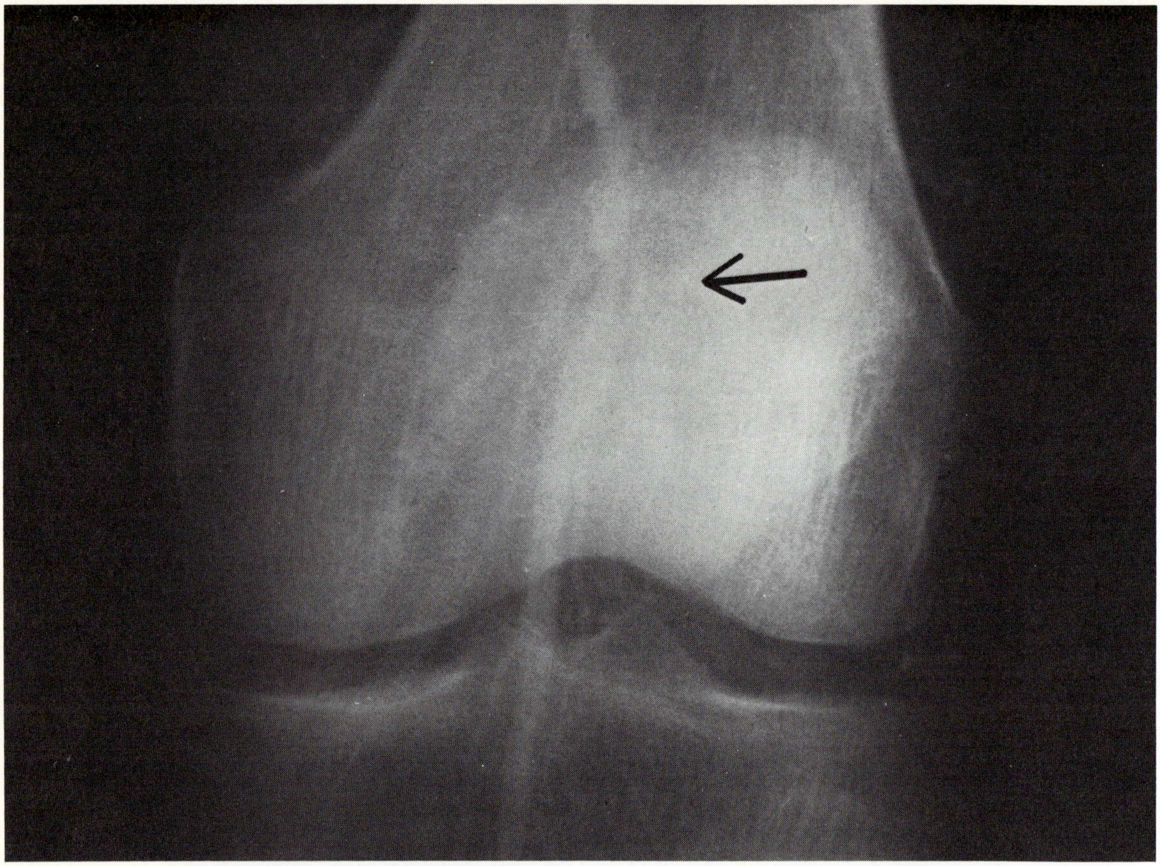

FIGURE 27-12 A postoperative arteriogram demonstrates the patent popliteal artery (of the patient shown in Figure 29-11) after angioplasty.

may eventually rule against that indication, leaving fibromuscular dysplasia as the chief reason to perform PTA upon the renal artery.[30]

Current information therefore suggests that experienced operators produce over 90 percent initial successes in selected patients and that 80 to 90 percent of those with lateralizing renin study results are improved. Restenosis occurs in 10 to 15 percent; secondary PTA or an operation can subsequently correct some of these.

PTA is not useful for completely occluded renal arteries and is not likely to help those with ostial lesions or nonlateralizing renin studies results.[31]

Figure 15-18 demonstrates a recent successful case.

Celiac and Mesenteric Lesions

These appear to be good candidates for PTA if the stenosis is intrinsic. Roberts noted relief of pain by PTA in five persons.[12] I have had no personal experience.

THE ROLE OF ANGIOPLASTY

PTA offers the advantages of ease, relatively low risk, and low cost. Its disadvantages are several: (1) Not all lesions can be managed thus. Roberts estimated that only a third of his patients were candidates.[12] (2) High-quality x-ray equipment is needed. (3) Experienced interventional radiologists are needed. They will not continue to be critical as experience accumulates. (4) There is radiation exposure, but it is small. (5) Finally, there is the ultimate question of how long a good result will continue. If necessary, angioplasty can usually be repeated.

On balance, angioplasty is here to stay, is better than an operation for some lesions (Figure

FIGURE 27-13 *Upper left,* stenosis of the common femoral artery just proximal to a patent femoropopliteal vein graft. *Upper right,* after PTA the femoral artery is widely patent. *Below,* the pre-PTA pressure gradient is considerably but not completely relieved.

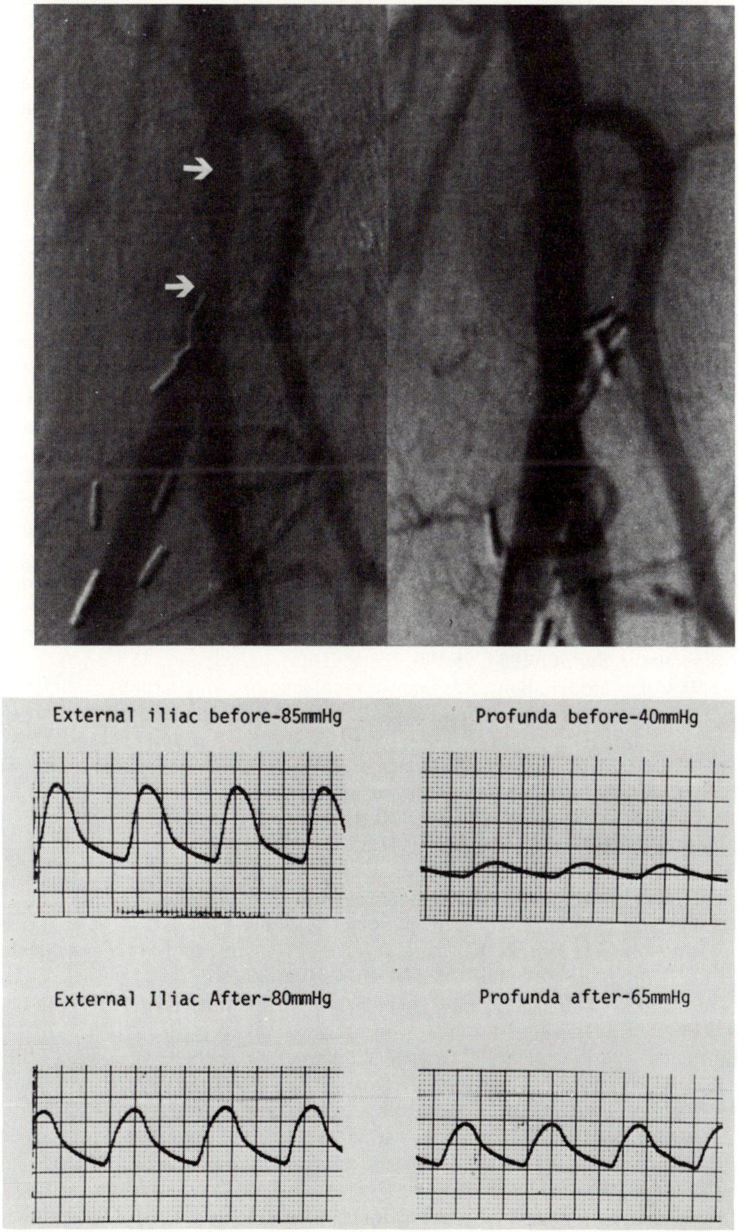

27-13), and requires a cooperative effort by the surgeon and radiologist.[10] The number of patients who are optimally managed by angioplasty is still controversial. Montarjeme's group estimated this at over 50 percent,[32] although the Toronto group thought that 5 to 10 percent was a better estimate.[7] The latter seems realistic.

Of interest to all physicians and surgeons is the recent comparison by Doubilet and Abrams of results and costs of three different strategies of managing symptomatic peripheral vascular disease, namely, (1) by angioplasty alone, (2) by surgery alone, and (3) by a combined angioplasty-surgery program. After surveying the pertinent literature between 1970 and 1981, they estimated that the recommended combined approach might save 352 lives, 5006 patent limbs, and $82 million yearly. The statistics and their mathematical management may be modified, but their general thesis of present underutilization of angioplasty is sound.[33]

Whether the outpatient use of angioplasty will become common is not clear yet. The 81 patients so managed by Manashil, Thunstrom, Thorpe, and Lipson were discharged 4 hours after the procedure unless a complication occurred. There were four—one contrast reaction and two reocclusions requiring surgical repair—but no later complications which could have been prevented by a longer stay in the hospital.[34]

REFERENCES

1 Dotter CT, Judkins MP: Transluminal treatment of arteriosclerotic obstruction: Description of a new technique and a preliminary report of its application. *Circulation* 1964, 30:65.

2 Dotter CT, Rosch J: Transluminal angioplasty—the catheter treatment of peripheral arterial obstruction, in Dale WA (ed): *Management of Arterial Occlusive Disease,* Year Book Medical Publishers, Chicago, 1971, chap 15.

3 Gruntzig A, Hopff H: Percutane Rekanalisation chronischer arterieller Verschlusse mit einem neuen Dilatationskatheter. Modification der Dotter-technik. *Dtsch Med Wochenschr* 1974, 99:2501.

4 Fogarty TJ, Chin A, Shoor PM, Blair GL, Zimmerman JJ, Adjunctive intraoperative arterial dilation: Simplified instrumentation technique. *Arch Surg* 1981, 116:1391.

5 Fogarty TJ, Kinney TB: A new approach to transluminal angioplasty. *Vasc Diag Treat* January–February 1984, p 26.

6 Chin A, Kinney T, Rurik, G, Shoor P, Fogarty T: A physical measurement of the mechanisms of transluminal angioplasty. *Surgery* 1984, 95:196.

7 Johnson KW, Colapinto RF, Baird RJ: Transluminal dilation: An alternative? *Arch Surg* 1982, 117:1604.

8 Zeitler E, Richter EI, Roth FJ, Schoop W: Results of percutaneous transluminal angioplasty. *Radiology* 1983, 146:57.

9 Zeitler E: Drug treatment before and after percutaneous transluminal recanalization, in Zeitler E, Gruntzig A, Schoop W (eds): *Percutaneous Vascular Recanalization,* Springer-Verlag, New York, 1978, p 73.

10 Glover JL, Bendick PJ, Dilley RS, Becker GJ, Richmond BC, Yune HY, Holden RW: Balloon catheter dilation for limb salvage. *Arch Surg* 1983, 118:557.

11 Sprayregen S: The current status of percutaneous transluminal angioplasty, in Veith FJ (ed): *Critical Problems in Vascular Surgery.* Appleton-Century-Crofts, New York, 1982, chap 5.

12 Roberts B, Ring EJ: Current status of transluminal angioplasty. *Surg Clin North Am* 1982, 62:357.

13 Ameli FM, St. Louis EL, Provan JL, Legrand JL: Percutaneous transluminal angioplasty without coagulation. *J Cardiovasc Surg* (Torino) 1983, 24:416.

14 Gruntzig A, Kumpke DA: Technique of percutaneous transluminal angioplasty with the Gruntzig balloon catheter. *AJR* 1979, 132:547.

15 Simonetti G, Rossi P, Passariello R, Faraglia V, Spartera C, Pistolese R, Fiorani P: Iliac artery rupture: A complication of transluminal angioplasty. *AJR* 1983, 140:989.

16 Samson RH, Sprayregen S, Veith FJ, Gupta SK, Ascer E, Scher LA: Inadequacy of the noninvasive hemodynamic evaluation of percutaneous transluminal angioplasty. *Am J Surg* 1984, 147:212.

17 O'Mara CS, Neiman HL, Flinn WR, Herman RJ, Yao JST, Bergan JJ: Hemodynamic assessment of transluminal angioplasty for lower extremity ischemia. *Surgery* 1981, 89:106.

18 Schuler JJ: Discussion of Schuler JJ, Flanigan DP, Ryan TJ, Buchbinder D, Castronuovo JJ: Crossover

femoropopliteal sequential bypass for combined ipsilateral iliac and femoropopliteal occlusive disease. *Arch Surg* 1984, 119:461.

19 Katzen BT: Percutaneous transluminal angioplasty for arterial disease of the lower extremities. *AJR* 1984, 142:23.

20 Heeney D, Bookstein J, Daniels E, Warmath M, Horn J, Rowley W: Transluminal angioplasty of the abdominal aorta. *Radiology* 1983, 148:81.

21 Kumpe DA: Percutaneous dilatation of an abdominal aortic stenosis, three balloon technique. *Radiology* 1981, 141:536.

22 Arbona GL, Van Aman ME, Smead WL: Percutaneous transluminal angioplasty of the abdominal aortic bifurcation. *South Med J* 1983, 76:22.

23 Kadir S, White RI, Kaufman SL, Barth KH, Williams GM, Burdick JF, O'Mara CS, Smith GW, Stonesifer GL, Ernst CB, Minken SL: Long-term results of aortoiliac angioplasty. *Surgery* 1983, 94:10.

24 Youkey JR, Clagett GP, Cohen AJ, Huggins M, Olson DW, Nodalo L, Salander Jm, Rich NM, Hutton JE: Percutaneous transluminal balloon angioplasty of the iliac artery for contralateral ischemia. *Surgery* 1983, 94:100.

25 Zarins CK, Lu C, McDonnell AE, Whitehouse WM: Limb salvage by percutaneous transluminal recanalization of the occluded superficial femoral artery. *Surgery* 1980, 87:701.

26 Rush DS, Gewertz BL, Ball DG, Zarins CK: Limb salvage in poor-risk patients using transluminal angioplasty. *Arch Surg* 1983, 118:1209.

27 Sos TA, Pickering TG, Sniderman K, Saddenki S, Case DB, Silane MF, Vaughan ED Jr, Laragh JH: Percutaneous transluminal renal angioplasty in renovascular hypertension due to atheroma or fibromuscular dysplasia. *N Engl J Med* 1983, 309:274.

28 Tegtmeyer CJ, Kofler TJ, Ayers CA: Renal angioplasty: Current status, *AJR* 1984, 142:17.

29 Levin DC: Percutaneous transluminal angioplasty of the renal arteries. *JAMA* 1984, 251:759.

30 Dean RH: Renovascular hypertension, in Moore WS (ed): *Vascular Surgery: A Comprehensive Review.* Grune & Stratton, New York, 1983, chap 16.

31 Gomes AS: Principles of angiography, digital subtraction angiography and international radiology, in Moore WS (ed): *Vascular Surgery: A Comprehensive Review.* Grune & Stratton, New York, 1983, chap 7.

32 Motarjeme A, Keifer JW, Zuska AJ: Percutaneous angioplasty as a complement to surgery. *Radiology* 1981, 141:341.

33 Doubilet P, Abrams HL: The cost of underutilization. Percutaneous transluminal angioplasty for peripheral vascular disease. *N Engl J Med* 1984, 310:95.

34 Manashil GB, Thunstrom BS, Thorpe CD, Lipson SR: Outpatient transluminal angioplasty, *Radiology* 1983, 147:7.

Invited Commentary

Thomas J. Fogarty, M.D.
Redwood City, California

Improved instruments, advanced techniques, and a conscious effort for cost containment in the medical field have provided the impetus for less-invasive therapeutic procedures.

In vascular surgery the concept of a therapeutic balloon catheter was first introduced in 1963 and was used for the performance of arterial embolectomy.[1] Its intent was to improve the efficiency of embolectomy, reduce the magnitude of the operation, and avoid general anesthesia. The first dilation of an artery by means of a balloon catheter was performed by Dotter in 1964. He utilized a standard Fogarty catheter to dilate an iliac artery.[2] Gruntzig reported in 1974 the successful use of a fixed-volume or noncompliant balloon catheter for dilation of peripheral arteries.[3] This improved instrumentation gained widespread acceptance in Europe and is gaining increasing acceptance in the United States. At present, the vast majority of dilations are done percutaneously and represent a primary therapeutic intervention. The procedure is performed by radiologists and is best done in the angiographic suite with heavy reliance on fluoroscopic control.

The concept of an improved catheter design that would allow simple catheter placement and dilation in the operating room without heavy reliance on fluoroscopic control was reported by Fogarty.[5] The catheter system, termed linear extrusion, was initially employed to dilate a lesion as an adjunct to a primary surgical procedure. Further experience was reported in 1981, and along with continuing use and follow-up, it has documented the efficacy of the catheter system when used in properly selected patients by surgeons trained in the technique. The linear extrusion concept has been extended to percutaneous use and has significant advantages over conventional coaxial systems in situations of total occlusion, stenosis greater than 10 cm in length, and tandem lesions.

The application of the dilation concept to additional anatomic areas and nonatherosclerotic pathology in and outside the vascular system is on the increase. This is easily documented by even a casual review of the medical literature and is presently most evident in the cardiology journals.

The impact of an effective dilation program on standard surgical procedures and practice is substantial. Dilation has replaced some standard operations and will continue to do so, and the necessity for reoperation can be avoided in some circumstances. In other situations a successful dilation can make a standard operation possible or extend the benefit of a planned surgical intervention.

The thoughtful surgeon has come to accept dilation as an effective therapy that may benefit certain patients. To exclude a therapeutic intervention simply because one cannot do it or lacks proper training is not morally acceptable. The alternatives available to the surgeon include learning the procedure and/or establishing a working relationship with properly trained interventional radiologists and cardiologists.

This cooperative interaction has been hampered by the existence of separate departments at training institutions, which fails to engender an atmosphere of cooperation among specialties. Such problems are clearly evident in the field of cardiovascular diseases. The attitudes of the cardiologist, radiologist, cardiac surgeon, and peripheral vascular surgeon toward one another would be quite different had their origins been from programs where such disciplines were more closely integrated. It is important for the surgeon to recognize that cardiologists and angiographers need no longer limit themselves to diagnostic procedures and that their integrated therapeutic efforts can be invaluable to overall patient care.

COMMENTARY REFERENCES

1 Fogarty TJ, Cranley JJ, Krause RJ, Strasser ES, Hafner CD: A method of extraction of arterial emboli and thrombi. *Surg Gynecol Obstet* 1963, 115:241–244.

2 Dotter CT, Judkins MP: Transluminal treatment of arteriosclerotic obstruction: Description of a new technique and a preliminary report of its application. *Circulation* 1964, 30:654–670.

3 Gruntzig A, Hopff H: Perkutane Rekanalization Chronischer Arterieller Venschlusse Mit Einem Neven Dilatations Katheter. *Dtsch Med Wochenschr* 1974, 99:2502–2505.

4 Beebe HG, Stark R, Freeny PC: Indications for transluminal angioplasty: A surgical view. (Discussion.) *Am J Surg* 1980, 140:31–39.

5 Fogarty TJ, Chin A, Shoore PM, Blair GL, Zimmerman JJ: Adjunctive intraoperative arterial dilatation: Simplified instrumentation technique. *Arch Surg* 1981, 116:1391–1398.

28 VARICOSE VEINS: MODERN MANAGEMENT PRODUCES GOOD RESULTS

The patient with varicose veins should be welcomed, since good results can be achieved that provide satisfaction with a minimum of risk. That such is not universal suggests unfamiliarity with the pathologic physiology by some physicians, the disinterest of others, and surgical attempts by occasional operators; it also reflects the minority of patients, who present complicated varicosities secondary to other lesions. In truth, many such limbs are treated by "Tom, Dick, and Harry" whether or not there is expertise. The recent statement that "varicose veins are beneath the vascular surgeon" reflects a concept of elitism, which, fortunately, represents only an unrealistic minority of surgeons. Varicose veins are common, they cause much disability, and they fully deserve our thoughtful attention.*

It is, however, evident that widespread knowledge of the modern management of varicose veins lags behind more dramatic and popular advances in arterial surgery.

ETIOLOGY

Primary varicose veins occur more commonly in females, are aggravated by pregnancy, and are often familial, but their actual cause is unknown, although a generalized weakness of the venous walls may be presumed.

Secondary varicose veins due to venous hypertension may complicate the postphlebitic syndrome, arteriovenous fistulas of several sorts, and proximal venous occlusion due to tumor or trauma. Recognition of their secondary nature is important, since their removal is often unnecessary or may even worsen the situation if the deep veins are occluded. Deep venous anomalies and valve failures may also produce secondary varicosities (Table 28-1).

Clinical Appraisal

History and examination usually allows determination of whether varicosities of the lower extremity are primary or secondary. In the absence of a history of venous thrombosis ("milk leg," phlebitis) or swelling after a previous illness, operation, trauma, or childbirth, and without signs of such (edema, induration, pigmentation, ulcer), the varicosities are usually primary. In the later stages there may be slight edema, some pigmentation, and even ulcers. Such usually require phlebography to allow differentiation of cause.

Sometimes the differentiation between symptoms due to the varicosities and those due to some other coexisting lesion is obvious. Table 28-2 summarizes symptoms which may be con-

*Dodd and Cockett's discussion of varicose veins[1] is encyclopedic, and George Johnson's new chapter[2] is excellent.

fusing. Specific therapy directed toward a concomitant problem may help decide which lesion is primary. Thus, it may be helpful to have the patient wear an elastic bandage, toes to knee, for a week, to learn if this relieves the discomfort (associated with varicosities) or does not (if it is caused by arthritis).

Unilateral varicosities should especially trigger suspicion of an underlying lesion, because primary varicose veins are generally bilateral, although often more pronounced on one side.

TABLE 28-1 CAUSES OF VARICOSE VEINS

Primary
Heredity
Pregnancy
Secondary—venous hypertension due to
Postphlebitic syndrome
Congenital deep vein anomalies
Arteriovenous malformations
Proximal occlusion from
Surgical ligation
Trauma

Tests

Tourniquet Tests These were at one time popular, along with various maneuvers whereby the leg was elevated and the suspected communicating perforating veins were temporarily occluded with another tourniquet or with the fingertip.[1] This had some validity at a time when the usual operation consisted of only high and low venous ligation with additional perforator ligations; it was then important to find out exactly where the perforating veins were located. At present this has no practical value, because the modern operation removes all varicosities and interrupts perforators regardless of their location. It is simpler to view the patient in a good light and mark all the veins which are varicose and remove them along with their perforators (Figure 28-1).

Phlebography Phlebography for primary varicose veins has little usefulness. Twenty years ago a series of 50 such showed that it had no diagnostic value or therapeutic usefulness, so it was abandoned and is now used only for "unusual" varicose veins (and of course for secondary ones). Unusual varicose veins include those in (1) the patient who has had recurrences after surgery (to look for unsuspected deep venous causes), (2) the patient with unilateral varicose veins, (3) the patient below the age of 20 (for whom the probability of deep venous anomalies is high), and (4) the patient suspected to have had a deep venous thrombosis, where knowledge of the deep venous system is important.

A simple technique for ascending phlebography is illustrated in Figure 28-2. The patient reclines in a 45° position on the radiologic table with a tight venous tourniquet in place just above the malleoli. Sixty milliliters of a suitable contrast medium (currently Hypaque-43) are slowly injected into a foot or ankle vein. Rapid injections produce unnecessary pain and are not needed,

TABLE 28-2 DIFFERENTIAL DIAGNOSIS OF SYMPTOMS ASSOCIATED WITH VARICOSE VEINS

Pain in the leg	Edema	Unilateral varicosities
Varicose veins	Venous obstruction	Deep venous occlusion
Thrombophlebitis	Deep vein thrombosis	Thrombosis
Arthritis	Pressure by a tumor	Tumors
Ischemia due to arterial occlusion	Lymphedema	Arteriovenous fistulas
Static foot problems	Trauma	Hemangiomas
Nerve root pressure	Infection	Deep venous anomalies
Functional problems	Systemic causes	
	Cardiac	
	Renal	
	Nutritional	

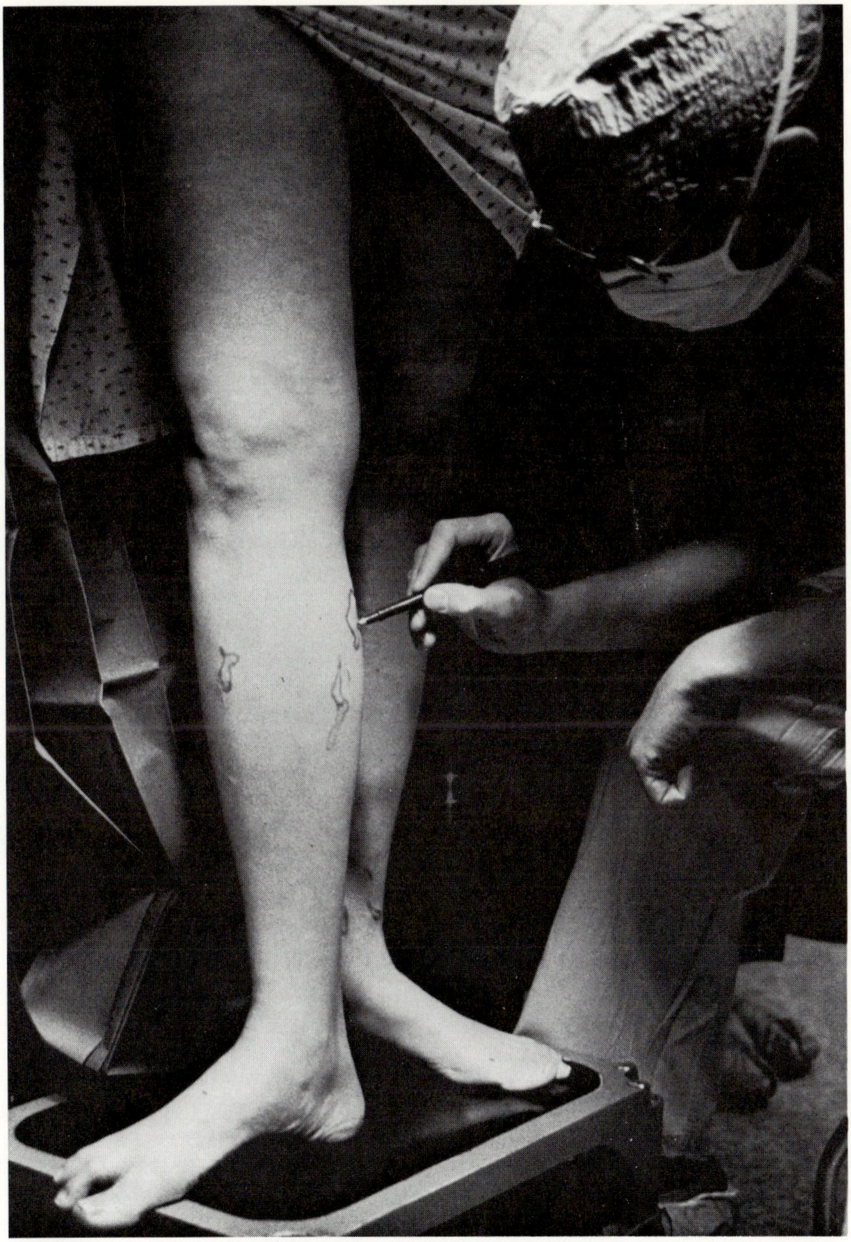

FIGURE 28-1 Marking the varicosities preoperatively.

because the material pools in the veins so long as no exercise occurs. Films are exposed in the anterior-posterior position and then in the lateral position (with the extremity rotated outward). The patient then rises on the toes 10 times, and another two films are exposed in the anterior-posterior and lateral positions. These latter films give some indication of the clearance of blood up the leg.

This often allows adequate visualization of the iliac veins. If it does not occur, a secondary

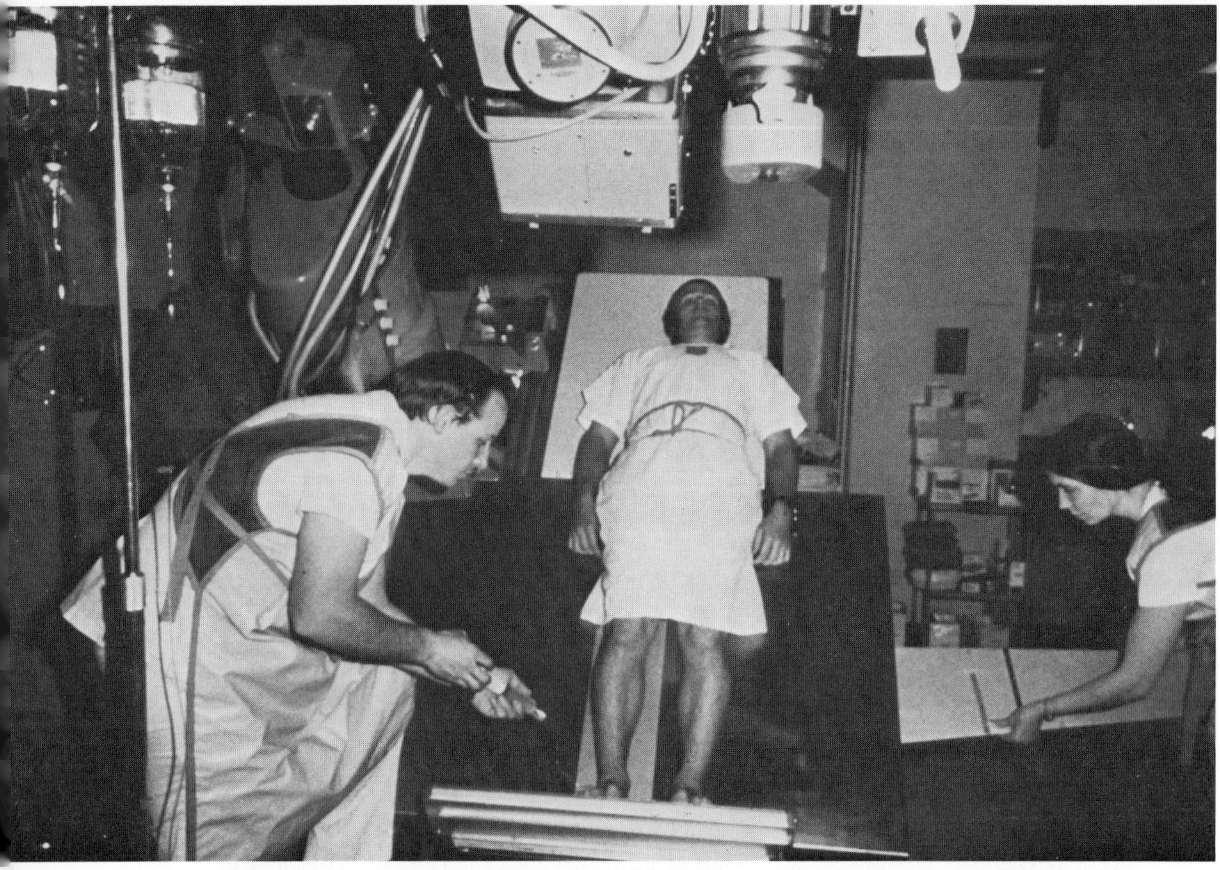

FIGURE 28-2 Technique of ascending phlebography showing the semierect position at 45° for injection of radiopaque material into a foot or ankle vein distal to a tight venous tourniquet on the ankle. Anterior-posterior and lateral films are made before and after exercise.

injection of 60 mL is made with a tight tourniquet placed high on the thigh to cause pooling of the material during its injection over a period of 20 to 30 seconds. The proximal tourniquet is then suddenly released, and the leg is elevated 45°, following which a single film lying underneath the pelvis is exposed. This provides excellent visualization of the iliac vein and the distal portion of the vena cava.

Some fear has been expressed regarding possible postphlebogram phlebitis. This has not been a particular problem in my experience, probably because all such patients either have been already receiving intravenous heparin for one reason or another or have had 5000 U.S.P. units of aqueous heparin injected into the intravenous line just prior to the radiopaque material. A retrospective study of 200 consecutive patients by Malcolm Lewis and myself disclosed only one known instance of postphlebogram phlebitis.[3] Since a single injection of heparin is virtually harmless, this precaution is strongly recommended to allow safe phlebography.

Arteriography An important part of the physical examination of each varicose vein patient should be directed toward the peripheral arteries, to avoid the tragedy of stripping veins from a patient with ischemia due to arterial insufficiency, in whom healing of the incisions is apt to be delayed or impossible. It has been observed on occasion and emphasizes the great importance of *absolutely confirming the peripheral arterial supply* either by detecting pulses or by an arteriogram. Arteriography is rarely needed.

Varicose veins and peripheral arterial occlusions are not commonly associated lesions. While it cannot be documented, there appears to be a negative correlation, because both are common yet not often seen in the same individual. When they do occur together, a proper plan of management emphasizing initial arterial repair is essential.

Venous Pressure Venous pressure studies are of no practical value in primary varicose veins. They do allow some understanding of the pathologic physiology of the postphlebitic venous hypertension which occurs with secondary varicose veins.

CHOICE OF TREATMENT

There are four alternatives for patients with varicose veins. First, is no treatment, in which case the varicosities will slowly increase. Second, external elastic support may be used as a temporary measure. Stockings are uncomfortable in hot weather and do not correct the underlying problem. Third, sclerotherapy may provide temporary relief. Finally, surgical removal is the optimal management of the otherwise healthy patient in modern America.

External Elastic Support

A variety of commercially available elastic stockings may be used to support the varicose veins while the patient sits or walks. When more support is necessary, one of several custom-fitted stockings may be prescribed. Despite the claims of their makers, there is little difference between them.

Most patients eventually end their dependence upon such stockings by operative correction. Pregnant patients are a notable exception, since their varicosities spontaneously recede after delivery.

Sclerotherapy

There is considerable interest among both laypersons and physicians regarding the treatment of varicose veins by injection therapy. This method has been tried and generally abandoned in North America but continues in England and on the Continent, probably because hospitalization, anesthesia, and surgical treatment are considerably less available and the overall cost of sclerotherapy is less to the ordinary individual there.

W. G. Fegan of Dublin[4] and John Hobbs of London[5] have described their methods of sclerotherapy. These experienced British sclerotherapists have documented low morbidity but also have admitted an increasing number of recurrences as the years pass.

John Hobbs, a consistent advocate of sclerotherapy, summarized his own 6-year results, at which time there was a failure rate of 21 percent following surgery versus 65 percent following injection. This emphasizes the temporary nature of sclerotherapy. The 6-year cure rate by the modern American surgical technique consistently produces a much higher instance of complete relief, with less than 5 percent recurrence in my experience.

The second problem of sclerotherapy is local complications: painful thrombi with slow resolution, permanent brown staining of the skin, sensitivity reactions to the injected material, and skin sloughs where the material has escaped from the intended vein into the subcutaneous tissue.

Dodd and Cockett summarized the situation very well in their opinion that "where skilled surgery is unavailable or unobtainable . . . injection therapy may be pushed." They commented further on the importance of an experienced staff and careful attention to the details of technique and said that the worst occurs when varicose vein patients are "herded into injection clinics, seen by junior or temporary staff . . . and injections are given to all who attend; there is little attempt at real diagnosis and minimal follow-up."[1]

Jack Cranley of Cincinnati commented after his visit to Fegan's clinic in Dublin that each varix must be injected and the site compressed continually for 6 weeks by a tight wrap and a bandage that are not removed at all during that period. This must be followed by another series of injections and rebandaging for another 6 weeks. He ended his discussion by saying that "there are very few Americans who would accept that type of treatment if they have any alternative."[6] Perhaps an alternative is an office procedure where a bit of local anesthetic allows removal of the offending vein if it is small, with repetitions over a period of weeks. This at least solves the problem of minor recurrences (Figure 28-3).

Surgical Treatment

Evolution of the Modern Operation Some knowledge of the history of varicose vein surgery is helpful in understanding the modern operation and its variations. Thomas Myers, dean of varicose vein surgeons after his experience at the Mayo Clinic, has noted that varicose veins were discussed by Hippocrates 2500 years ago and that numerous ancient methods of treatment included puncturing, avulsion, excision, cauterization, ligation, injection, and removal by stripping. In 500 B.C. Hippocrates recommended multiple punctures. In the second century Galen advocated their removal with a hook. In the sixteenth century Ambroise Paré discussed their ligation and excision.

After general anesthesia became available, more extensive surgery was performed. Madelung in 1884 made a long incision over the inner aspect of the thigh and leg to remove the greater saphenous vein. An excessive rate of infection discouraged this operation.

Keller in 1905 first attempted stripping by passing a twisted wire through the lumen and tying one end of the vein to it. Babcock in 1907 described a rodlike stripper with an acorn-shape tip, and in 1906 Charles Mayo used an extraluminal curettelike stripper which surrounded the vein with a loop and freed the main channel from the subcutaneous tissue. The main difficulty with all these techniques and instruments was incomplete removal of varicosities outside the main saphenous system.[6]

In the 1940s the usual procedure was division of the saphenous vein near its junction with the femoral vein, to which was soon added a lower ligation just above the knee, followed by other ligations at the sites of identified perforators. There followed a plan to inject a sclerosant into the distal segment of the divided saphenous vein in the hope that the entire distal segment would become obliterated. Difficulties with deep venous thrombosis and pulmonary embolism soon ended this.

Preparation The patient is instructed to scrub the legs, lower abdomen, and femoral regions with chlorhexidine (Hibiclens) and water on a washcloth for 5 minutes twice daily for 5 days preceding hospitalization, as prophylaxis of infection. Many patients prefer to shave themselves on the morning of hospital admission.

Each varicosity should be carefully marked by the operating surgeon on the day before operation, to ensure that none are overlooked (Figure 28-1), with the patient standing on a stool and the surgeon seated opposite with a goosenecked lamp to allow eye-level visualization of the legs. A variety of marking solutions such as brilliant green or carbol-fuchsin may be used. The Codman skin pencil is as satisfactory as any of these and is a readily available disposable marker. Pajama or scrub pants should be worn until the patient reaches the operating room, to ensure that cross-marking does not occur.

Technique Over the years a technique for the removal of varicose veins has evolved which is efficient as well as complete. I have used it during the past 15 years for 983 cases.

The lower extremities are elevated approximately 30° upon a padded Zimmer rack attached to the operating table (Figure 28-4). This allows easy access to every aspect of the legs for preparation and for the surgical procedure. The elevation also reduces venous bleeding so that subcutaneous ligatures are unnecessary; there is no necessity to turn the patient in most instances.[7]

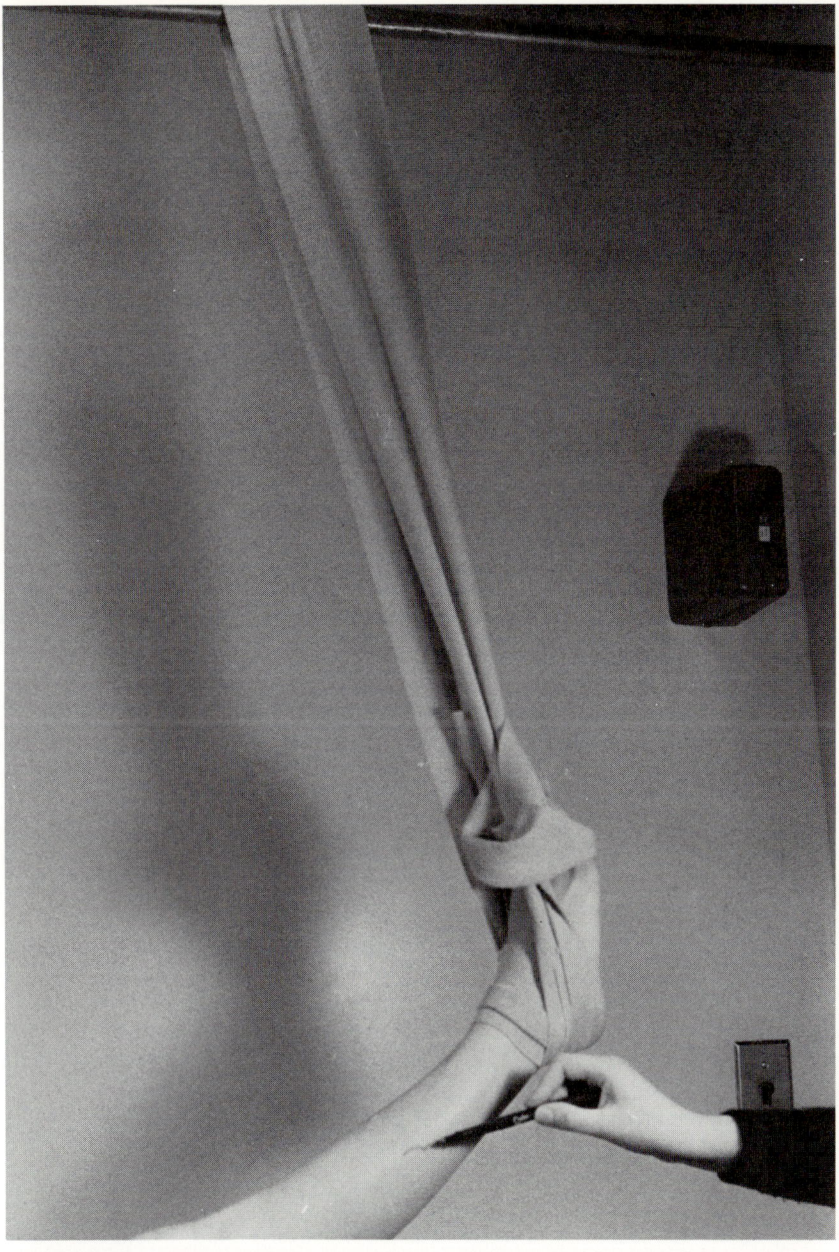

FIGURE 28-3 Minor residual varicosities are easily removed as an office procedure with the leg elevated to an overhead rack to aid control of bleeding.

Seven important points may be stressed:

1 All incisions (except in the groin) are made longitudinally to obtain optimal cosmetic results. The groin incision is often described 2 cm or more below the flexion crease of the thigh. Actually, it should be made in the hair-bearing area just at the groin crease or even higher; there

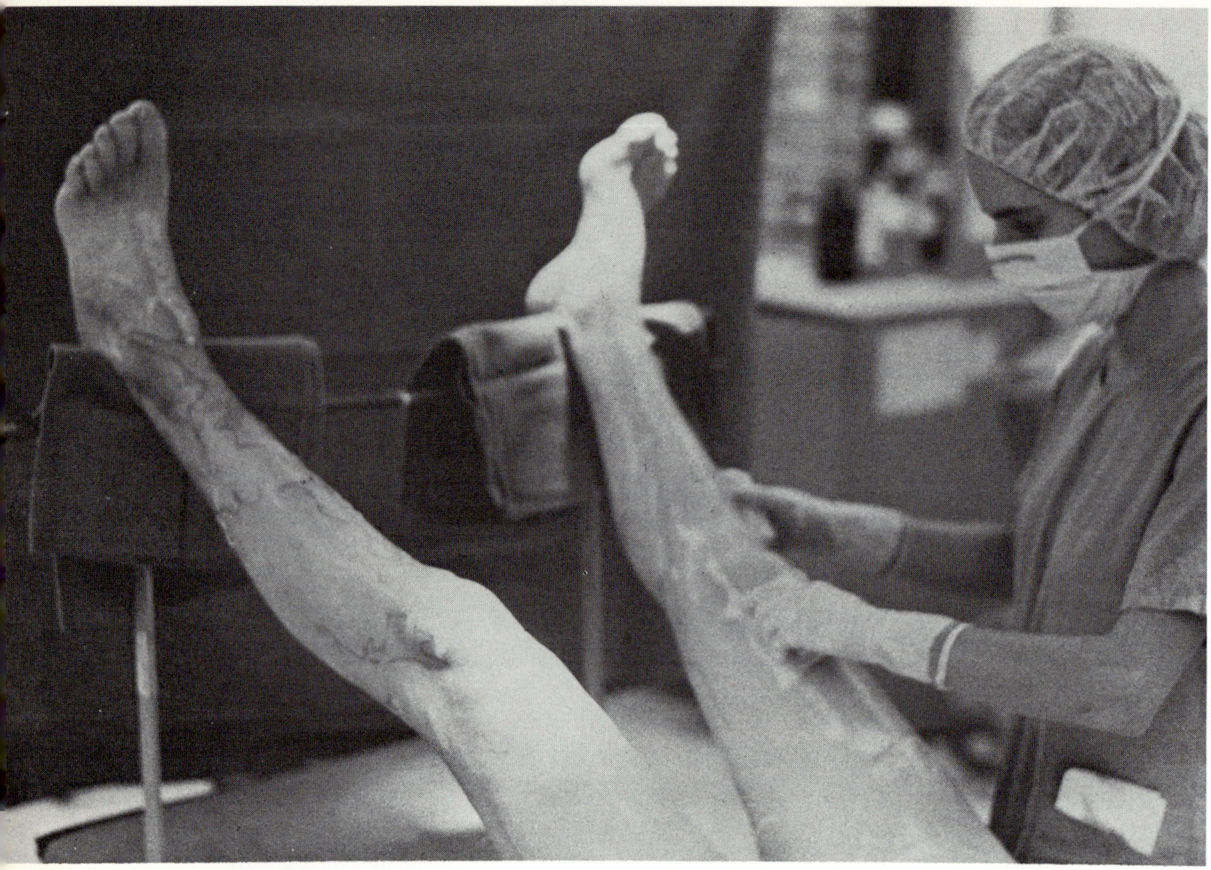

FIGURE 28-4 Elevation of the legs to a 30° angle allows easy preparation, draping, and operation.

it produces a relatively invisible scar. This high exposure leads directly to the saphenofemoral junction.

2 The stripper is placed initially into the saphenous vein at the ankle and thereafter is passed proximally so that there is no hang-up due to valves. The proximal incision is created in the groin directly over the easily palpable stripper tip, thus avoiding extensive dissection in searching for the saphenous vein. The stripping from above downward is less likely to damage the saphenous nerve in the lower leg.

3 While the stripper lies in place in the greater saphenous vein, all marked varicosities outside its line are removed. Avulsion by a clamp placed through a 5-mm incision is often possible (Figure 28-5), but a longer incision and direct dissection may be necessary for large varicosities. These wounds are closed, and a firm elastic bandage is placed before the stripper is pulled through, thereby preventing subcutaneous hemorrhage. The tight bandage is later removed and the rewrapping done less firmly.

4 If the saphenous vein is normal, it need not be stripped and indeed should be saved for possible later reconstructive use. Sometimes only the distal portion of the vein need be removed. Conservation of the saphenous vein is in order, but radical removal of all other marked varicosities should be carried out.

5 Closure is conducted as simply as possible with interrupted nonabsorbable sutures. Subcutaneous sutures are avoided except in unusually long incisions.

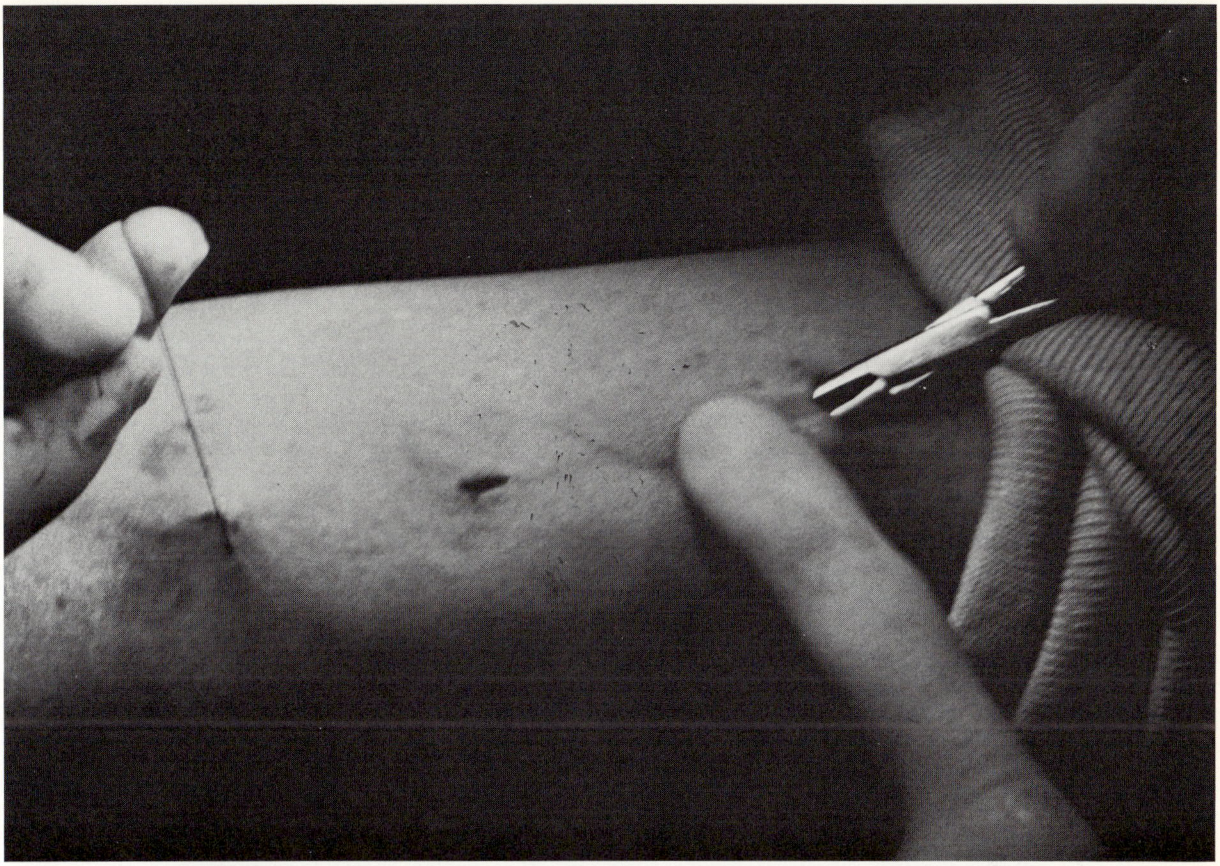

FIGURE 28-5 The previously marked varicosities are avulsed with a clamp through a small longitudinal skin incision, which is later closed with a single suture. The index finger guides the superficial varicosity into the jaws of the clamp.

6 Absolute hemostasis is achieved in the groin, where it is not possible to place external pressure. Firm elastic dressings prevent hematomas in the thigh and calf. If a large incision with considerable dead space exists, there should be no hesitation to place a suction drain through a stab wound.

7 The saphenous vein should be suture-ligated flush with the common femoral vein at their junction. Proper identification is mandatory and depends upon two things: first, the stripper should appear in the presumed saphenous vein as it is pushed up from below, and second, the vein should appear to be the expected size and in the expected position of the saphenous vein. Any doubt about the size or position of the vein should lead the surgeon to extend the incision and make absolute identification to avoid the sad error of division of the common femoral vein. If that technical error occurs, there should be immediate repair by the appropriate end-to-end anastomosis. Two such errors made personally have been immediately corrected without long-term complications.

Postoperative Care Postoperative care stresses simplicity. The patient is out of bed the day of the operation and thereafter walks as much as desired but is asked to refrain from sitting with the legs in a dependent position. Little pain is expected, because the elevated position and the placement of firm wraps during the stripping prevent hematoma formation, which is the cause of most of the postoperative pain. The dressings remain without change for 7 days, at which time all the sutures are removed and replaced by strips of adhesive paper tape. After the first week the elastic bandages are reapplied only from the toes to the knee and are maintained that way for approximately 2 more weeks or until all edema ceases.

COMPLICATIONS

Complications are unusual following a properly conducted varicose vein operation (Table 28-3). In my experience there has been no mortality, nor has any patient been returned to the operating room for control of postoperative bleeding. One patient required placement of a skin clip in her room to control a bleeding point in the dermis.

The low incidence of clinically significant infection requiring antibiotic administration seems remarkable. It is believed to be due to prevention of seromas and hematomas by elevation of the limbs and by the firm elastic wraps applied while the legs are elevated so that there is no dead space or bleeding. No patient in this series received prophylactic antibiotic therapy. A suction drain was placed wherever the wound was large.

The reported 2 percent of patients who developed venous thromboembolism represent a minimum, since other cases perhaps were not recognized. These deep venous thrombosis patients all received heparin for a minimum of 10 days; some were thereafter placed on warfarin for periods up to 3 months. There were no deaths due to pulmonary embolism.

Many patients complained of postoperative headache and tightness in the muscles of the neck, believed to be secondary to the spinal anesthesia. With modern technique using a fine needle, this complication has diminished. No patient required a surgical procedure to stop the symptoms. Spinal anesthesia remains my choice for the operation.

Neuritis A common complaint during the postoperative period is burning pain or lightning pain along the course of the greater saphenous nerve in the lower leg and ankle following stripping of the vein which lies alongside it. The patient may be reassured that such sensations will gradually disappear, although some medication may be temporarily required.

Rarely the pain persists and may require surgical correction. Search for a neuroma is usually worthless. A better result is obtained by severing all the nerve filaments at the ankle. Through a transverse incision, dissection is carried down to the periosteum of the tibia with the intent to completely sever all sensory nerves in that area (Figure 28-6). It produces a numb area just distal to the incision and relief of pain.

RECURRENCES

Varicose vein surgery has achieved a bad reputation among some patients because of so-called recurrences or the belief that the operation makes the varicose veins worse. This is the opposite of the results of a well-conducted modern operation, where the recurrence rate is about 3 to 4 percent.

The myth that varicose vein surgery tends to produce more varicosities and that recurrences are common is probably based upon persistence of existent varicosities which simply have not been removed. If such a residual varicosity is discovered at the first postoperative dressing, it should be immediately corrected by removal under local anesthesia. Figure 28-3 illustrates how

TABLE 28-3 COMPLICATIONS AMONG 983 RECENT VARICOSE VEIN OPERATIONS

Complication	No.	Percent
Infection	4	0.4
Deep venous thrombosis	18	1.8
Bleeding requiring return to the operating room	0	
Death	0	

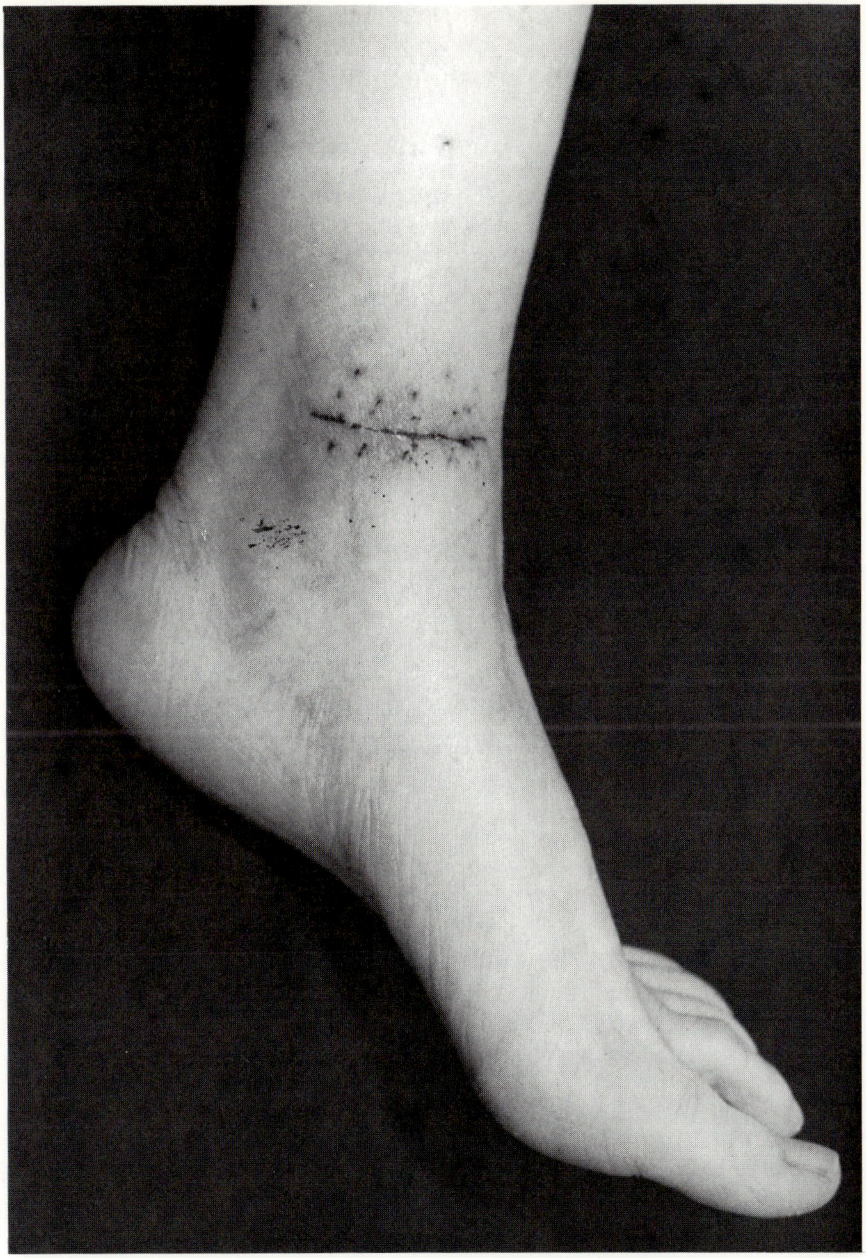

FIGURE 28-6 A transverse incision proximal to the medial malleolus is carried to the periosteum to sever all the sensory nerve fibers of saphenous distribution and relieve postoperative neuritis.

such a limb is elevated with an elastic bandage sling holding the foot over a metal bar. The error is thus at once rectified without prolonging the patient's total disability time or requiring further hospitalization.

Genuine recurrences do appear in a few patients and require repetitive procedures, whose conduct is no different from the original except that vein stripping is not required. Operation for recurrent varicose veins should be preceded by phlebography to determine whether there is a lesion of the deep venous system which was not previously recognized and which caused the recurrence, as illustrated in Figure 28-7.

VARICOSE VEINS IN CHILDREN

Varicose veins most commonly occur and become symptomatic in early and middle adulthood; they rarely occur prior to the age of 20. This age predilection indicates that the development of varicosities in a young person is unusual and that it should be investigated by tests designed to discover unsuspected arteriovenous fistulas as well as congenital anomalies of the deep venous system. Both of these have their own special indications for treatment.

The large communicating vein seen in Figure 28-8 was found in a 12-year-old boy. Its phleborgraphic demonstration led to surgical removal and relief of symptoms of pressure and pain.

Varicosities which are secondary to various arteriovenous malformations are better treated by external elastic support than by immediate excision, since that is usually followed by prompt recurrence. Sometimes one or another form of hemangioma forces an early operation because of ulceration, infection, or invasion of a joint, in which case some of the varicosities may be removed along with whatever procedure is otherwise indicated.

PREGNANCY

Pregnant women frequently develop varicosities of the lower extremities, which are usually troublesome, sometimes require elastic stockings, occasionally demand periods of rest and elevation, and rarely require a surgical procedure during the pregnancy. They are caused by hormonal changes secondary to the pregnancy and not by pressure of the enlarging uterus upon the pelvic veins, as was supposed at one time. Their regression is to be expected and ordinarily is complete by 6 weeks postpartum, so plans for surgical treatment should be delayed for at least that period of time.

A subsequent pregnancy will once again stimulate the formation of varicose veins, so it is preferable for women in the childbearing age group to delay operative correction until their families are completed (Figures 28-9 to 28-12).

A pregnant patient may occasionally have bleeding from a varicose vein, which may require a local procedure and occasionally may require surgical interruption to alleviate severe symptoms. This may be simple high ligation and interruption of the saphenous vein near its entry into the femoral vein. The complete removal of all varices has never been necessary in my experience.

ACUTE SUPERFICIAL PHLEBITIS

Acute thrombosis of any part of the deep venous system is a contraindication to operation upon varicose veins, because bad as they are, they may serve as useful collaterals if the deep venous system is occluded.

Superficial phlebitis is a different matter, since if allowed to persist untreated, it may progress into a more severe form and even involve the deep venous system. Anything beyond the most minimal superficial phlebitis should be at once treated by intravenous heparinization for a period of days to prevent propagation or, alternatively, should be removed surgically.

The contrast between the prompt recovery of patients whose acutely thrombosed superficial veins are surgically removed and the slow resolution of those treated by anticoagulation therapy recommends surgical treatment for most patients. The technique should be modified to initially ligate the saphenous vein in the groin rather than push up the stripper from below, which con-

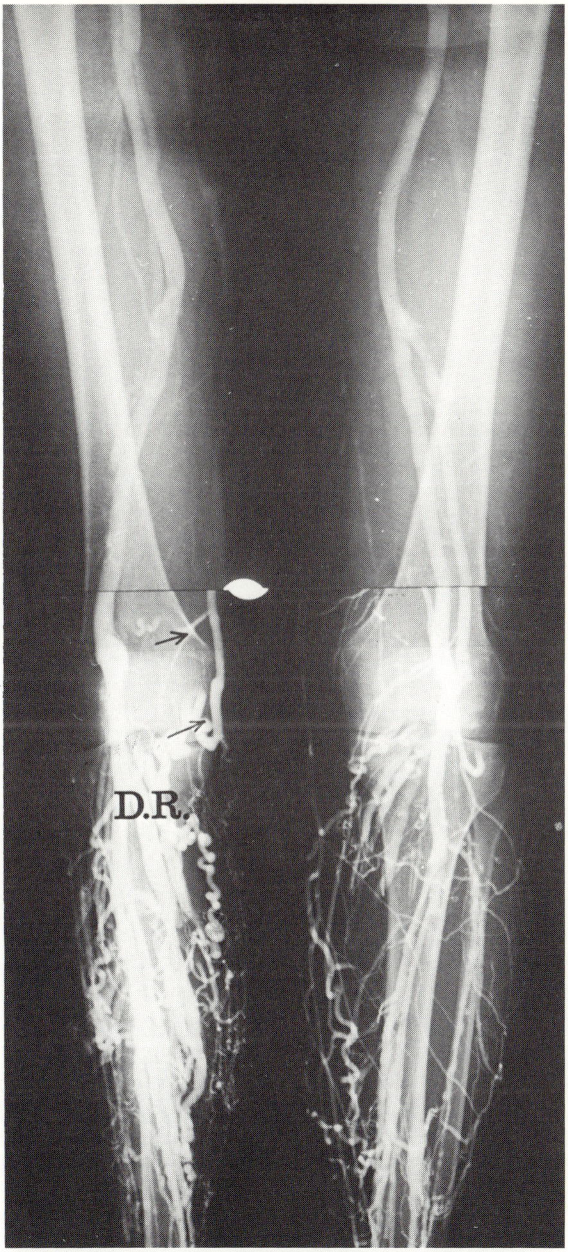

FIGURE 28-7 Phlebography demonstrates that a segment of saphenous vein remains connected to the deep venous system and explains the so-called recurrence after operation.

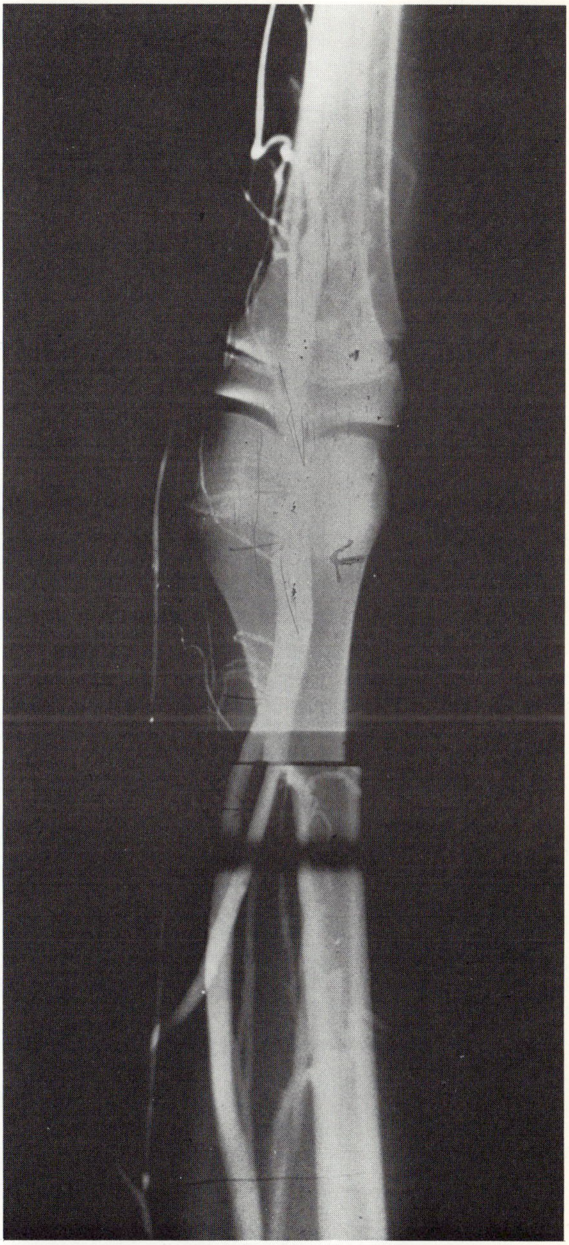

FIGURE 28-8 A prominent superficial varicosity in a teenager proved to be a congenital anomalous deep venous connection, whose removal relieved symptoms.

ceivably might force thrombus into the femoral vein, with resultant occlusion there or even embolization. Operation upon acutely thrombosed veins has not resulted in either of these complications in my experience.

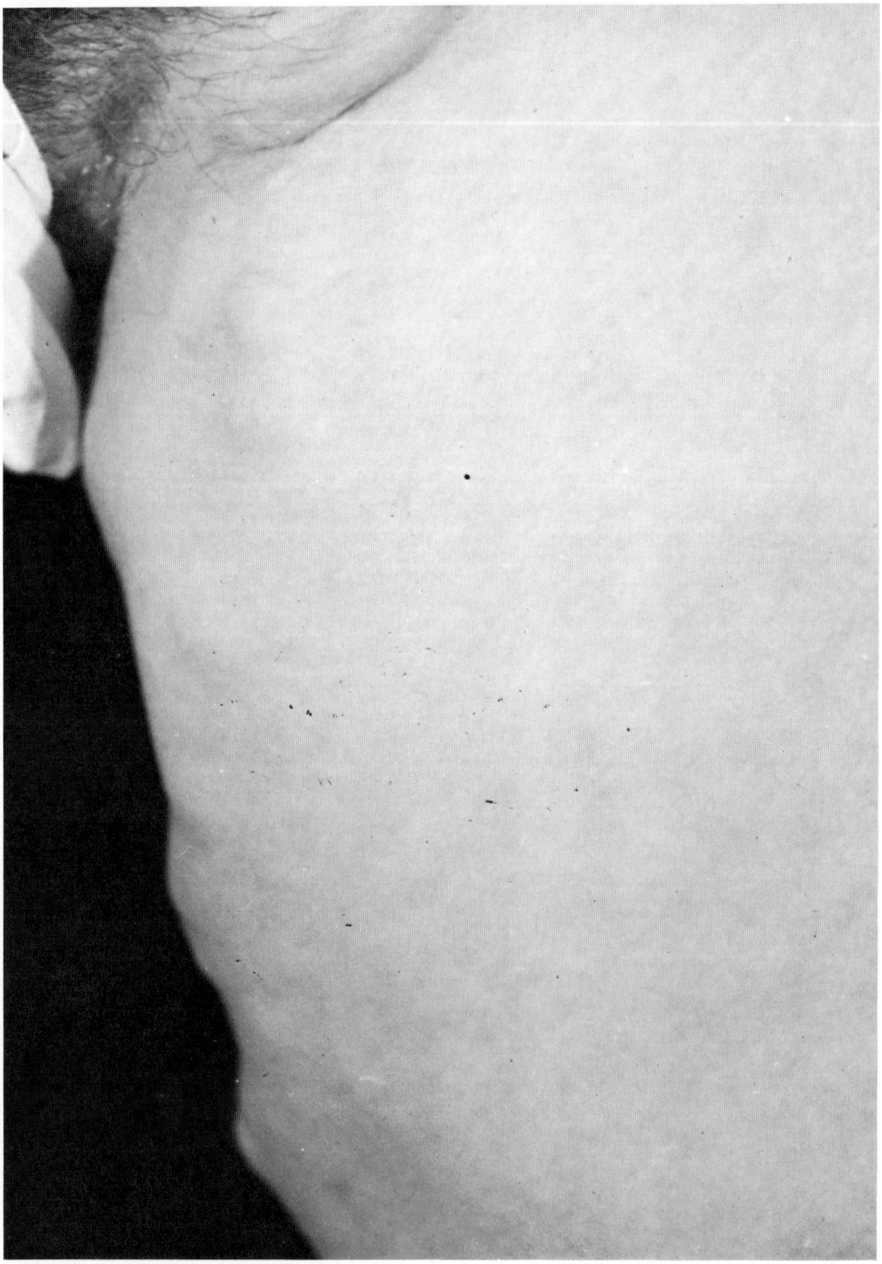

FIGURE 28-9 Severe varicosities of the thigh in an 8-months-pregnant female.

VARICOSE VEINS IN THE POSTPHLEBITIC LIMB

Varicosities secondary to valvular destruction and dysfunction along with deep venous occlusion must be sharply differentiated from primary varicose veins, which are the main subject of this chapter. Any suspicion that the varicosities are secondary ones should at once lead to suitable investigation to determine the proper diagnosis. Phlebography is invariably needed.

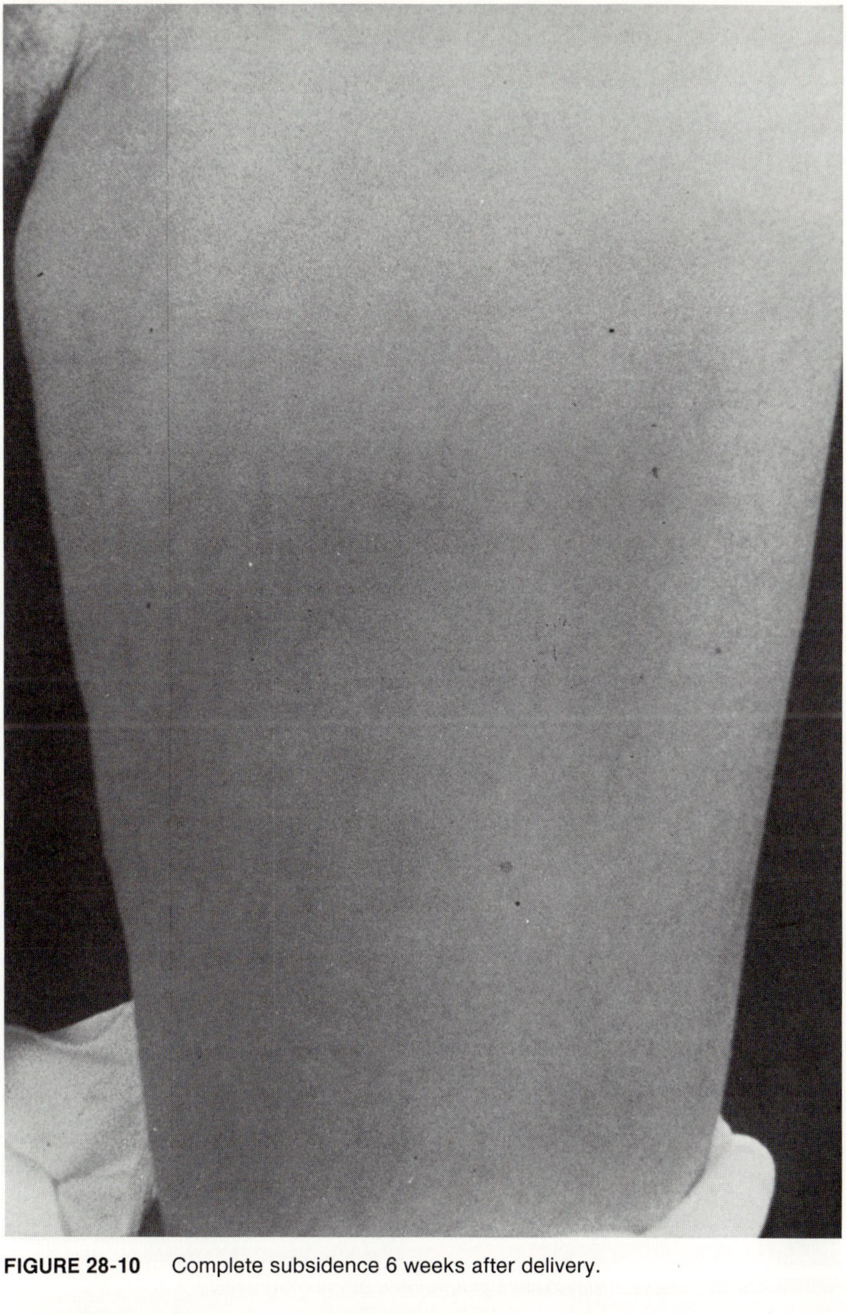

FIGURE 28-10 Complete subsidence 6 weeks after delivery.

A minority of secondary varicose veins require correction. Their routine removal, as practiced in the past, is not valid. Indeed, a survey of such routine removals of secondary varicose veins shows that most recur within a relatively short time and leads to the estimate that only about 15 percent of secondary varicose veins need radical removal as is done for the primary type. Plans for removal of secondary varicose veins should be based on the phlebogram and ambulatory venous pressure studies, which may indicate removal of varicosities up to the midcalf or to the

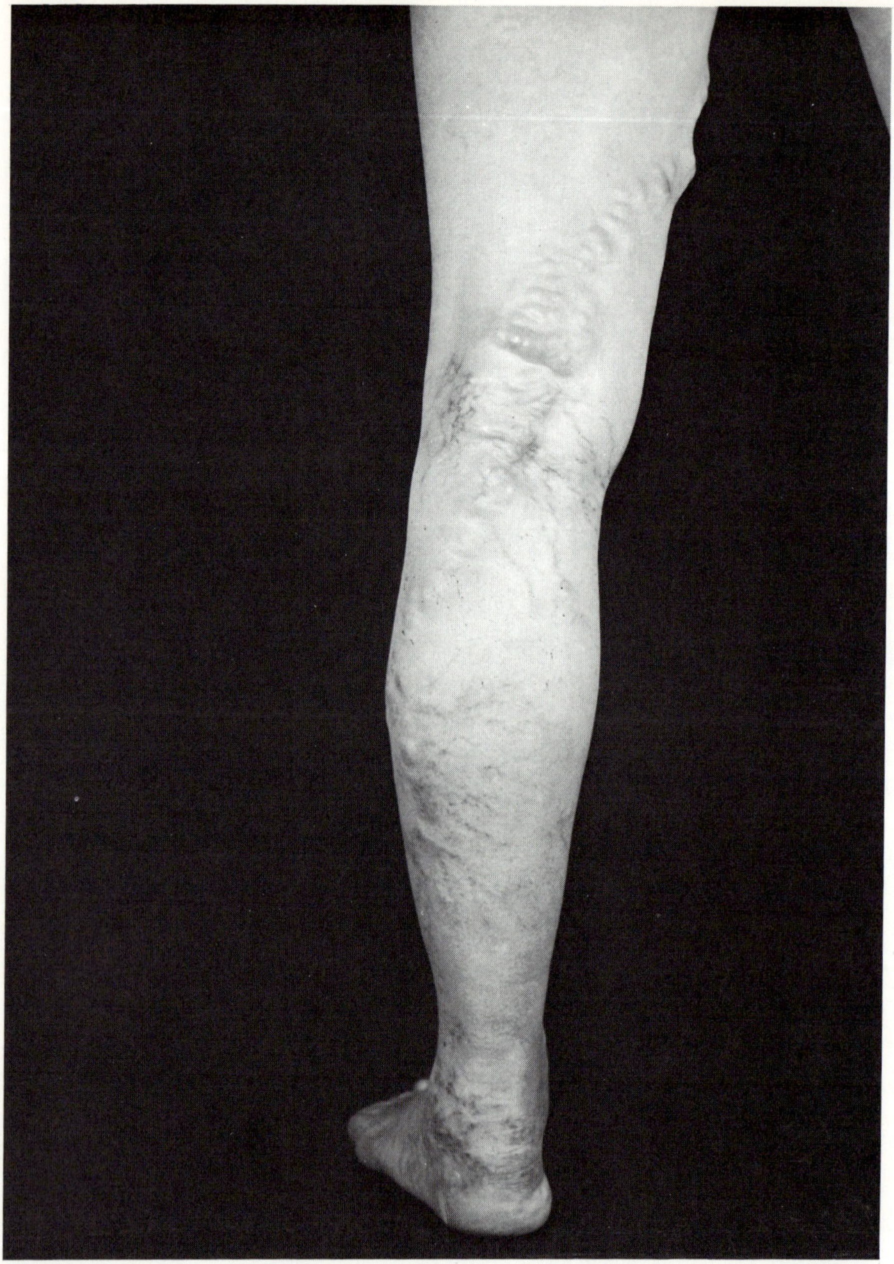

FIGURE 28-11 Severe varicosities at 8 months of the pregnancy.

knee or the low thigh but retention of even badly distorted veins which appear to be serving a functional purpose (Figure 28-13). Control is often best done by external elastic support, while removal of the veins may be disastrous.

Chronic leg ulcers do require consideration of removal of varicose veins, but removal often

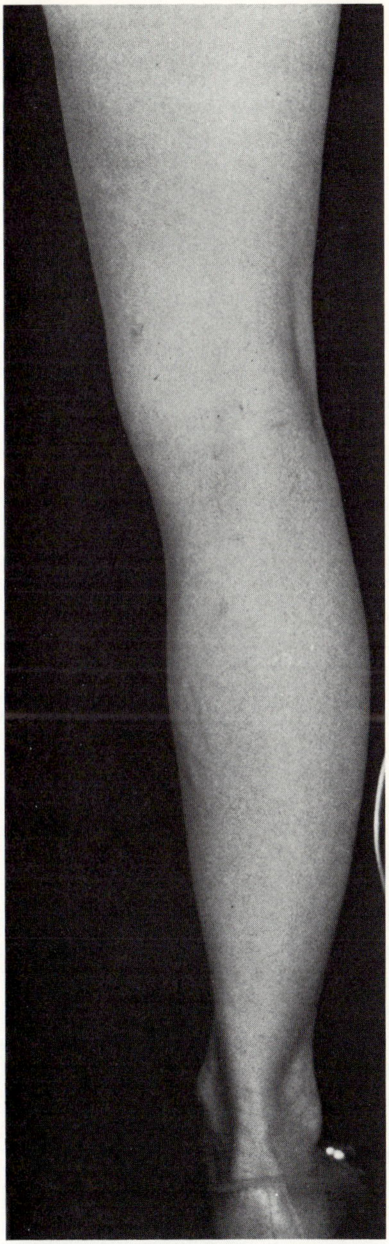

FIGURE 28-12 Subsidence of varicosities 6 weeks postpartum.

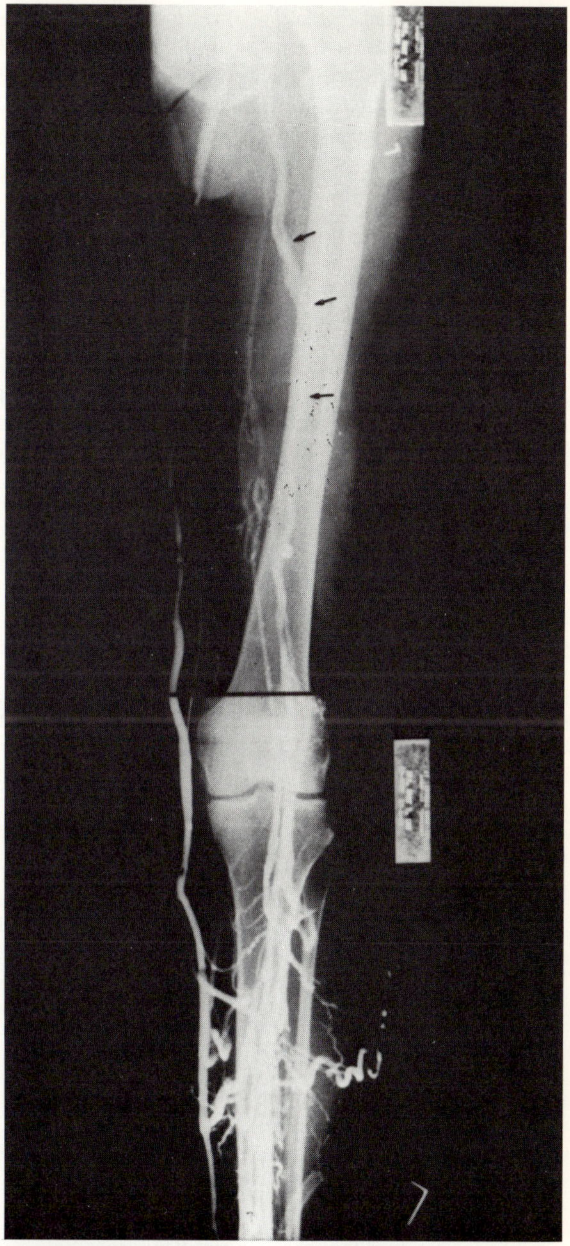

FIGURE 28-13 Saphenous varicosities in a postphlebitic patient with occlusion of the superficial femoral vein, at the *arrows,* should not be removed because the vein is serving as a channel for proximal blood flow.

should be limited to those veins near the area of the ulcer, rather than a widespread stripping and radical removal. This is discussed in more detail in Chapter 29.

The discovery of a deep venous anomaly immediately suggests its correction, particularly if there is a large communication between the deep and superficial venous systems. Such a perforator, or connection, allows the ordinarily high deep venous pressure to be transmitted to the ordinarily low-pressure superficial system, resulting in the creation of varicose veins. Correction of such communications, as seen in Figure 28-8, along with the removal of the already developed varicose veins, ordinarily solves the problem.

REFERENCES

1 Dodd H, Cockett FB: *The Pathology and Surgery of the Veins of the Lower Limb.* Livingstone, Edinburgh and London, 1956.
2 Johnson G: Varicose veins, postphlebitic syndrome and chronic venous insufficiency, in Moore WS (ed): *Review of Vascular Surgery—Preparation for the Vascular Board Examination.* Grune & Stratton, 1984.
3 Lewis MR, Dale WA: Phlebography as a clinical tool. *Surg Gynecol Obstet* 1971, 133:301.
4 Fegan WG: Treatment of varicose veins by injection as practiced in Dublin, in Hobb JT (ed): *Treatment of Venous Disorders of the Lower Limb.* MTP Press, Lancaster, 1976.
5 Hobbs, JT: The treatment of varicose veins by sclerosing therapy, in Rutherford RB (ed): *Vascular Surgery.* Saunders, Philadelphia, 1977, p 1166.
6 Dale WA, Cranley JJ, DeWeese JA, Myers TT: Symposium, management of varicose veins. *Contemp Surg* 1975, 6:86.
7 Dale WA: Ligation, stripping and excision of varicose veins. *Surg Rounds,* July 1978.

Invited Commentary

George Johnson, Jr., M.D.
Chapel Hill, North Carolina

This is an excellent review of the evaluation and therapy of varicose veins. My remarks are based on our experience, which we have interpreted differently in some cases.

The introductory paragraph eloquently sets the stage for a discussion of this common but not necessarily simple clinical problem. Even so, the author inadvertently expresses the same view that he criticizes the "Tom, Dick, and Harry" surgeon for making, by speaking of varicose veins as if they were a single entity, instead of dividing them, as he does elsewhere throughout this chapter, into primary and secondary veins. As emphasized later, secondary varicose veins, whether a result of congenital or acquired valvular incompetence or obstruction, have poorer results from operative treatment than do primary superficial varicose veins.

I agree that removal of secondary varicose veins is usually not indicated, but in certain unusual situations, their excision is warranted for the temporary improvement in venous circulation that is accomplished. This is especially true if the varicosities are the source of marked venous stasis and do not function as collateral bypasses around a deep venous occlusion.

It is suggested that secondary varicosities can be identified by signs such as edema, induration, pigmentation, and ulcer; my personal experience leads me to believe that this is not always the case. At times the differentiation between primary and secondary varicose veins is difficult. The author suggests that congenital deep vein anomalies, listed in Table 28-1 as a cause of secondary varicose veins, may be more frequent than had previously been thought. The studies of Folse in 1970, demonstrating some degree of deep vein valvular incompetence in most patients with varicose veins, support this.[1] Thus, some patients thought to have primary varicose veins in reality have varicose veins secondary to localized congenital deep valvular incompetence.

I certainly agree that several of the clinical tests used to appraise the status of varicose veins are obsolete and are only of value in teaching about pathophysiology.

The technique for phlebography is accurately described. The ascending venogram may not reveal the valvular incompetency secondary to venous anomaly, especially if it is localized; moreover, the descending venogram as usually performed is a test of the competency of the highest femoral vein valve only. The functional phlebograms recommended for appraising the efficiency of the venous pump are certainly superior. It is obvious that results from this set of pictures might well combine the anatomic accuracy of the venogram with an expression of physiologic function.

There is proper emphasis upon the importance of the arterial circulation in patients with varicose veins. Several years ago we were interested in the influence of arteriovenous malformations on the venous circulation and performed a series of arteriograms on patients with unusual manifestations of varicose veins, e.g., location, size, number, appearance. In none of these did we see any evidence of arteriovenous communication as supported by early filling of the venous system.

The choice of treatment is outlined very well. External elastic support stockings with less than 20 mmHg pressure at the ankle are probably of no value. It is best to use the stockings with 20 to 30 mmHg—or, perhaps even better, 30 to 40 mmHg—if this type of therapy is recommended. Above-the-knee stockings serve little purpose.

The facts concerning sclerotherapy are presented well in an eminently fair appraisal of the technique. It is predicted that this form of therapy will have little place in the treatment of varicose veins in the future unless newer techniques become available.

It is difficult to criticize the operative techniques described, since the author contributed extensively to the now standard technique for the operative therapy of this disease. A few minor variations may be worthy of mention. We think it is important to use permanent, water-indelible marking pencils, such as are available in garden centers, for marking the varicose veins. Our approach to partial involvement of the saphenous vein differs. Although our experience is limited, we have had little success in leaving portions of the saphenous system that did not appear to be involved. In several years, most of these patients develop varicose veins in the remaining segment. We suspect that, although we have been unable to demonstrate valvular incompetence in these veins at the time of the first operation, the increased flow from the incompetent valves associated with varices causes the saphenous system to develop irreversible changes. Partial devascularization is certainly an advantageous one and should be considered in smokers, especially if they are male or diabetic; the saphenous vein in these patients should be preserved for subsequent arterial bypass surgery.

Finally, we are hesitant to teach our residents to divide the saphenous vein flush with the femoral vein. We have seen only one patient who had a pulmonary embolus following a high saphenous ligation. Therefore, we do not think a 1-cm stub of saphenous vein is of any consequence. We do think that it is important to identify the saphenofemoral junction to be certain that all tributaries to the saphenous system have been divided.

One valuable procedure has not been mentioned. We follow a specific skin closure approach, although it takes a few extra minutes. This involves using a subcuticular absorbable suture and adhesive skin closure strips. These techniques facilitate early discharge and subsequent clinic visits, since no sutures have to be removed.

The reported recurrence rate is probably due to the inclusion of some varicose veins with occult secondary causes. If methods of evaluation were more precise, operative therapy for primary varicose veins should have a recurrence rate approaching zero. In our practice we infrequently see patients requiring 30 to 40 incisions to completely remove the varicosities. In these patients, varicose veins frequently persist postoperatively. We excise these using a local anesthetic or we use sclerotherapy. Although we have been unable to document that these are secondary varicose veins, I suspect that they are due to congenital valvular incompetency of some portion of the deep venous system which will be demonstrated with improved techniques of evaluation.

This discussion on varicose veins in childhood, pregnancy, acute superficial thrombosis, and varicose veins in the postphlebitic limb is in keeping with our philosophy and understanding. We do think that in rare instances there is an indication for removal of secondary varicose veins. The recurrence rate will be high, but we afford these patients considerable relief from venous stasis during the interval until recurrence. We have several patients whom we have operated upon on two or three occasions, and each alleges to be markedly benefited by the procedure.

COMMENTARY REFERENCE

1 Folse R: The influence of femoral vein dynamics on the development of varicose veins. *Surgery* 1970, 68:974.

29 CHRONIC LEG ULCERS

The occurrence of lower leg ulcers is widely known and indeed is so generally recognized as commonplace that there is at times acceptance of their chronicity and pessimism regarding their cure. Although there are no hard facts to determine the actual number,[1] it has been estimated that there are 300,000 to 400,000 such cases in the United States.[2]

HISTORICAL BACKGROUND

Earliest medical history indicates concern with these, Hippocrates supposedly having first noticed the association of varicose veins with leg ulcers. Writings of Roman physicians about the time of Christ dealt with roller bandages and plasters of various types for leg ulcers and with methods of management of varicosities by blunt hook avulsion as well as by the actual cautery. During the period of Galen's theory of humors in the first 15 centuries A.D., it was generally believed that a leg ulcer permitted noxious materials to escape and that healing would therefore be risky to the patient's general health. An occasional patient today expresses a similar belief!

During the early nineteenth century increasing emphasis on the associated varicose veins led to general use of the term varicose ulcer. However, in 1867, John Gay wrote that "ulceration is not a direct consequence of varicosity but of other conditions of the venous system of which varicosity is not infrequently a complication" and introduced the term *venous ulcer.*[3] Little further advance occurred until John Homans presented his studies of the pathology of deep venous thrombosis and showed that recanalization with destruction of valves was very common following such thrombosis. The later introduction of phlebography and venous pressure studies in the leg and foot at rest and during exercise have more recently added to our knowledge of the pathologic physiology of these lesions.

ETIOLOGY

The occurrence of trauma or minor infection to an area of poorly nourished abnormal ankle skin is usually associated with poor healing and often with continued ulceration. While there are several common, as well as many rare, causes of chronic ankle ulcers (Table 29-1), it is particularly pertinent to discuss briefly the development of these following venous thrombosis.

The occurrence of leg complications many years after a bout of deep venous thrombosis is widely recognized. Serial phlebograms show that almost all deep veins recanalize later, although evidences of wall and valvular damage are common. Furthermore, delayed films made after leg exercises often show failure of passage of the dye on up toward the heart as an indication of

TABLE 29-1 CAUSES OF LEG ULCERS

Type	Common causes	Rare causes
Venous	Postphlebitic syndrome Varicose veins	Arteriovenous fistula Postinjection reaction Pressure Valve anomaly
Arterial	Atherosclerotic block	Pernio
Lymphatic		Lymphedema precox
Infectious	Pyogenic	Synergistic gangrene Syphilis Tuberculosis Fungus
Bone		Osteomyelitis Adherent fracture site Paget's disease
Tumor		Primary tumor Leukemia
Burn	Radiation Heat	Marjolin's indolent ulcer
Systemic Disease		Anemia Ulcerative colitis Diabetes Neurogenic lesion Pellagra

functional insufficiency of the deep veins. Venous pressure studies document the ambulatory venous hypertension (AVH).

Careful historical inquiry often brings out swelling of the leg or pain after childbirth, operation, or injury that may not have been specifically ascribed at the time to phlebitis. Phlebographic studies of some ulcer patients without history of previous phlebitis indicate that either the patient has forgotten when such occurred or it was of no clinical significance and went unrecognized. These considerations make the true incidence of postphlebitic complications difficult to assess.

Severe primary varicose veins may also lead to ulceration. Other less common causes of ulceration of the lower leg may be overlooked chiefly because they are not considered. For instance, the pain associated with the ulcer may override symptoms of arterial insufficiency and therefore lead to incorrect management until the arterial lesion is recognized. Unilateral leg signs should lead to consideration of local causes of ulceration, such as unusual infections, arteriovenous fistulas, congenital valve anomalies of deep veins, and underlying osteomyelitis. The occasional development of epidermoid carcinoma in the skin surrounding an old ulcer should be recalled along with the occurrence of dermatitis due to local radiation therapy, which may go on to malignant change if the damaged skin remains for periods of many years. Table 29-1 may therefore serve as a checklist of common as well as some unusual causes of ulceration of the lower leg, whose identity is chiefly dependent upon consideration of the disease as a diagnostic possibility.

Most lower leg ulcers are venous in origin. In the series of 110 patients studied earlier, 69 percent were of either postphlebitic or varicose vein origin while 31 percent were due to various nonvenous causes. Among the venous ulcers, 75 percent were postphlebitic and 25 percent were due to severe primary varicose veins.[4] This latter figure was similar to the 30 percent reported by Cranley's group.[5]

PATHOPHYSIOLOGY

It is not completely clear why edema and ulcers develop in postphlebitic legs. Phlebographic study has proved incorrect the earlier belief that continued thrombotic obstruction of the deep calf and thigh veins causes these changes. Indeed, long-standing occlusion of calf veins is rare, and superficial femoral vein blocks in the thigh are not the rule and, when they do occur, are usually well-collateralized.

Leg ulcers ordinarily begin from a break in the skin due to minor trauma. Healing in abnormal skin is often retarded further by the patient's well-meaning but faulty management of the local lesion so that an increasing area of skin becomes necrotic. The relation of the skin ulcer to previous damage of the vein by thrombosis is generally accepted, although the exact mechanism is far from clear. Postthrombotic studies in animal veins by direct examination and in human veins by phlebographic examination indicate that the early thrombus begins to organize and eventually recanalizes in most instances. This is a major difference between the end results of thrombosis in the venous and arterial systems, since thrombosis in the latter is usually permanent in the particular vessel involved and the new blood supply is determined by collateralization. On the venous side, the early-forming collaterals tend to disappear gradually as recanalization of the thrombosed vein occurs.[4] The majority of thrombosed veins do recanalize and become patent, as evidenced by phlebograms. Complete persistence of thrombosis of the deep veins of the calf is unusual despite many previous statements to the contrary. Only an occasional phlebogram shows such failure to recanalize.

The critical functional lesion leading to postphlebitic skin changes has never been completely isolated. There is little doubt that most of these patients have varying degrees of anatomic damage associated with functional insufficiency of the deep veins. This is demonstrated on phlebograms by a failure of clearing of the contrast medium into the proximal venous system following the exercise test, which uniformly clears the contrast medium from the legs of normal subjects. For some time there has been the widespread belief that this is the essential lesion and that an increase in the pressure in the distal deep vein leads to the difficulty in the skin. However, phlebograms also show that some postphlebitic extremities with ulcers have little or no valve or wall damage in the deep venous system and that a few actually clear the contrast agent very well following exercise. Recently, this has led to the concept that the basic lesion is in the communicating, perforating veins, which are damaged to the extent that they transmit an excessive pressure from the deep venous system into the superficial system via faulty valves.* It is also possible that both these lesions are implicated to varying degrees in different people and that a combination of effects causes the ambulatory venous hypertension which results in the postphlebitic syndrome.[7]

The deep lymphatics are normal, although the superficial lymphatics are often obliterated locally about an ulcer. In this connection, it should be noted that a major characteristic of primary lymphedema is the absence of ulcers of the skin. This lack of ulceration in the presence of lymphedema also rules against the importance of lymphatic dysfunction in the development of ulcers. The obliteration of superficial lymphatics about leg ulcers found by Moyer and Butcher was probably the effect rather than the original cause of the ulceration.[8]

The factor of abnormal arteriovenous communications with increased venous oxygen content near an ulcer noted by Fontaine[9] and by Gius[10] is not well understood at present, although ulcers due to such fistulas are well-known. Such lesions certainly result in persistent venous hypertension in the extremity.

Deep venous valvular damage has also been said to cause the postphlebitic syndrome. Though

*The discussion of the importance of perforator vein incompetence, rather than femoral and saphenous insufficiency, presented by Dodd and Cockett in Chapter 17 of their book[6] should be read by everyone interested in leg ulcers.

many of these limbs do show paucity or absence of valves in the phlebogram, others show a reasonable number of valves.

The pressure within the deep veins of the leg reflects the distance between the heart and the site of measurement. During walking there are dynamic changes, but mean pressure with the deep veins is essentially unchanged. Mean pressure within the superficial veins during walking does change, however, by decreasing. The differences in venous pressure of the superficial veins between normal, varicose, and postphlebitic veins are shown in Figure 29-1. Pressure within the normal superficial veins is reduced during walking. When there are varicose veins, the reduction is less. The postphlebitic limb shows a great difference from normal. Often there is no reduction of superficial venous pressure, or even some elevation. When exercise ceases, there is a gradual return to the preexercise level of pressure.

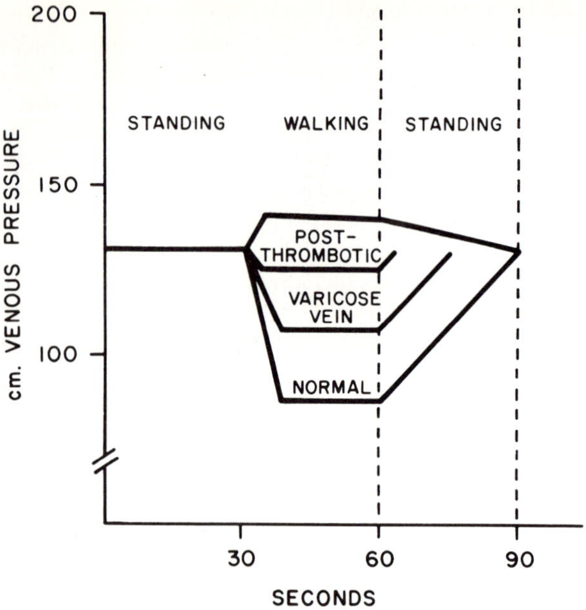

FIGURE 29-1 Superficial venous pressure measured in the saphenous vein with the patient standing quietly usually equals the distance from the heart to the needle position. When the normal patient walks, the peripheral muscle pump reduces superficial venous pressure, which slowly rises again when walking ceases. When pressures are measured in the postphlebitic limb, there is little reduction or even some increase, so there recurs ambulatory venous hypertension. Varicose veins produce measurements somewhere in between.

The failure of venous pressure to decrease during walking is termed *ambulatory venous hypertension* and appears to be an important physiologic defect in the leg with a damaged venous system. AVH is apparently due to constant transmission of the high deep-vein pressure through damaged perforating veins into the superficial venous system, probably because the perforating venous valves have been made incompetent.[4] Kinmonth, Rob, and Simeone, however, pointed out that other conditions with venous hypertension, such as arteriovenous fistula, do not often form skin ulcers.[11]

Ambulatory venous hypertension eventually dilates venules as well as larger veins, so all sizes of varicosities begin to appear. Edema follows the pressure change. Areas of fat necrosis appear as firm, tender, red areas and are believed to be caused by impaired venous return secondary to local thrombosis or venous hypertension.

Further evidence of the validity of the AVH mechanism is the well-known healing effect of rest and elevation, as well as of external pressure dressings by elastic wraps or hose. Indeed, these measures will heal most ulcers without recourse to operation unless the size is so large as to make impossible complete ingrowth of skin from the edges.

However, many, including myself, are not quite satisfied that abnormal perforating veins are the only factor involved in the postphlebitic syndrome, because in many people their complete eradication by subfascial ligation does not cure the postphlebitic syndrome completely. It is likely that deep venous valvular abnormalities, failure of the muscle pump due to atrophy, and persistent deep venous obstruction also play some role. Despite vein stripping, perforator ligation, and ulcer excision and grafting, *it is usually necessary to maintain external elastic support postoperatively* to prevent recurrent ulcers, indicating persistence of the postphlebitic problem despite surgical efforts. Part of the reason for this is the permanent scarring of fat and skin that follows healing; this diminishes arterial perfusion. The lymphatic plexuses of the skin are destroyed, although the deeper lymphatics are not affected. The situation was well stated by Kinmonth, Rob, and Simeone: "It follows that the healed area . . . is most vulnerable and likely to break down under the ordinary stresses of life."[11] It is a good trick to heal an ulcer, but a better one to maintain healing!

DIAGNOSIS

Recognition of the variety of causes of leg ulcers is important, since an improper diagnosis usually leads to incorrect therapy, with failure the result. More than once it has become apparent that failure to take a proper history has led the previous physician to treat the ulcer patient on an incorrect basis, such as two patients with radiation dermatitis who were being treated for postphlebitic ulcers. Similarly, previous management of an ulcer which was also associated with atherosclerotic thrombosis of the femoral artery resulted in failure until the true cause was recognized and treated by arterial reconstruction.

A careful history must be centered on the possibility of previous phlebitis, which may be partially or completely forgotten until the symptoms associated with the episode are brought to the patient's attention. Careful inquiry often brings out a history of previous swelling of the leg or pain after childbirth, operation, injury, or illness that may not have been specifically ascribed at the time to phlebitis. A previous episode of phlebitis may be denied but an episode of "milk leg" readily acknowledged. The history should also cover episodes of trauma, previous operations, and other therapy and the current method of management used by the patient.

Physical examination of the ulcer, the venous system in the legs, the arterial pulses, and oscillometric findings often themselves point immediately to the cause of the ulceration.

Cultures are made to determine the organism and its sensitivity only if there appears to be an unusual degree of surrounding cellulitis or lymphangitis. Routine cultures are not critical in determining treatment, since infection is not ordinarily the primary cause of the skin breakdown but is a secondary event. If the ulcer is long-standing or is in any way suspicious of carcinoma, biopsies should be made from several points on the edge. If an ulcer has been present for more than a year, a biopsy should invariably be done.

Suitable roentgenographic bone examinations and blood studies for anemia, diabetes, and other systemic diseases are undertaken.

In the event that pulse examination and oscillometric studies indicate any degree of arterial insufficiency, angiograms are performed to ascertain the status of the arterial supply to the extremity.

Functional Phlebography

While the practical significance of phlebographic examination of the veins is not yet completely settled, it is a valuable adjunct to management, since it clarifies the diagnosis and permits evaluation of anatomic as well as functional characteristics of the deep and superficial veins of the lower extremity.

Indications are (1) the postphlebitic state and (2) unusual varicose veins. All patients with leg symptoms as sequelae of previous venous thrombosis are examined by this technique in order to clarify the anatomy and function of the deep veins, which are otherwise inaccessible to study. More rational selection of surgical and nonsurgical forms of treatment is possible with this knowledge of the deep venous circulation. Run-of-the-mill varicose veins are not subjected to phlebography; it is reserved for (1) unusual varices, including unilateral ones, (2) those recurrent after surgery, and (3) those occurring at an early age.

Our technique of functional phlebography is a consolidation of a variety of practices described by others.[12–14] It consists of the injection of 60 mL of Conray-43 via a no. 19 or no. 21 needle placed in a vein of the foot or ankle. A tourniquet is firmly applied distally so that the contrast medium is forced from the superficial into the deep venous circulation. The technique, illustrated in Figure 29-2, includes positioning of the patient at the 45° angle to prevent layering of the contrast medium, which might result in diagnostic error.

Fears that the contrast medium injection results in needless complications have proved essentially groundless in 200 such examinations, after which only a single episode of postphlebographic venous thrombosis occurred. We attribute this safety, greater than that often reported by others, to the preexamination injection of 5000 U.S.P. units of aqueous heparin placed through the needle in the ankle vein. There also have been no heparin complications.[15] This experience has led to boldness in performing phlebography in the postphlebitic leg.

PLAN OF MANAGEMENT OF LEG ULCERS

Correct etiologic diagnosis combined with an understanding of the physiologic and pathologic changes occurring in ulceration of the leg leads to a general plan of management which is individualized in particular patients (Figure 29-3). Not only is it essential that the physician furnish detailed care to the patient, but also teaching the patient about the lesion enables considerably better cooperation. There is a well-recognized difference in the results of treatment between clinic

FIGURE 29-2 Phlebography is conducted through a small needle placed in an ankle or foot vein with the patient in the 45° position. A distal ankle tourniquet is placed to force the radiopaque material into the deep venous circulation. Five thousand U.S.P. units of heparin are initially injected, followed by the bolus of the 60 mL of Conray 43. Films are exposed in both anterior-posterior and lateral positions before and after exercise.

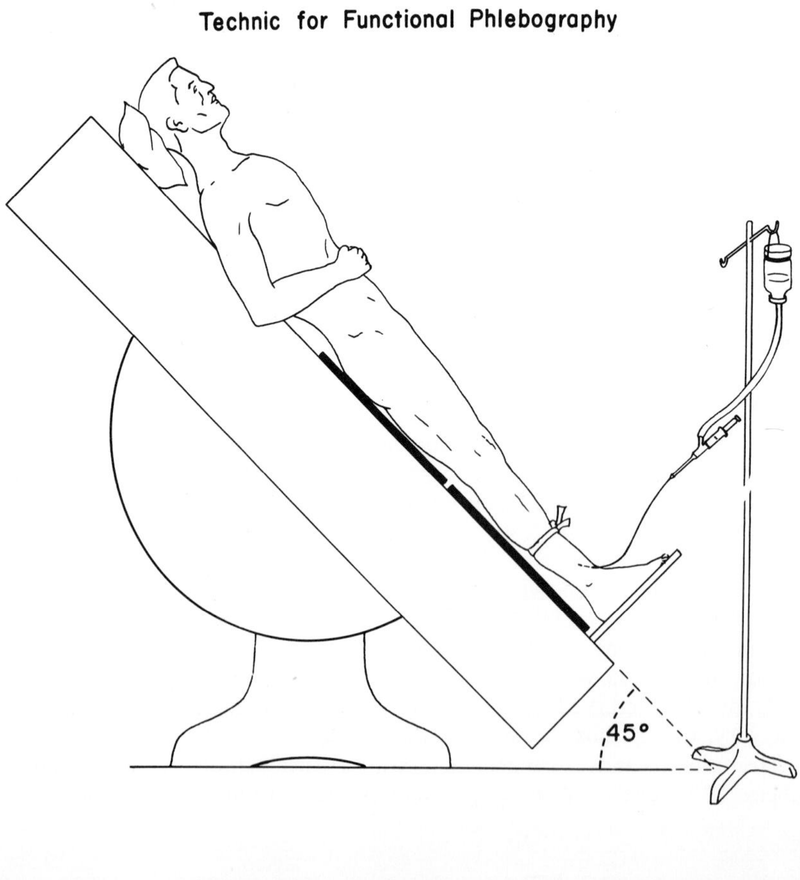

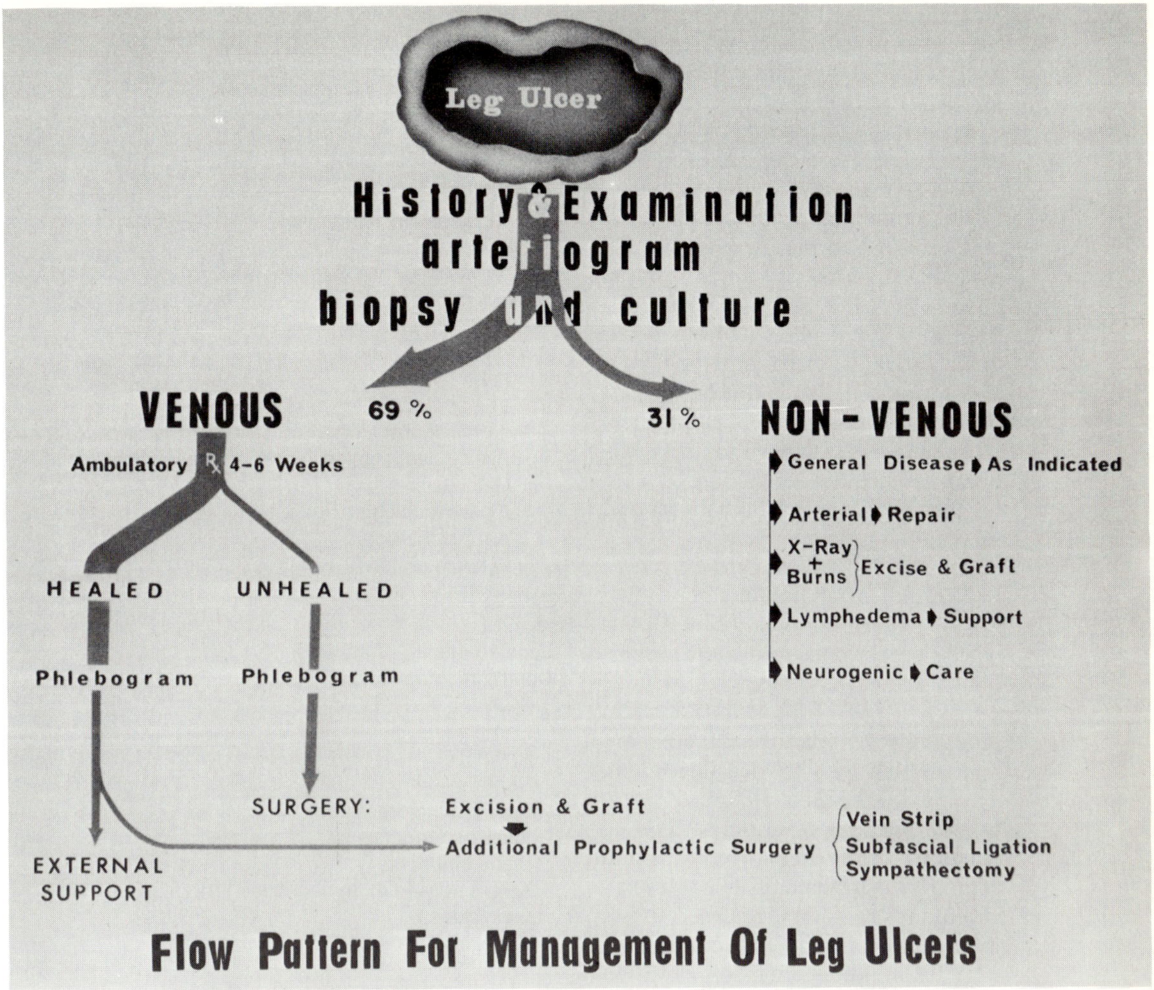

FIGURE 29-3 Summary of the plan of management of leg ulcers which is described in the text.

patients and private patients, which is undoubtedly based to a considerable extent on this understanding or the lack of it.

An essentially nonoperative program is aimed at healing the skin. Operations are done only in those patients whose ulcers cannot otherwise be healed and maintained that way. Approximately 66 percent have therefore had no operation, while a third have required one or another surgical procedures. The program outlined in Table 29-2 has proved simple and practical.

First is an attempt to heal the ulcerated leg on an outpatient, ambulatory basis for 4 to 6 weeks, unless the presenting ulcer is so large (with its least diameter over 3 cm) that it obviously requires excision and grafting. Patients are started on a program of elevation, rest, and external pressure, and a compress with saline is applied to the ulcer itself twice daily.

Elevation

Reduction of edema by elevation of the part has been understood by laypersons and physicians for centuries. It continues to be an important treatment and should be stressed as an easy and inexpensive method. Most patients attempt to achieve elevation by placing folded blankets or pillows beneath the foot and ankle. This is ineffective, either because the extremity rolls off the pad or because the pad is crushed down. A considerably better method is to elevate the foot of the bed approximately 6 in by placing newspapers, magazines, books, or wooden blocks under it. It is remarkable to see the difference in reduction of edema when this method is used compared with attempts to elevate the feet on pillows. Most people learn to sleep with the feet elevated to this extent without any particular difficulty. When the spouse occupies the same bed, both must learn to sleep with the feet elevated or they must change to separate beds.

The patient shown in Figure 29-4 was referred for amputation of a postphlebitic leg swollen to gigantic proportions. There were ulcers as well as actual splitting of the skin. Elevation produced severe pain, and the patient was sleeping with the leg dependent. Treatment consisted of forced elevation (with heavy opiate and barbiturate sedation) until edema receded and comfort was restored. The leg was salvaged and the patient returned to her usual life, wearing an elastic stocking.

A 15-minute period of elevation midmorning and midafternoon while at home or at work can usually be arranged (perhaps in a rest room or even by lying on the floor of a garage and placing the feet up on the wall!). Some patients with venous edema and its complications need even longer periods of elevation.

TABLE 29-2 MANAGEMENT OF LEG ULCERS

- General
  - Treatment of reversible disease
    - Edema of other causes (heart failure, low protein levels)
    - Obesity
    - Diabetes
    - Arterial lesions (atherosclerotic occlusions, arteriovenous fistulas)
    - Specific infections (syphilis, tuberculosis, fungus)
  - Reduction of ambulatory venous hypertension and control of edema by
    - Rest with leg elevation
      - In bed
      - In a tip-back chair
    - External support
      - Elastic bandages with over sponge-rubber pads
      - Gelocasts
      - Elastic stockings
      - Aero-pulse boots
      - Jobst intermittent-compression units
    - Diuretics
- Specific
  - Local treatment of the ulcer
  - Control of infection by
    - Rest
    - Compresses
    - Antibiotics
    - Debridement
    - Nonirritating dressings
  - Control of dermatitis by
    - Bland ointments
    - Antipruritics [e.g., trimeprazine tartrate (Temaril)]
    - Fungicides
  - Surgical treatment by excision and graft
- Prophylactic
  - Avoidance of trauma with shin guards
  - Elevation of the leg
    - During rest periods at work
    - At home
  - External support with elastic stockings
  - Weight control
  - Surgical treatment by
    - Removal of varicose veins
    - Subfascial ligation of perforating veins
    - Sympathectomy (for hyperhidrosis)

External Pressure

There are available a variety of elasticized cloth materials ranging from inexpensive elastic wraps to custom-fit two-way stretch hose. The elastic bandage has the virtue of low cost, ready availability, and adaptability to changes in the degrees of edema. It has the disadvantage of constant slipping; it is hot and wrinkles, with consequent discomfort. It is useful in initial treatment until the size of the leg has become stabilized, at which time stockings are prescribed.

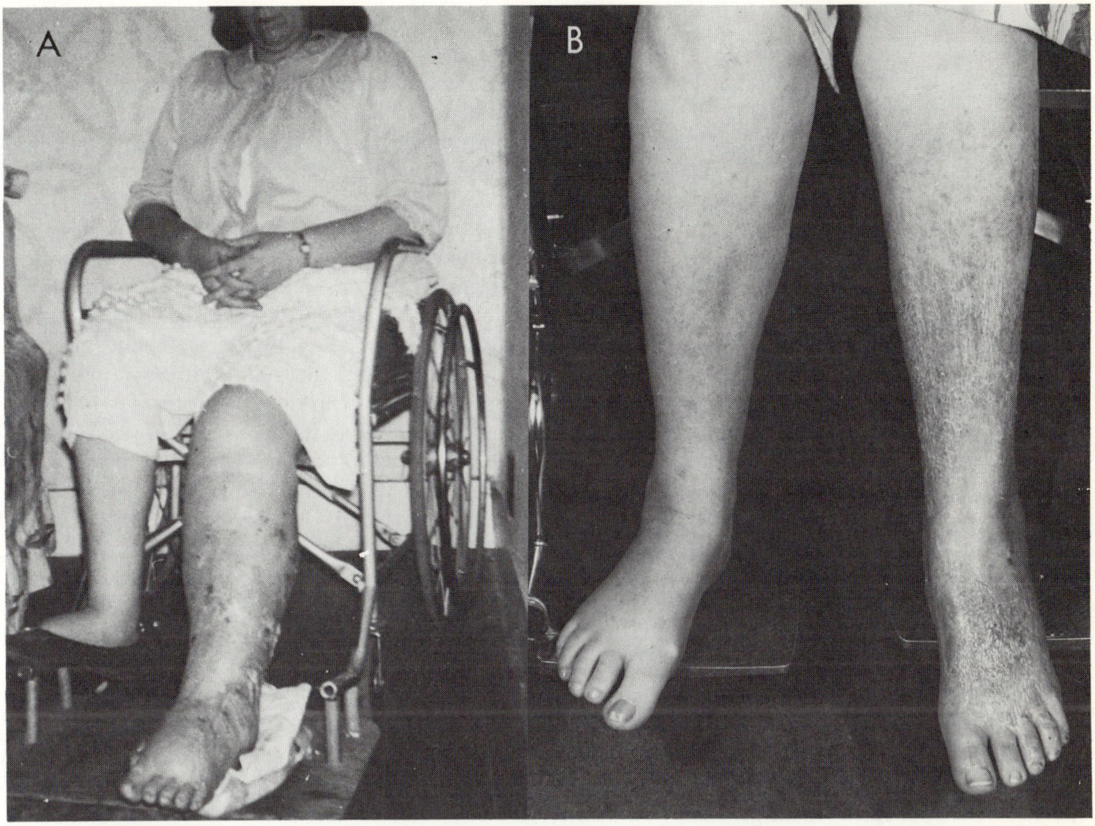

FIGURE 29-4 (*a*) This severely swollen postphlebitic leg was so painful that the patient would not allow elevation without narcotic medication. The skin had split and she was referred for amputation. (*b*) Following elevation and compression a properly fitting elastic stocking was placed. This photograph taken 6 months later shows residual pigmentation but excellent control of edema and rehabilitation, with the patient wearing a 40-mmHg elastic stocking.

Elastic hose should be measured when the patient's edema is minimal. This may occur at the end of a brief period of hospitalization or may be produced by 48 to 72 hours of bed rest combined with diuretics at home. In the latter event, the patient should place firm elastic bandages before arising and sit in the back of an automobile with the feet elevated on the way to the office for measurement.

A variety of elasticized stockings are available. Ordinarily there is no skin difficulty above the knee, and thigh-length stockings are difficult to support, so these have been largely abandoned and the stocking is usually prescribed to a point just below the patella. It is ordered at 40 mmHg pressure for the ordinary patient, although it is available in both 30 and 50 mmHg tensions. A reinforced heel is advantageous in adding to the life of the hose, which under ordinary conditions is approximately 3 to 4 months. The stocking exerts a greater pressure at the ankle than at the calf. A unilateral leotard and one with a cutout for the pregnant abdomen are also available.

More elaborate forms of external support, such as the Aero-pulse boot,[16] have been devised and are occasionally needed. The intermittent-pressure apparatus,[17] which functions to milk edema from the periphery toward the heart, is not usually needed for venous edema.

Local Treatment

The advice of Hume in 1801 is sound: "It must appear obvious that there is no probability that any one medicine can ever be discovered which, internally administered or locally applied, shall have powers adapted to the cure of all ulcers on the leg; and it would appear, the idea that such a medicine may exist has retarded very considerably the advancement of our knowledge and the treatment of ulcer." Although it is to be hoped that some accelerator of healing will eventually be discovered, there does not yet appear to be any real evidence that such is available. This leads to the concept that nothing harmful should be placed directly in any wound, and to my use of normal saline. The patient is strongly cautioned not to place antiseptics, unguents, or other medications directly on the wound. While antiseptic solutions undoubtedly destroy organisms, they also cause necrosis of tissue and delay the healing of the tissues. It is to be emphasized that there is no evidence that there is any material that hastens healing by external application.

The patient is asked to apply a saline compress to the ulcer for 30 to 60 minutes twice daily and to replace it by a sterile dry gauze pad dressing placed directly on the wound. Over this is placed a piece of foam rubber $\frac{1}{2}$ in thick, and both are held in place by an elastic bandage. At the next dressing the gauze pad removes the necrotic debris and exudate as it is taken off (by soaking if painful) and thereby accomplishes debridement twice daily. This pressure dressing is maintained by night also. A bland ointment or oil may be advised for dryness. An antifungal agent may be useful after bathing, as prophylaxis and treatment of interdigital fungus infection.

Most leg ulcers can be healed with this or some other program,[1] but long-term cure is less successful and recurrences are common. Careful continued follow-up care is mandatory.

Surgical Treatment

Varicose Vein Surgery While excision of primary varicose veins produces excellent results (Chapter 28), the old concept that the same is true for varicosities secondary to the postphlebitic syndrome is incorrect. Indeed only about 15 to 20 percent of patients with secondary varicosities benefit from surgery directed at the veins alone. Most do better with elastic compression, and varicosities simply recur if treated surgically. They are a manifestation of and not the cause of the ambulatory venous hypertension. Their correction alone is usually doomed to failure.

Cranley has contrasted the good results (95 percent of 174) of the surgical removal of primary varicosities which led to ulcers with the poor results (33 percent recurrence among 205) when the ulcers were secondary to deep venous insufficiency. He also noted that "swelling is never eliminated in such extremities so that heavy elastic hose are necessary after operation."[18]

Operation on the veins is sometimes needed if the varicosities have become severe to the point of contributing further to venous stasis. The physician must then carefully analyze the state of the deep venous system to decide whether the saphenous systems may be sacrificed or whether they should be left in place beneath a constantly applied elastic stocking. At times it may be good judgment to remove varicosities below the knee but leave the saphenous vein in the thigh as a collateral when the superficial femoral vein is occluded. Functional phlebography helps in this decision. If the veins are to be removed, it is done along with whatever excision and grafting is needed for the ulcer.

Subfascial Ligation of Perforating Veins The interruption of communicating, perforating veins advocated by Linton in the United States[19] and by Dodd and Cockett in England[6] aroused hope that venous insufficiency and its attendant problems, including leg ulcers, could be successfully treated by a surgical procedure. Unfortunately, the hypothesis of cause was misunderstood, the operation was poorly conceived, and its clinical failures have led to general abandonment.

The operation originally proposed by Robert Linton included (1) ligation of the superficial femoral vein, (2) stripping of the saphenous veins, (3) excision of a wide strip of deep fascia, and

(4) subfascial ligation of venous perforators.[19] He continued to perform this procedure and toward the end of his illustrious career stated that a long-lasting cure of postphlebitic ulcer would be achieved only "if you interrupt the deep venous circulation just distal to the profunda femoris vein."[20]

Other interested clinicians have noted the failure of any operative technique to cure postphlebitic leg ulcers and suggested one or another concomitant procedure. Linton's pupil—and later authority—John Cranley of Cincinnati believed "the patient with the true postphlebitic leg to be incurable, although manageable" in view of his own recurrence rate of 36 percent. A young Bostonian, Thomas O'Donnell, has stated that "subfascial ligation does not correct the problem."[21]

Since then, deep venous ligation (either of the superficial femoral or the popliteal vein) has been generally abandoned because it further damages the deep venous circulation by interrupting it.

Simplification of the Linton procedure by omission of fascial excision,[6,22] which is unnecessary, led to Dodd and Cockett's operation, whereby subfascial ligations of the communicating (perforator) veins between the deep and superficial veins of the lower leg were performed in the belief that their incompetence was a major factor in the persistence of leg ulcers. This too is doubtful. Burnand, O'Donnell, Thomas, and Browse later (in 1977) reported a 50 percent recurrence rate after ligation of perforators alone and questioned the entire concept on the basis of venous pressure studies. They concluded, "Our management is nonoperative for postthrombotic patients."[23]

Hyde's retrospective study in 1981 of 109 patients after subfascial ligation showed not only a high infection rate of 15 percent but also a recurrence rate of 25 percent and the necessity for further operative procedures in 17 percent. He further noted that "wearing supportive pressure graded hosiery is also essential."[24] Removing varicose veins may be helpful, but they occasionally furnish the chief route of venous return and should be studied preoperatively with that in mind.

Whether subfascial venous ligation or some other procedure is done, it remains a general rule that external pressure by some form of elastic hose is still necessary to prevent recurrences of skin ulcers. I performed some subfascial ligations in the early 1960s (Figures 29-5 and 29-6) and learned that these could be carried out without a high risk, but I was not convinced that this procedure offered any more than did lesser procedures (removal of indicated varicose veins, excision and grafting of ulcers) and continued to find that external stocking support was invariably necessary.

In some reports the use of the subfascial ligation operation appears forced and unnecessary. If the operation is postponed until the ulcer is healed (even by excision and skin grafting when necessary),[22] it is probable that subfascial ligation is unnecessary if external elastic support is used and that the operation will not necessarily allow the omission of elastic hose. In one enthusiastic report of 31 operations on 28 patients it was finally stated that "the crural fascia was not incised in 12 of our patients." Thus, only 57 percent of the cited patients had the advocated subfascial ligation; the rest apparently had only removal of the saphenous veins plus ulcer excision and delayed grafting.[25]

The complication rate, delayed healing time, and failure to prevent recurrent ulcers appear to me to be no better than with my policy of excision of the ulcer, immediate skin grafting, and simultaneous ligation and stripping of veins and perforators in the area. The addition of the distant perforator ligations under the fascia is probably not necessary and should not be done in most patients. Meyers's statement that "going behind the fascia to get perforators is unnecessary"[26] represents the opinion of an experienced venous surgeon. Linton's associate Darling has stated that of the two ways to manage a healed postthrombotic ulcer (first, a subfascial operation, and second, an elastic stocking), "the majority of patients I see can be managed with the latter."[27] Wylie also has suggested that, since elastic hose are needed after operation, the same results can be obtained by hose without operation.[28]

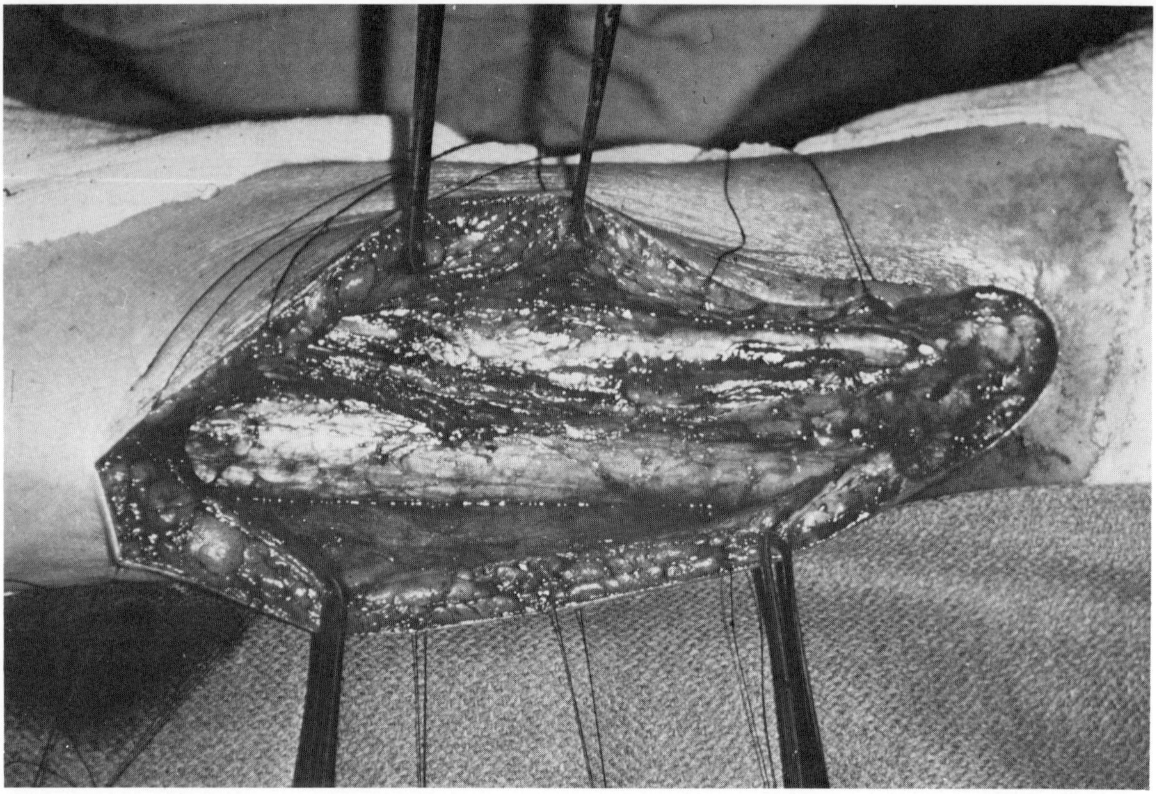

FIGURE 29-5 Subfascial ligation of perforating veins. Silk stay sutures retracted the skin so that it was not needlessly damaged. Allis clamps elevated the fascia, which had been split to allow subfascial interruption of the perforating veins.

FIGURE 29-6 The medial wound of the lower leg was closed following subfascial ligation. The chronic malleolar ulcer was excised and a split-thickness skin graft applied.

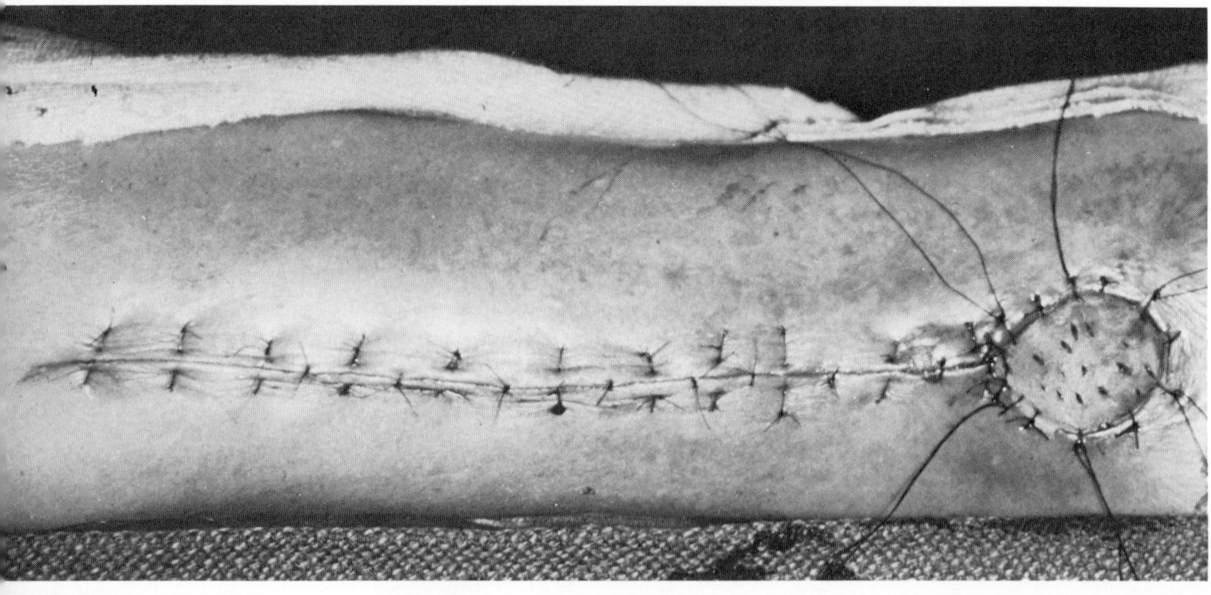

The procedure of subfascial ligation has thus not been widely accepted, nor can it be advocated as useful for most individuals. It is not the widely applicable curative procedure that was hoped for at the time of its introduction. The same result can be accomplished more simply, and subfascial ligation should be abandoned.

Excision and Skin Grafting of Ankle Ulcers The principal indication for excision and grafting is chronicity, which may be defined as failure to heal or to make visible progress during a 4- to 6-week course of ambulatory therapy. The other indication is size—an ulcer whose area is such that solid continued healing does not seem likely (Figure 29-7). Experience indicates that if the least diameter of the ulcer is over 3 cm, complete and continued healing is unlikely and early excision and skin grafting should be advised.

Once the decision has been made to remove the ulcer and apply a split-thickness graft, there need be no particular delay to prepare the wound. The vast majority of chronic ankle ulcers have been present for a long time, so the local situation is static and there is neither advancing cellulitis nor lymphangitis, nor is there much tendency toward healing. Pockets of infection should be drained, but these are uncommon. Antibiotic preparation is unnecessary, and the only reason for obtaining a culture for sensitivities is to have this information available in the early postoperative period in the event that the edges of the graft begin to succumb rapidly to spreading infection.

The patient is asked to continue saline compresses regularly until the time of hospital admission and is scheduled for operation on the day after admission, without any prolonged prepara-

FIGURE 29-7 Large chronic malleolar ulcers were excised and closed with split-thickness skin grafts, shown 10 days postoperatively.

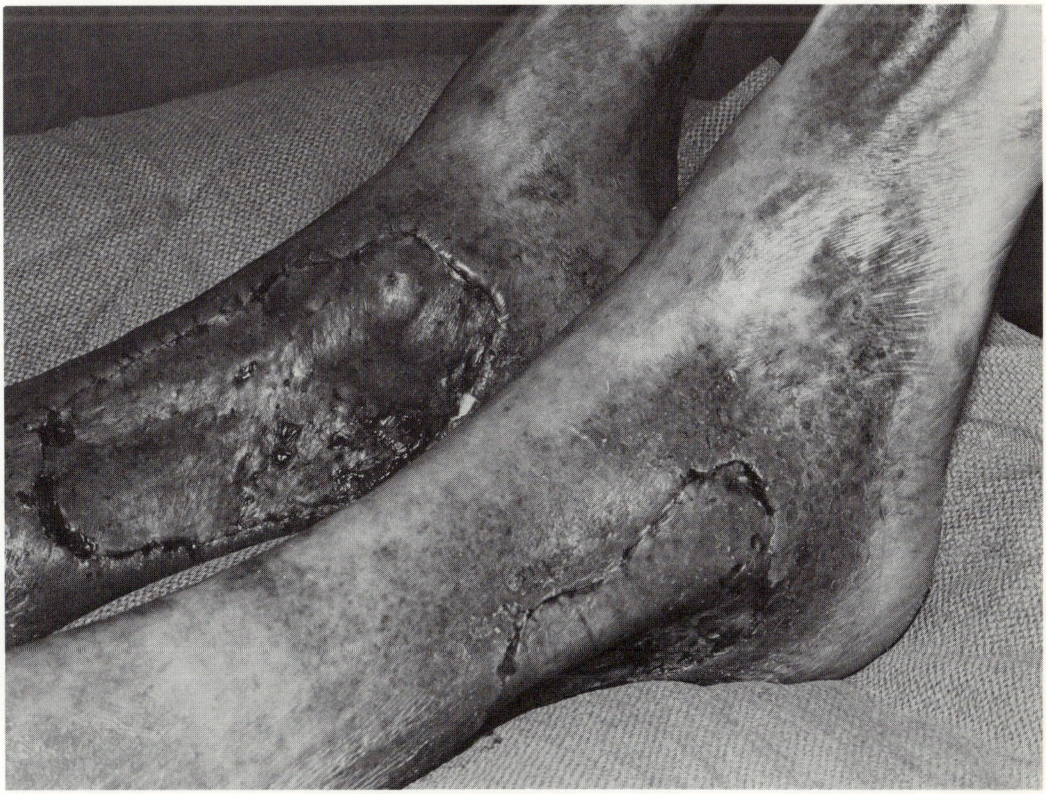

tion. While some have stated that ulcers should be excised primarily and the skin grafting should be delayed to a secondary operation, our policy of immediate excision and grafting has given excellent results, so staging is not necessary. Table 29-3 indicates that, among the 55 patients having excision of ulcer and immediate split-thickness skin grafting, only 9 percent had failure of viability of the graft which required a formal secondary procedure. Many of the successful grafts had sloughing of some part of the edge or even a small portion of the center of the graft, but 91 percent progressed to final healing following primary grafting. Figure 29-7 shows the results of such an operation, where four extremely large ulcers occupied both sides of both ankles and required three dermatome drums of split-thickness grafts. This patient was subsequently followed until his death 7 years later without recurrence and with perfectly healed ankles. He faithfully wore stockings as advised.

TABLE 29-3 TREATMENT OF 153 CONSECUTIVE LEG ULCERS

Excision and primary skin graft (36%)	
Did not need a secondary graft	50
Required a secondary split graft	5
Total	55
No surgical treatment (64%)	98

Excision of scarred, fibrotic tissue, which comprises the ulcer bed, is as important as is the skin graft. Incomplete excision of fibrotic scar tissue invites recurrence of ulceration. It is tempting simply to scrape the top of the granulation and place the graft on this. Such a procedure often allows immediate take of the graft, but with later recurrence of ulceration (Figure 29-8). The

FIGURE 29-8 A chronic malleolar ulcer was not excised but merely scraped, and a fitted split-thickness graft was placed. The initial viability shown here changed 6 weeks later, when the graft gradually became necrotic and sloughed away as the underlying fibrous tissue healed and contracted so that the graft no longer had a sufficient blood supply.

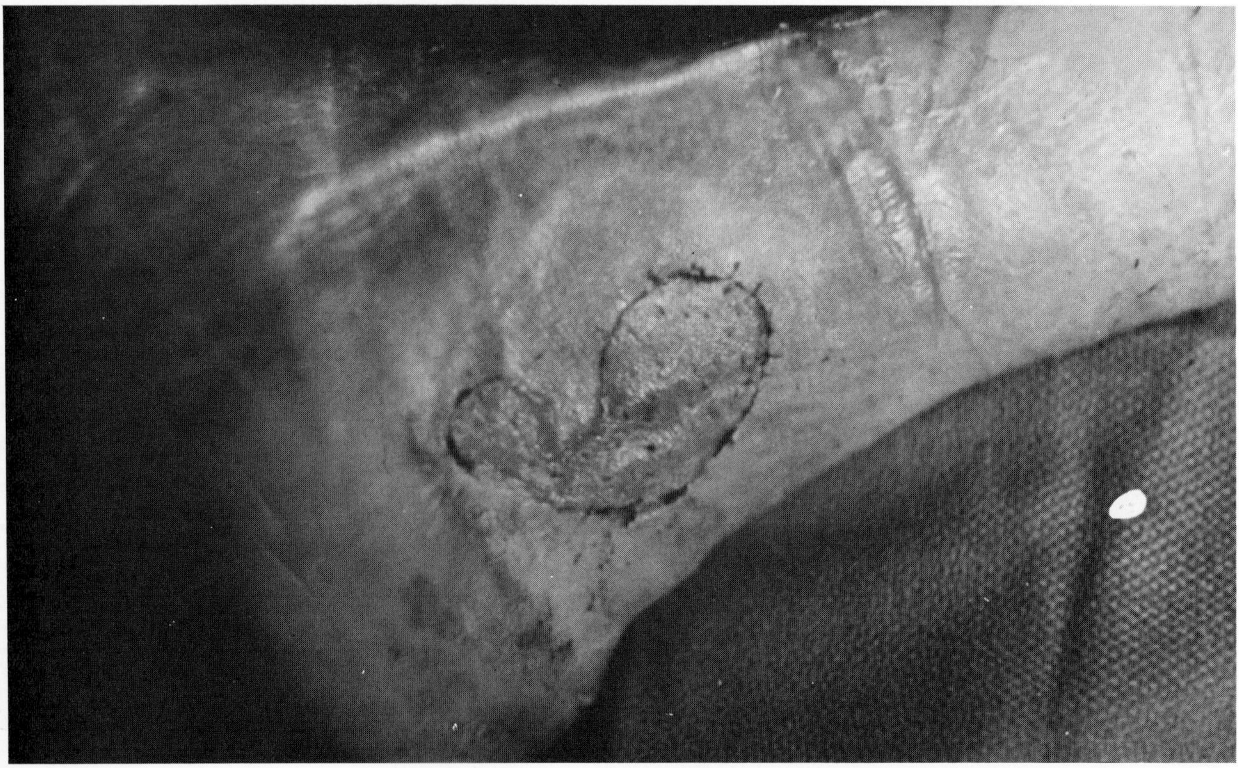

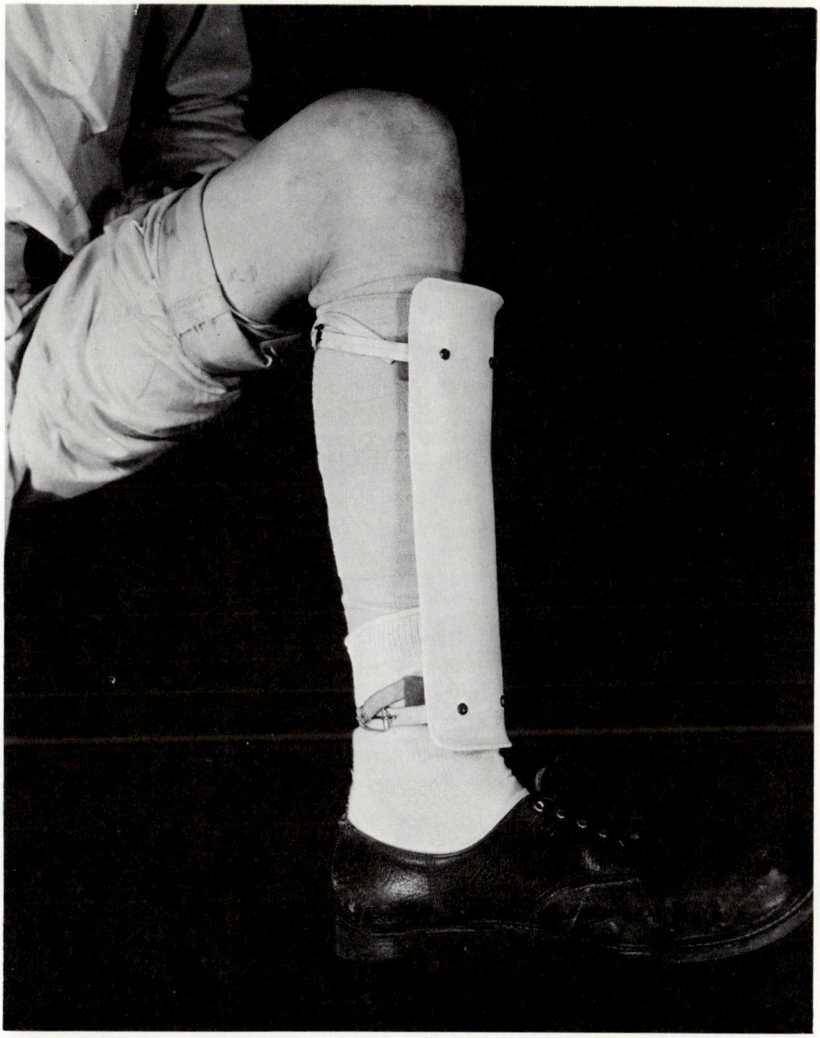

FIGURE 29-9 A shin guard protects the leg of this worker following excision and grafting of a chronic malleolar ulcer.

probable explanation for failure is that the vascular supply that initially nourishes the graft through the granulation is later fibrosed as the scar tissue matures, so eventually ischemia of the grafted skin occurs. Complete excision of scar and fibrotic tissue removes this thick bed of contracting, fibrosing, collagenous tissue.

The technical details of placing and dressing the split-skin graft have been described,[29] are well-known, and will not be repeated here.

After the fresh graft is solidly healed, a knee-length 40-mmHg stocking replaces the elastic bandage. It is worn for a minimum of 1 year, at the end of which time the patient may be allowed to remove it for a gradually increasing time period daily. Any evidence of edema or recurrent ulceration signals the need for return to its constant use. Most patients must wear it for a lifetime to prevent recurrent ulcers.

Some patients need a skin-protective device to prevent trauma to the legs and ankles while at work (Figure 29-9).

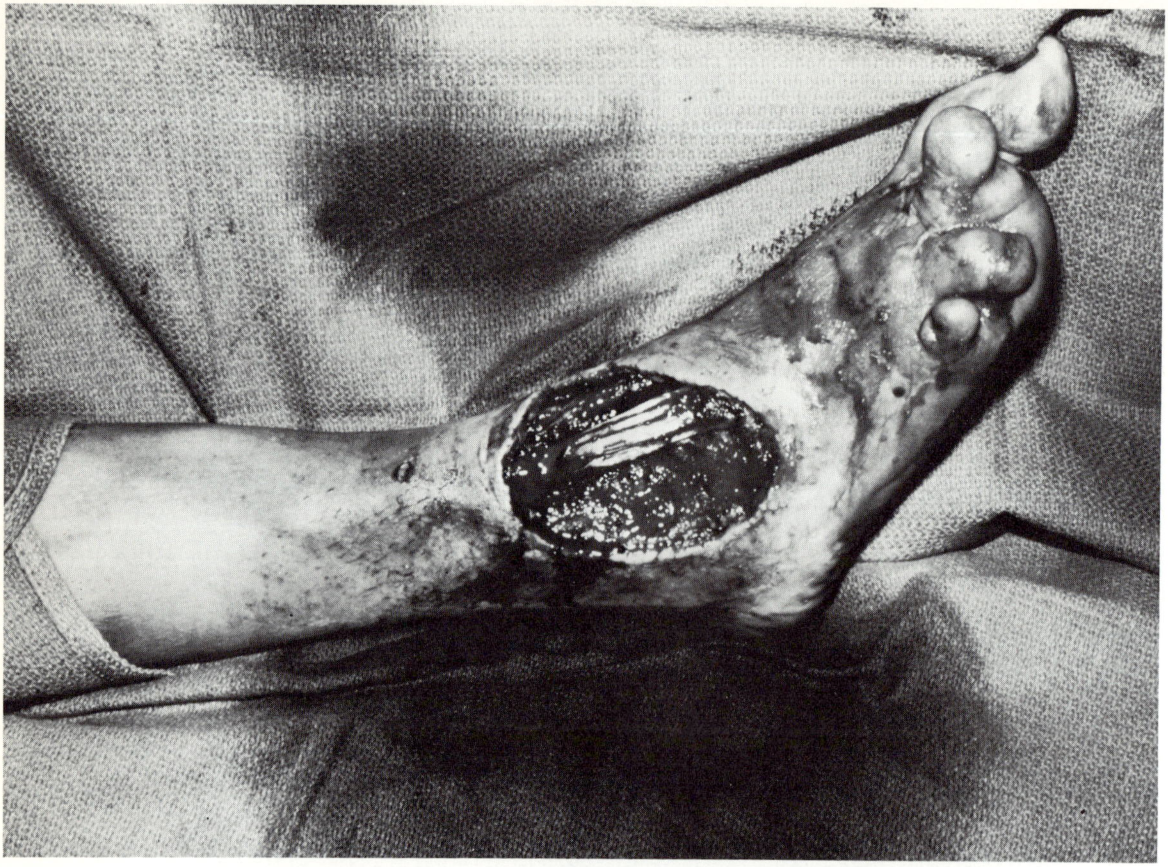

FIGURE 29-10 A recurrent ankle ulcer incapacitated this 25-year-old woman for many months. Multiple excision and split-thickness grafts by three different surgeons failed. The final successful operation began with this extensive debridement of scarred tissue to the extent that tendons lay bare in the base of the wound.

Flap Transplants Plastic surgeons and knowledgeable microvascular surgeons have developed useful techniques of transplanting tissue to cover a wound. This extreme resort is sometimes necessary in chronic leg ulcers. Figures 29-10 to 29-12 illustrate a cross-leg flap placed by Dr. Glenn Buckspan which finally solved the chronic unrelieved ulcer of a 25-year-old woman with severe postphlebitic disease after multiple excision and skin graftings by three different surgeons had failed.

Lumbar Sympathectomy Recently Patman has revived interest in the virtues of sympathetic ablation as a specific procedure for leg ulcers, citing healing of such in patients who had proved refractory to other methods.[30] Sympathectomy does prevent hyperhidrosis and thereby dries the surrounding skin. Whether there are other benefits seems doubtful.

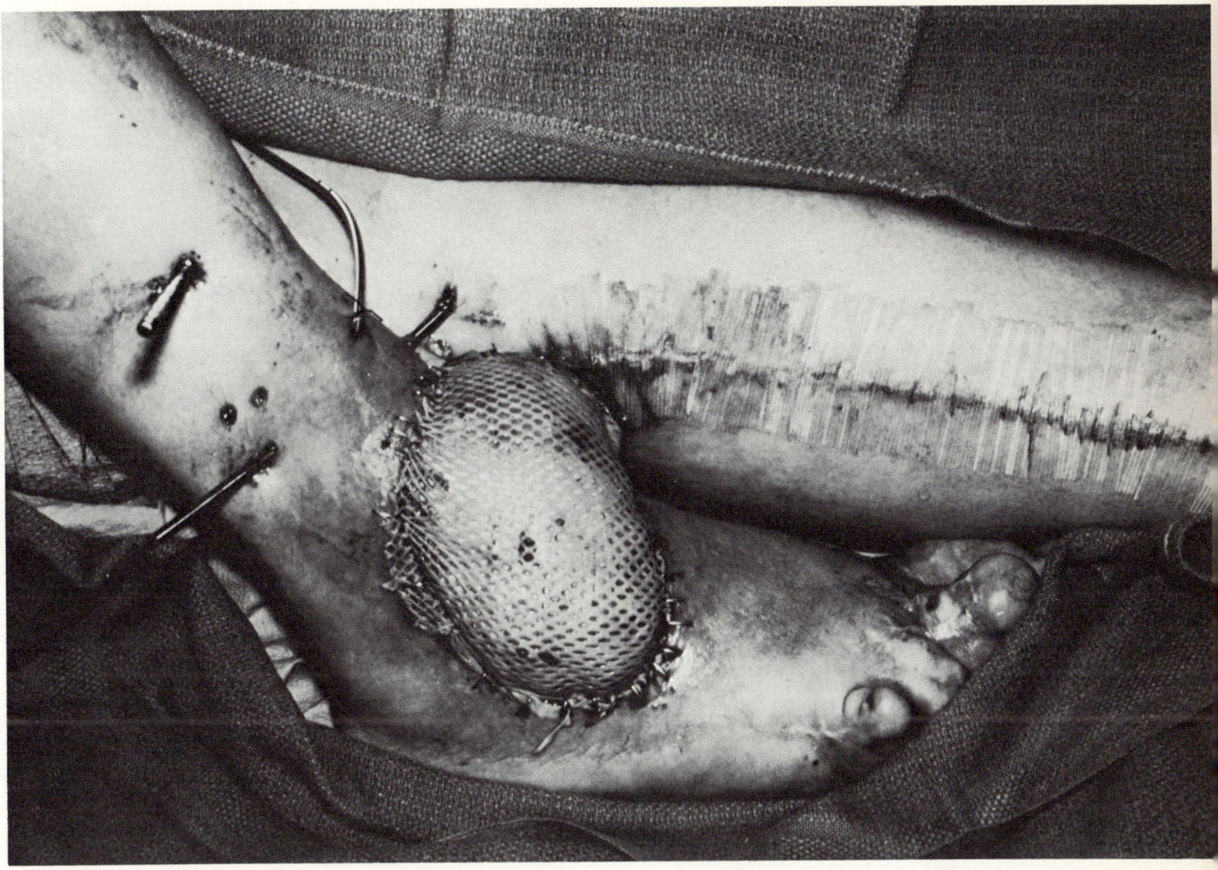

FIGURE 29-11 The ankle was pinned to the contralateral tibia and a cross-leg flap placed.

SUMMARY

It should be recognized that neither healing the ulcer by conservative measures nor doing any combination of surgical procedures will restore a postphlebitic leg to a normal state. After the ulcer has healed and active measures are no longer needed, the patient should continue to follow a regimen of care of the leg which has been learned during the course of healing of the ulcer. Luke in 1951 not only commented upon certain irrational operations being done at that time but also set up a group of instructions for care of the postphlebitic leg which he termed the "new way of life."[31] These instructions include proper use of external support, periods of elevation of the legs during the day, and proper foot care and hygiene. Considerable time should be spent in going over every detail of these continuing methods of care, to be certain that the patient understands how to live as well as possible with a damaged leg. The physician can teach and advise the patient, but in the final analysis the individual must learn to care for his or her own leg from day to day.

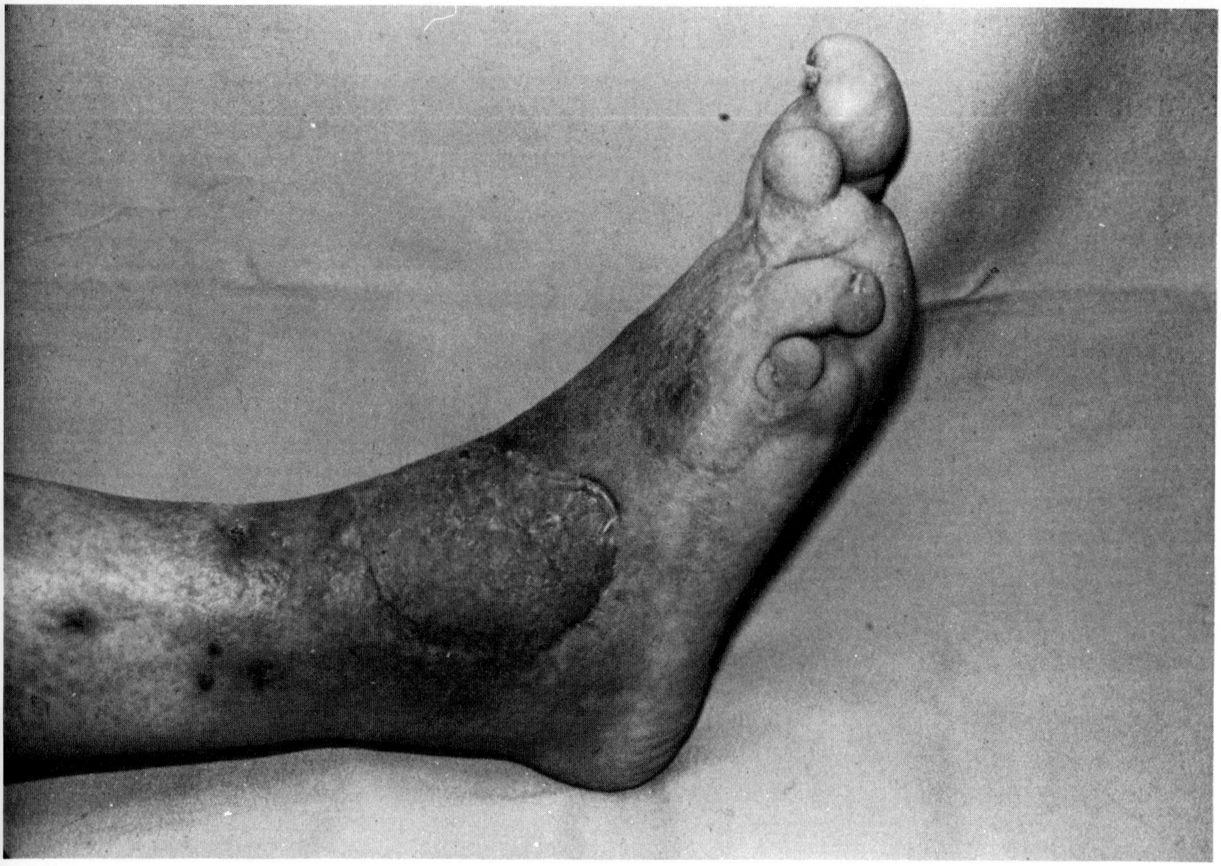

FIGURE 29-12 Three months later the cross-leg flap was detached and was completely healed. The patient was ambulatory and returned to work.

REFERENCES

1 Kitahama A, Elliott, LF, Kerstein MD, Menedez CV: Leg ulcer: Conservative management or surgical treatment? *JAMA* 1982, 247:197.
2 Dale WA: Managmeent of chronic leg ulcers. *J Tenn Med Assoc* 1960, 53:463.
3 Gay J: *On Varicose Diseases of the Lower Extremity.* The Lettosomian Lectures of 1867, Churchill, London.
4 Dale WA, Foster JH: Leg ulcers. *Trans South Surg Assoc* 1964, 75:399.
5 Cranley JJ, Krause RJ, Strasser ES: Chronic venous insufficiency of the lower extremity. *Surgery* 1961, 49:46.
6 Dodd H, Cockett FB: *The Pathology and Surgery of the Veins of the Lower Limb.* 2d ed. Churchill Livingston, New York, 1976.
7 DeCamp PT, Schramel, RJ, Ray CJ, Feibleman ND, Ward JA, Oschsner A: Ambulatory venous pressure determinations in postphlebitic and related syndromes. *Surgery* 1951, 29:44.
8 Moyer CA, Butcher HR: Stasis ulcers. *Ann Surg* 1955, 141:577.
9 Fontaine R: Remarks concerning venous thrombosis and its sequelae. *Surgery* 1957, 41:6.
10 Gius JA: Arteriovenous anastomoses and varicose veins. *Arch Surg* 1960, 81:299.
11 Kinmonth JB, Rob CG, Simeone FA: *Vascular Surgery.* Williams & Wilkins, Baltimore, 1963.
12 DeWeese JA, Rogoff SM: Functional ascending phlebography of the lower extremity by serial long film technique. *AJR* 1959, 81:841.

13 Scott HW, Roach JF: Phlebography of the leg in the erect position. *Ann Surg* 1951, 134:104.
14 Shumacker HB, Moore TC, Campbell JA: Functional venography of the lower extremities. *Surg Gynecol Obstet* 1954, 98:257.
15 Lewis MR, Dale WA: Phlebography as a clinical tool. *Surg Gynecol Obstet* 1971, 133:301.
16 Scott WMJ: Postphlebitic and varicose vein stasis. *Postgrad Med* 1953, 14:494.
17 Brush BE, Wylie JH, Benison J: Some devices for management of lymphedema of the extremities. *Surg Clin North Am* 1959, 39:1493.
18 Cranley JJ: Venous stasis (letters to the editors). *Surgery* 1975, 77:730.
19 Linton RR: The post-thrombotic ulceration of the lower extremity: Its etiology and surgical treatment. *Ann Surg* 1953, 138:415.
20 Linton RR: Discussion of Kwaan JHM, Jones RN, Connelly JE: Simplified technique for the management of refractory varicose ulcers. *Surgery* 1976, 80:746.
21 O'Donnell T: Discussion of Kwaan JHM, Jones RN, Connelly JE: Simplified technique for the management of refractory varicose ulcers. *Surgery* 1976, 80:746.
22 Field P, Van Boxel P: The role of the Linton flap procedure in the management of stasis dermatitis and ulceration in the lower limb. *Surgery* 1971, 70:920.
23 Burnard KG, O'Donnell TF, Thomas ML, Browse NL: The relative importance of incompetent communicating veins in the production of varicose veins and venous ulcers. *Surgery* 1977, 82:9.
24 Hyde GL, Litton LC, Hull DA: Long term results of subfascial vein ligation for venous stasis disease. *Surg Gynecol Obstet* 1981, 153:683.
25 Silver D, Gleysteen JJ, Rhodes GR, Georgiade NG, Anlyan WG: Surgical treatment of the refractory postphlebitic ulcer. *Arch Surg* 1971, 103:544.
26 Meyers TT: Discussion of Field P, Van Boxel P: The role of the Linton flap procedure in the management of stasis dermatitis and ulceration in the lower limb. *Surgery* 1971, 70:925.
27 Darling RC: Discussion of Field P, Van Boxel P: The role of the Linton flap procedure in the management of stasis dermatitis and ulceration in the lower limb. *Surgery* 1971, 70:925.
28 Wylie EJ: Discussion of Silver D, Gleysteen JJ, Rhodes GR, Georgiade NG, Anlyan WG: Surgical treatment of the refractory postphlebitic ulcer. *Arch Surg* 1971, 103:560.
29 Dale WA: The swollen leg. *Curr Probl Surg* Sept 1973.
30 Patman R: Sympathectomy in the treatment of chronic venous leg ulcers. *Arch Surg* 1982, 117:1561.
31 Luke, JC: The deep vein valves: A venographic study in normal and postphelebitic states. *Surgery* 1951, 29:381.

Invited Commentary

John J. Cranley, M.D.
Cincinnati, Ohio

In my experience, about 30 percent of ulcers of the leg are due to disease of primary varicose veins. This approximates the author's 25 percent. These ulcerations are curable, because after healing and removal of varicosities there will be a 94 percent cure. When ulceration is secondary to the postphlebitic syndrome, the ulcer is incurable but controllable.

The fundamental functional abnormality is ambulatory venous hypertension, which causes dilatation of the capillaries, leading to edema that permits some elements of the blood (proteins and red and white cells) to extravasate into the tissues. In some unknown way, the breakdown of these elements interferes with the normal physiology of the tissues and skin. Browse's suggestion seems the most plausible, namely, that layers of fibrin interfere with the transport of oxygen to the overlying epidermis and produce cellular death and venous ulceration.[1]

The first phase is swelling. Based on experience with 1300 patients with nonulcerative postphlebitic syndrome, 1800 others with ulceration, and another 4000 patients with deep venous thrombosis, I believe that the postphelbitic syndrome is entirely preventable if the swelling is controlled. This can be done in most cases by using a heavyweight elastic stocking, combined with elevation of the foot of the bed. A few patients describe varicosities or phlebitis; a greater number, however, recall a history of a fracture of the limb or great swelling following some illness. Recurrent ulcers are common. An experienced clinician can make the diagnosis quickly. The problem is a quantitative hydraulic deficit in the venous system (not in the lymphatics). Antimicrobial drugs are rarely needed. Infection in not the problem. Treatment of venous ulcers can be divided into two phases—the first, initial healing, and the second, prevention of recurrence. It is axiomatic that a venous ulcer will heal if the limb is maintained above heart level. There are no exceptions to the rule, although it may be impossible to elevate the limb of a patient with cardiac disease or advanced obliterative arterial disease.

Approximately 89 percent of patients treated in our office are healed while ambulatory. This can be accomplished in any patient who can walk normally and on whom a compressive type of bandage can be applied from the metatarsal heads to the tibial tubercles. My choice is Gelocast,[1] which in turn is covered by plain gauze and a 4-inch-wide elastic bandage. Hospitalization is reserved for patients who cannot walk normally or who must travel a long distance to the office, and on occasion it is necessary because of the foulness of the ulcer. After initial healing, the patient whose ulcer is due to primary varicosities is offered an elective operation, with the recommendation that it will probably make the limb feel better and may eliminate the need for an elastic stocking. Those who choose not to have the operation are advised to wear elastic stockings for life.

On the other hand, patients with a postphlebitic syndrome are advised that their condition is "incurable but generally controllable." They must wear a heavyweight elastic stocking for life whether or not an operation is performed. Approximately 80 percent of our postphlebitic patients are treated conservatively. Operation is recommended to those whose limbs fail to remain healed with heavyweight stockings and elevation of the foot of the bed. Thus, the patients treated surgically are preselected, so the results are better than the statistical report. Approximately 34 percent will have recurrent ulceration, often many years after the operation. This is frequently the result of not wearing the stocking or of wearing one that is worn out. The recurrent ulcer can usually be managed by applying a litt'e additional pressure. Sixty-six percent of the patients remain healed.

Skin Grafting

Skin grafting is a good operative procedure. A good result does depend on total excision of the scar tissue. We have performed 102 skin-grafting procedures, usually in combination with excision of the incompetent veins; 90 were done for deep venous disease. Relatively few grafts are performed on our service, because by far the greatest number of our patients are managed without hospitalization. The recurrent rate has been 35 percent after 30 years. This rate is very close to that following the Linton vein patch procedure, 35 percent versus 34 percent respectively.

Summary

The postphlebitic syndrome represents a quantitative hydraulic deficit. It is incurable but controllable by diligent and continuous conservative management. It is aided by surgical treatment in those cases that prove refractory to conservative measures.

The physician must accept the fact that there is a certain hard core of patients who can be treated only by repeated management of the limb over a period of years, the sole alternative being a life at bed rest. This group is composed of those patients who cannot walk, who live alone, or who cannot bend to wrap their limbs or put on elastic stockings because of severe arthritis, obesity, or fused hip or knee joints. Occasionally, a patient is too mentally incompetent to follow instructions. The physician must willingly accept these chronic "incurables" and treat them with patience and understanding.

COMMENTARY REFERENCE

1 Burnard KG, Whimster I, Naidoo A, Browse NL: Pericapillary fibrin in the ulcer-bearing skin of the leg: The cause of lipodermatosclerosis and venous ulceration. *Br Med J* 1982, 285:1071–1072.

30 ILIAC VEIN COMPRESSION SYNDROME

Among the causes of chronic edema of the lower extremity is an internal derangement of the left common iliac vein, whereby intraluminal scarring and the formation of webs and scars result from extrinsic pressure (Table 30-1). The clinical syndrome of edema of the thigh with associated discomfort and with collateralization of veins (Figure 30-1) has become well-recognized in Europe and Great Britain but has attracted little notice in North America.

It has been termed *venous spur, iliac vein compression, internal iliac adhesions, May-Thurner syndrome,* and *Cockett syndrome.* Let us consider a typical case.

ILLUSTRATIVE CASE

M.D., a 38-year-old female, presented with measurable left-thigh edema and discomfort both there and in the calf. A phlebogram showed narrowing of the left common iliac vein with cross-pelvic collateralization (Figure 30-2). At laparotomy the aorta and right iliac artery were elevated off the distal inferior vena cava and left common iliac vein, disclosing a whitish constricted area in the vein which, when opened, contained interior webs and scars. These were trimmed away, and the iliac vein was closed with a venous patch taken from the right forearm. A phlebogram 6 months postoperatively showed a patent repair. The patient was asymptomatic. She was last seen 8 years postoperatively in good condition.

ETIOLOGY

Adhesions within the common iliac vein were described in 1908 by McMurrich,[1] who reported such in 34 of 105 autopsies, with the suggestion that they were congenital. A later study by Erich and Krumbharr cast doubt upon this congenital theory, since only a few were found in infants among the 24 percent present in 412 autopsied bodies.[2]

Extrinsic pressure rather than a congenital lesion was further established by May and Thurner, who in 1957 reported cicatricial thickening and webs within the lumen of the left iliac vein in 22 percent of 430 autopsies.[3] They believed the changes resulted from the overlying crossing right iliac artery's repetitively pressing the underlying vein against the bony vertebra. They used the term *venous spur* because of the lession's similarity to the whirls of a river flowing past a bridge support.[4,5]

The lesion was later termed *iliac vein compression syndrome* by Cockett and Thomas in their discussion of 35 patients in 1965.[6] Ellis and del Rosario added four cases and the term *left iliac vein adhesions* in 1968.[7]

Extrinsic pressure by entrapment of the common iliac vein between the overlying artery and the underlying vertebra does now appear to be the cause of the intravenous lesions. Whether both sources of pressure are necessary or whether one may cause the problem is unknown. A recent personal case suggests that posterior pressure from the vertebra may be responsible for the problem. In that patient the bony vertebral eminence was at once related to the venous cicatrix. The crossing artery did not overlie the area at any point (Figures 30-3 to 30-6). This suggests that perhaps too much has been made of the arterial pressure and too little of that due to the underlying bone.

The inflammatory response evoked by an aortic aneurysm occasionally compresses the venous system. The aneurysm in Figure 30-7 appeared so relatively benign that the left iliac venous occlusion raised the question of an unrecognized tumor rather than pressure of the aneurysm, which later proved to be the case. Another rare cause is retroperitoneal fibrosis.

TABLE 30-1 CAUSES OF CHRONIC EDEMA OF THE LOWER LIMB

1 Venous
Postphlebitic syndrome
Extrinsic pressure from
A tumor
Retroperitoneal fibrosis
An overlying iliac artery
An underlying vertebra
Trauma (surgical ligation, plication or IVC filter)
An arteriovenous fistula
2 Lymphatic
Primary iliopathic lymphedema
Secondary causes
Infections
Tumors
Radiation
Bites
3 General causes of bilateral edema

DIAGNOSIS

Females predominate both in reported experiences and among my own cases (Table 30-2).[19] The lesion usually occurs in a relatively young or middle-age woman in good health who complains of slight to moderate edema with pain secondary to that. Severe edema is usually due to complete thrombosis of the iliac vein.

Phlebography Ascending phlebography by injection of radiopaque material into a foot or ankle vein may suggest the iliac venous lesion either by defects seen in the iliac vein itself or by collateralization of pelvic veins via crossover channels or ascending collaterals. This ascending technique is usually only suggestive because of lack of definition.

Direct injection into the femoral vein through a needle or catheter is a better radiographic technique. Various patterns of stenosis and occlusions have been described, notably by Weber.[8] The injection catheter may also be used to compare venous pressure superior and inferior to the site of compression.[9]

TREATMENT

The symptoms of some of these patients are minimal and require little if any treatment. Those whose swelling is more constant may benefit from external compression of the extremity by properly fitted elastic hose; a few lesions require surgical correction. The statement that "early operation is recommended . . . before sequelae ensue"[9] is an overreaction, since serious consequences have not occurred in most patients followed on a nonoperative basis. Only those who are incapacitated or are seriously troubled by their symptoms require operation.

Thus, a 9-year observation of a 9-year-old girl with phlebographically proven stenosis of the left common iliac vein has indicated that while external venous collateralization has increased, the appearance of the phlebogram has improved in terms of apparent stenosis as well as cross-pelvic collateralization. Her symptoms have continued to be minor.

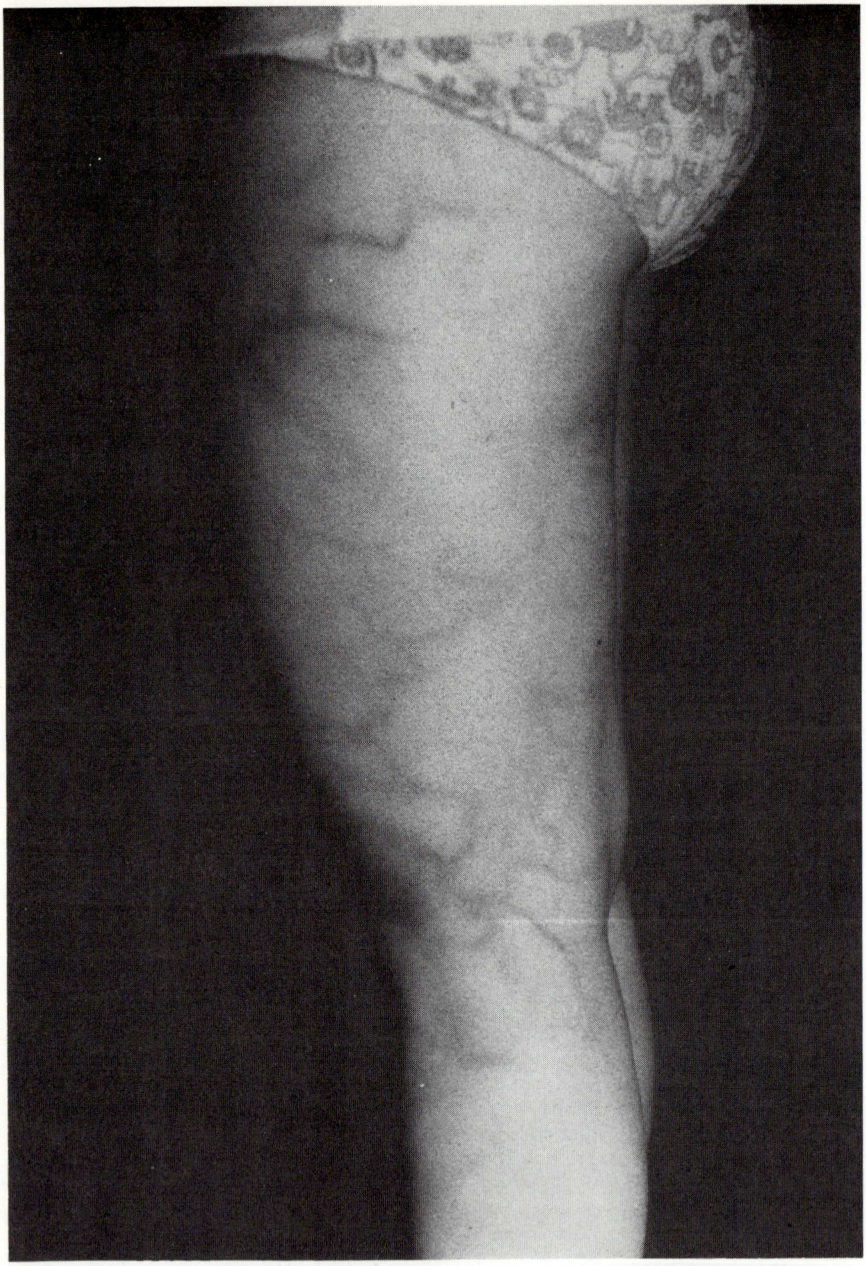

FIGURE 30-1 This infrared photograph demonstrates collateralization of veins in a 19-year-old woman with compression of the left iliac vein.

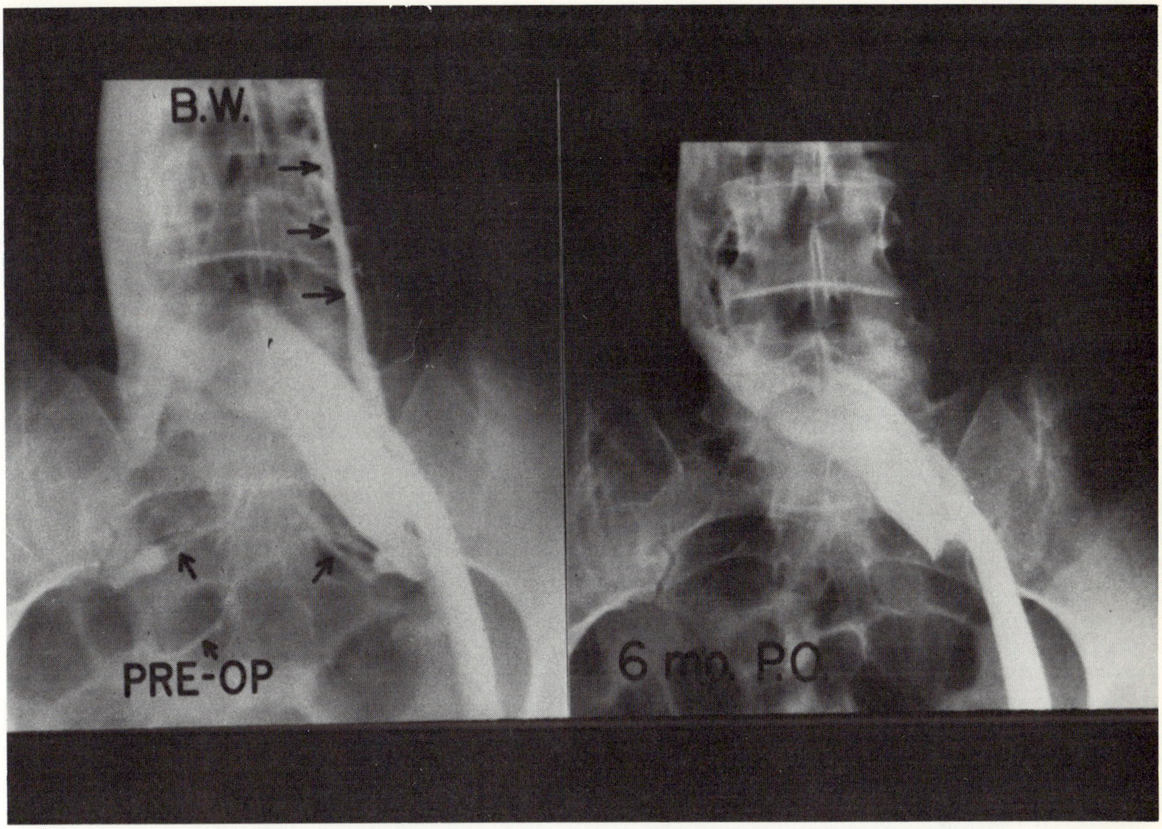

FIGURE 30-2 *Left,* collateralization at the *lower arrows* as well at the stenosis at the iliocaval venous junction shows the preoperative phlebographic situation. *Right,* 6 months postoperatively the venous collateralization has disappeared and the opaque material opacifies the wide iliac lumen.

OPERATION

Should surgical relief be required it may be sought via a *femorofemoral bypass* using a cross-pelvis transplanted saphenous vein (as described in Chapter 31). This indirect approach recommends itself for the occasional male patient,[10] in whom retroperitoneal dissection at the level of the aortic bifurcation may cause sexual problems. Thus the 18-year-old male in Table 30-2 and Figure 30-8 had this operation. The crossover vein graft is a considerably less hazardous procedure than is a laparotomy and direct venous repair, with less morbidity and more rapid convalescence.

As yet there has been no personal experience, but a more direct *bypass from the external iliac vein to the inferior vena cava* may also be considered, especially in light of our recent favorable experiences with polytetrafluorethylene (PTFE) grafts for vena cava reconstructions[11] (Chapter 31) and the successful iliac-to-cava Dacron graft reported by Jacob and his associates in 1980.[12]

Traditionally, the direct approach of a laparotomy with *venotomy and patch vein grafting* has been used (Figure 30-9). This should not only relieve the stenosis by appropriate excision of webs and scars but also allow an expanded lumen at the time of closure. A small vein patch serves this purpose. It should be removed from the hand, arm, or ankle in order to leave the main saphenous vein intact. Figures 30-4 to 30-6 illustrate this.

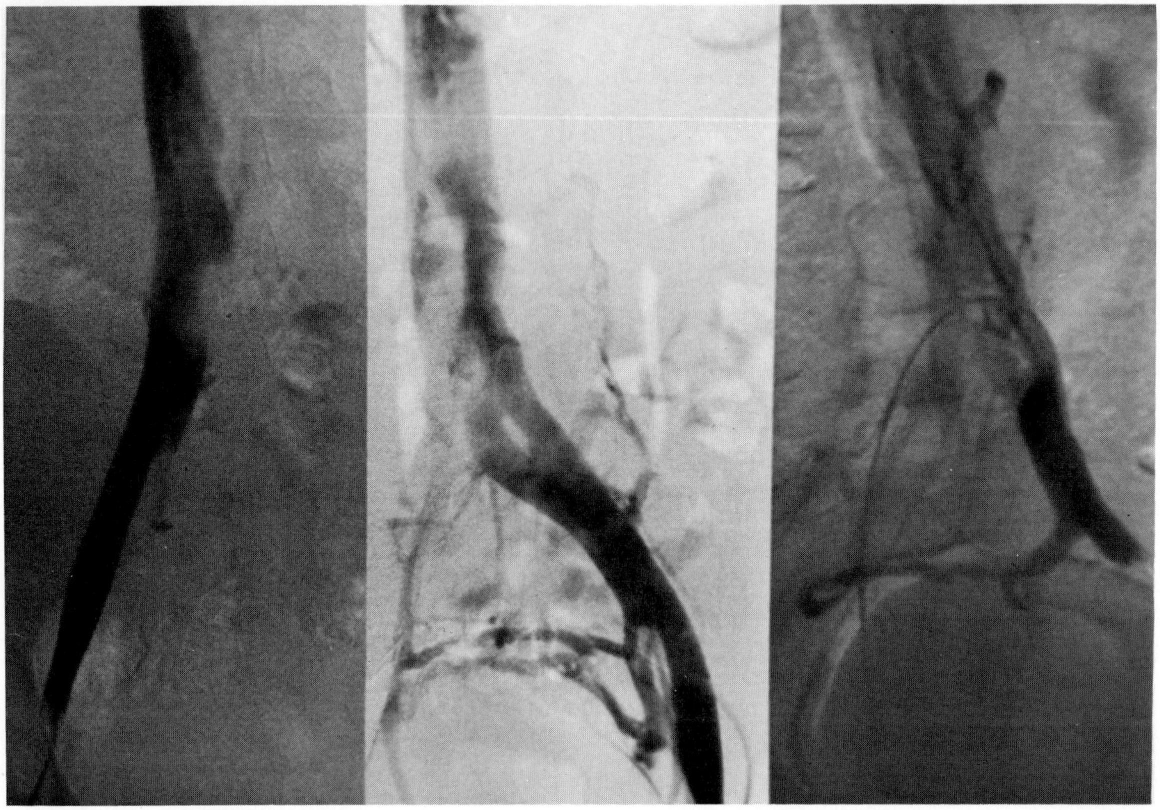

FIGURE 30-3 *Left,* the normally patent right common iliac vein flows into the patent inferior vena cava with a defect at their junction suggested by the inflow of nonopacified blood. *Center,* the collateralization of the left iliac venous system is apparent, along with the defect in the iliac vein which ultimately proved to be due to complete obliteration of the central portion of the lumen by scarring at that point. *Right,* a catheter passed through the right iliac vein across the bifurcation into the left again demonstrates the iliac venous stenosis on that side.

An unresolved problem is relief of the cause of the extrinsic pressure which originates the problem. This has been attempted by placement of a sling of fascia to pull the artery away[12] or a plastic bridge to lift it off the vein.[5] Neither of these is really attractive, because of the undesirable long-term effects of pressure upon an artery.

Lengthening the iliac artery by inserting a short plastic graft is feasible, yet the long-term effects of a synthetic tube placed in a young woman with 40 to 50 years to live are dubious.

Another tactic suggested by Dick[14] but as yet untried personally is to remove bone from the point of posterior pressure. This deserves further trial.

Another method of relieving the pressure of the overlying iliac artery is transposition of the common iliac artery to the side of the contralateral hypogastric artery. Cormier has reported successful use of this technique for iliac venous compression syndrome as well as trauma problems.[15]

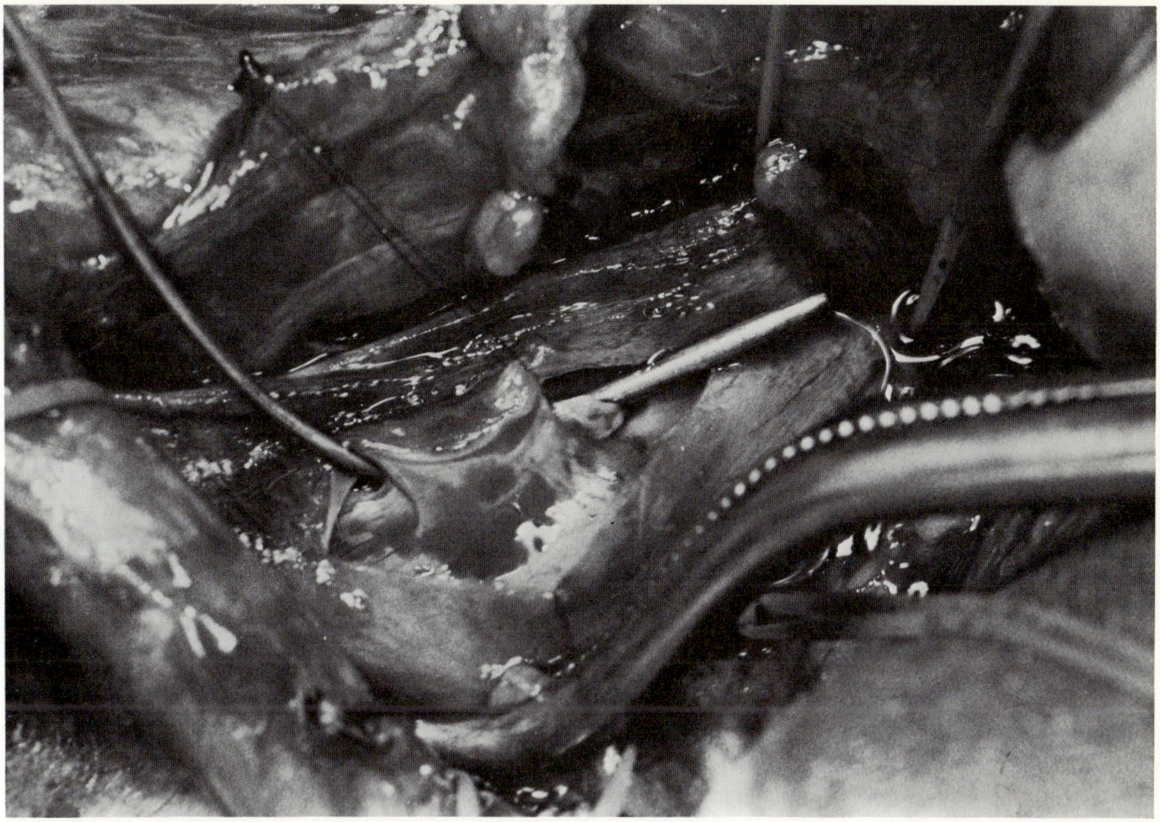

FIGURE 30-4 The operative view of the opened left common iliac vein with a probe passed behind the central cicatrix.

TABLE 30-2 ILIAC VEIN COMPRESSION SYNDROME

Patient	Age/sex	Procedure	Follow-up
K.D.	9/F	No operation	9 yr—improved
S.S.	43/F	No operation	4 mo—no change
H.W.	46/F	No operation	NA*
B.R.	38/F	Patch venoplasty	13 yr—relief
M.D.	38/F	Patch venoplasty	8 yr—relief
B.W.	37/F	Patch venoplasty	Persistent edema
R.S.	43/F	Patch venoplasty	Failure
W.D.	43/F	Previous vein decompression, no new treatment	None
E.W.	18/M	Saphenous crossover graft	No patency, no change

*Not available.

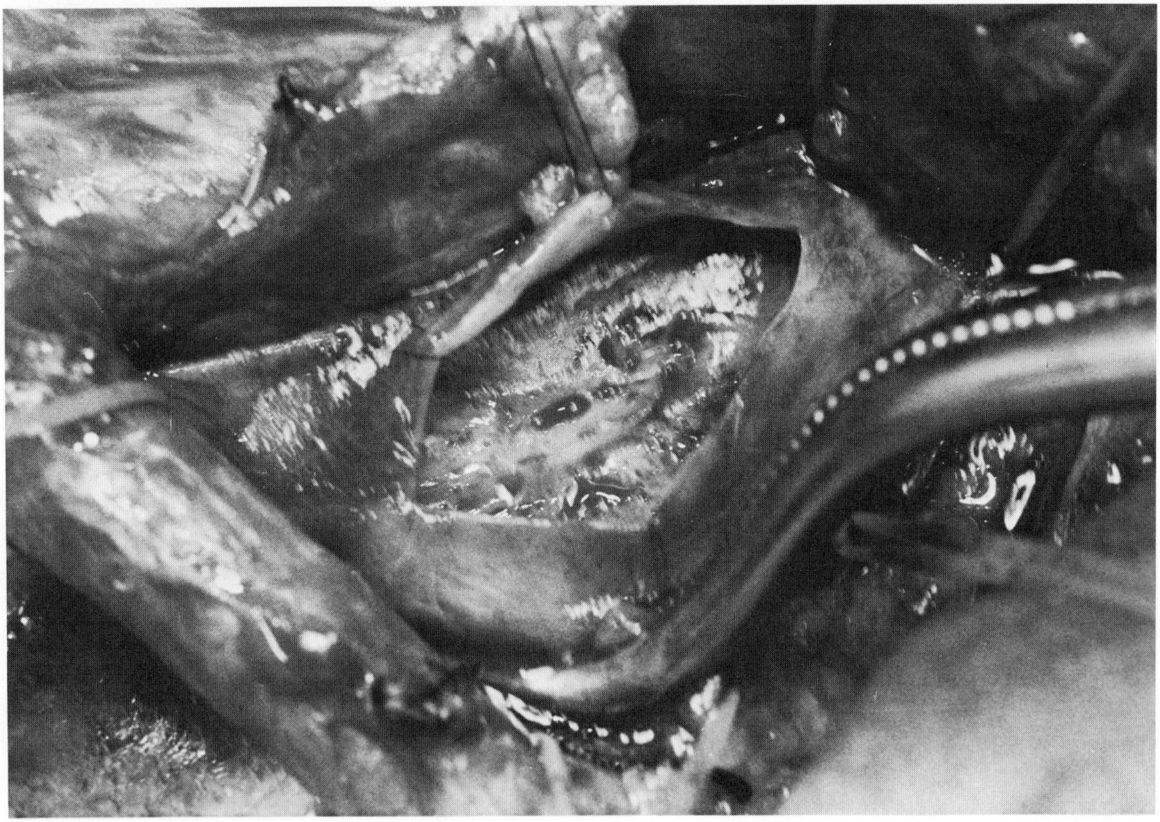

FIGURE 30-5 The internal cicatrix and webs have been trimmed out of the opened left common iliac vein, leaving an irregular posterior intimal surface. At *left* appears the aortic bifurcation and iliac arteries with a tape placed about the right.

SUMMARY

It is safe to say that the diagnosis of iliac venous compression syndrome will become more frequent as knowledge of it spreads and as definitive phlebograms are performed for edema of the lower extremity. The few operative experiences recorded to date (Table 30-3) allow no definite recommendations for surgical therapy. Each patient's care must be individualized.

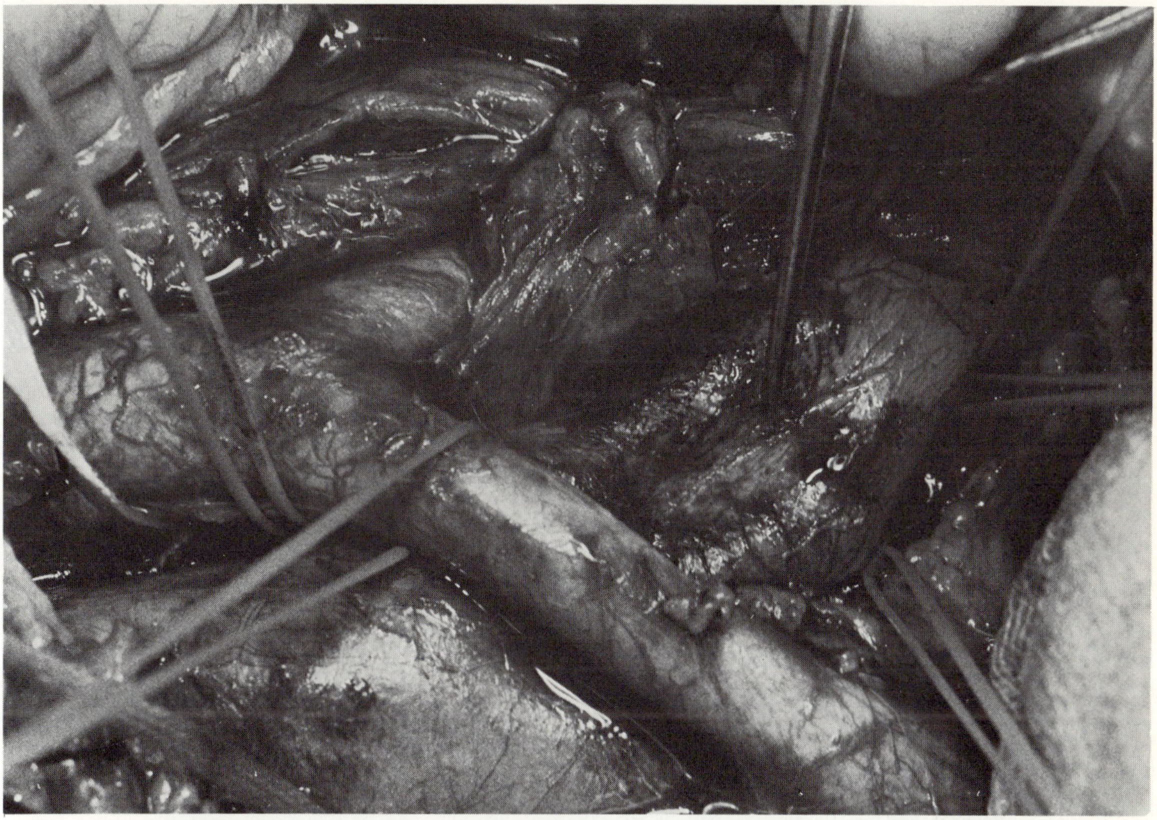

FIGURE 30-6 Forceps point to the patch graft used to enlarge the lumen of the left common iliac vein. The crossing right common iliac artery clearly does not overlie the point of obstruction, which overrode a bony spur of the vertebral body underneath.

TABLE 30-3 RESULTS OF TREATMENT OF ILIAC VEIN COMPRESSION

Author	Year	Procedure	No. done	No. improved
Cockett[5]	1965	Decompression alone	17	13
		Venoplasty	13	12
Connett[16]	1974	Decompression alone	3	3
Rigas, Vomvoyannis, Tsardakas[13]	1970	Venoplasty and fascial sling	8	8
Smith, Trimble[9]	1977	Venoplasty and Silastic bridge	14	11
Ferris, Lim, Smith, Casali[17]	1983	Venoplasty	2	2
Welter, Becker[18]	1980	Rectus sling	4	0
Dale (this text)	1985	Venoplasty and patch	4	2
		Saphenous crossover	1	0

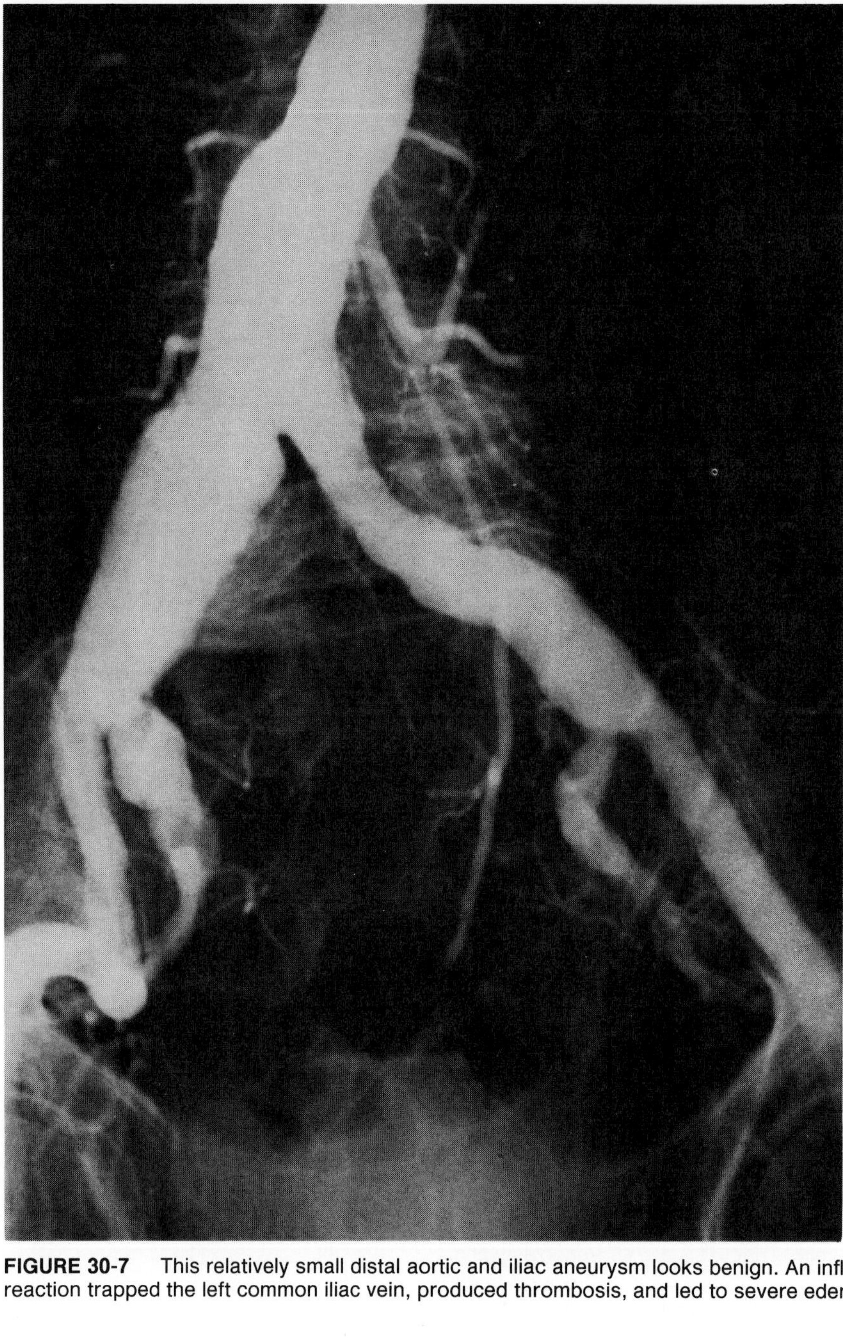

FIGURE 30-7 This relatively small distal aortic and iliac aneurysm looks benign. An inflammatory reaction trapped the left common iliac vein, produced thrombosis, and led to severe edema and pain.

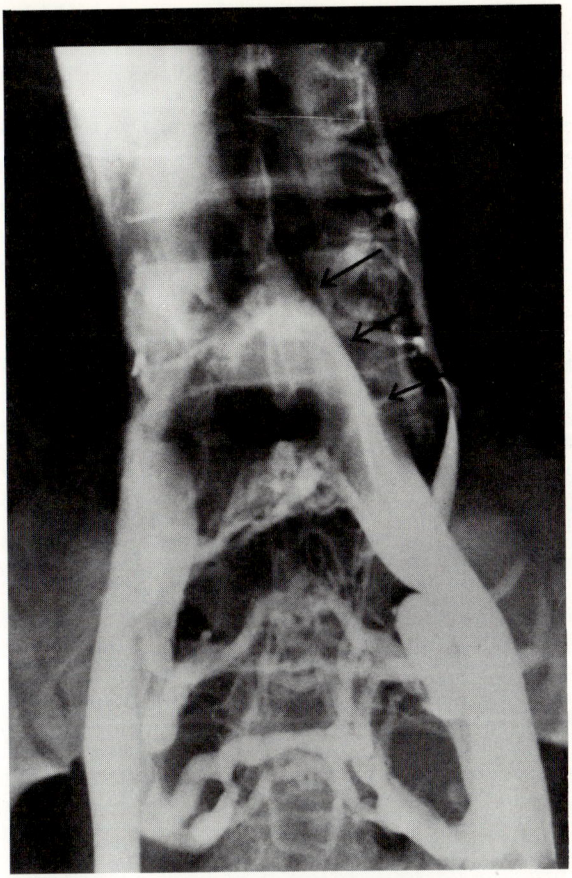

FIGURE 30-8 An 18-year-old male with compression of the left common iliac vein. Laparotomy was performed to rule out tumor, but aortic dissection and elevation were avoided to prevent sexual dysfunction. A crossover vein graft was done.

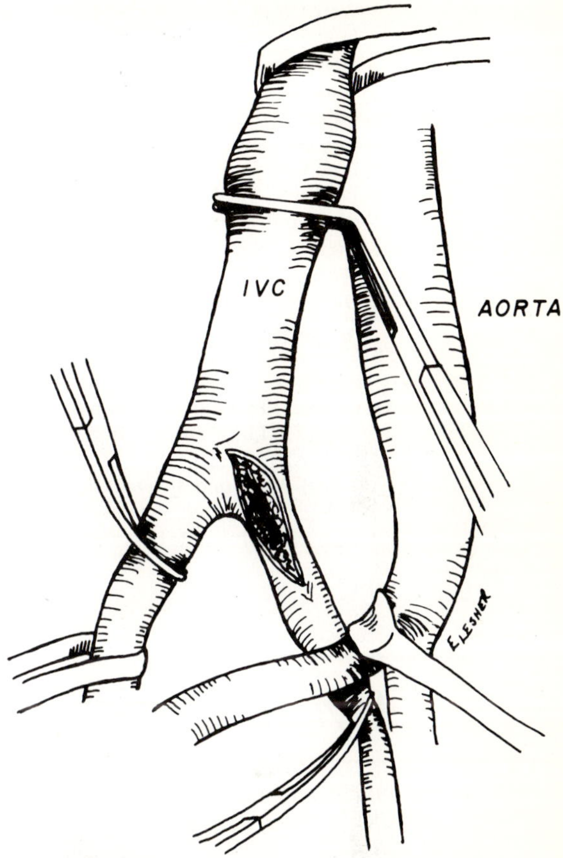

FIGURE 30-9 After elevation of the crossing right common iliac artery, the underlying left common iliac vein is opened and interior webs and bands removed. The venotomy is closed with a venous patch graft.

REFERENCES

1 McMurrich JP: The occurrence of congenital adhesions in the common iliac veins and their relation to thrombosis of the femoral iliac veins. *Am J Med Sci* 1908, 135:342.
2 Erich WE, Krumbhaar EB: A frequent obstructive anomaly of the mouth of the left common iliac vein. *Am Heart J* 1943, 26:737.
3 May R, Thurner J: The cause of the predominately sinistral occurrence of thrombosis of the pelvic veins. *Angiology* 1957, 8:419.
4 May R, Thurner J: in May R, Weber J (eds): *Pelvic and Abdominal Veins: Progress in Diagnostics and Therapy.* International Congress Series 550. Excerpta Medica, Amsterdam, 1981, p 119.
5 May R: in May R, Weber J (eds): *Pelvic and Abdominal Veins: Progress in Diagnostics and Therapy.* International Congress Series 550. Excerpta Medica, Amsterdam, 1981, p 115.
6 Cockett B, Thomas ML: The iliac compression syndrome. *Br J Surg* 1965, 51:816.
7 Ellis PR Jr, del Rosario VC: Left iliac vein "adhesions," *Surgery* 1968, 63:166.

8 Weber J: in May R, Weber J (eds): *Pelvic and Abdominal Veins: Progress in Diagnostics and Therapy.* International Congress Series 550. Excerpta Medica, Amsterdam, 1981, p 135.

9 Smith DE, Trimble C: Surgical management of obstructive venous disease of the lower extremity, in Rutherford R (ed): *Vascular Surgery.* Saunders, Philadelphia, 1977, p 1259.

10 Miller IW, Eickhoff JH, Hansen HJ, Lindewald H: The iliac vein compression syndrome: A case report with a review of the literature. *Acta Chir Scand,* 1980, 502:141.

11 Dale WA, Harris J, Terry RB: PTFE reconstruction of inferior vena cava. *Surgery* 1984, 95:625.

12 Jacob ET, Bar-Nathan N, Heim M, Moras B, Rubistein Z: The iliac vein compression syndrome and lower limb vascular access for hemodialysis. *J Cardiovasc Surg* (Torino) 1980, 21:155.

13 Rigas A, Vomvoyannis A, Tsardakas E: Iliac compression: Report of ten cases. *J Cardiovasc Surg* (Torino) 1970, 11:389.

14 Dick W: Dlinik und Therapie der Venensperre am Confluens der beiden gemeinsamen Iliacaclavene. *Langenbeck's Arch Chir* 1962, 301:573.

15 Cormier JM: Transposition of the common iliac artery onto the contralateral hypogastric artery [Author's transl]. *Nouv Presse Med* 1980, 29:2015.

16 Connett FB: An anatomical basis for unilateral leg edema in adolescent girls. *West J Med* 1974, 121:324.

17 Ferris EJ, Lim, WN, Smith PL, Casali R: May-Thurner syndrome. *Radiology* 1983, 147:29.

18 Welter HF, Becker HM: Therapy of the pelvic venous spur in postoperative follow-up, in May R, Weber J (eds): *Pelvic and Abdominal Veins: Progress in Diagnostics and Therapy.* International Congress Series 550. Excerpta Medica, Amsterdam, 1981, p 171.

19 Dale WA, Allen TR: Unusual problems of venous thrombosis. *Surgery,* 1975, 78:707.

Invited Commentary

Robert W. Hobson II, M.D.
Newark, New Jersey

This chapter summarizes clearly the essential features of the iliac vein compression syndrome. Of perhaps greater importance, it clarifies the multiple terms used to describe the clinical syndrome of thigh edema associated with discomfort and collateralization of the superficial venous system. I suspect that its lack of recognition in this country may be related to the beneficial response to venous support hose and the tendency to avoid phlebography in patients experiencing a favorable response to conservative therapy. In those patients who, due to persistence of lower extremity edema, are ultimately diagnosed, I agree that a direct exploration of the iliac vein, excision of the web or scar as necessary, and vein patch angioplasty will produce the best results. My experience consists of two cases. In both, patients were managed in this manner and improvement was observed.

A more liberal use of phlebography is appropriate in efforts to identify patients with iliac vein compression syndrome. The natural history of the disease may thereby be better defined. Conservative management is satisfactory in the majority of these patients. Direct surgical intervention should be reserved for those with more severe symptomatology. Using this diagnostic and theraputic plan, excellent clinical results may be anticipated.

31 PERIPHERAL VENOUS RECONSTRUCTION

Reconstruction of the peripheral venous system has lagged far behind arterial revascularization, not only because of lack of understanding of the pathologic physiology involved but also because of poor results and the general disinterest evoked by them.

Inability to produce deep venous thrombosis experimentally has seriously limited investigation of the basic pathologic physiology, to the extent that current concepts are generally based upon clinical observations of the disease and its response to a variety of measures aimed at altering its natural course; recognizably, these changes are quite variable. The general uncertainty has been further confused by lack of accurate diagnostic methods, to which may be added a widespread apathy toward a process which, while disabling, is not often lethal or dramatic enough to create an emotional response.

In every area of vascular surgery, the animal experiments of Carrel and Guthrie form a background; 75 years ago they investigated grafts in the venous system. It is not likely that the Parisian surgeon Doyen knew of these studies when he successfully used the jugular vein of a sheep to replace a human vein in 1909, with known patency for 6 months.[1] In any event, it was a quantum leap, which went unnoticed and unrepeated.

After a long hiatus, isolated reports of successful venous repairs in humans began to appear in the 1950s. Thus, Kunlin[2] in 1952 reported success with a saphenous vein used to bypass an obstructed iliac vein, and Warren and Thayer in 1954[3] described saphenopopliteal bypass for the postphlebitic limb. Hardin,[4] Cerino and associates,[5] and Kenawai[6] in the 1960s added their experiences.

My interest in this field began in the late 1950s and led to the 1963 report of results in over 100 animals and several humans, along with an attempt to formulate general principles in this area of surgery.[7]

Palma's success[8] in crossover saphenous-to-femoral vein bypasses in Montevideo, Uruguay, came to my attention in 1960 and led to a series of animal experiments that indicated probable success in humans; this was reported in 1968.[9]

From these investigations evolved the conclusions that (1) properly constructed venous anastomoses and grafts remain patent for long periods, (2) a refined, delicate surgical technique is mandatory, (3) an autogenous graft is quite superior to a prosthetic, and (4) venous graft patency is affected more by internal pressure and flow than by external pressure.[9] Recently the last conclusion has become doubtful.[10]

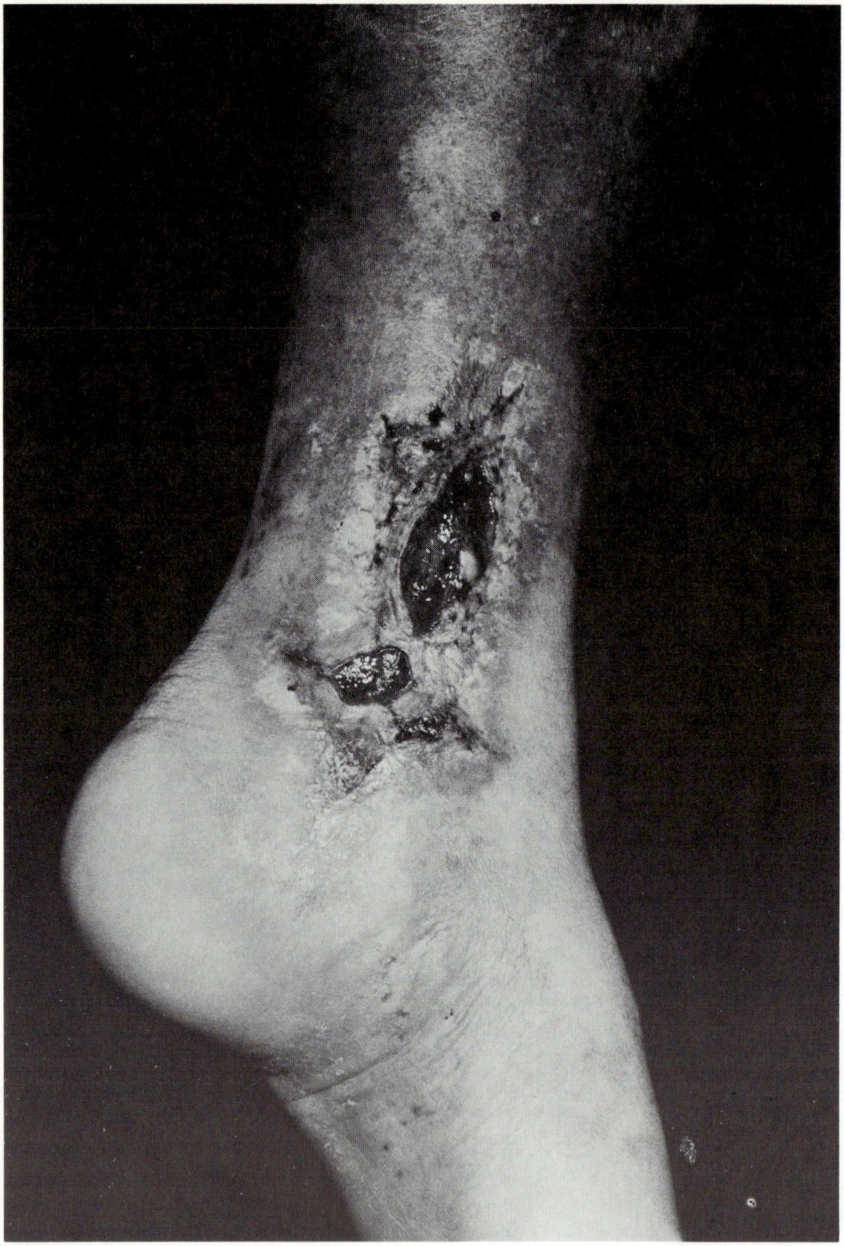

FIGURE 31-1 Typical chronic ulcer of the ankle due to the postphlebitic syndrome with iliac venous occlusion.

DIAGNOSIS

Currently there are recognized two states of altered venous function; first, postphlebitic obstruction, and second, venous reflux due to valvular dysfunction. Diagnostic measures are designed to detect and differentiate these.

Clinical Syndrome

Edema, secondary varicose veins, skin pigmentation, ulcers, and pain are all due to venous obstruction and valvular dysfunction of one or another sort (Figure 31-1). Most are postphlebitic in origin, a few are congential, and some are due to occluding tumors or to injury.

Whether venous reflux due to valve failure alone explains the pain and swelling of some patients remains to be determined. Raju believes it does,[11] yet previous attempts to explain all the symptoms by one lesion have failed. Thus the perforator operation alone has been little better than ligation and stripping or venous ligation. It is likely that the syndrome is associated with a number of defects: valvular, perforator, and muscular weakness.

Noninvasive Studies

Experience has not yet fully delineated the virtues and disadvantages of the various noninvasive tests which are suggested by many authors as well as the advertisements of manufacturers, each of whom claims the most critical aid to clinical diagnosis and the most efficient and least expensive way to replace phlebography. Many of the tests find their chief use as scouting procedures. Phlebography of one type or another remains the "gold standard." Further description and the controversy concerning noninvasive techniques will be left to their advocates.

Venous Pressure Studies

Nicolaides's group in 1982 discussed the prognostic and therapeutic implications of ambulatory venous pressure assessments in 124 limbs.[12] Their results follow the classic diagram (Figure 31-2) of the effect of walking, which normally reduces the superficial venous pressure, while intact valves in the perforating communicating veins do not permit the high back pressure of the deep venous system to be transmitted. When valvular insufficiency exists, whatever its cause, there is failure of this reduction during walking and the occurrence of ambulatory venous hypertension (AVH).

A simple, inexpensive method of studying the superficial venous pressure may be done at the time of phlebography (Figure 31-3). A long segment of sterile tubing is supported upright beside the standing patient, attached by a three-way stopcock to the needle in the ankle vein. Heparinized saline is allowed to flow until the pressure head is determined (at the atrial level). The patient then walks in place, and the diminution in venous pressure is noted. A typical study recently showed the results in Table 31-1. The normal decrease of 81 cm during walking contrasts sharply with the 5-cm fall in the postphlebitic limb, which denotes

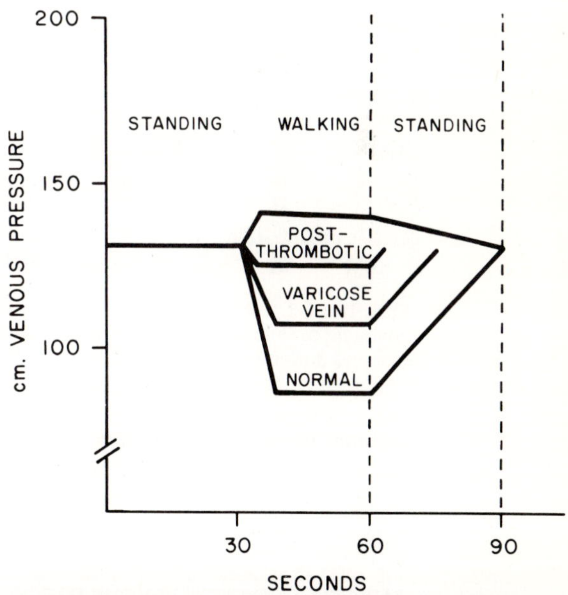

FIGURE 31-2 Superficial venous pressure measured through an indwelling needle in the saphenous vein or a foot vein normally demonstrates considerable diminution during walking. If the deep venous system is obstructed due to the postphlebitic syndrome, the pressure decreases very little or occasionally rises slighty. Varicose vein patients fall in between.

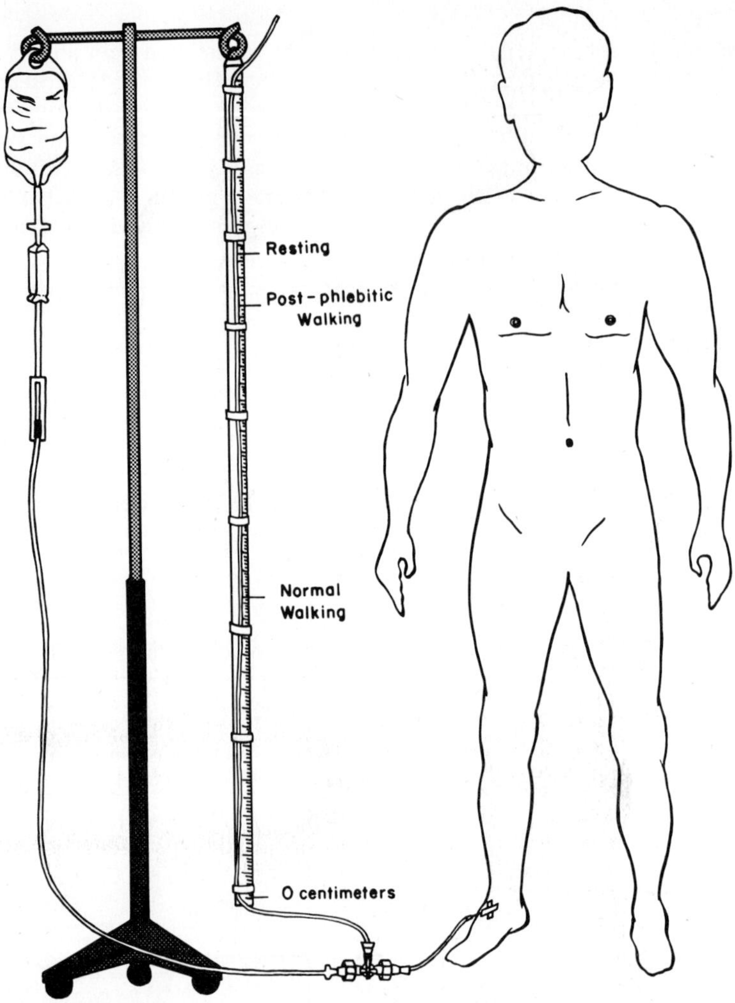

FIGURE 31-3 A no. 19 needle is placed in a foot or ankle vein to allow a three-way manometer connection. Pressure within the superficial venous system may thus be measured while the patient is at rest and during and after exercise.

ambulatory venous hypertension. This simple test can be extended by a studying of the time for return of the pressure to the prewalking level, but that adds little critical information.

This test can easily be made complex and expensive by use of transducers, computer printouts, and trained technicians to report the results.

TABLE 31-1 TYPICAL VENOUS PRESSURES

	Pressure standing, cm	Pressure walking, cm
Postphlebitic limb	114	109
Normal limb	109	28

Phlebography

Angiography of the venous system is considerably older than generally realized, extending back into the 1930s. That early experience failed because of toxicity of the available radiopaque materials and poor techniques of visualization. Those early efforts were largely abandoned until standardization began to emerge in the 1950s.

Presently a relatively large amount (60 mL to as much as 120 mL) of relatively nontoxic radiopaque material is slowly injected into a vein of the foot or ankle through a small indwelling needle while the patient rests in the 45° semiupright position (Figure 31-4). Whether the patient bears weight on the leg or not is not important. A tourniquet placed just above the ankle forces the injected material into the deep venous system. It also allows the superficial system to be well visualized through perforating communicating veins. If the tourniquet is omitted, the distal portion of the deep system may not be seen, which may lead to an erroneous diagnosis of its absence. The addition of films made after the patient exercises by heel lifts, to force the material proximally allows better visualization of the thigh and pelvic veins. Even so, the iliac venous system is so often poorly defined so that an additional examination is necessary. This is easily accom-

FIGURE 31-4 Techniques of phlebography. (*a*) The patient reclines in a 45° position. The no. 21 needle is placed in a foot vein or the saphenous vein, with a venous tourniquet proximal to this. (*b*) The iliac venous system is better visualized by injection of 60 mL of the contrast material, with a very tight tourniquet placed at *X* to prevent passage of the material proximally. The less tightly applied tourniquet at *Y* helps force the material into the deep venous system. After 60 mL is placed, the *X* tourniquet is suddenly removed and the leg elevated just prior to exposure of the film. (*c*) Iliac and vena caval opacification may be obtained by placement of a needle or a catheter into the common femoral vein in the groin. Descending phlebography is performed by the same technique, but with the patient elevated to the standing position after placement of the catheter. (*Reprinted courtesy Surg Gyn Obstet 1971, 133:301.*)

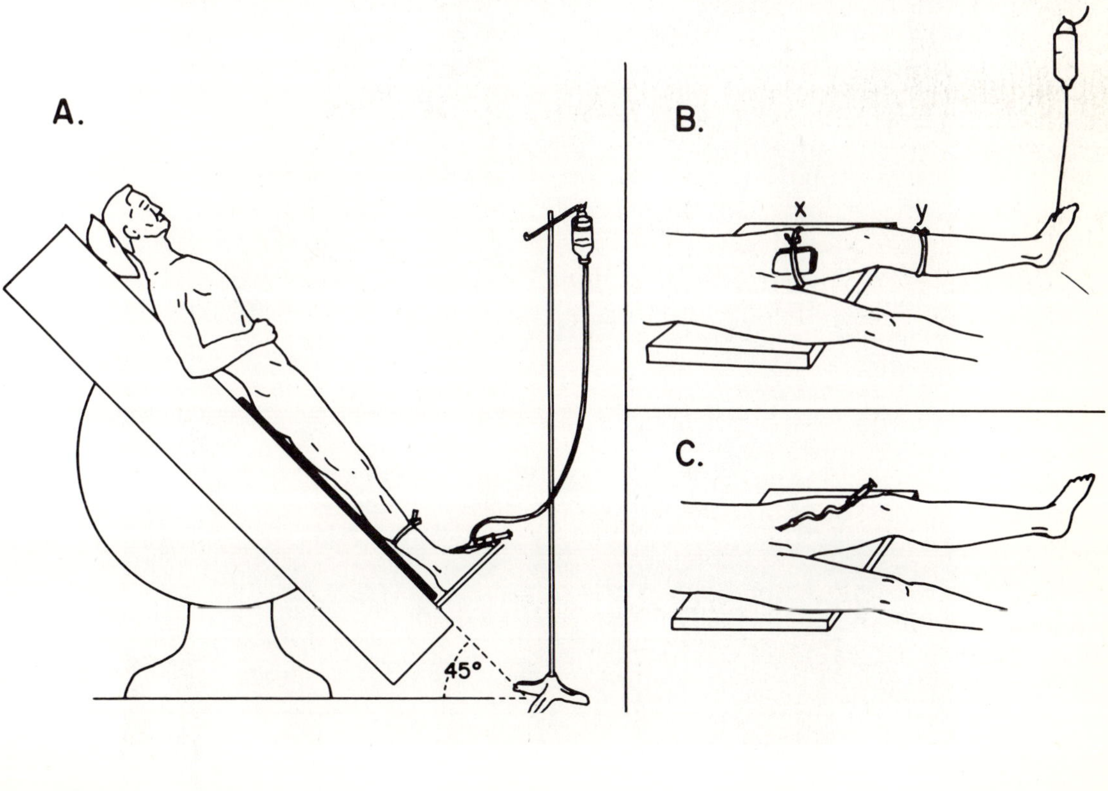

plished by injection of 60 mL of radiopaque material distal to a tight thigh tourniquet so that it pools until sudden release of the tourniquet allows flow into the iliac veins and the inferior vena cava. This flow is aided by recumbency of the patient during this particular examination (Figure 31-5).

FIGURE 31-5 This phlebogram showing a patent crossover vein graft 6 months after operation was obtained by injection of radiopaque material into the saphenous vein and subsequent elevation of the extremity.

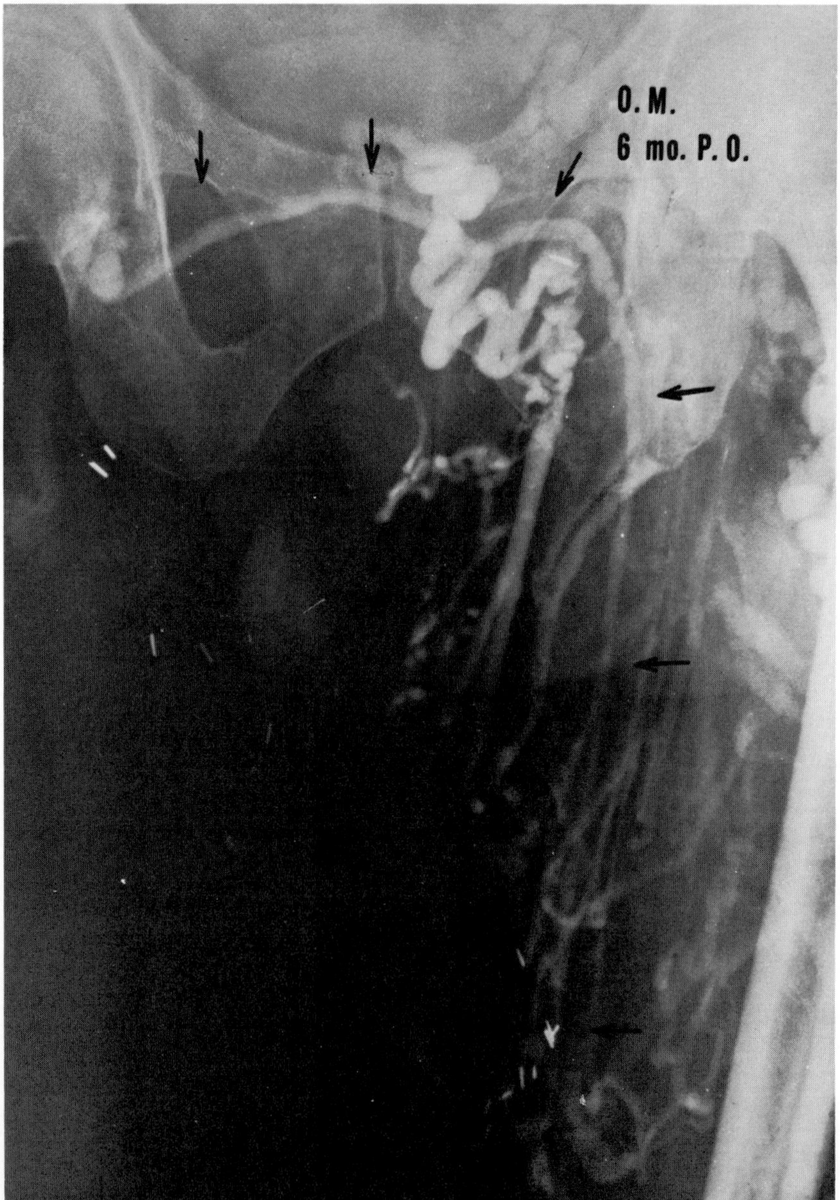

Descending phlebography is performed via a catheter passed from an arm vein through the heart into the inferior vena cava or, more simply, by placement of a catheter directed proximally into the common femoral vein for visualization of the iliac and caval system. Following this, the patient is changed to an upright position and a slow injection is made to determine whether there is reflux of the material through the valvular system of the femoral veins distally.

The radiologic literature contains references to postphlebogram thrombosis in the venous system due to the irritating radiopaque material. Some of my patients have also complained of the pain associated with phlebograms done elsewhere. Both of these problems can be eliminated by injection of 5000 U.S.P. units of aqueous heparin prior to the phlebogram and thereafter by injection of the radiopaque material slowly over a period of 60 to 120 seconds. The rapid injection required in arteriography is not needed in the venous system, where the material will pool quietly until the patient begins to exercise. Apparently, this is not recognized by a number of physicians, who make forcible injections. Our retrospective analysis of 200 patients showed only 1 who developed clinical evidence of venous thrombosis after a phlebogram.[14] Phlebography is safe and painless when done properly.

The commonly performed ascending phlebography provides information concerning patency of the veins and the anatomic state of the venous valves, along with their number. The less commonly performed descending phlebography provides further functional information. Kistner's proposal that all retrograde flow is abnormal and that such can be categorized into four grades dependent upon how far distally the material flows[15] is arbitrary and unworkable. Normally there is some reflux as the material drifts distally through the valve cusps, which are not forced together unless there be proximal pressure (by the Valsalva maneuver or walking). We term the examination *normal* or *abnormal* without an attempt to specify *how* abnormal it is. The Bergan group raised serious objections to the valvular reflux theory when they found "reflux to the ankle level in the apparently normal, asymptomatic opposite leg."[16] Raju has also noted reflux in normal asymptomatic volunteers.[11] The significance of reflux is therefore not clear.

MANAGEMENT PROGRAM

The studies outlined in Table 31-2 are designed to determine the cause of the venous obstruction and to delineate its extent. Recently the computerized tomography (CT) scan has become important in finding small tumors (lymphomas or metastases) which previously required an operative exploration.

The etiology and anatomic distribution of the lesion must be well understood before a rational plan of management is begun.

INDICATIONS

In obstructive disease impeded egress of blood from the lower extremity due to occlusion of the iliac or common femoral vein results in collateralization of venous flow across the pelvis to the contralateral iliac venous drainage system. If any part of the femoral or saphenous venous system in the groin or thigh is patent, it is feasible to cross the contralateral saphenous vein over to it, attach it to this open portion, and thereby decompress the extremity.

Occlusion of the venous system by tumor furnishes an excellent indication

TABLE 31-2 PLAN OF MANAGEMENT OF THE POST-PHLEBITIC SYNDROME

1 Diagnosis: tumor or phlebitis?
- Examination, including pelvis and rectum
- Visceral x-rays, intravenous pyelogram, barium enema, CT scan
- Cystocopy, sigmoidoscopy
- Exploration

2 Delineation of venous block by phlebography
- Site and extent
- Contralateral patency

3 Treatment: crossover vein graft for
- Stable, nonrecanalizing venous thrombosis
- The tumor patient who has a life expectancy of 6 months

for a crossover graft, whose results are particularly gratifying. Postphlebitic obstruction is more common; an occasional indication is a posttraumatic or an iatrogenic occlusion.

An extension of this principle is the saphenous-to-popliteal venous anastomosis to bypass femoral occlusion.

The indications for surgical correction of pure reflux problems are not well understood at present. They are discussed below.

SURGICAL PROCEDURES

A variety of operations have been advocated, often based more on hope than rationale. Fortunately for the patient (and the semiscientist), the adjunctive measures which accompany an operative procedure for the postphlebitic syndrome usually improve the situation, whether or not the procedure "works." If the limb is elevated, pressure applied, and the rudiments of hygiene followed, there will be improvement.

The improvement due to ancillary treatments obscures the results of any operation to correct the problem so much that proof of a procedure is dependent upon later phlebographic evidence of success and, of even more importance, improvement of symptoms to the extent that external elastic support is no longer necessary. Anything less than relief without a stocking must be viewed with suspicion. Let us examine the several available procedures in the light of these remarks.

Varicose Vein Operations

Ligation and stripping of varicosities, along with ligation of perforators, is an ablative rather than a reconstructive procedure. When done for varicose veins secondary to the postphlebitic syndrome, the recurrence rate is high, since the basic cause has not been corrected. Indeed, only about 15 to 20 percent of postphlebitic patients need a varicose vein procedure; most do better with hose support. The minority who benefit are those with large varices which are nonfunctional. After operation they require continued long-term support with elastic hose.

On the other hand, when used in connection with reconstructive operations, the removal of nonfunctioning veins may be useful. The results of concomitant procedures are difficult to assess. A series illustrating this is the six patients with congenital venous valvular aplasia treated by Plate and associates in Sweden. Their clinical and ambulatory venous pressure results were excellent over the short (9-week median) follow-up period.[17] Whether this will continue over the years may be doubtful, but the paper does illustrate how one procedure may influence the results in the evaluation of another procedure done concomitantly.

Femoral or Popliteal Vein Ligation

Venous ligation is actually a destructive rather than a reconstructive procedure. It is briefly discussed because knowledgeable surgeons continue to revive a procedure which should be of historical interest only.

The rationale of venous interruption procedures has been that reflux of blood through nonfunctional or valveless veins causes the symptoms, which can be stopped by a venous ligation. Since ligation of the superficial (but not the common femoral) vein is tolerable such procedures are often associated with improvement, probably because of the treatment associated with them, including rest, elevation, and elastic support.

Buxton's advocacy of superficial femoral vein ligation in 1944[18] attracted the attention of Linton, who followed his advice,[19] as well as Bauer, who changed the ligation site to the popliteal vein.[20] The skepticism of Decamp[21] and of Boyd[22] to some extent checked this trend when they demostrated that venous pressure curves during exercise always deteriorated after such ligations. More recently May and Nissl found "no case in which the venous pressure curve improved after ligation of the femoral or popliteal vein."[23] On the other hand, Kistner and Sparkuhl reported "marked relief" for 2 to 8 years in four of five patients who had femoral vein ligations.[24]

Main-channel venous ligations are outmoded and useless. The burden of proof rests heavily upon a surgeon who performs one.

Venous Valve Operations

Venous valvular insufficiency following deep venous thrombosis has been believed to be the chief cause of the postphlebitic syndrome of the lower extremities for many years. The illustrious venous pioneer John Homans noted this in 1917,[25] Luke again reemphasized it in 1941,[26] and Dodd and Cockett discussed valvular problems at length in their classic book, with particular emphasis upon the role of the communicating perforating veins of the calf.[27] Recently Raju has proposed that valvular dysplasia, rather than the postphlebitic syndrome, is the usual original venous lesion.[11] Whether this is a leap forward or a mere heresy remains to be seen.

Extrinsic "Valve" Operations

A completely different approach to the control of venous reflux has been advocated by Psathakis of West Germany during the past 20 years.[28] The 1984 version of his substitute-valve procedure uses a Silastic band attached to the gracilis tendon to occlude the popliteal vein intermittently during walking. He found clinical improvement, along with reduction of ambulatory venous hypertension, in the 131 limbs reported in 1984.[29]

Attractive as these results may be, there has not yet been satisfactory confirmation. Berger and Brucke in 1970 had 8 good results in 10 patients.[30] Haeger's pessimistic report of improvement from only 4 of 48 operations contradicts this to the extent that he "could not find that this procedure had any value at all."[31]

The procedure is generally unknown and its value unconfirmed despite the 20-year period since the original report.

Femoral Valvuloplasty

In the belief that prevention of the reflux of blood down the femoral venous system would be helpful for the syndrome of venous insufficiency, Robert Kistner introduced superficial femoral valvuloplasty in 1975.[32] Again in 1982 he discussed its results in 32 patients. Initially there developed some misunderstanding of the good results (78 percent), which were believed to be due to valvuloplasty alone. Later it was recognized that concomitant procedures (such as removal of varicose veins and ligation of incompetent perforating veins) had been done, so that the results could not be ascribed to any one procedure. The most recent report noted the importance of concomitant ligation of incompetent venous perforators along with the valvuloplasty. There were "excellent" results after 48 percent of the double procedures, while only 5 percent of the results were excellent when the perforator operation was not done at the same time. However, the figures can also be summarized to show 80 percent "good" and "excellent" results after the first procedure and 81 percent after the second, which suggest no difference.[33] This illustrates the difficulty in understanding and assessing these results.

Few valvuloplasties have been reported by others. Fogarty had two successes.[34] The single patient reported by Huse and associates developed recurrence of leg ulcers and failure to maintain hemodynamic competence 6 months later[35] Schanzer and Peirce reported three valvuloplasties with "improvement," but postoperative venous pressure studies showed little change after the procedure and no phlebograms were reported.[36]

The most optimistic confirmation was that of Raju, whose 15-patient series suggested to him that valvuloplasty was more durable than either venous segment transfers or transplants. All except two of his patients returned to full-time work. Only one required a support stocking. The repaired valves retained competency, while four of the five phlebograms done showed correction of reflux.[11]

No personal cases can be added to the meager reported experience because the few candidates found have been treated by venous transfer, transplants, or crossover grafts. The ultimate role of valvuloplasty remains in doubt.

Femoral Vein Transfer

Kistner also described the transfer of a functional venous valve within the femoral system by division and appropriate anastomosis of the veins in the groin (Figure 31-6). Again the concomitant procedures made it difficult to attribute improvement to any single one of the multiple treatments. Seven of his fourteen patients undergoing vein transfers had phlebograms 3 to 6 years later. Four showed no change, but in three there was worse function.[33]

Minimal experience has been documented by others. Fogarty reported good clinical, angiographic, and hemodynamic results in eight venous transfer patients.[34] The results of the Huse group's five limbs at 12 to 22 months were not remarkable in clinical terms.[35] Kempczinski was more optimistic after his experience with five patients.[37] In an attempt to separate the effects of venous valve transposition from those of multiple simultaneous procedures (removal of varicosities and ligation of perforators), Bergan's group studied 12 limbs of 10 patients* who had femoral venous transposition of functional valves. At 12 to 18 months none attained a normal venous pressure and all required elastic support. The researchers concluded that "femoral valve reconstruction performed alone for venous stasis is not sufficient."[38] Kistner himself has agreed that chronic venous insufficiency requires multiple operative procedures.[39] Like valvuloplasty, the future of femoral vein transfers seems questionable.

Thus, the concept of transfer of a valve-bearing segment at best rests on shaky ground and at worst may be just another good idea which has proved useless. My own small experience (two

FIGURE 31-6 The valveless superficial femoral vein has been transferred to the profunda distal to a competent valve to prevent venous reflux.

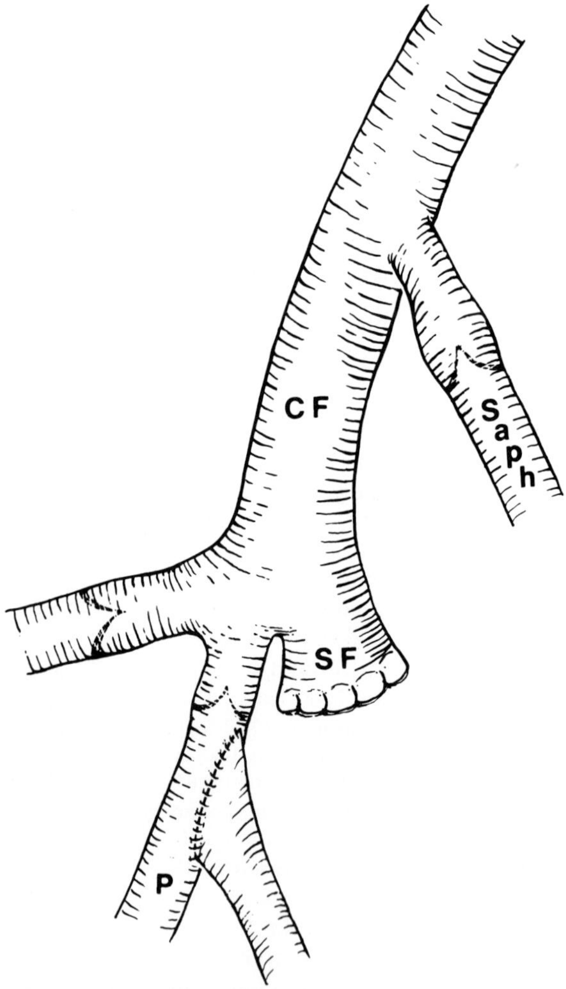

*Nobel laureate George Whipple of Rochester often commented on the virtues of a few experiments personally studied with care as opposed to large numbers followed poorly by subordinates.

brachial transplants, one profunda transfer, no valvuloplasties) is due partly to inability to find suitable candidates and partly to skepticism. These few patients have "improved" and phlebograms show patency, but whether the result is due to operation or to the continued use of a stocking is unknown. Raju's three patients improved, but the results tended "to deteriorate with time."[11]

Venous Valve Transplants

Taheri and associates in 1983 reported 30 transplants of a 2-cm segment of a valve-bearing brachial vein into the superficial femoral vein, with excellent short-term (24-month) clinical results. Nine of these were studied postoperatively and were found to have patent grafts. None of the four patients whose venous pressures were determined had improvement, suggesting either that a simple functional valve is not enough to normalize the venous pressure or that perhaps that pressure is not critical to clinical success.[40] The experience of others with free grafts of valve-bearing veins is not extensive. Raju reported 23 in 21 patients. Primary symptom relief in only 13, improved laboratory study results in only 10, and continued phlebographic reflux in 5 of the 6 studies[11] are not impressive results, especially in view of the fact that only 10 of the 21 were "cured" by the operation. One does as well as or better than that by grafting ulcers and using stocking support thereafter.

The operation whereby a valve-bearing segment of the brachial vein is transplanted to the femoral vein is illustrated in Figures 31-7 to 31-10. My experience with this and another phlebographically successful case is too small to allow sweeping conclusions. The two successes do encourage further efforts.

The effect of arteriovenous fistulas of increasing the patency rate of transplanted valve-containing vein grafts was studied in dogs by Kroener and Bernstein. There was little difference in the actual patency rates whether or not a fistula was used (80 percent versus 100 percent among 10 dogs each), but

FIGURE 31-7 Preoperative descending phlebography demonstrated reflux peripheral to the ankle.

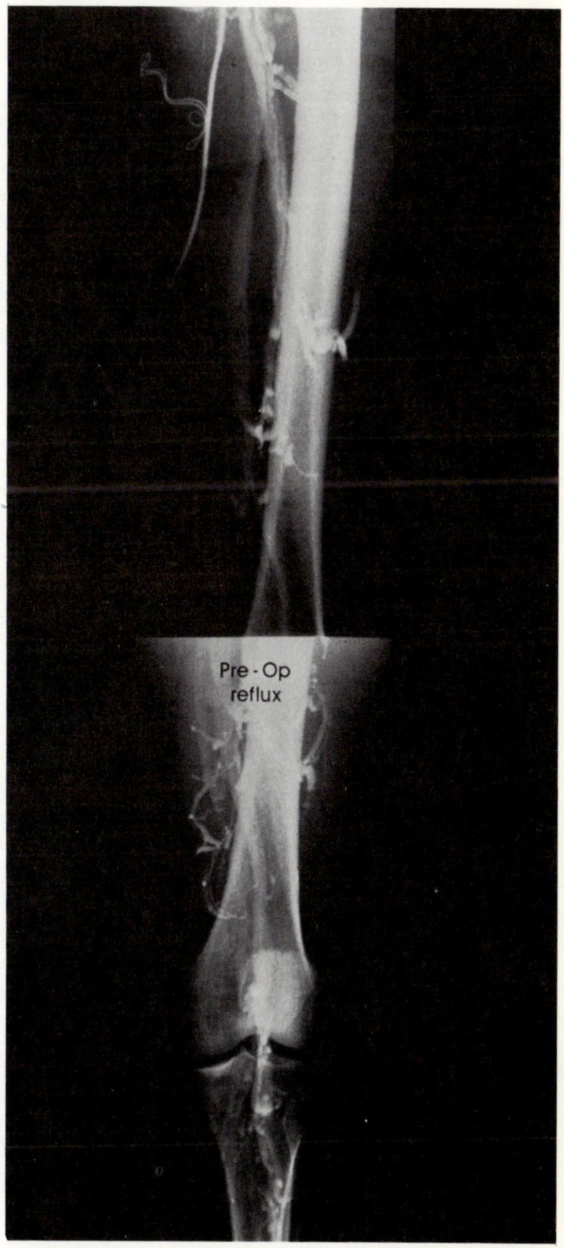

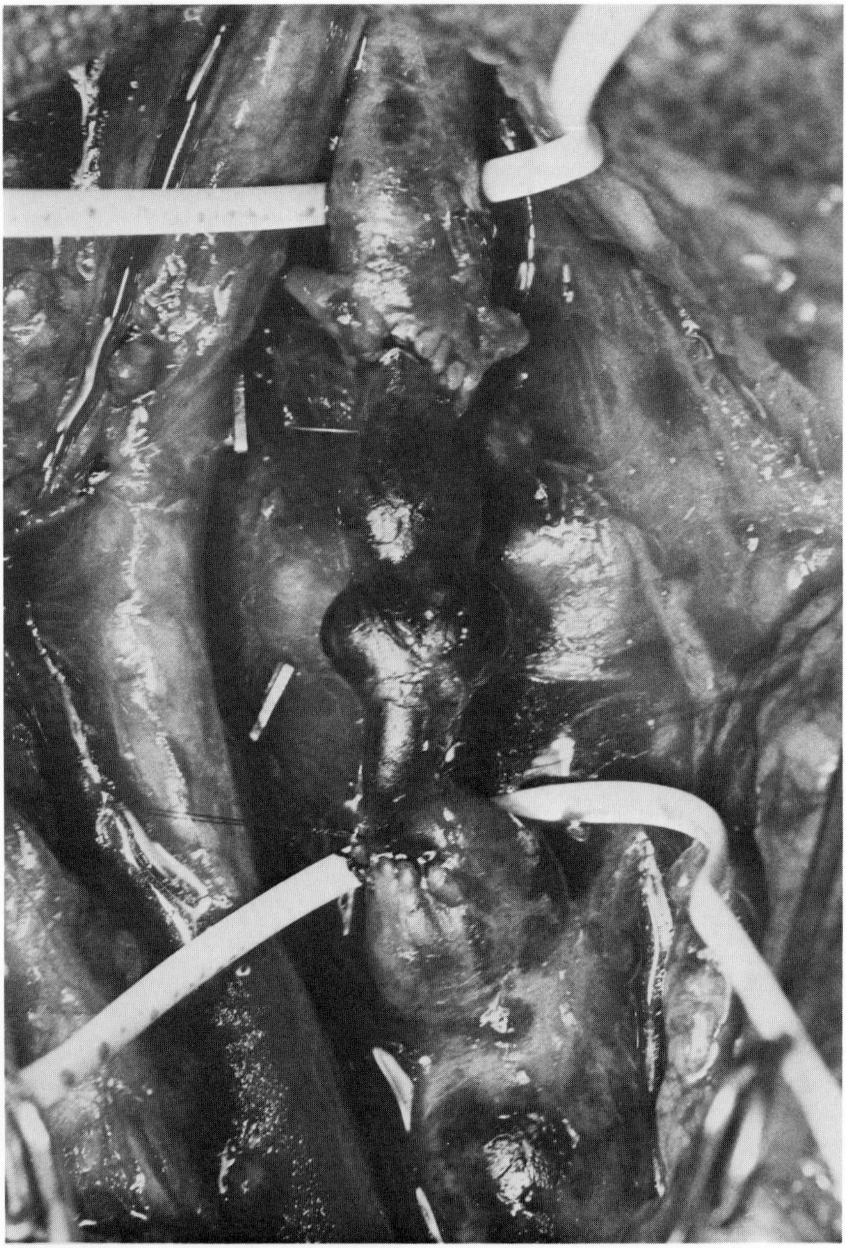

FIGURE 31-8 A segment of brachial vein with a competent valve was transplanted to the superficial femoral vein in the groin.

a considerable effect on the intraluminal appearance (and presumably the valve function) occurred.[41] Sterling Edwards's simplified technique to construct an arteriovenous fistula was used. The distal end of the crossover saphenous vein graft was attached as an extension to the adjacent femoral artery. A loop of suture left about this could be pulled up and tied later to obliterate the fistula.[42]

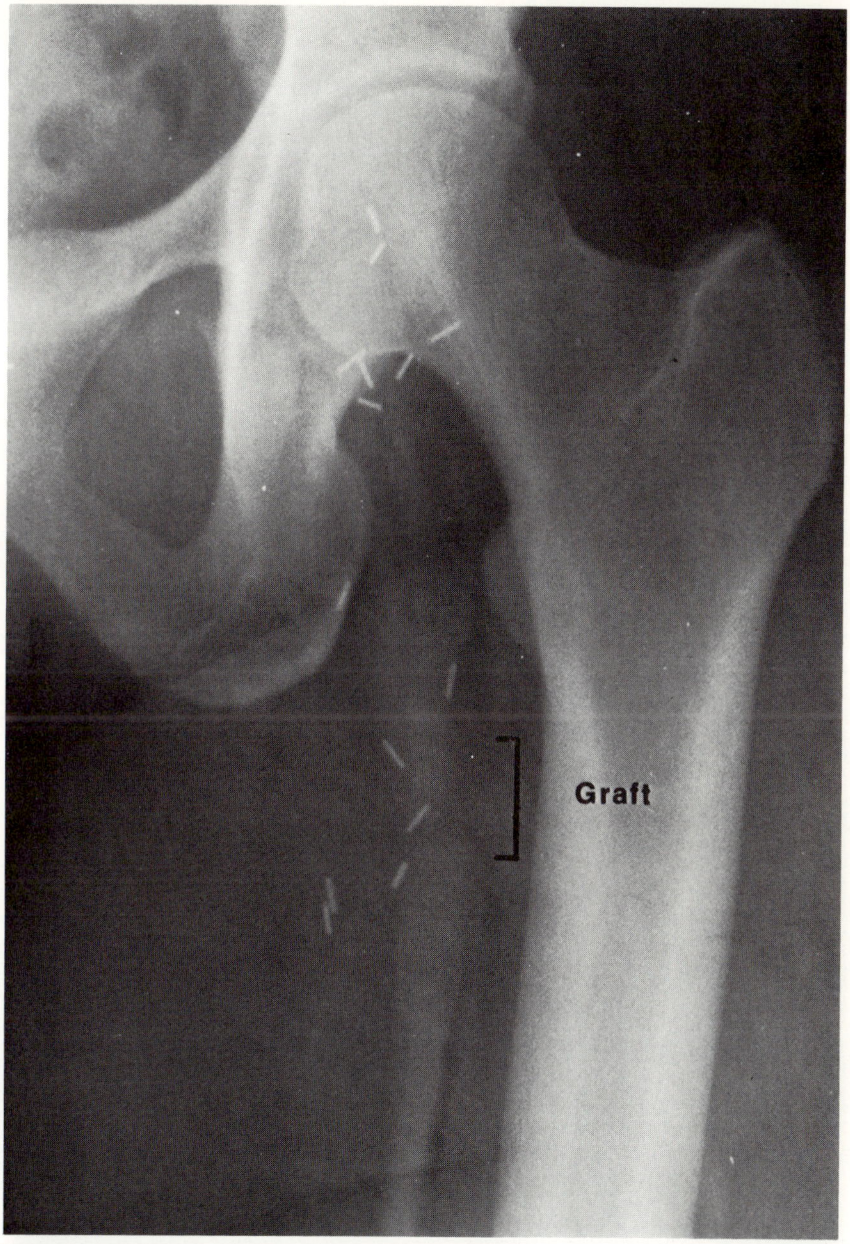

FIGURE 31-9 Postoperatively an ascending phlebogram demonstrates patency of the transplanted venous segment.

Venous Bypass Grafts

The natural history of veins after thrombosis is recanalizaton and ultimate patency. Although extensive damage to the valves and intraluminal webs and scarring are usual (Figure 31-11), sometimes there is also failure of recanalization to the extent that complete occlusion of portions

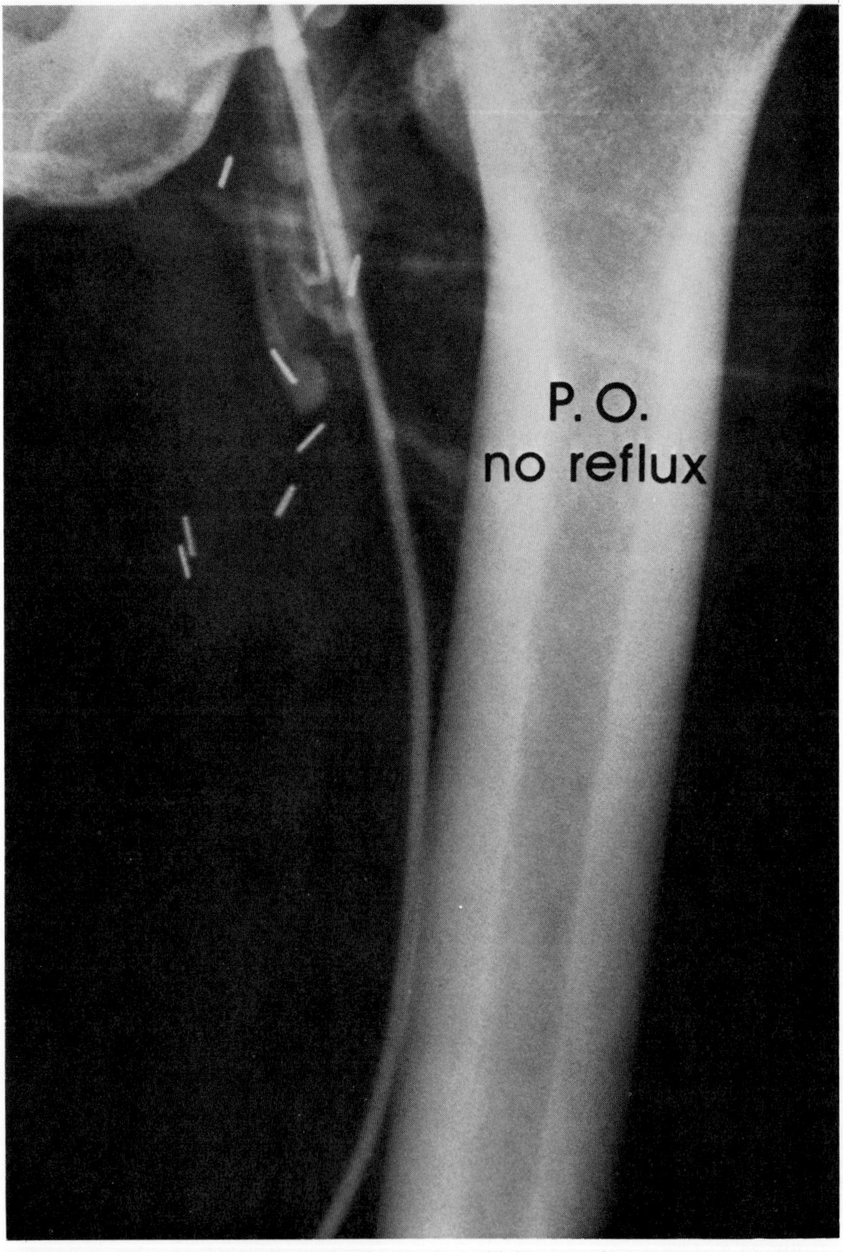

FIGURE 31-10 Postoperatively the descending phlebogram demonstrates that the radiopaque material no longer refluxes through the transplanted venous segment bearing a competent venous valve.

of the deep venous system persist. There are no reliable statistics concerning patients with such residual venous occlusions. Estimates of 10 percent seem high;[43] 1 percent is more reasonable. In any event, the edema, pain, and varicosities and ulcers due to the venous hypertension are quite troublesome to the patient.

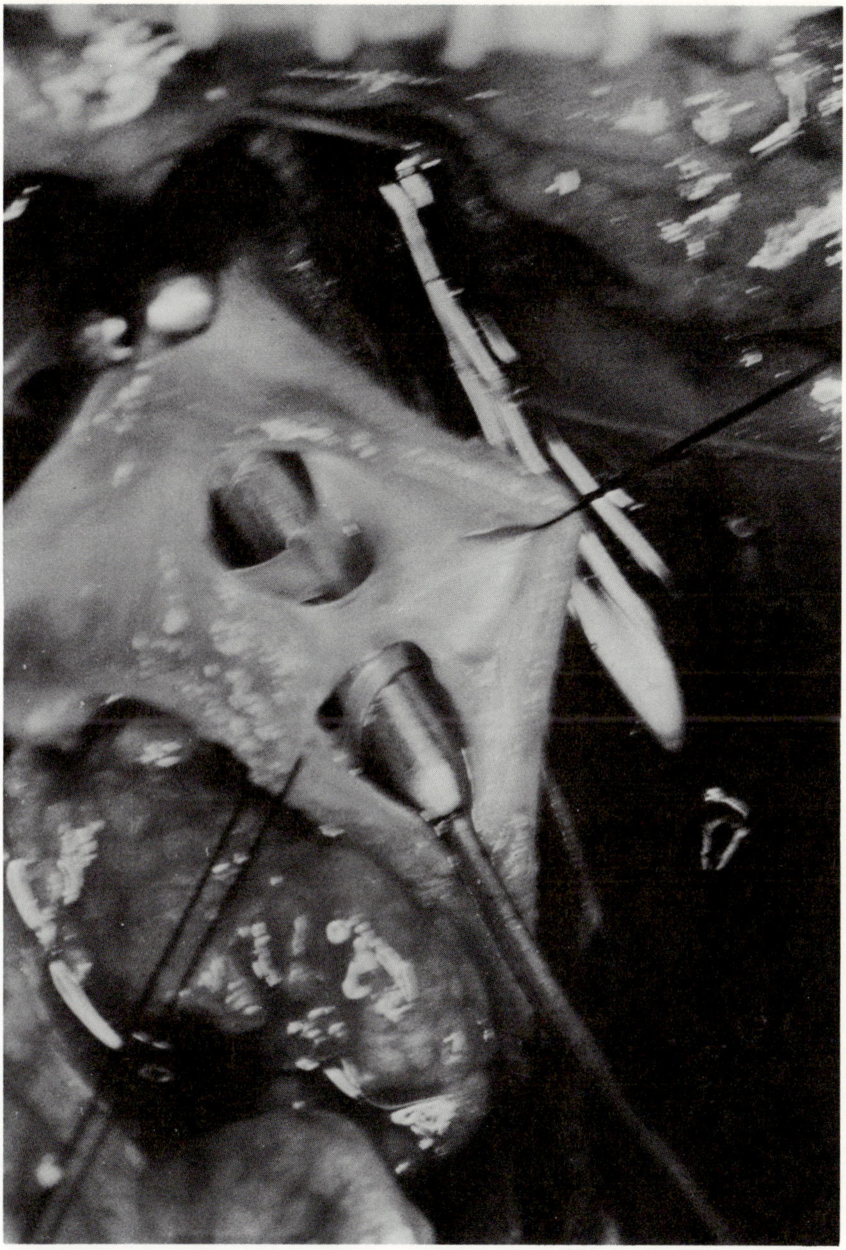

FIGURE 31-11 Femoral venotomy often discloses the sequelae of deep venous thrombosis with webs and bands traversing the lumen.

Traditionally the postphlebitic syndrome has been treated by elevation, rest, and external compression, along with removal of varicose veins and skin grafting for a selected group. The addition of bypass grafting to decompress the venous hypertension has become an important addition to the management scheme, although it is not yet well known.

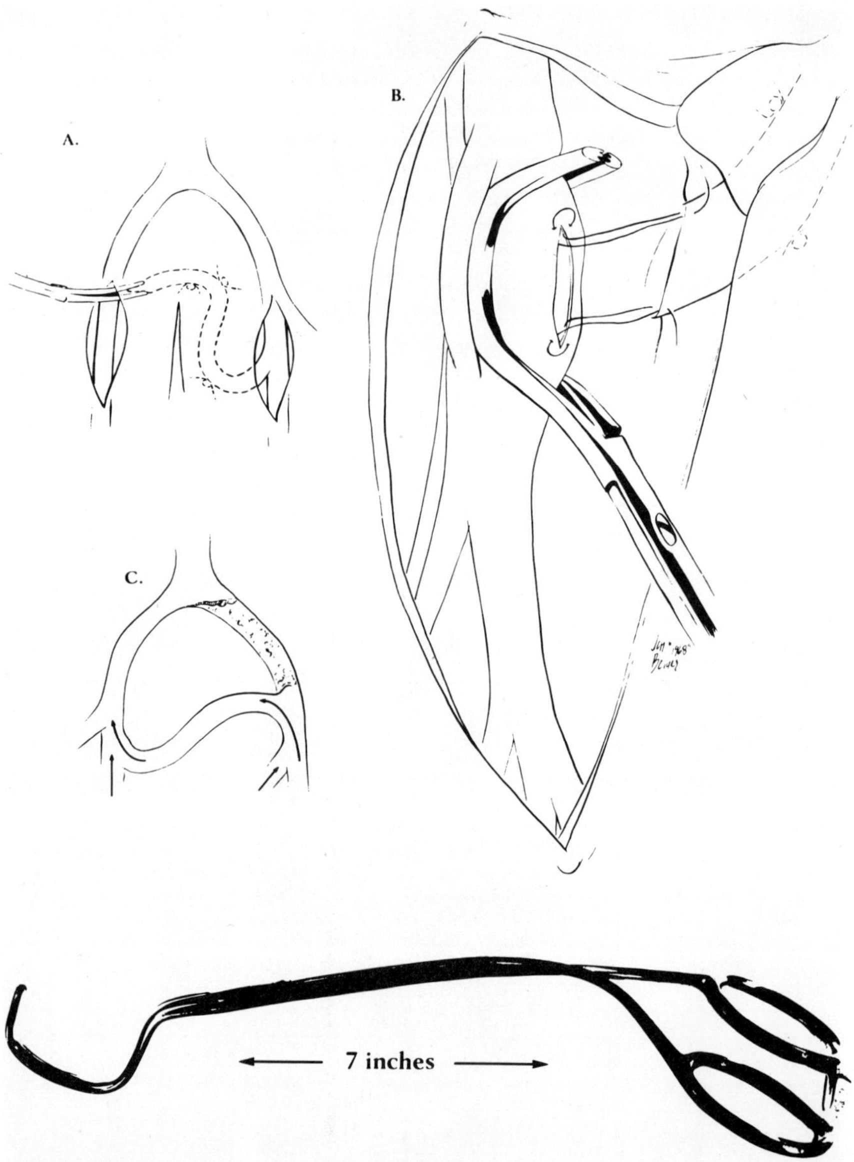

FIGURE 31-12 A "U"-shaped vascular clamp allows the anastomosis to be done without complete dissection of the posterior aspect of the common femoral vein, where several large tributaries lie. *(Reprinted courtesy Ann Surg 1968, 168:319.)*

The plan of management is summarized in Table 31-2. It begins with a search for the cause, goes on to complete delineation of patent as well as occluded veins, and thereafter considers the time of the operation. In practical terms the diagnosis generally is either tumor or venous thrombosis, although occasional instances of venous ligation for trauma or during an operation do occur. Rarely the inflammatory reaction about an aneurysm or retroperitoneal fibrosis may incite the thrombosis.

Crossover Saphenous-to-Femoral Vein Graft

The crossover saphenous-to-femoral vein transposition to bypass iliac venous occlusion described by Eduardo Palma of Montevideo in 1960 was an important milestone in peripheral venous reconstruction.[8] Our canine experiments confirmed the feasibility of this bypass, and its clinical use was reported in 1968,[9] with updates to present experience. Long-term patency rates of approximately 75 percent have been reported by several vascular surgeons, including myself.[44]

Principles of the crossover saphenous-to-femoral venous bypass may be summarized as follows. First, the desired length of saphenous vein is prepared as for an arterial bypass, but the proximal end is left attached to the femoral vein in the groin. Second, the recipient common femoral (or occasionally saphenous) vein of the symptomatic limb is dissected to expose only its anterior 180°, thus preserving every possible collateral. The special anastomosis clamp (Figure 31-12) allows an end-to-side anastomosis through the limited dissection field. Third, the freed saphenous vein is tunneled across the suprapubic region in the fat. Fourth, after systemic heparinization a long anastomosis is constructed with 6-0 continuous monofilament suture.

This simple operation requires ninety-odd minutes under spinal anesthesia.

Sometimes the patent graft may be demonstrated in the early postoperative period by an isotope phlebogram (Figure 31-13). Patency may also be ascertained by Doppler study. The most

FIGURE 31-13 An isotope phlebogram demonstrates a patent crossover vein graft during the early postoperative period.

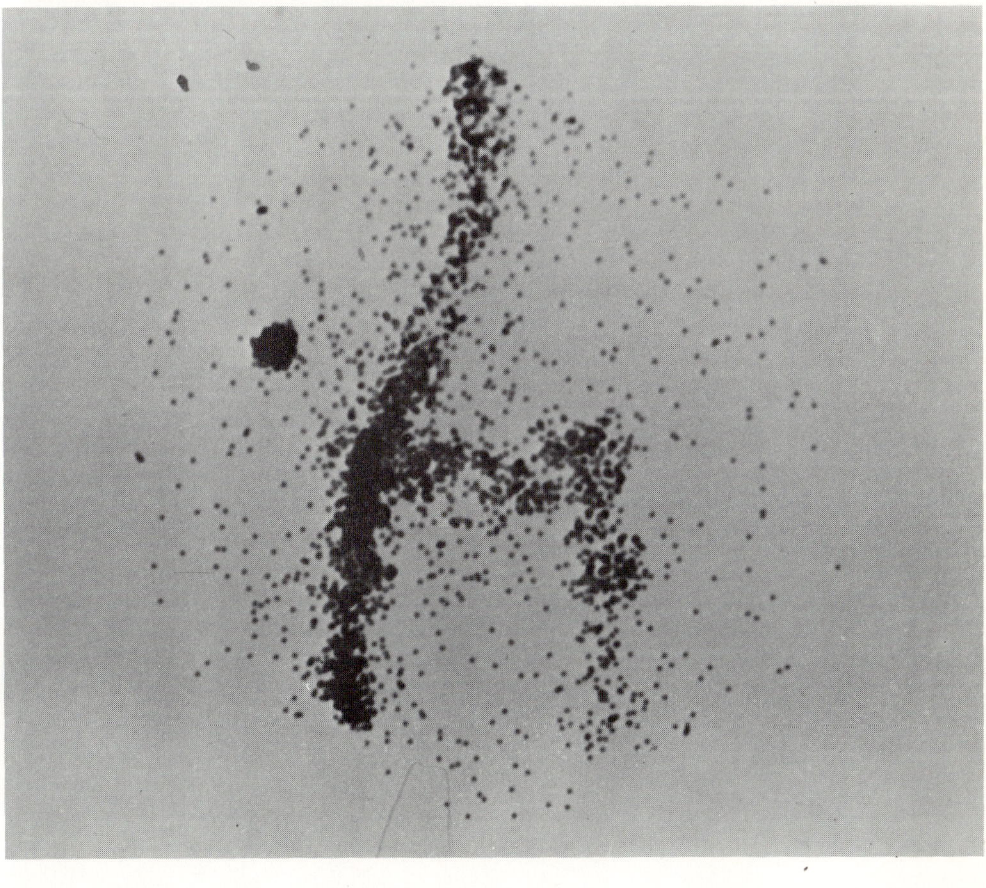

reliable documentation of the result is a phlebogram made several months later (Figures 31-5 and 31-14). All our patients agree to this postoperative plan prior to the procedure.

Saphenopopliteal Anastomosis

Sometimes the superficial femoral vein remains occluded in the postphlebitic state. If this is persistent and the patient has considerable symptoms, a bypass may be constructed by dissection of the saphenous vein along the medial aspect of the lower thigh and knee region and anasto-

FIGURE 31-14 A patent crossover saphenous vein graft 7 months after operation.

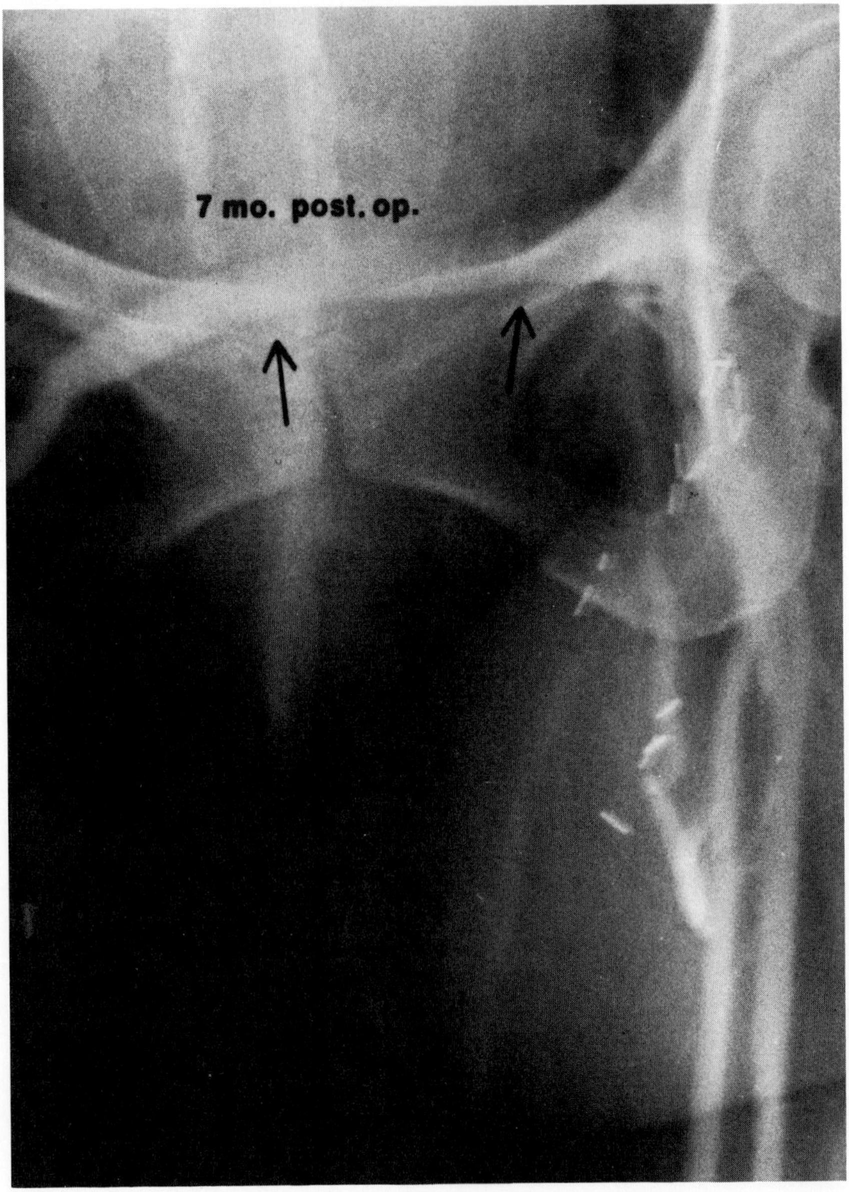

mosis of it through a medial approach to the deeply lying popliteal vein, again with 6-0 polypropylene. The anastomosis may be construction as a side-to-side operation or an end-to-side operation (Figure 31-15). The side-to-side anastomosis has theoretic advantages, since it does not interrupt flow through the saphenous vein, but it requires more dissection and may result in angulation. The end-to-side anastomosis is easier to perform. The number of performances of either operation is insufficient to allow a choice based on follow-up material.

The saphenopopliteal operation may be combined with a proximal crossover saphenous-to-femoral vein graft (Figures 31-16 and 31-17). The double operation requires approximately 2½ hours and is easily done under spinal anesthesia.

The results of these venous bypasses have continued to be encouraging. There have been no deaths, nor has an infection occurred. My patency results are 75 percent for the 85 saphenous crossover grafts and 60 percent for the 14 superficial femoral bypasses.

It is important to note that graft failure has not worsened the symptoms, which simply remain unchanged. These procedures may therefore, within the statistics noted above, be recommended to patients.

Synthetic Tubes for Venous Reconstruction

Occasionally the saphenous vein is not available or not suitable for use in a bypass. Earlier this problem led to abandonment of the procedure, since animal as well as clincal experience indicated that synthetic tubes used to replace peripheral veins would not long remian patent. The situation was summarized by Scherck, Kerstein, and Stansel after their exhaustive review in 1974 as "replacement of venous segments has still not been nearly successful enough to be realistically applied to any but the most desperate clinical situation."[45] It also meant that occluded vena cavas and iliac veins could not be helped.

Developments during the past 12 years have altered the outlook, so today it may be possible to reconstruct large veins with a synthetic material. Polytetrafluoroethylene (PTFE) is currenctly the choice, not only because of its characteristics but also because it is available with external stenting, which resists the weight of the overlying tissues that tends to collapse the graft.[10]

In 1972 there appeared two studies of the PTFE graft in the venous system which, hardly noticed then, led on to our present use. Soyer, Lempinen, Cooper, Norton, and Eiseman reported that 89 percent of 25 small PTFE prostheses used to replace various veins in dogs were patent 2 weeks to 6 months later.[46] Two portal veins were thereafter replaced in humans by PTFE grafts and remained patent for the short time of those cancer patients' survival. In the same year Heydorn, Zajtchuk, Miller, and Schuchmann studied the effects of pore size, the covering, and the external spiral support of PTFE tubes.[47] There were only six animals in each of their groups, and the similarity in patency rates did not really justify their conclusions but did confirm the promise of PTFE.

Further evidence suggesting that PTFE might be useful in the venous system came from Fujiwara, Cohn, Adams, and Collins, who in 1974 reported grafts in dogs of both the superior vena cave (SVC) and inferior vena cava (IVC) which remained patent over 7 months in 78 percent of the survivors.[48] The next year saw the article of Smith, Hammon, Anane-sefah, Richardson, and Trimble, who found PTFE grafts to be superior to homologous veins as well as to autogenous collagenous tubes for the suprarenal inferior vena cavae, 83 percent being patent at 3 months.[49] An experimental comparison of PTFE, venous allografts, and bovine heterografts by Wilson, Jabour, Stone, and Stanley in 1978 again suggested PTFE's superiority.[50] In 1981 Husfeldt reported another successful experimental series, in which 87 percent of 23 PTFE grafts remained patent in the canine inferior vena cava for periods up to 9 months.[51]

Occasional reports of the successful clinical use of PTFE grafts have begun to accumulate, several being described briefly at the Pelvic Vein Symposium in Igls-Innbruck, Austria, in October 1980.[52] These cases are summarized in Table 31-3.

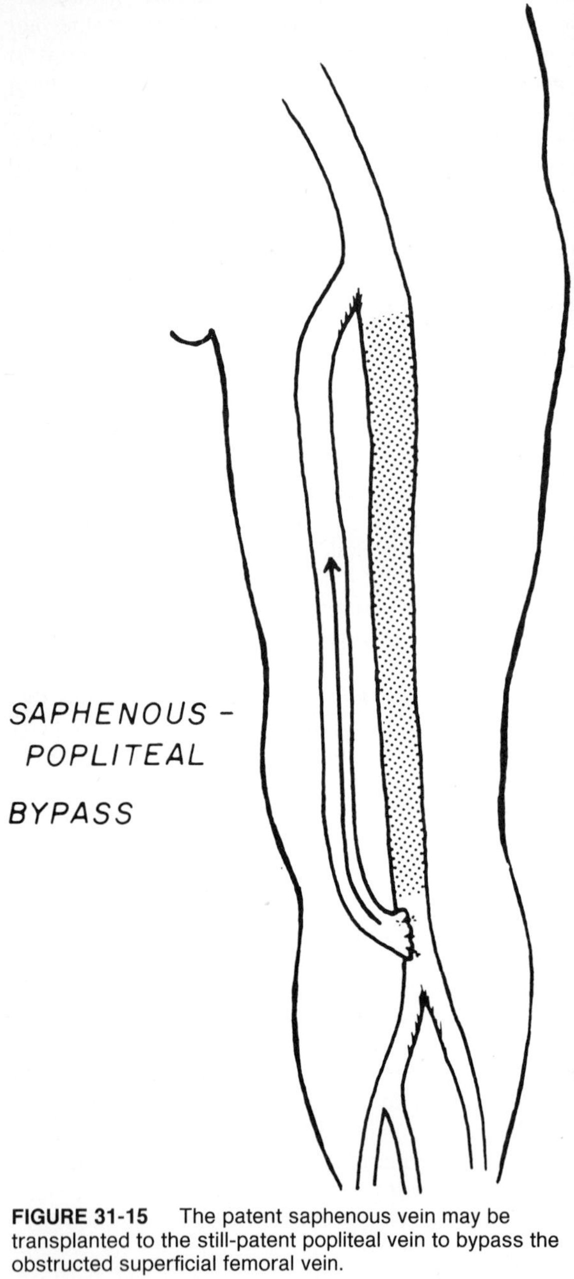

FIGURE 31-15 The patent saphenous vein may be transplanted to the still-patent popliteal vein to bypass the obstructed superficial femoral vein.

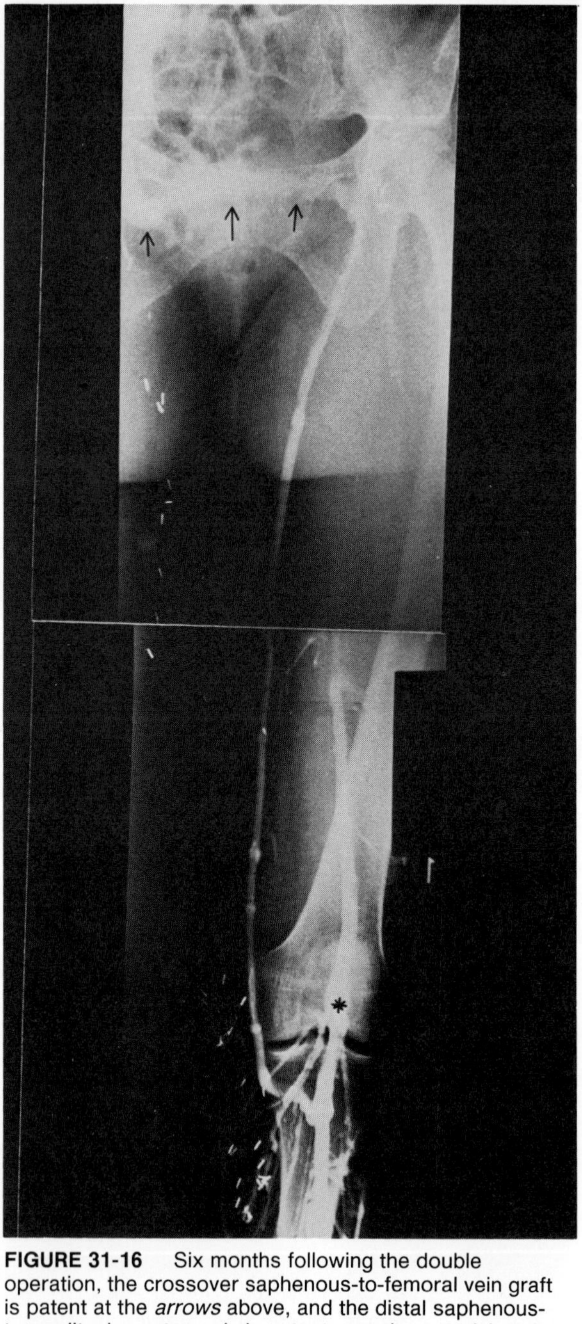

FIGURE 31-16 Six months following the double operation, the crossover saphenous-to-femoral vein graft is patent at the *arrows* above, and the distal saphenous-to-popliteal anastomosis is patent near the *asterisk* at the knee.

Reconstruction of the Inferior Vena Cava

Reconstruction of the infrarenal inferior vena cava has remained an unsolved problem and has continued to thwart the skill of vascular surgeons. Although occasional successful grafts were

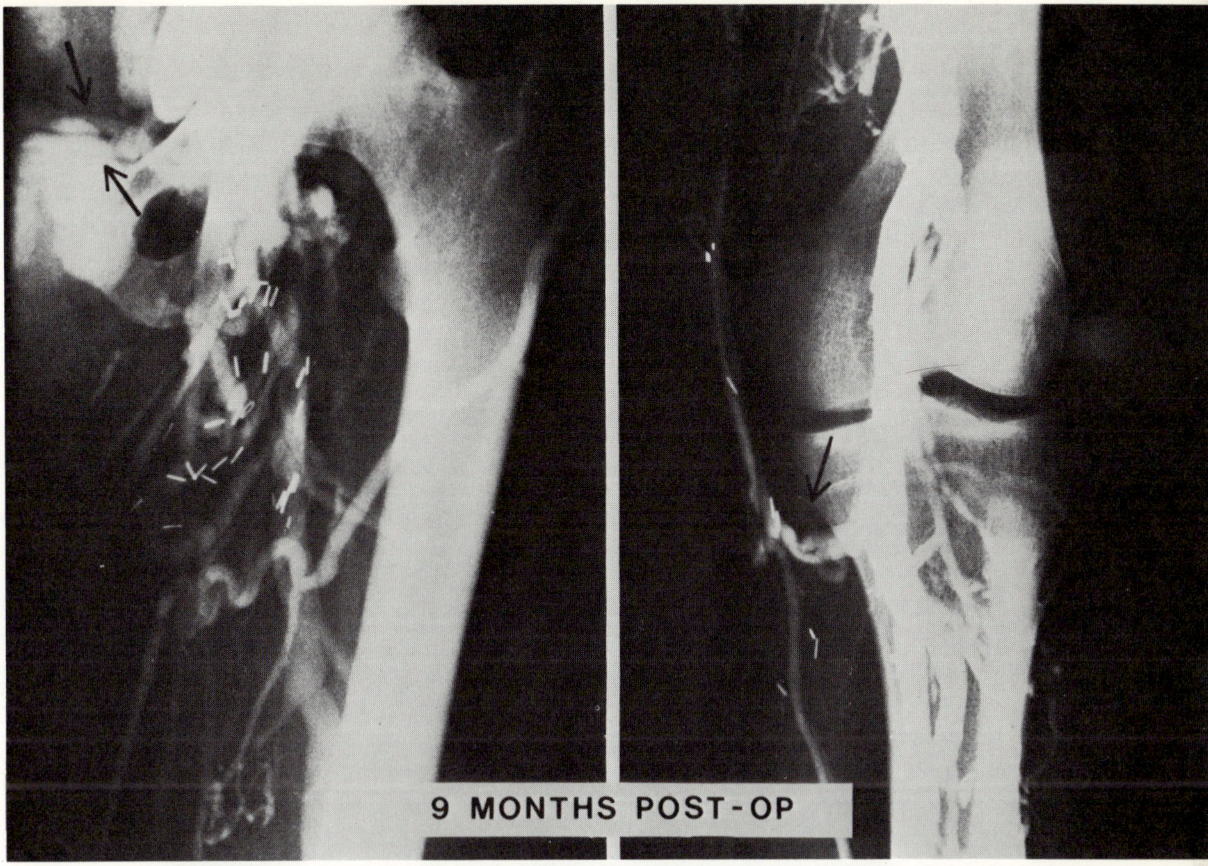

FIGURE 31-17 Nine months after the double operation, *left,* the crossover saphenous-to-femoral vein graft is patent at the *arrows,* and *right,* the saphenous-to-popliteal anastomosis is patent at the *arrow.*

TABLE 31-3 CLINICAL REPORTS OF PTFE GRAFT RECONSTRUCTION OF LARGE VEINS

Author	Year	No. of grafts	Site	Patent/ total	Remarks
Rosenthal[56]	1979	7	Portal shunt	7/7	
Clowes[54]	1980	1	Femorofemoral	1/1	Patent 1 yr
Vollmar[55]	1981	4	Femorofemoral	4/4	Patent 6–36 mo
		4	Iliac-IVC	1/4	3 failed after AVF* closure
Gruss[57]	1981	5	Iliac-IVC	4/5	4 patent
Husfeldt[51]	1981	2	SVC graft	2/2	2 patent 12–30 mo
		4	Femoral-IVC	1/4	1 patent 4 mo
		1	Internal jugular	1/1	1 patent 4 mo
Eklof[58]	1981	5	Iliocaval (after thrombectomy)	4/5	4 patent 14–22 mo
Ijima[59]	1981	4	Femorofemoral	3/4	3 patent
Fiore[60]	1982	1	SVC graft	1/1	1 patent 9 mo

* AV fistula.

TABLE 31-4 RESULTS OF PTFE REPAIRS OF THE VENA CAVA AND ILIAC VEINS

Patient's age/sex	Indication	Graft placed	Remarks
1 14 yr/F	IVC trauma	14-mm PTFE tube	Patent 48 mo*
2 46 yr/F	IVC ligation	12-mm PTFE "Y"	Patent 25 mo*
3 52 yr/M	IVC thrombosis	14-mm iliac-IVC tube	Patent 21 mo*
4 39 yr/M	Iliac thrombosis	10-mm PTFE tube	Occluded early

*To date.

FIGURE 31-18 Following inferior vena caval ligation for pulmonary embolism, the distal iliocaval system became completely thrombosed, with ensuing severe symptoms of venous hypertension in the lower limbs.

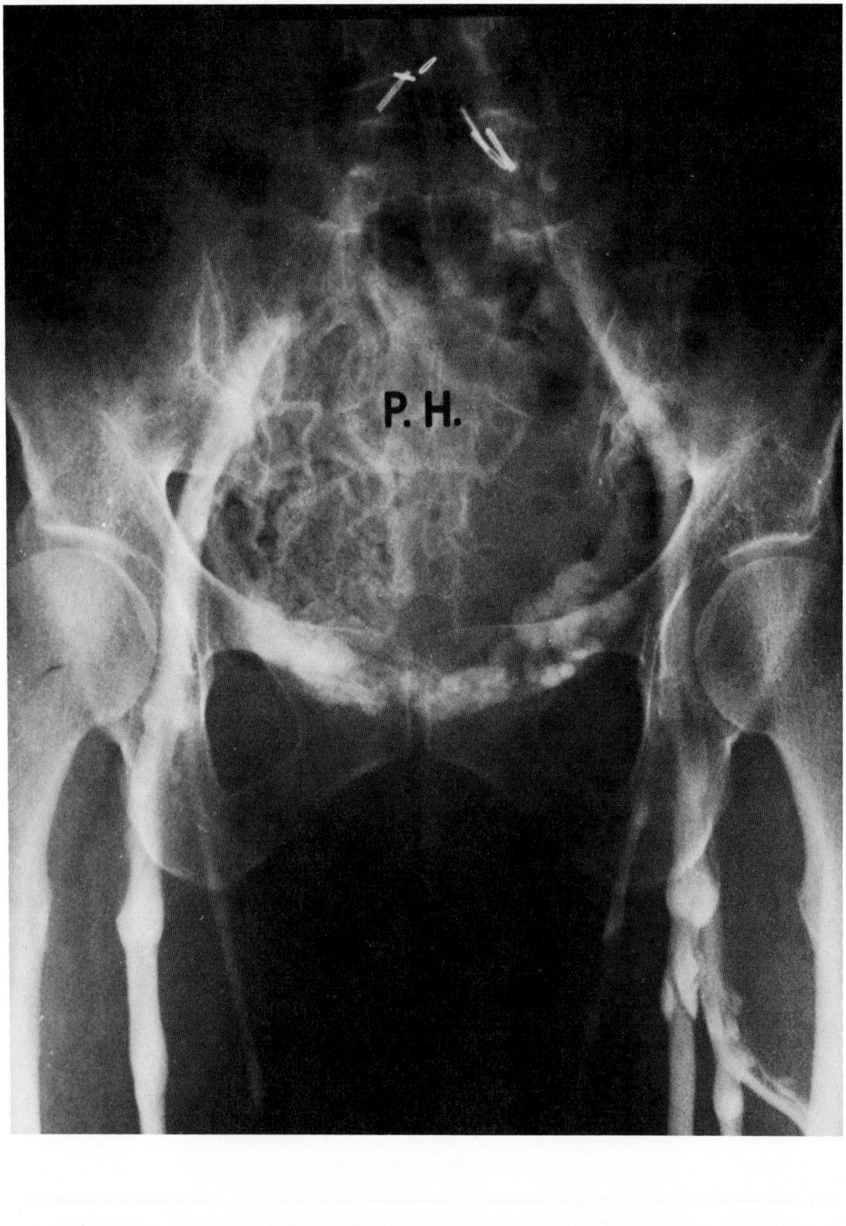

reported, the situation until recently did not change much after our report in 1963, which summarized the results of ourselves and others, finding a 33 percent patency rate in dogs along with 63 successful operations in humans.[7] Most of the clinical reports were based upon observation; few cavagrams were done. The published cases were the best; no doubt many failures were unreported.

A spiral vein graft long enough to extend from the external iliac veins to the IVC just distal to the renal veins would require a long segment of saphenous vein, placement of undesirable incisions in the already symptomatic thigh, and robbery of a vein which would possibly be needed as a collateral. That reconstruction would be impractical for the IVC although useful for the SVC.[53]

A slowly accumulating series of experiments and a few successful grafts in humans encouraged the idea that the inferior vena cava might be successfully reconstructed by a PTFE graft. Initially PTFE was used in femorofemoral crossovers, when the saphenous vein was not available. Clowes's 1980 report of three patencies at 1 year[54] was a remarkable change from the earlier trials of Dacron, which had usually failed. Vollmar and associates confirmed these results,[55] followed by other small series (Table 31-3). Concomitant, surgically created arteriovenous fistulas aided some of these.

The addition of external rings to PTFE tubes has made them resist collapse from the pressure of the overlying tissues or viscera. Presently we have used four PTFE grafts to replace the inferior vena cava or one of the iliac veins, of which three have remained patent, as shown by phlebography, over moderately long periods.[10] These cases are summarized in Table 31-4. None of these patients received postoperative heparin, nor did any have a concomitant arteriovenous fistula.

Illustrative Case A 46-year-old female had edema and pain of both lower extremities due to venous hypertension produced by inferior vena caval ligation done 2 years earlier for posthysterectomy pulmonary embolism. Phlebography demonstrated patent external iliac veins (Figure 31-18) as well as patency of the cava proximal to the site of its ligation (Figure 31-19).

A "Y" graft was formed from 12-mm externally stented PTFE and placed to form a new caval bifurcation (Figure 31-20). This has remained patent for the 19 months which have elapsed (Figure 31-21). Her symptoms have been relieved dramatically.

The postoperative phlebogram of another of the cited cases is shown in Figure 31-22.

I have never used a concomitant fistula because of (1) the additional operative time and dissection needed, (2) the necessity for a later procedure to close the fistula, and (3) the eventual requirement that the graft remain patent without a fistula, whether it be early or late. Our three successful IVC cases demonstrate patency without a fistula. Whether failure in the fourth might have been prevented by a fistula is speculative.

Whether external stenting is preferable to a nonsupported graft has not yet been finally determined. Perhaps stenting prevents the weight of the overlying viscera from closing the graft and therefore has particular merit within the abdomen.

It has been stated that the PTFE graft develops a thin but incomplete neointima which is thrombosis-resistant. Examination of such grafts recovered from the arterial system shows some to be covered within by a thin neointima, yet this is not always true. Whether there is a difference in the venous system is not known, but communication with one investigative team recently revealed that some of their canine PTFE grafts at 3 months were almost devoid of any neointima. Vollmar and Hutschenreiter, after reviewing the experimental and clinical evidence, stated: "There is little doubt that the micro-porosity of PTFE prostheses is not sufficient to build up a protective neo-intima in a six months' period."[55]

These favorable results suggest that further trials of PTFE for venous reconstructions are in order. In the single instance in which a stented PTFE tube was used as a femorofemoral graft (in the absence of a suitable saphenous vein), it did not remain patent, yet others will be needed.

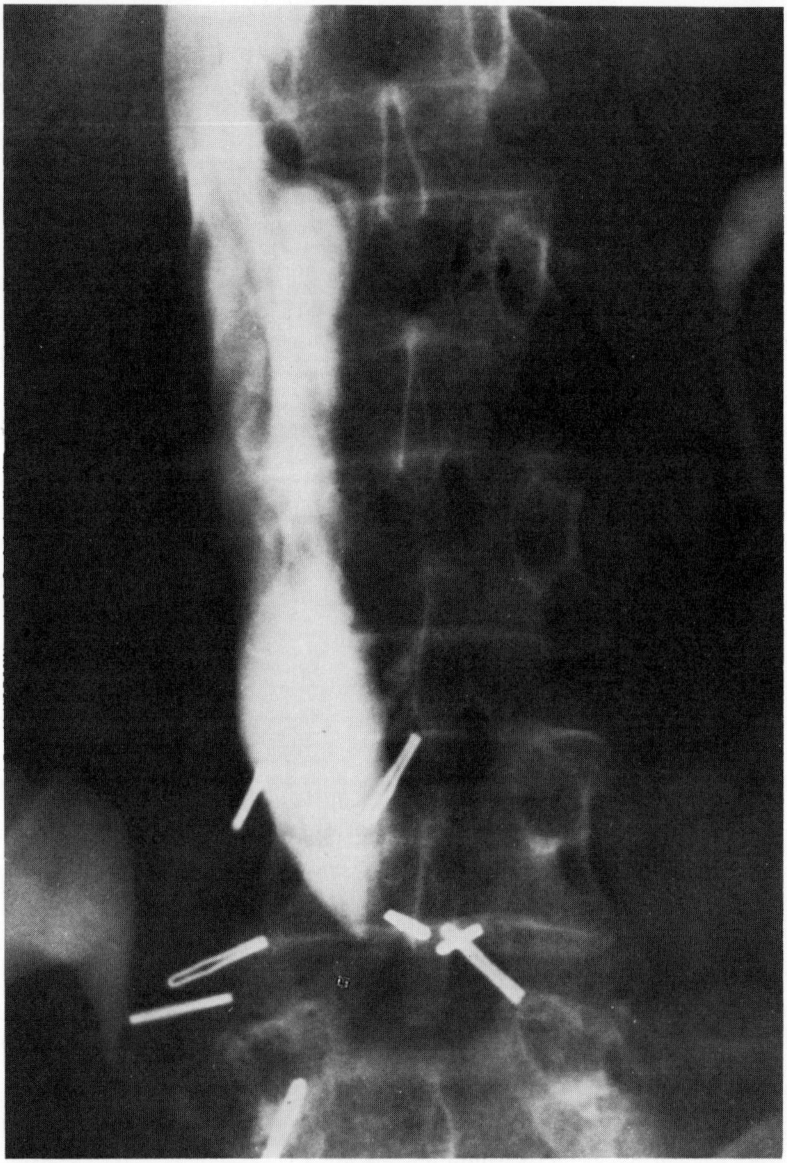

FIGURE 31-19 The infrarenal portion of the inferior vena cava was shown to be patent by a phlebogram obtained by a catheter passed through the heart.

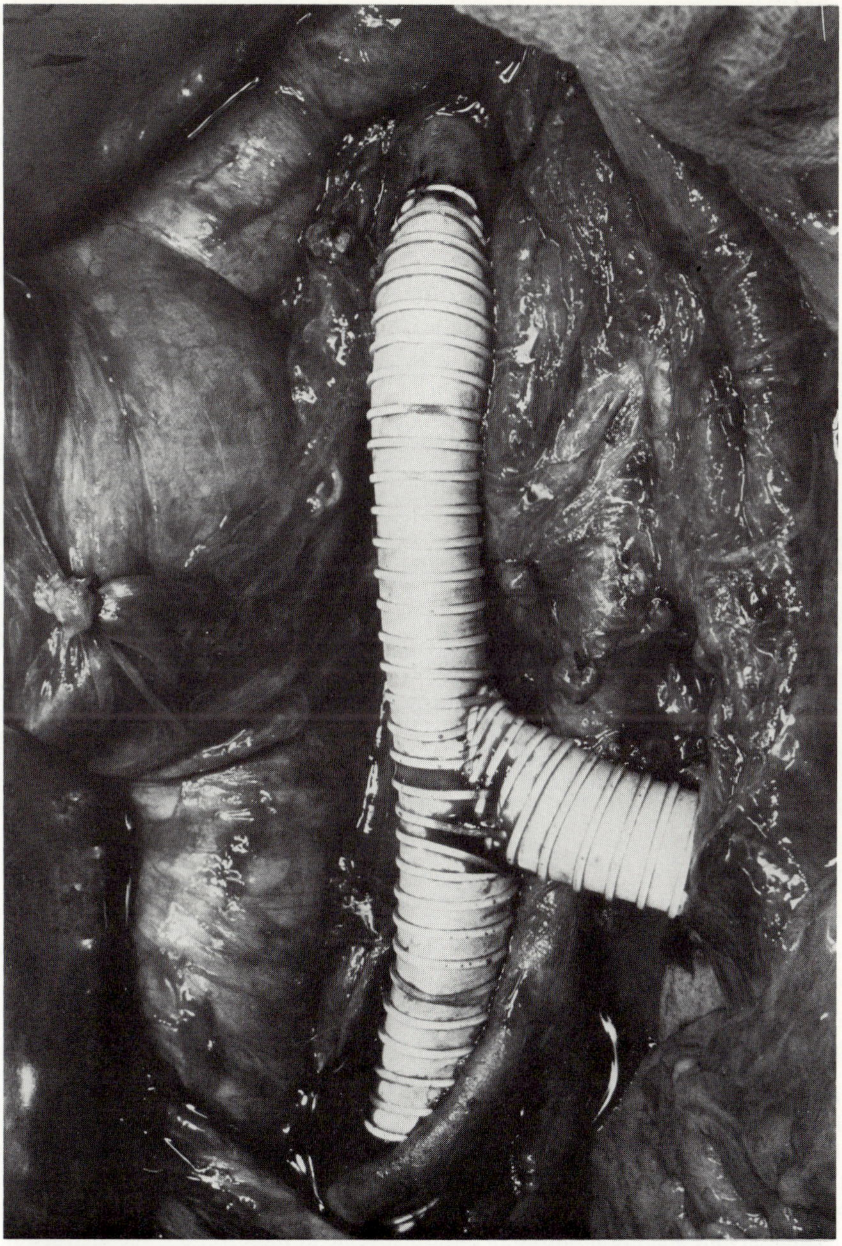

FIGURE 31-20 A "Y" graft was fashioned from a 12-mm stented PTFE tube and placed as a bypass between the patent iliac veins and the infrarenal portion of the inferior vena cava. The aortic bifurcation appears in the lower portion of the picture.

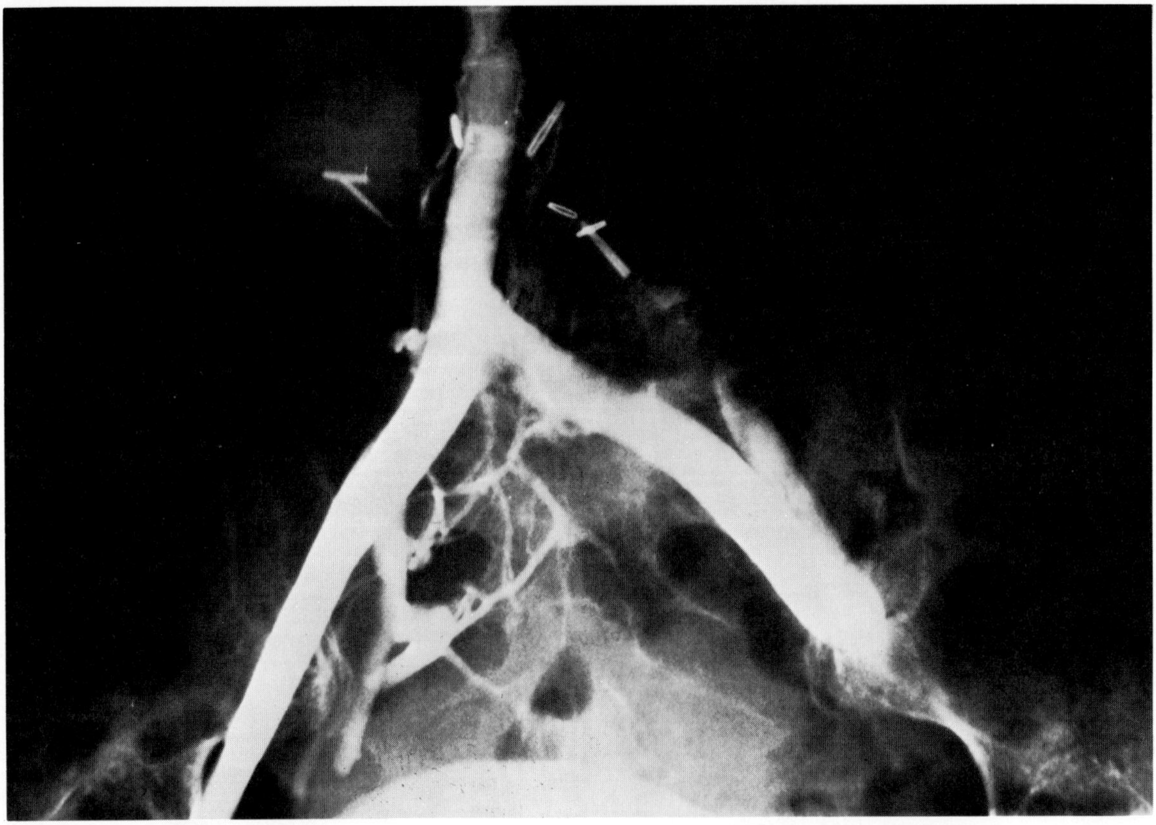

FIGURE 31-21 Six months postoperatively there is continued patency of the PTFE "Y" graft replacing the bifurcation of the inferior vena cava.

The evidence is small, the cases are few, but stented PTFE is presently the most promising substitute for an autogenous vein graft. It deserves further trials.

COMPLICATIONS

The low morbidity rates of these operations allow their classification as low-risk procedures. There have been no deaths and no infections among 112 patients. There has been one hematoma. There have been two temporary lymphorrheas. While it was earlier feared that deep venous thrombosis might be a real hazard, it has occurred only four times, once in the extremity operated upon and three time contralaterally. This suggests that deep venous thrombosis is a risk of anesthesia and operation but not a hazard specific to these venous reconstructions.

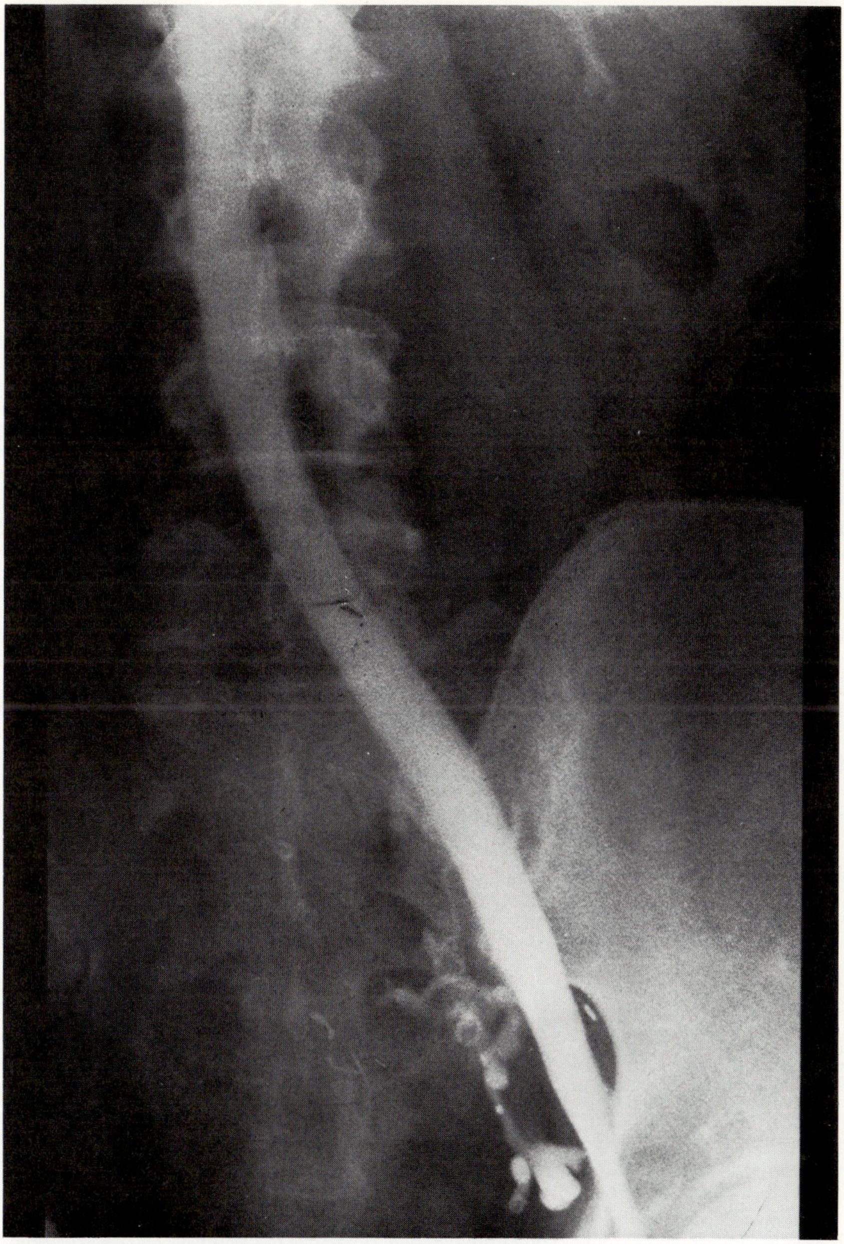

FIGURE 31-22 The PTFE bypass from the left iliac artery to the inferior vena cava is demonstrated to be patent 16 months postoperatively.

REFERENCES

1 Doyen E: *Surgical Therapeutics and Operative Technique.* Wood, New York, 1917, vol 1, p 363.
2 Kunlin J: The re-establishment of venous circulation with grafts in case of obliteration from trauma or thrombophlebitis. *Mem Acad Chir* 1953, 79:109.
3 Warren R, Thayer TR: Transplantation of the saphenous vein for postphlebitic stasis. *Surgery* 1954, 35:867.
4 Hardin CA: Bypass saphenous grafts for the relief of venous obstruction of the extremity. *Surg Gynecol Obstet* 1962, 115:709.
5 Cerino M, McGraw JU, Luke JC: Autogenous vein graft replacement of thrombosed deep veins. *Surgery* 1964, 55:123.
6 Kenawai MM: Venous grafting in the treatment of phlebosclerosis. *J Egypt Med Assoc* 1960, 1:480.
7 Dale WA, Scott HW: Grafts of the venous system: Correlatiom of previous reports with 100 experiments and 7 clinical cases. *Surgery* 1963, 53:52.
8 Palma EC, Esperon R: Vein transplants and grafts in the surgical treatment of the post-phlebitic syndrome. *J Cardiovasc Surg* (Torino) 1960, 1:94.
9 Dale WA, Harris J: Cross-over vein grafts for iliac and femoral venous occlusion. 1968, *Ann Surg* 168:319.
10 Dale WA, Harris J, Terry RB: Polytetrafluoroethylene reconstruction of the inferior vena cava. *Surgery* 1984, 95:625.
11 Raju S: Venous insufficiency of the lower limb and stasis ulceration: Current concepts and management. *Ann Surg* 1983, 197:688.
12 Nicolaides A, Hoare M, Miles C, Schull K, Fernandes JF: The value of ambulatory venous pressure in assessment of venous insufficiency. *Vasc Diag Ther* January 1983, p 41.
13 Arndt RD, Grollman JH Jr, Gomes AS, Boss CJ: The heparin flush: An aid in preventing post-venography thrombophlebitis. *Radiology* 1979, 130:249.
14 Lewis MR, Dale WA: Practical value of phlebography. *South Med J* 1980, 73:9.
15 Kistner RL: Transvenous repair of the incompetent femoral valve, in Bergan JJ, Yao JST (eds): *Venous Problems.* Year Book, Chicago, 1978, p 493.
16 Herman RJ, Neiman HL, Yao JST, Egan TJ, Bergan JJ, Malave SR: Descending phlebography: A method of evaluating lower extremity venous valvular function. *Radiology* 1980, 137:73.
17 Plate G, Brudin L, Ekof B, Jensen R, Ohlin P: Physiologic and therapeutic aspects in congenital vein valve aplasia of the lower limb. *Ann Surg* 1983, 198:229.
18 Buxton RW, Farris JM, Moyer CA, Coller FA: Surgical treatment of long standing deep phlebitis of leg. *Surgery* 1944, 15:749.
19 Linton RR: The postthrombotic ulceration of the lower extremity: Its etiology and surgical treatment. *Ann Surg* 1953, 138:415.
20 Bauer G: Indications for popliteal vein ligation. *J Cardiovasc Surg* (Torino) 1963, 4:18.
21 DeCamp PT: Ambulatory venous pressure studies in postphlebitic and other disease states. *Surgery* 1951, 29:365.
22 Boyd AM: Major vein ligation in the treatment of postphlebitic sequelae. *Lancet* 1953, 2:113.
23 May R, Nissl R: The post-thombotic syndrome, in May R (ed): *Surgery of the Veins of the Legs and Pelvis.* Thieme, Stuttgart, 1979, chap 6, p 142.
24 Kistner RL, Sparkhul MD: Surgery in acute and chronic venous disease. *Surgery* 1979, 85:31.
25 Homans J: The etiology and treatment of the varicose ulcer of the leg. *Surg Gynecol Obstet* 1917, 24:300.
26 Luke JC: Diagnosis of chronic enlargment of the leg with description of a new syndrome. *Surg Gynecol Obstet* 1941, 73:742.
27 Dodd H, Cockett FB (eds): *The Pathology and Surgery of the Veins of the Lower Extremity.* 2d ed. Churchill Livingstone, New York, 1976.
28 Psathakis ND: A new rational operative treatment for the insufficiency syndrome of the deep veins of the lower extremity. *Vasc Dis* 1964, 1:261.
29 Psathakis ND: The substitute "valve" operation by technique II in patients with postthrombotic syndrome. *Surgery* 1984, 95:542.
30 Berger A, Brucke, P: Zur chirurgischen Behandlung der insuffizienz tiefer Beinvenen. *Acta Chir Aust* 1970, 2:97.
31 Haeger K: The treatment of the severe post-thrombotic state. *Angiology* 1968, 19:439.
32 Kistner R: Surgical repair of the incompetent femoral vein valve. *Arch Surg* 1975, 110:1336.

33 Ferris EB, Kistner RL: Femoral vein reconstruction in the management of chronic venous insufficiency: A 14 year experience. *Arch Surg* 1982, 117:1571.

34 Fogarty TJ: Discussion of Ferris EB, Kistner RL: Femoral vein reconstruction in the management of chronic venous insufficiency: A 14 year experience. *Arch Surg* 1982, 117:1578.

35 Huse JB, Nabseth DC, Bush HL, Widrich WC, Johnson WC: Direct venous surgery for venous valvular insufficiency of the lower extremity. *Arch Surg* 1983, 118:719.

36 Schanzer H, Peirce EC: A rational approach to surgery of the chronic venous stasis syndrome. *Ann Surg* 1982, 1953:25.

37 Kempezinski, RF: Discussion of Johnson ND, Queral LA, Flinn WR, Yao JST, Bergan JJ: Late objective assessment of venous valve surgery. *Arch Surg* 1981, 116:1465.

38 Johnson ND, Queral LA, Flinn WR, Yao JST, Bergan JJ: Late objective assessment of venous valve surgery. *Arch Surg* 1981, 116:1461.

39 Kistner RL: Discussion of Johnson ND, Queral LA, Flinn WR, Yao JST, Bergan J: Late objective assessment of venous valve surgery. *Arch Surg* 1981, 116:1465.

40 Taheri SA, Lazar L, Elias S, Marchand P, Heffner R: Surgical treatment of postphlebitic syndrome with vein valve transplant. *Am J Surg* 1982, 144:221.

41 Kroener JM, Bernstein EF: Valve competence following experimental autotransplantation. *Arch Surg* 1981, 116:1467.

42 Edwards WS: Letter. *Ann Surg* 1983, 198:118.

43 Nissil R: Acute thrombosis: Roentgenologic aspects, in May R (ed): *Surgery of the Veins of the Leg and Pelvis.* Thieme, Stuttgart, 1979, chap 5, p 96.

44 Dale WA: Crossover vein grafts for iliac and femoral venous occulsion. *Resident and Staff Physician,* March 1983, p 58.

45 Scherck JP, Kerstein MD, Stansel HC Jr: The current status of vena cava replacement. *Surgery* 1974, 76:209.

46 Soyer T, Lempinen M, Cooper P, Norton L, Eiseman B: A new venous prosthesis. *Surgery* 1972, 72:864.

47 Heydorn WH, Zajtchuk R, Miller J, Schuchmann GF: Gore-Tex grafts for replacement of the superior vena cava. *Ann Thorac Surg* 1977, 23:539.

48 Fujiwara Y, Cohn LH, Adams D, Collins JJ: Use of Gore-Tex grafts for replacement of the superior and inferior venae cavae. *J Thorac Cardiovasc Surg* 1979, 67:774.

49 Smith DE, Hammon J, Anane-sefah J, Richardson RS, Trimble C: Segmental venous replacement: A comparison of biological and synthetic substitutes. *J Thorac Cardiovasc Surg* 1975, 69:589.

50 Wilson SE, Jabour H, Stone RT, Stanley TM: Patency of biologic and prosthetic inferior vena cava grafts with distal limb fistula. *Arch Surg* 1978, 113:1174.

51 Husfeldt KJ: Venous replacement with Gore-Tex prosthesis: Experimental and first clinical results, in May R, Weber J (eds): *Pelvic and Abdominal Veins: Progress in Diagnostics and Therapy,* International Congress Series 550. Excerpta Medica Amsterdam, 1981, p 249.

52 May R (ed): *Surgery of the Veins of the Leg and Pelvis.* Thieme, Stuttgart, 1979.

53 Faro RS, Watson WD, Roberts AJ, Knauf DG, Alexander JA: Superior vena cava obstruction: Use of the spiral saphenous vein graft. *Contemp Surg* 1983, 23:15.

54 Clowes W: Extra-anatomical by-pass of iliac vein obstruction: Use of a synthetic (expanded polytetrafluoroethylene ⟨Goretex⟩ graft. *Arch Surg* 1980, 115:767.

55 Vollmar JF, Hutschenreiter S: Vascular prosthesis for the venous system, in May R, Weber J (eds): *Pelvic and Abdominal Veins: Progress in Diagnostics and Therapy.* International Congress Series 550. Excerpta Medica, Amsterdam, 1981, p 234.

56 Rosenthal D, Deterling RA, O'Donnell TF, Callow AD: Interposition grafting with expanded polytetrafluoroethylene for portal hypertension. *Surg Gynecol Obstet* 1979, 148:378.

57 Gruss JD, Bartels D, Kawai S, Karadedos C, Tsafandakis E: Application of plastic material in the Palma operation. *Angiology* 1981, 1:51.

58 Eklof B, Broome A, Einarsson E: Venous reconstruction in acute iliac vein obstruction using PTFE grafts, in May R, Weber J (Eds): *Pelvic and Abdominal Veins: Progress in Diagnostics and Therapy.* International Congress Series 550. Excerpta Medica, Amsterdam, 1981, p 259.

59 Ijima H, Sakurai J, HJori M, Kodama R: Temporary arteriovenous fistulae for venous reconstruction using a synthetic graft: Clinical and experimental evaluation. *J Cardiovasc Surg* (Torino) 1981, 22:480.

60 Fiore AC, Cromartie RS, Peigh PS, Deschner WP: Prosthetic replacement for the thoracic vena cava. *J Thorac Cardiovasc Surg* 1982, 84:560.

Invited Commentary

John J. Bergan, M.D.
Chicago, Illinois

In this chapter the author has been scholarly and complete. His opinion of the work of others is informed, candid, and even blunt. It is a remarkable summation of the current status of direct venous reconstruction.

My own beliefs about direct venous reconstruction have recently been summarized.[1] They differ very little from the author's. There are four elements to chronic venous stasis. These are venous obstruction (for which ascending venography is diagnostic), deep venous valvular reflux (for which descending venography is helpful), superficial venous incompetence due to intrinsic venous wall or valvular deficit (for which the physical examination supplemented by photoplethysmographic evaluation with the tourniquet test is diagnostic), and perforator incompetence (for which physical examination is requisite). Any of these four features may exist alone or in combination to produce the final picture of venous stasis disease.

Once the clinical picture is defined, treatment may be determined. For example, stasis produced by superficial incompetence alone is best treated by superficial vein stripping; this is true whether the indication is external hemorrhage, recurrent superficial thrombophlebitis, dermatitis, or simply ill-defined discomfort. Venous obstruction caused by venous thrombosis or poorly recanalized thrombus is well treated by crossover grafting, with or without arteriovenous fistula, or saphenopopliteal bypass, in which two-thirds of the procedures remain patent. It is interesting in respect to the latter procedure that the initial suggestion of Richard Warren[2] to perform transplantation of the saphenous vein to the subsartorial position has not been followed by subsequent surgeons interest in this problem.

With regard to direct venous reconstruction, I believe that direct reconstruction should be performed only in patients with severe, intractable, and incapacitating venous stasis. Treatment of the stasis syndrome must include conventional methods of therapy before newer, less-proven surgical procedures are applied.

With this in mind, I select patients whose outpatient care has failed for admission to the hospital for noninvasive evaluation with impedance plethysmography and photoplethysmography, and invasive evaluation by ascending and descending phlebography utilizing videotape recordings. When surgery is planned, the first-choice procedures include removal of superficial varicosities if the photoplethysmography tourniquet test shows that there is superficial venous incompetence, and superficial varicose vein removal combined with subfascial interruption of perforating veins is a major contributing factor to the venous stasis. In the latter situation, *lifetime graded elastic compression remains the keystone of therapy.* If a patient does not benefit from such surgical procedures and the possibility exists for venous segment transfer, valve reconstruction, valve transplantation, proximal bypass, then one of these is done as a secondary procedure.

Thus, the interesting new reconstructive procedures are reserved for the 15 to 20 percent of patients who fail to benefit from conventional surgical therapy. Adherence to this attitude avoids the situation which is being seen with increasing frequency, in which a patient with severe chronic venous stasis and intractable ulceration is subjected to a proximal venous valve transplantation as the primary surgical procedure and, when this fails, the procedure is discredited and the patient is not improved.

Finally, the experience detailed by the author with externally reinforced PTFE grafts to replace major segments of the venous system has been corroborated by us. This is a significant surgical advance, despite the fact that there are few patients who need such operations.

COMMENTARY REFERENCES

1 Bergan JJ: Overview of potential benefits of direct venous reconstruction. *Int Angiol* (in press).
2 Warren R, Thayer TR: Transplantation of the saphenous vein for postphlebitic stasis. *Surgery* 1954, 35:867–876.

32 CONTROL OF THE INFERIOR VENA CAVA TO PREVENT PULMONARY EMBOLISM

VENA CAVAL LIGATION, CLIPS, AND FILTERS

Despite efforts at prophylaxis venous thromboembolism continues to be a major clinical problem. Its standard treatment by heparin is designed to prevent propagation of the thrombus, to minimize damage to the lumen and valves of the veins, and to avoid pulmonary embolism. Despite repeated efforts to carry the theoretic advantages of enzymatic dissolution of clot into clinical practice,[1] the complexity of management, bleeding complications, and occasional reactions of streptokinase and urokinase therapy have weighed against their general acceptance. Anticoagulation with intravenous heparin remains the standard, backed by continued oral administration of warfarin for some time thereafter. Control of venous thromboembolism by this regimen has been repeatedly documented. Our statistics for 159 episodes in 133 consecutive such patients showed a 3 percent recurrence of pulmonary embolism and 1.5 percent mortality.[2]

Occasionally heparin fails or cannot be used and a mechanical method must be substituted to prevent pulmonary embolism. The two usual indications for this change in strategy include failure of heparin therapy to prevent recurrent embolism and contraindications to the anticoagulant. Rare indications include septic emboli and prophylactic control of the inferior vena cava (IVC) following operations in high-risk patients or after pulmonary embolectomy.

The diagnosis of pulmonary embolism is suggested by the clinical syndrome and supported by perfusion and ventilation lung scans and phlebograms. If control of the inferior vena cava is considered, the diagnosis should be confirmed by pulmonary angiography, which if positive may be followed immediately by placement of a filter.

LIGATION OF THE INFERIOR VENA CAVA

Surgical occlusion of the inferior vena cava became known as a bad operation because of postoperative problems with the legs. It was labeled a life-saving procedure done at the expense of permanent damage to the lower extremities. There were two reasons for this idea. First was poor postoperative care by surgeons who ignored the early venous hypertension because they had little interest in the patient once the operation was done. Second, it was not recognized that the leg problems were often due to deep venous obstruction, which would have produced the postphlebitic syndrome regardless of a caval ligation.[3]

The pessimism of the majority was not universal. Forty years ago Alton Ochsner concluded from a large experience with caval ligation that it was not necessarily done at the expense of function of the lower extremities.[4] The venous hypertension gradually subsided over a period of many months as the venous collateral circulation developed. Animal experience showed how the myriad small venous collaterals gradually changed to fewer more direct ones.[5] This pointed clearly to the importance of careful management of the legs during the period of development of these byways. Two contrasting groups of patients in Atlanta emphasized a difference in postoperative care. The 25 patients followed at a free clinic almost universally developed leg problems of pain, edema, and ulcers.[6] On the other hand, in the 11 private patients of Poer there was only 1 such problem.[7] The difference between patients whose postoperative care was at best indifferent and patients receiving personalized management of their venous hypertension demonstrated that postoperative management was considerably more important than the technical performance of the ligation.

Postoperative care of the lower extremities still is important, whether the vena cava be tied, clipped, or filtered (Figure 32-1).

FIGURE 32-1 The legs are normal 18 months after ligation of the inferior vena cava. Skin pallor is seen where knee-length elastic hose have been worn.

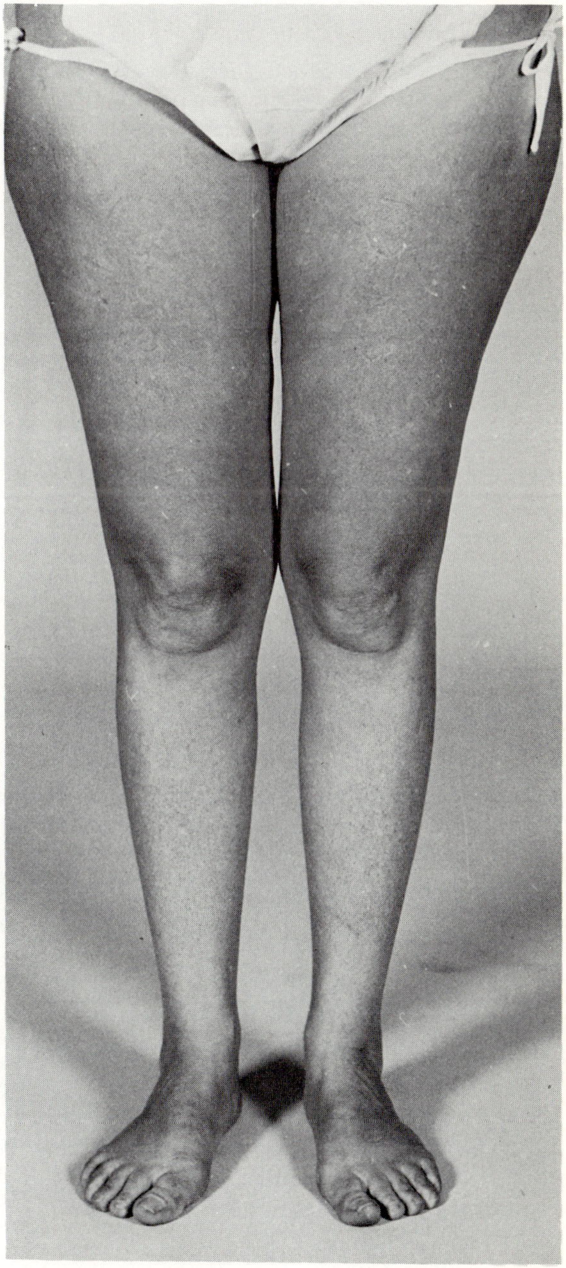

Current Indications

Ligation of the inferior vena cava presently may seem to be of historical interest only,[8] but it does have a place. First, it is the simplest of all methods of caval control and may be useful in an isolated environment where fluoroscopy screens and multiple helpers are not available. A knowledgeable surgeon can tie the IVC without a sophisticated laboratory or skilled assistants.

Second, for one reason or another, a filter cannot be passed and placed in occasional patients. The informed consent to operation should recognize these few and allow an immediate change to ligation or plication of the cava.

Third, there are the occasional patients who embolize after a clip or filter is placed. These few may be managed by transabdominal ligation of the infrarenal vena cava plus both gonadal veins. Only two such have occurred in my experience.

Technique

The inferior vena cava may be approached transperitoneally (which allows concomitant ligation of the gonadal veins) or, preferably, via a right retroperitoneal approach, as for lumbar sympathectomy (Figure 32-2). Writers usually suggest double ligation of the vein with 0-0 silk. Why two ties is better than one is uncertain, except to comfort an insecure surgeon. A single umbilical tape tie does as well. There is no need to divide the cava.

Descriptions of IVC ligation usually recommend that the tie be placed here or there. Practically, one finds the cava and ties it superior to the iliac vein bifurcation. It is a 20-minute procedure for a quite ill patient.[9]

Anatomic Anomalies

Misplaced left-sided inferior vena cavas as well as double veins have been described.[10] When pulmonary embolism occurs after any form of control of the cava, the possibility of an anomaly should be investigated at once. Variations should be in mind whenever the cava is visualized with radiopaque material. Anomalies may also be first found in the operating room, in which event the technique must be modified accordingly.

FIGURE 32-2 The inferior vena cava and both gonadal veins may be ligated via an upper midline or paramedian incision. Most patients do without the gonadal venous occlusion. The tranverse incision *(insert)* provides adequate exposure of the cava via a retroperitoneal approach.

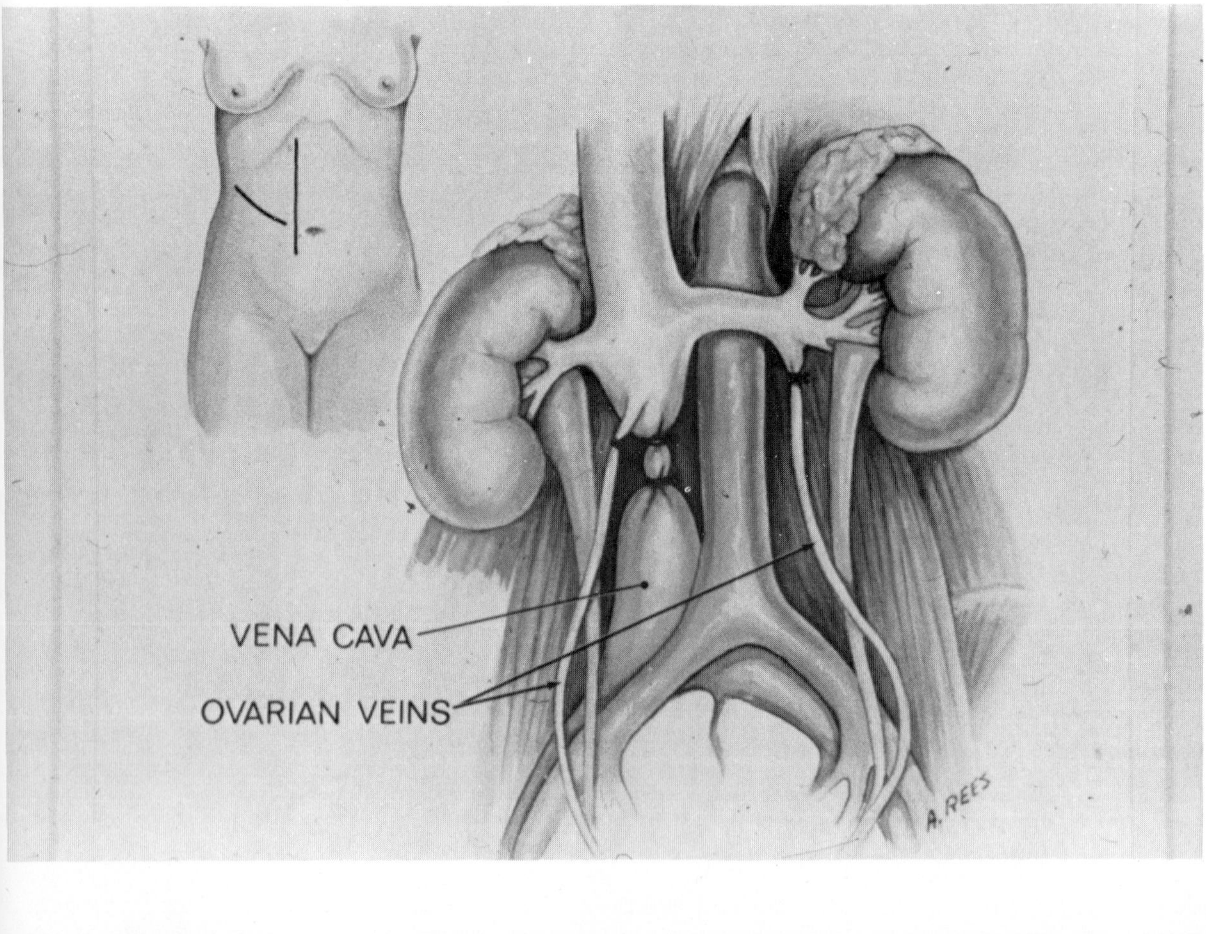

Complications

Complications of caval ligation or plication include intraoperative injury to the vein. Local pressure will stop hemorrhage while lights, assistants, and instruments are assembled. In fact, all else failing, a pack may be left to control the situation until another day. Ordinarily, however, a "U"-shaped vascular clamp should be placed and the laceration (often a torn tributary) sutured.

Occasional instances of distal pooling of venous blood with inadequate return to the heart have occurred. This may be tested by temporary placement of a vascular clamp upon the IVC for 5 minutes prior to its actual ligation. Unfortunately, this brief test is not always definitive.

Retroperitoneal bleeding is not expected unless the patient is heparinized. Anticoagulation is theoretically useful to diminish the likelihood of immediate extensive thrombosis of the pelvic and leg veins. Such occlusion is uncommon (although it may already be present) and does not usually justify the risk of bleeding incurred with heparin use.

Results

Among 32 ligations of the inferior vena cava there was a single death, 2 hours later, probably due to blood pooling distally. There were no known instances of recurrent pulmonary embolism. All patients except two returned to their former occupation and life-style, although there was some degree of leg symptoms in several. No primary caval ligations have been done since the filters became available.

PLICATION AND CLIPPING OF THE INFERIOR VENA CAVA

Recognition of venous hypertension resulting from caval ligation led to various attempts to modify the procedure to reduce this pressure. Thirty years ago we studied absorbable gut ligation of the IVC in 45 dogs, finding that 85 percent became reconstituted.[11] Experiments continued and in 1956 five patients underwent gut ligation without difficulty.[5]

About that time others developed methods of partially occluding the cava, some by placing a series of compartmentalization sutures and others by enclosing the vein in a clip with serrations, which accomplished the same (Figure 32-3).[12,13] Initially it was hoped that such plication procedures would control embolism while not producing venous hypertension in the legs. This promise was not fulfilled, because many plicated or clipped cavae become occluded, because of either local thrombosis or trapped emboli (Figure 32-4).[14]

The "plicators" and the "ligators" discussed their preferences without either side achieving a clear decision.[15,16] After tabulating the statistics and claims, it appeared that the debate merely emphasized personal bias and that no rational differentiation was possible.[17] If so, the simplest method should be used, which to me was ligation. The argument became moot when the filter was developed.

The clip is still useful for prophylactic control of the inferior vena cava when the abdomen is already open in a high-risk patient. The Adams-DeWeese or the Miles clip may be placed more easily than sutures to plicate the vein.

IVC FILTERS

Ligations and plications of the cava did prevent pulmonary embolism but required general anesthesia and a major operation for patients who often were already critically ill. The next progression was control of the caval route of embolization from a distant point of access using local anesthesia.

The development of a method to prevent pulmonary embolism through the inferior vena cava by an indwelling filter device was a sizable step forward. Currently there are available three filters and one balloon device which can be placed under local anesthesia through the jugular or femoral vein (Table 32-1 and Figure 32-5). The characteristics to be considered in choosing one or

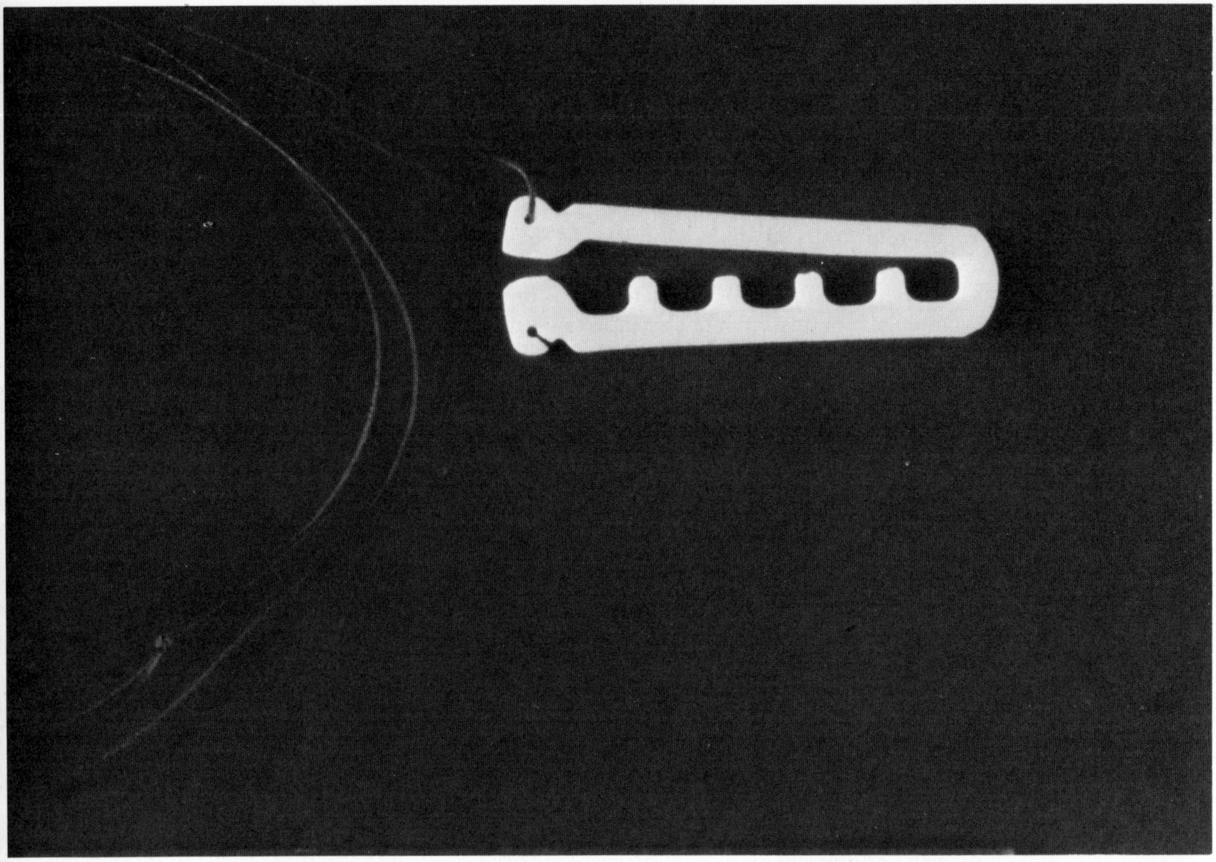

FIGURE 32-3 The Adams-DeWeese serrated clip may be slipped around the inferior vena cava. The suture binds its ends together.

another of these for a patient include (1) the ease of placement, (2) the likelihood of misplacement, (3) the possibility of intravascular migration, (4) the rate of long-term patency of the cava, (5) the incidence of recurrent embolism, and (6) the incidence of complications due to the device itself. Each of the devices will be discussed in their order of appearance upon the surgical scene.

Mobin-Uddin Filter

The first of the intraluminal devices was introduced in 1967 as a Silastic umbrella with metal vanes. The initial dimension of a 23-mm diameter proved too small for most cavas. Improper placement and migration accompanied early efforts. The change in diameter to 28 mm solved the size problem, while experience allowed safe and secure placement for most patients (Figure 32-6).

The results after placement of the Mobin-Uddin filter are reminiscent of the controversy which occurred between the plicators and ligators. One Boston group in 1980 reported no recurrent embolisms among 128 patients. Only 16 percent had severe leg edema.[18] Another Boston group a year later had different results and expressed dissatisfaction with the Mobin-Uddin filter. Their retrospective study of 41 patients showed recurrent embolism in 12 percent and occlusion of the vena cava in 85 percent.[19]

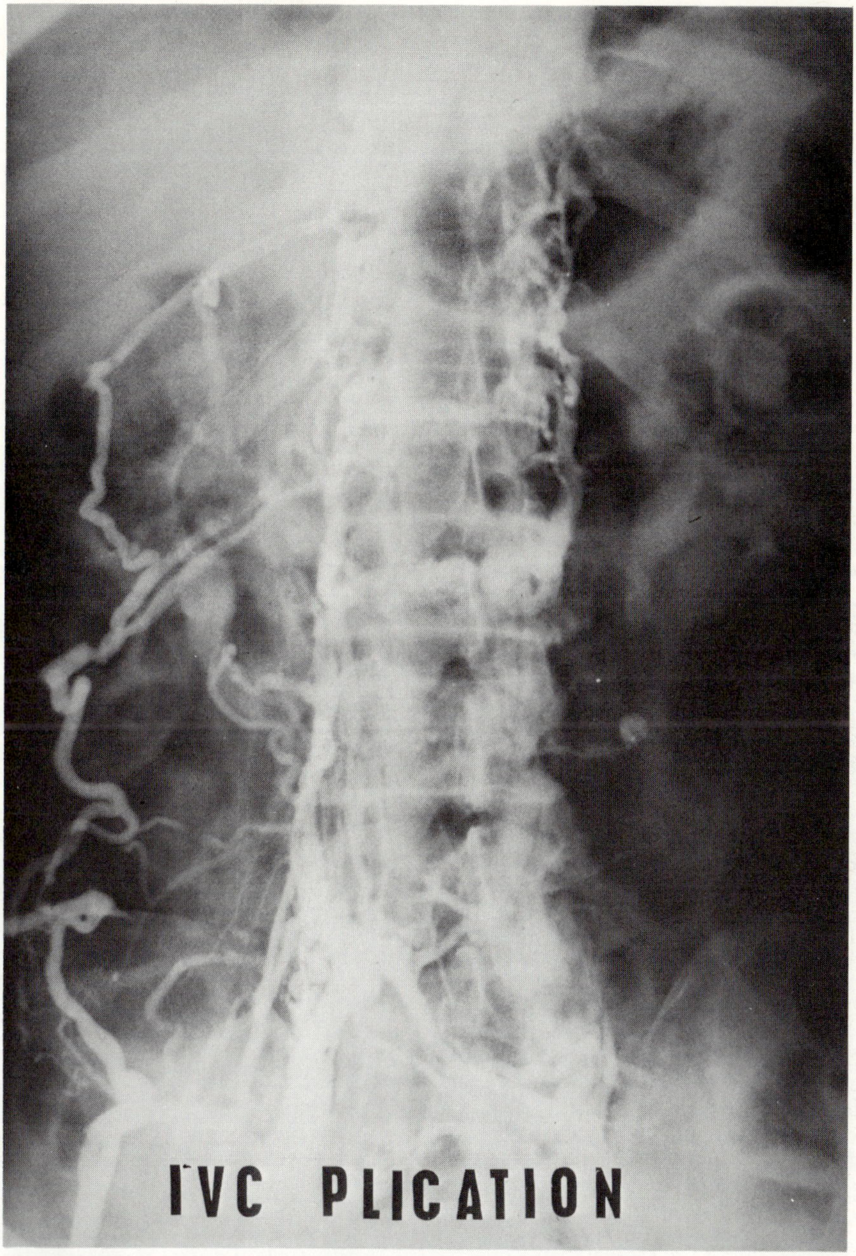

FIGURE 32-4 Caval thrombosis occurred after a clip was applied.

Personal experience with 33 placements of the Mobin-Uddin filter was better. There were no instancces of incorrect placment or of migration (Figures 32-7 and 32-8). Two patients had later embolism, one of which was treated by ligation of the inferior vena cava and ovarian veins. The other refused another operation. One patient died suddenly as the carrier passage was begun, suggesting massive embolism. This episode triggered reevaluation and a shift to general anesthesia with an endotracheal tube in place.

TABLE 32-1 DEVICES TO CONTROL EMBOLISM THROUGH THE INFERIOR VENA CAVA

Device	Technique			Recurrent embolism, %	Long-term patency, %	Limb venous stasis, %	Caval occlusion, %
	Percutaneous	Transjugular	Transfemoral				
Hunter balloon[30]	No	Yes	No	2	0	30	100
Mobin-Uddin filter[18]	No	Yes	Yes	3	28	9	73
Greenfield filter[23]	No	Yes	Yes	2 to 3	98	0	5
Roehm filter[28]*	Yes	Yes	Yes	0	100	0	0

*Statistics based upon only 28 cases.

Venous stasis of the legs was not a problem, probably because of intense prophylactic efforts to prevent edema. The incidence of total caval occulsion is unknown because most patients have not had later cavagrams.

FIGURE 32-5 *Left,* a Greenfield filter; *center,* Roehm's bird's nest; *right,* a Mobin-Uddin filter.

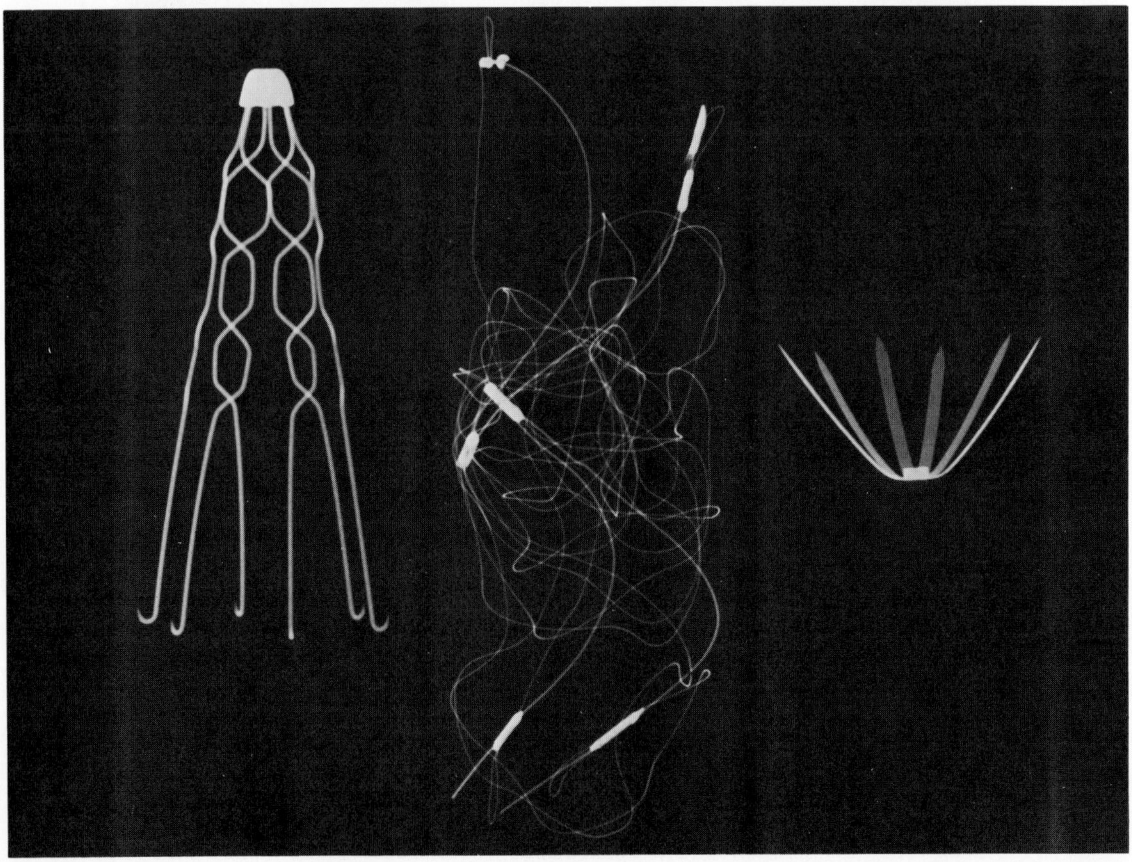

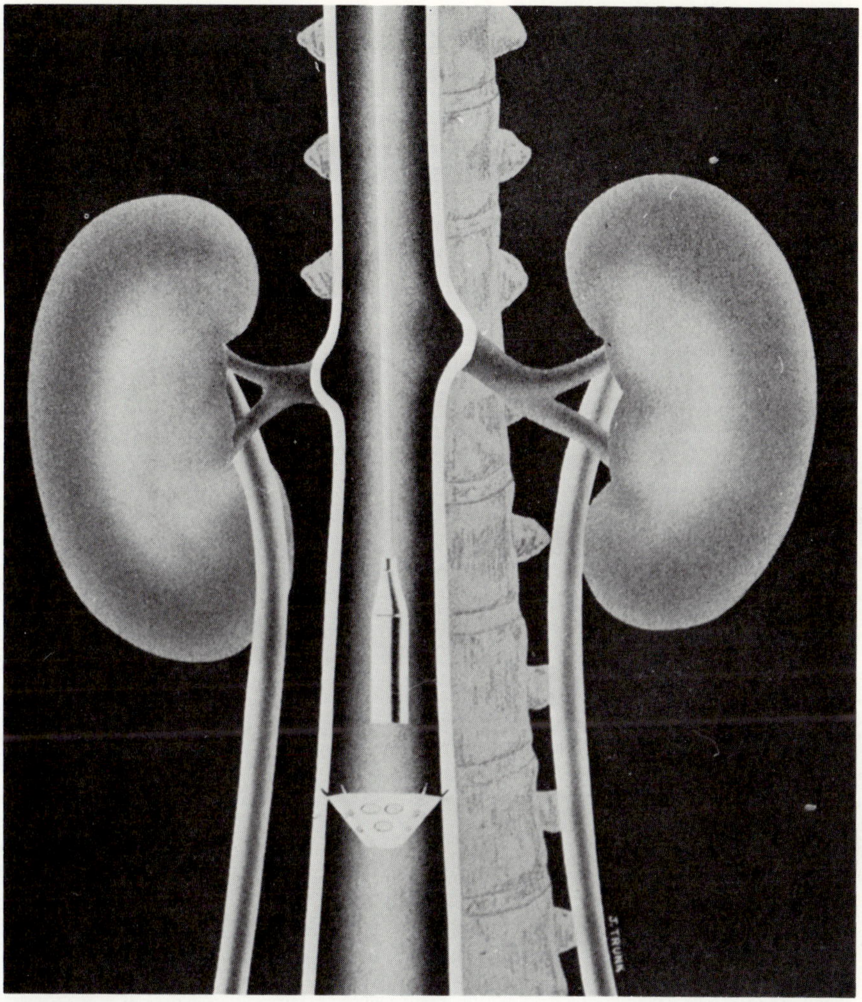

FIGURE 32-6 The Mobin-Uddin umbrella filter is ejected from its carrier after it is lodged in the infrarenal vena cava.

Greenfield Filter

The most popular of such devices currently offers a higher rate of continued caval patency than its predecessor (Figure 32-9). Cimochowski and associates in 1980 retrospectively studied the autopsy and phlebographic results of 65 Mobin-Uddin (28 percent caval patency) and 32 Greenfield filters (95 percent caval patency). The better patency results of the Greenfield device were attested by no clinical evidences of venous stasis, while 9 percent of patients developed this after a Mobin-Uddin device was placed.[20] Gomez's group similarly reported a 97 percent patency rate and only one patient with severe venous stasis syndrome.[21]

The Greenfield filter placed over an indwelling but removable guide wire may be passed through either the jugular or femoral vein. The inventor reported 260 patients, without death due to the procedure and with only 5 instances of recurrent thromboembolism. Some 98 retained

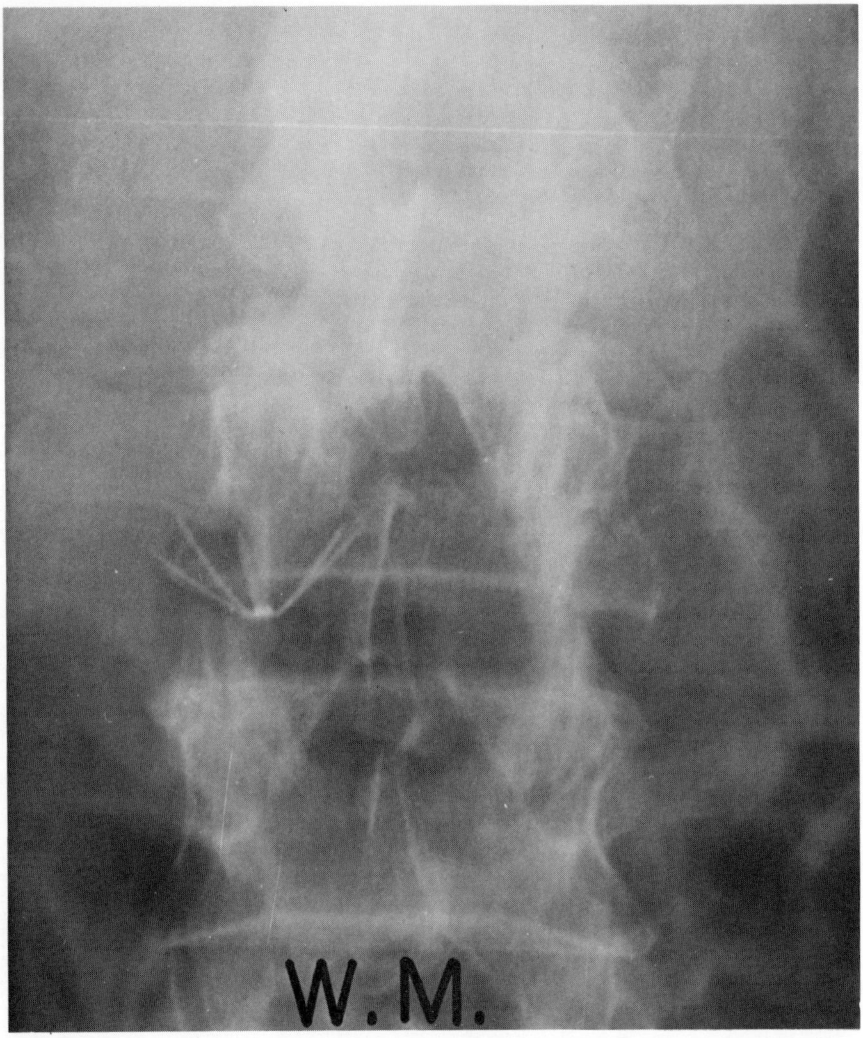

FIGURE 32-7 The Mobin-Uddin filter position is documented by a plain roentgenogram immediately after it is placed.

caval patency,[22,23] a figure similar to the 95 percent reported by Wingerd and associates.[24] The rate of recurrent embolism was 2 percent.

Since caval occlusion is unlikely after the Greenfield filter is placed, the filter may be used in the suprarenal position if the caval thrombosis extends proximally, as well in the gonadal veins. Orsini and Jarrell's nine such patients had no problems during their 1- to 14-month follow-ups.[25] Greenfield's 10 patients also did well.

It should be recognized that the hooks of the filter often completely penetrate the wall of the vena cava,[22] although this does not usually cause any problem.[20,26,27]

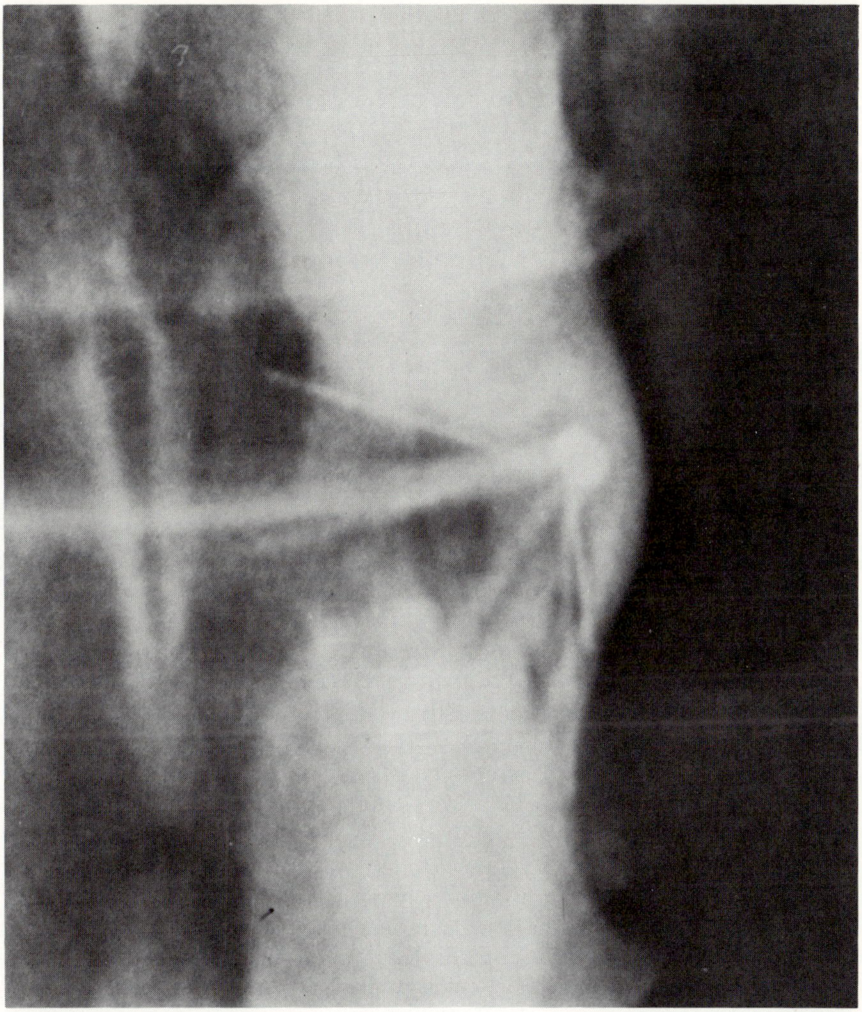

FIGURE 32-8 A year after insertion this Mobin-Uddin filter is tipped but has not migrated within the still-patent inferior vena cava.

Roehm Filter

The "bird's-nest" filter introduced recently has been used successfully in 40 patients by Roehm and in another 20 by others. The filter does not require a cutdown or open operation, and this appears to be a real advance.[28] As of August 1984 it had not ben released for general use.

The Hunter Balloon

This total occlusion absolutely blocks the IVC by placement of a detachable balloon filled with 25 percent Hypaque, which allows it to be followed radiographically (Figure 32-10). Hunter has

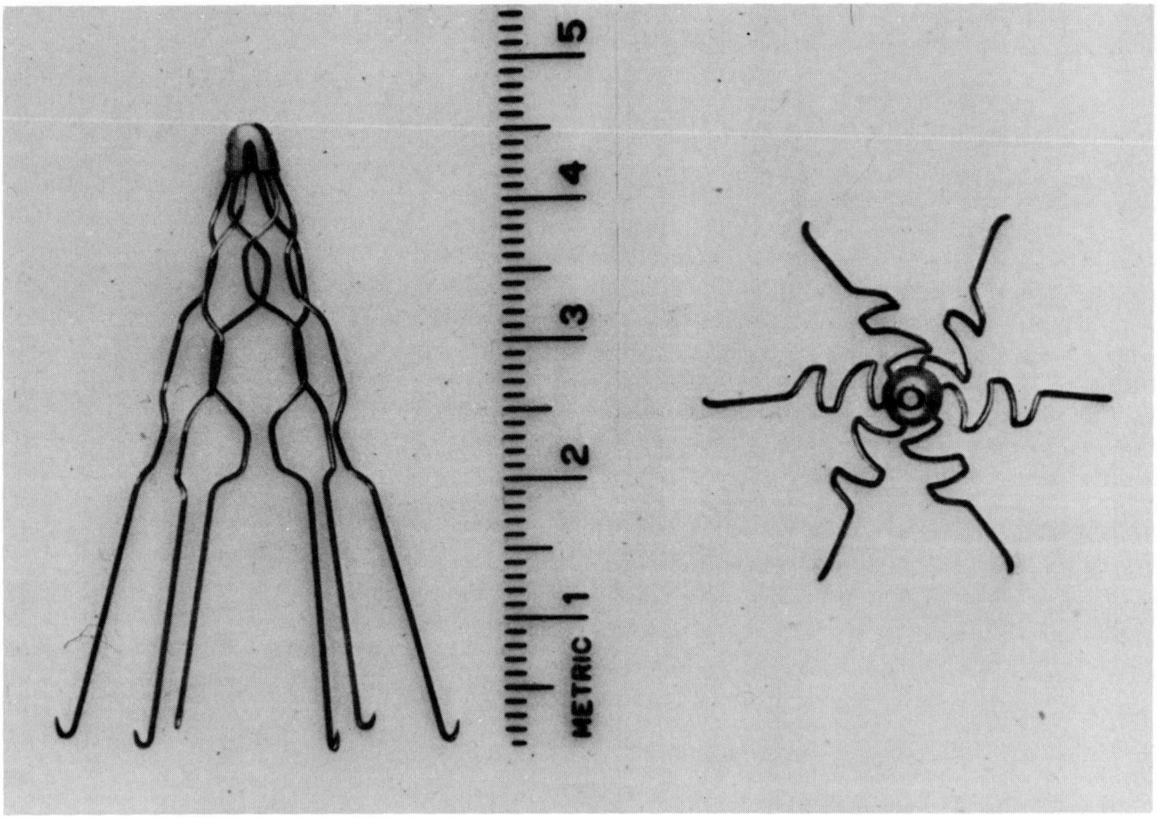

FIGURE 32-9 A Greenfield filter.

placed this in 135 patients since 1970 [29] without early reembolization and with 2 late instances (2 percent) of pulmonary embolism. Leg results have been similar to those expected after actual ligation of the inferior vena cava and have depended considerably upon whether or not significant deep venous thrombosis is present as well as upon postoperative care.[29]

CHOICE OF DEVICE

Personal experience and the reports of others have led to these conclusions. First, the incidence of error is so high that the diagnosis of pulmonary embolism should be confirmed by pulmonary arteriograms prior to any vena caval procedure. Ordinarily we schedule arteriography and then filter placement, so one follows the other if the diagnosis is confirmed.

Second is the necessity of a team accustomed to dealing with large vessels and with critically ill patients. Rather than attempt to place a filter alone in a setting without experienced help and video screen visualization, it would be safer to ligate or clip the cava.

Third, a filter can be placed more safely in an anesthetized patient, who is receiving oxygen through an endotracheal tube with indwelling "lines" where needed, than in one receiving local anesthesia, which often requires undesired doses of sedatives, resulting in hypoxia. The new Roehm filter may change this, since it is placed percutaneously.

Fourth, if the filter is placed properly, it does not usually migrate or cause complications.

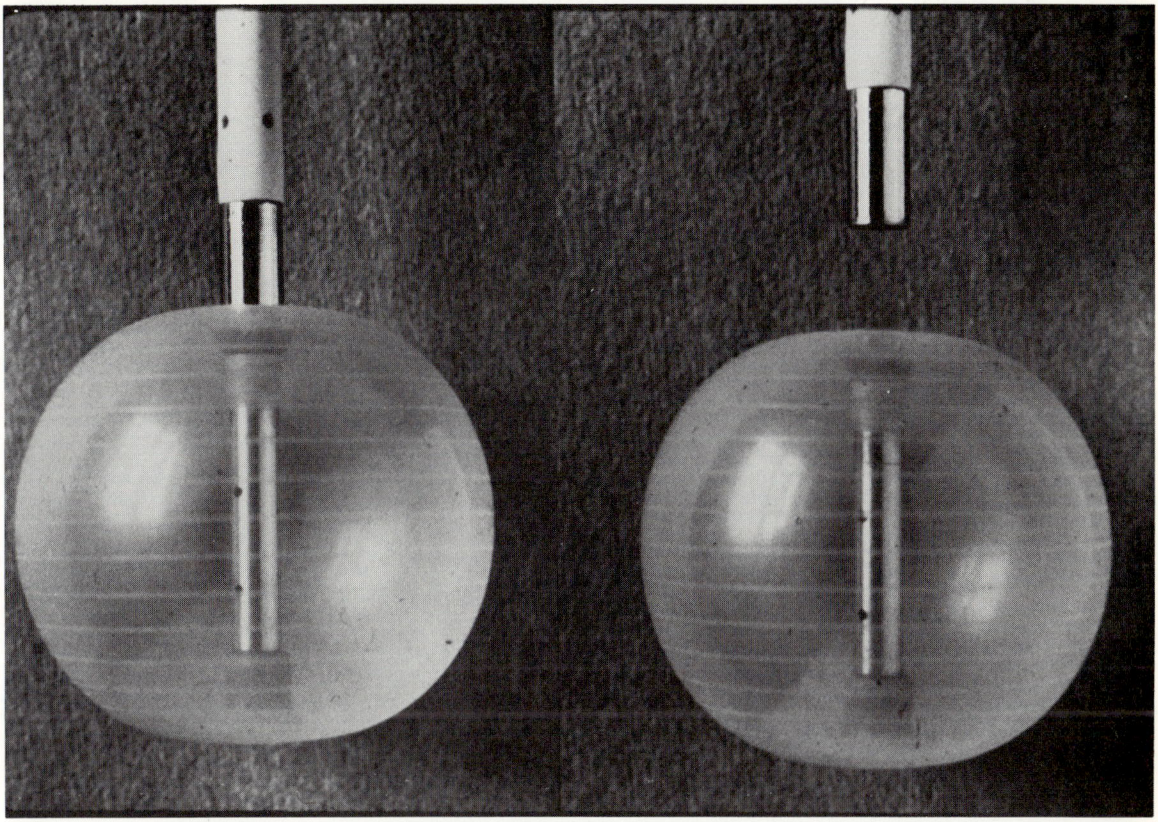

FIGURE 32-10 A Hunter balloon on a carrier, *left,* and ejected from the carrier, *right,* to lie within the vena cava.

Fifth, the correct timing as well as the duration of postoperative anticoagulation is uncertain. If the patient has no flank pain or tenderness and if the hematocrit has not decreased 18 hours after placement of the filter, it is reasonable to resume systemic heparinization, which may be continued for 5 days. If that is contraindicated, warfarin is begun and continued for 3 months on an outpatient basis.

Sixth, custom-fitted elastic hose are used for at least a year after the filter is placed, longer if edema becomes persistent.

Postoperative Management After Ties, Clips, or Filters

Elevation of the extremities along with external pressure form the basic plan to encourage venous flow and prevent edema during a period when venous hypertension is likely (Table 32-2). As shown in Figure 32-11, the "venous

TABLE 32-2 MANAGEMENT AFTER INFERIOR VENA CAVAL PROCEDURES

1	Prevent edema
	Elevation of feet
	External elastic compression
2	Prevent further thrombosis
	Heparin Intravenously
	Warfarin by mouth
3	Exercise
	Early walking, but no sitting
	Continued program of leg exercise

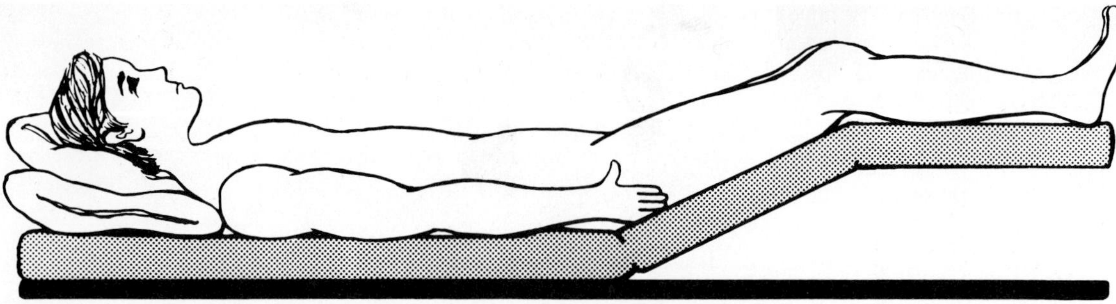

FIGURE 32-11 The venous position in bed elevates the lower legs and feet above heart level.

position" in bed provides elevation of the legs above heart level. The hip and knee flexion is considerably more comfortable than simple elevation of the foot of the bed. Early ambulation is required, but sitting is prohibited, so for the first 5 to 7 days the patient either lies in the venous position or walks. She or he does not stand without walking in place. Brief visits to the toilet are allowed.

Both lower extremities are wrapped snugly with wide elastic bandages extending from the toes to the high thigh. These require changes at each nursing shift, or by the patient or family as required. Custom-fitted elastic hose replace the wraps at 7 to 10 days. These are prescribed only to the knee level. Higher, thigh-length hose are uncomfortable, difficult to maintain in position, and not needed after the early several days. The knee-length hose are used for a year, at which time most patients may be allowed gradually to taper off until they no longer wear hose. If any edema occurs thereafter, the hose are at once replaced.

A regular exercise program to prevent loss of muscle tone and mass in the legs is mandatory. It is started several weeks after the operation. This may consist of rapid walking (13 to 15 minutes per mile) twice daily or, better, swimming. Running during the first year often causes problems so is not advised. Biking is similar.

To be reiterated is the importance of preventing edema at any time so that the patient returns to a level of work and play equivalent to the preoperative state. This has been generally true of the patients having IVC ligation as well as those having filter placement. Three patients did have postoperative leg problems. One was a truck driver whose legs were constantly dependent while at work, another was an alcoholic who would not wear hose, and the third was uncooperative for other reasons. With proper postoperative care the life-saving potential of a caval filter need not be accompanied by limb disability.

REFERENCES

1 Cairols MA, Marco-Luque MA, Caralt MT, Ballon H, Aced S, Capdevila JM: A phlebographic and ultrasonic evaluation of fibrinolytic therapy. *Vasc Diag Treat* May–June 1983, p 37.
2 Dale WA, Lewis MR: Heparin control of venous thromboembolism. *Arch Surg* 1970, 101:744.
3 Kirtley JA, Riddell DH, Hamilton EC: Indications and late results of ligation of inferior vena cava. *Ann Surg* 1955, 141:661.
4 Ochsner A: Discussion of Kirtley JA, Riddell DH, Hamilton EC: Indications and late results of ligation of inferior vena cava. *Ann Surg* 1955, 141:661.
5 Dale WA, Pualwan F, Bauer FM: Ligation of inferior vena cava with absorbable gut. *Surg Gynecol Obstet* 1956, 102:516.
6 Shea PC, Robertson Rl: Late sequelae of inferior vena cava ligation. *Surg Gynecol Obstet* 1951, 93:153.
7 Poer DH: Postoperative thromboembolism. *Ann Surg* 1952, 135:687.
8 Dale WA: Ligation of the inferior vena cava for thromboembolism: Comprehensive discussion with 16 illustrative cases. *Surgery* 1958, 43:24.

9 Dale WA: Inferior vena caval ligation for venous thromboembolism. *Rev Surg* 1962, 19:1.
10 Edwards EA: Clinical anatomy of lesser variations of the inferior vena cava and a proposal for classifying the anomalies of this vessel. *Angiology* 1951, 2:85.
11 Pualwan F, Jones G, Bruny S, Dale WA: Effects of ligation of the inferior vena cava with absorbable ligature. *ACS Clin Congr Forum* 1954, 1:179.
12 Miles RM, Elsea PW: Clinical evaluation of the serrated vena caval clip. *Surg Gynecol Obstet* 1971, 132:581.
13 Adams JT, DeWeese JA: Partial interruption of the inferior vena cava with a new plastic clip. *Surg Gynecol Obstet* 1966, 123:1087.
14 Bergan JJ: Discussion of Lindenauer SM: Prophylactic staple plication of the inferior vena cava. *Arch Surg* 1973, 107:669.
15 Adams JT, Feingold BE, DeWeese JA: Comparative evaluation of ligation and partial interruption of the inferior vena cava. *Arch Surg* 1971, 103:272.
16 Lindenauer SM: Prophylactic staple plication of the inferior vena cava. *Arch Surg* 1973, 107:669.
17 Kersten T, Varco RL: Vena caval interruption: The why, the how, the uncertainties, in Norjarian JS, Delaney JP (eds): *Vascular Surgery.* Symposia Specialists, Miami, 1978.
18 Menzoian JO, LoGerfo FW, Qeitzman AF, Ezpeleta M, Sequeira JC: Clinical experience with the Mobin-Uddin vena cava umbrella filter. *Arch Surg* 1980 115:1179.
19 Adelson J, Steer ML, Glotzer DJ, Skilman JJ, Simon M, Salzman EW: Thromboembolism after insertion of the Mobin-Uddin caval filter. *Surgery* 1980, 87:184.
20 Cimochowski GE, Evans, RH, Zarins CK, Lu CT, Demeester TR: Greenfield filter versus Mobin-Uddin umbrella. *J Thor Cardiovasc Surg* 1980, 79:358.
21 Gomez GA, Cuttler BS Wheeler HB: Transvenous interruption of the inferior vena cava. *Surgery* 1983, 93:612.
22 Greenfield LJ, Stewart JR: Improved technique for insertion of Greenfield vena cava filter. *Surg Gynecol Obstet* 1983, 156:217.
23 Greenfield LJ: Current indications for and results of Greenfield filter placement. *J Vasc Surg* 1984, 1:502.
24 Wingerd M, Bernhard VM, Maddison F, Towne JB: Comparison of caval filters in the management of venous thromboembolism. *Arch Surg* 1978, 113:1264.
25 Orsini RA, Jarrell BE: Suprarenal placement of vena cava filters: Indications, techniques and results. *J Vasc Surg* 1984, 1:124.
26 Greenfield LJ: Discussion of Hunter JA, DeLaria GA, Goldin MD, Javid H, Najafi H, Serry C: Requirements for a method of transvenous inferior vena cava interruption. *Arch Surg* 1980: 115:1324.
27 Phillips MR, Widrich WC, Johnson WC: Perforation of the inferior vena cava by the Kim-Ray Greenfield filter. *Surgery* 1980, 87:233.
28 Roehm JOF Jr: The bird's nest filter: A new percutaneous transcatheter inferior vena cava filter. *J Vasc Surg* 1984, 1:498.
29 Hunter JA, Session R, Buenger R: Experimental balloon obstruction of the vena cava. *Arch Surg* 1970, 171:315.
30 Hunter JA, DeLaria GA: Hunter vena cava balloon: Rationale and results. *J Vasc Surg* 1984, 1:491.

another center, well-known for its interest in venous thromboembolism, only 3 operations were

Invited Commentary

James A. DeWeese, M.D.
Rochester, New York

This is a clear exposition of the management of patients who require something more than anticoagulation or thrombolytic therapy for the management of recurrent pulmonary emboli secondary to venous thrombosis of the lower extremity. It is a practical approach to the management of these problems based upon basic physiologic principles coupled with an extensive clinical experience. I would like to emphasize two points, disagree mildly with another point, and present experiences with an additional form of therapy, pulmonary embolectomy, which may be used for uncontrolled massive pulmonary emboli.

The first point worthy of emphasis is that the need for vena caval interruption is rare. With proper prophylaxis and the judicidous use of anticoagulant therapy, significant pulmonary embolism can be prevented. Less than 10 percent of patients who are being treated for deep venous thrombosis develop primary pulmonary emboli, and recurrent emobli are even rarer. Less than three vena caval interruptions per year are currently being performed in our institution,[1] and at another center, well-known for its interest in venous thromboembolism, only 3 operations were performed in 50 patients treated for thromboembolism over a 6-year period.[2] The author found vena caval interruption necessary in less than 3 percent of patients treated. In addition to excellent preventive therapy, insistence upon a positive pulmonary arteriographic diagnosis of pulmonary embolism before performing an unnecessary venous interruption is laudable.

The second point is the importance of controlling edema following venous interruptions. Edema is a result of venous hypertension which may result from preexisting or progressive venous thrombosis. It may also be caused by occlusion of the vena cava from ligation or from thrombus either forming at the site of a partial-interruption device or embolizing there from a peripheral venous thrombosis. The resulting edema not only contributes to early morbidity, but also sets the stage for a later secondary lymphedema, recurrent cellulitis, and prolonged disability. In the early postoperative period only elevation is effective in controlling edema. Daily monitoring is necessary to determine if elevation is adequate. Marked elevation and prolonged elevation may be necessary. When patients ambulate, it is important that they walk and not sit, except for the use of a commode. Elastic support should be used whenever a patient is not elevating his or her legs above the level of the heart. Strong elastic support must be used, preferably with a pressure gradient. The continued daily monitoring of ankle, calf, and thigh circumferences is necessary to determine if sufficient elevation and sufficiently strong elastic support are being used.

The author indicates that after an early preference for ligation as the procedure of choice for venous interruption, he now prefers the intracaval devices for routine use and suggests that clips can be used if the abdomen is already open. I do think that regardless of the approach it is important that a partial interruption, and not a total occlusion, be performed. A review of the literature on vena caval interruptions supports this thesis.[1] Following ligation of the cava, venous pooling and decreased venous return to the heart may result in sudden cardiovascular collapse, as occurred in 1 of 32 cases of vena caval ligation reported by Dr. Dale. This, of course, does not occur with partial interruptions. Partial interruption and ligation are equally effective in preventing fatal pulmonary emboli. Recurrent small pulmonary emboli can occur following both procedures. Thrombi may embolize through the partial interruption device or through collaterals which develop rapidly after ligation. When postoperative vena cavagrams have been performed, there has been a greater than 60 percent incidence of patency reported for all of the partial-interruption devices. The use of partial interruption, therefore, can decrease the risk of venous hypertension in both the immediate and late postoperative courses.

Fatal pulmonary emboli may still occur during the best of therapy. Autopsy series indicate that 25 percent of patients who ultimately die of their embolism live for more than 2 hours after onset of their symptoms. If cardiopulmonary bypass is readily available, pulmonary embolectomy can be successfully performed. Therefore, if the diagnosis is promptly established, there is a small group of patients whose lives might be saved by operative intervention. We have performed pulmonary embolectomy on cardiopulmonary bypass on 10 patients.[3] Of the five patients who had had cardiac arrest prior to institution of cardiopulmonary bypass, only two survived the procedure, and they died of complications secondary to cerebral anoxia. On the other hand, among the five patients in whom cardiopulmonary bypass was instituted when patients were hypotensive but had not yet arrested, four of the patients are long-term survivors.

COMMENTARY REFERENCES

1 Adams JT, DeWeese JA: Venous interruptions, in Haimovici H (ed): *Vascular Surgery: Principles and Techniques.* Appleton-Century-Crofts, Norwalk, Connecticut, 1984, pp 99–1005.

2 Silver D, Sabiston DC Jr: The role of vena caval interruption in the management of pulmonary embolism. *Surgery* 1975, 77:1–10.

3 DeWeese JA: The role of pulmonary embolectomy in venous thromboembolism *J Cardiovasc Surg* (Torino) 1976, 17:348–353.

33 LYMPHEDEMA

Little known by internists, rarely seen by pediatricians, shunned by technically oriented arterial surgeons, and referred elsewhere by general surgeons, lymphedema is a lesion in limbo whose effects have largely been treated by dermatologists and plastic surgeons, at times with little regard for its pathologic physiology. Nonetheless, lymphedema is a part of the vascular disease spectrum and certainly requires understanding and management by the qualified vascular surgeon.

CLASSIFICATION OF EDEMA OF THE LEG

Edema of the lower extremity may be due to venous, lymphatic, or systemic causes or to a combination of these, as outlined in Table 33-1. Unilateral swelling suggests that the etiology is venous or lymphatic obstruction and not a remote or general cause, which would be associated with bilateral edema of the lower extremities as well as of other soft parts of the body. General causes of edema are omitted from discussion, with the exception below.

Idiopathic Cyclic Edema

This deserves some comment because it is not well known or often recognized. It is a recurrent edema of the feet, hands, and face of women who are, usually, overweight and who often have obvious psychologic problems, which further confuse the diagnosis. The recurrent edema progresses as the day wears on, and the patient may change to larger clothes as water accumulates in the body.

Although it has been suggested that cyclic edema is caused by increased aldosterone production, this may be a secondary compensatory phenomenon, since normal individuals who experience an excess of aldosterone secretion do not long retain salt or swell excessively but escape these effects. Studies of the excretion of water and minerals may be helpful, but the basic diagnostic test consists of an accurate record of the patient's morning and evening weights to determine whether there is an actual increase greater than that seen in normal individuals.

Therapy is far from completely effective, but the use of a restricted-sodium diet coupled with dextroamphetamine and amobarbital (Amytal) and a low dose of spironolactone has been found helpful. Rovner has an excellent review of this problem.[1]

Cyclic edema affects both lower extremities, as well as other parts of the body, and should be differentiated from other causes of swollen leg.

TABLE 33-1 ETIOLOGY OF EDEMA OF THE LEG

General	Lymphatic
Hepatic cirrhosis	Primary lymphedema
Heart failure	Congenital lymphedema
Nephrosis	Lymphedema praecox
Hypoproteinemia	Lymphedema tarda
Allergic disorders	Acquired secondary edema
Venous	Infection
Acute thrombosis	Filariasis
Chronic postphlebitic syndrome	Lymphogranuloma venereum
Extrinsic pressure	Tuberculosis
Tumor	Syphilis
Retroperitoneal fibrosis	Radiation
Pressure of overlying iliac artery	Surgery
Interruption	Toxicity
Trauma	Snakebite
Surgery	Insect bite
Arteriovenous fistula	Miscellaneous
	Infection
	Inflammation after vascular repair

CLASSIFICATION OF LYMPHEDEMA

Lymphedema is swelling due to the collection of lymph in the interstitial tissues, resulting from anatomic abnormalities and/or functional overload. It may be primary or secondary (Table 33-2). Primary or idiopathic edema may be present at birth as a congenital form. More often primary lymphedema becomes manifest in the teens or twenties and is then termed lymphedema praecox.[2] Figure 33-1 shows a unilateral example. Occasionally, its appearance may be delayed until after age 35, and it is then termed lymphedema tarda.[3] The relative numbers of patients developing clinical evidence of lymphedema at various ages are shown in Table 33-3.

Elephantiasis

This was defined by Matas in 1913 as a "progressive histopathologic fibromatosis or hypertrophy of the hypodermal and dermal connective tissues"[4] but has been loosely used to describe several conditions in which severe chronic swelling and skin changes occur. It implies severe and grotesque deformation of a limb. Both lymphatic and venous causes have been included under this descriptive term, which refers not to a specific etiology but only to the clinical state of an extremity. Pratt suggested that the term originated during the campaign of the Roman army in Libya, when some of the natives captured had limbs resembling those of the pachyderm in size and texture.[5]

TABLE 33-2 CLASSIFICATION OF LYMPHEDEMA

1 Primary
- Congenital—present at birth*
- Praecox—begins at an early age
- Tarda—begins at a later age

2 Secondary (acquired)
- Inflammatory—granulomatous
  - Filarial
  - From lymphogranuloma venereum
  - Tuberculous
  - Syphilitic
- From recurrent lymphangitis
- Postphlebitic
- Postoperative
- Postradiation
- Tumor
- Toxic
  - From insect bite
  - From snakebite

*Milroy's disease is also familial.

Milroy's Disease

In 1890 Nonne described a family with lymphedema that was both hereditary and congenital.[6] Later this came to be known as Milroy's disease after he described its occurrence in 24 members of a 97-member family in 1892 (and an additional 30 in 1928). The ensuing literature is confusing because different authors have used the eponym to describe various syndromes. In Europe it is sometimes called Meige's disease.[7]

The 1966 summary of Ersek, Danese, and Howard noted that 22 percent of the original family described by Milroy were affected although later information increased the incidence to 28 percent. These authors believe the disease is transmitted in a sex-linked dominant pattern.[8] Kinmonth's 1957 report of 107 cases of primary edema showed that 17 percent had a positive family history.[9] This hereditary tendency fits the concept of the disease as an inborn error of development of the lymphatics. Whether lymphedema occurs at birth (Milroy's disease) or a few years later (lymphedema praecox) is probably dependent upon the degree of abnormality. The separation of the two forms of lymphedema is therefore an artificial one. Figure 33-2 shows a father and son with hereditary lymphedema, which was not present in either at birth, although there is little doubt the lymphatics were congenitally abnormal.

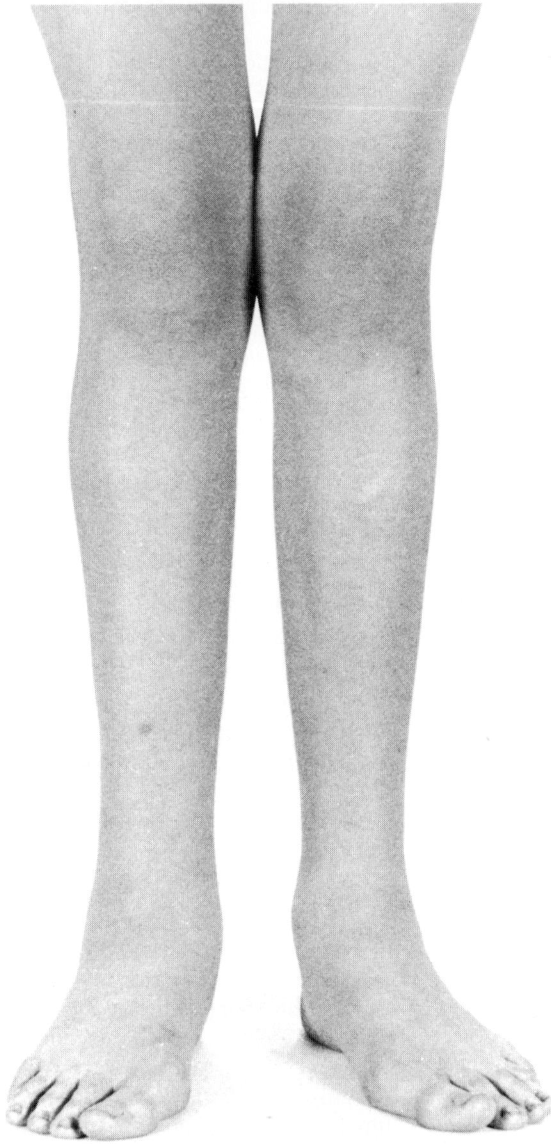

FIGURE 33-1 Early lymphedema praecox of the left lower extremity of an 18-year-old girl. (*Reproduced from* The Swollen Leg, *in the Current Problems of Surgery series, courtesy Year Book, 1973.*)

The incidence of primary, idiopathic versus secondary, acquired lymphedema varies with the reporter and is greatly influenced by factors such as geography (tropical filariasis) and the interest of the author (e.g., cancer). Allen's 1934 report listed 93 primary cases of a total of 300 cases seen at the Mayo Clinic.[2]

J. B. Kinmonth's 432-page monograph is recommended to anyone requiring detailed information on lymphedema.[10]

Pathologic Physiology

The valveless lymphatics of the superficial dermis drain into a valved subdermal system. Beneath this lies the subcutaneous lymphatic system, which classically has been thought to be

TABLE 33-3 INCIDENCE OF ONSET OF PRIMARY LYMPHEDEMA

	Incidence by source	
Onset	**Wolfe[16]**	**Gough[19]**
At birth—congenital lymphedema	10%	25%
Before age 35—lymphedema praecox	71%	61%
After age 35—lymphedema tarda	19%	14%
Total	(372 cases)	(44 cases)

separated from the deep system by the deep fascia except for some connections at the popliteal and inguinal node regions. The concept of separated subcutaneous and deep lymphatic systems has recently, however, been challenged by Crockett[11] and by others. The functional role of the connections in normal limbs is not yet clear. In any event, the fluid of lymphedema lies in the subcutaneous tissue and not in the deep muscle layers.

The lymph vessels are lined by endothelium and form a closed system, which on the outside is bathed by the tissue fluids. The permeable endothelium admits interstitial fluid, while the protein molecules apparently enter the terminal lymph capillaries through openings between cells. The return of albumen is of particular importance, for the "protein leak" from the capil-

FIGURE 33-2 Lymphedema of father and son.

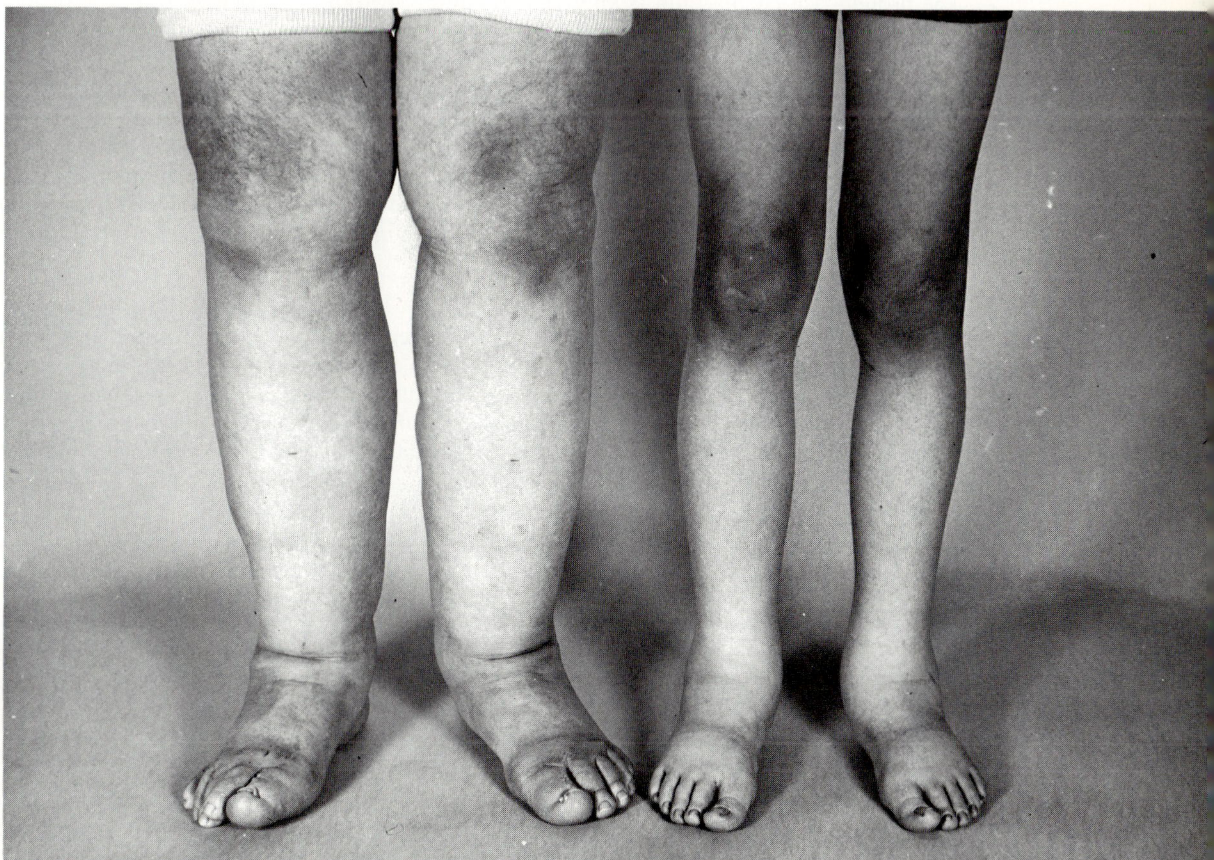

laries (by virtue of the excess of hydrostatic pressure over osmotic pressure) is large and involves over 50 percent of the total circulating albumen every 24 hours.[12]

Muscle contractions force lymph along toward the heart, the direction being determined by valves. The normal intralymphatic pressure is subatmospheric but becomes positive when lymphedema occurs.[13]

Lymphedema occurs when abnormalities exist in the lymphatic vessels or when an overload causes functional failure and resultant retention of fluid and protein molecules in the tissues. The abnormally high protein content of the retained fluid raises osmotic pressure and begins the vicious cycle of lymphedema. The protein content of 1.0 to 5.5 g/100 mL in lymphedema contrasts with that of edema due to venous stasis, cardiac failure, and hypoproteinemia, in which the level is 0.1 to 0.9 g.

The anatomic abnormalities were classified on the basis of lymphangiographic patterns by Kinmonth in 1957[9] as aplasia, hypoplasia, and hyperplasia, and others have followed this (Table 33-4). Some objection to this mechanistic explanation of lymphedema has recently been raised. Yune and Klatte[14] and Calnan[15] suggest that the varicose pattern of hyperplasia indicates a functional derangement rather than an anatomic block.

The continuing studies by Kinmonth of 372 patients for 5 to 20 years led to his conclusion that the eventual extent of the lymphedema could be assessed within the first year of management. While only 7 percent of patients showed an increase in the extent of involvement of the limb, there was increased girth in 30 percent as time passed.[16] The worst prognosis that might be expected occurred in patients with proximal pelvic lymphatic obstruction.

The protein-rich edema fluid is an excellent culture medium for bacteria from toe or foot lesions, and it may also cause fibrosis in the tissues, even without overt infection.

As swelling increases, the tissue tension, which normally is of little significance, rises and causes ultimate failure of elastic fibers as edema progresses and stretches the skin. Despite edema, diffusion of nutrients continues, and necrosis with ulcer is unlikely in lymphedema.

Efforts at reversal of the lymphedematous process may be aimed at (1) increased tissue tension by use of elastic wraps or a compression apparatus, (2) gravitational drainage of fluid, (3) dehydration by diuretics, (4) control of infections with antibiotics, (5) complete surgical removal of the diseased tissue, or (6) surgical reconstruction of the lymphatic drainage.

Differential Diagnosis

Although there often is doubt as to whether a swollen leg is due to venous obstruction or to a lympathic problem, the clinical differentiation of these two is usually easy because of certain differences (Table 33-5). First, lymphedma is usually harder and has less pitting than venous edema. Second, lymphedema does not tend to disappear overnight when the feet are elevated. Third, in lymphedema there is usually absence of associated postphlebitic signs, including varicosities, pigmentation, skin eczema, and ulcers.

TABLE 33-4 LYMPHANGIOGRAPHIC PATTERN IN PRIMARY LYMPHEDEMA

	Incidence by source		
Finding	**Kinmonth[9]**	**de Rooe[18]**	**Gough[19]**
Aplasia—no subcutaneous lymphatics	14%	9%	20%
Hypoplasia—decreae in size or number of lymphatics	55%	83%	74%
Hyperplasia—varicose, tortuous	24%	9%	6%
Dermal changes only	6%	——	——
Total	(87 cases)	(69 cases)	(66 cases)

TABLE 33-5 DIFFERENTIATION OF VENOUS AND LYMPHATIC EDEMA

	Venous	Lymphatic
1 History	Previous or present phlebitis	No phlebitis
2 Examination	Soft, later firm; decreases with overnight elevation	Firmer; does not decrease with elevation
3 Accompanying signs	Varicosities, pigmentation, ulcer common	Late skin changes; ulcer uncommon
4 Phlebography results	Positive	Negative
5 Lymphangiography results	Negative	Positive

If there is still uncertainty regarding the cause of edema, it may be resolved by phlebography and/or lymphangiography. Because of the ease of procedure and low risk, we usually perform phlebography as a part of the workup of the swollen limb, but we reserve lymphangiography for the occasional patient with greater diagnostic difficulty or for the patient who cannot be adequately managed by nonoperative therapy and who requires an operation for apparent lymphedema.

Primary Lymphedema

This is most common in females (Table 33-6). The actual cause of clinical symptoms developing in a leg whose lymphatics have probably been abnormal from birth is unknown. Inability of the abnormal lymphatics to carry the water load under conditions of increased need is a common explanation. Little is known of the triggering mechanism, although common onset in the teens has suggested hormonal changes associated with increased ovarian function. Earlier and later onset is also well known. The early development of edema heralds a more severe problem than the mild course of lymphedema occurring later in life. The most frequent age of development of swelling is the teens, but occurrence at birth and in the fifties is known. Statistics on age of onset are summarized in Table 33-6.

About half the patients with primary lymphedema eventually have bilateral swelling, but there is no way to predict its contralateral appearance. A splendid discussion of the clinical manifestations of lymphedema and its variations is given by Fairbairn, Juergens, and Spittell.[17]

Lymphangiograms of the apparently normal contralateral leg by de Rooe[18] and by Gough[19] have demonstrated lymphatic anomalies in some, even though no lymphedema has occurred.

Physical examination of the patient with primary lymphedema may show only a soft, pitting edema with normal skin in a young person whose disease has not been present for a long period. Ordinarily, the foot and often the toes as well as the ankle are edematous, and the thigh may be

TABLE 33-6 STATISTICS OF LYMPHEDEMA PRECOX

Source	Total no. of cases	Percent female	Percent unilateral	Age at onset
Allen[2]	93	87	70	65% 9 to 25 yr
Kinmonth, Tracey, Marsh[9]	95	74	47	80% $<$ 35 yr
Schirger, Harrison, Janes[20]	123	91	NA*	90% $<$ 30 yr
Calnan[15]	52	88	66	19.6 yr
Gough[19]	44	64	50	86% $>$ 35 yr

*Not available.

involved. The edema is worse in hot weather, just before and during the menstrual period, and following prolonged activity. Swelling decreases overnight with bed rest and after therapeutic elevation, but not so rapidly as in venous edema. Figure 33-1 shows early primary lymphedema precox in a young female. The originally soft edema often progresses to a firmer, nonpitting swelling. With the passage of time the skin tends to become thickened and horny, and warts may form lymphostatic verrucosis (Figure 33-3).

Ulceration is uncommon because the nutrition of the skin continues to be adequate despite the swelling. Bouts of cellulitis and lymphangitis may alter the otherwise relatively benign appearance of lymphedema. Such infections are common, since organisms from toes and feet enter the boggy tissues and the high protein content furnishes a good place for bacterial proliferation. Twenty-four percent of Kinmonth's patients[9] and 25 percent of those reported by Schirger's group[20] had definite bouts of cellulitis and/or lymphangitis.

In 1980 Kinmonth and Wolfe introduced the idea that chronic fibrosis of pelvic lymph nodes may bear an important relationship to primary lymphedema.[21] Biopsy of pelvic nodes of 74 patients with primary lymphedema disclosed fibrotic areas which were considerably more prominent in patients whose lymphangiograms showed proximal hypoplasia than in those with other types of lymphatic abnormality. The fibrosis was apparently not related to infection. The clinical importance of this finding is not yet certain.

There are no changes in the venous pattern in primary lymphedema. There may be associated patches of capillary hemangiomas in occasional patients. These represent developmental abnormalities of other vascular channels associated with the lymphatic abnormality. Of Kinmonth's 107 cases, 7 were found to have such skin anomalies.[9] In his report there were 14 patients (13 percent) with congenital anomalies, and Gough reported 32 percent.[19] Most involved the vascular system.

The rare condition known as chylous reflux occasionally allows intestinal chylous material to pass downward into the leg channels, where skin vesicles may occur. Kinmonth found nine such cases.[9]

No arterial changes are associated with primary lymphedema.

Secondary Lymphedema

This follows filarial infestation and is epidemic in some tropical areas. It has been estimated that there are 200 million such patients![22] In 1943, during World War II, 56,646 men were evacuated from the Pacific with lymphedema.[5] I have seen only one case, in a man recently returned form Africa. Tuberculosis and lymphogranuloma venerum are now rare as causes of lymphedema.

Lymphatic obstruction may occur in postphlebitic legs. The exact mechanism is not clear.

Postmastectomy edema of the arm was common in the past. It has been ascribed to various causes. Phlebography has ruled out venous thrombosis as the common cause, and it is now generally believed that this is a secondary lymphedema due to extensive excisional destruction of the lymphatics of the axillary region, including the deep system near the vessels. Similar swelling of the lower extremity may follow radical node dissection in the groin.

Even simple nodal excision may produce problems. Gough suggested that some of these lesser excisions may have involved a lymphangiomatous anomalous mass after which the lymphatic system decompensated.[19] Preoperative lymphangiography is recommended to investigate a thigh mass in a patient with edema or with a family history of it.

Secondary lymphedema due to radiation therapy is often difficult to differentiate from that due to recurrent tumor, and time itself may be the determining factor. Thus, swelling occurring during the first year after radiation therapy may be due to it, but that occurring later is likely to be due to recurrent tumor. There are no differences in the swelling itself.

The exact mechanism of the edema, often of long duration, which follows insect bites and snakebites is not known. It probably represents a lymphatic rather than a venous problem and eventually subsides, suggesting a temporary overload of the system.

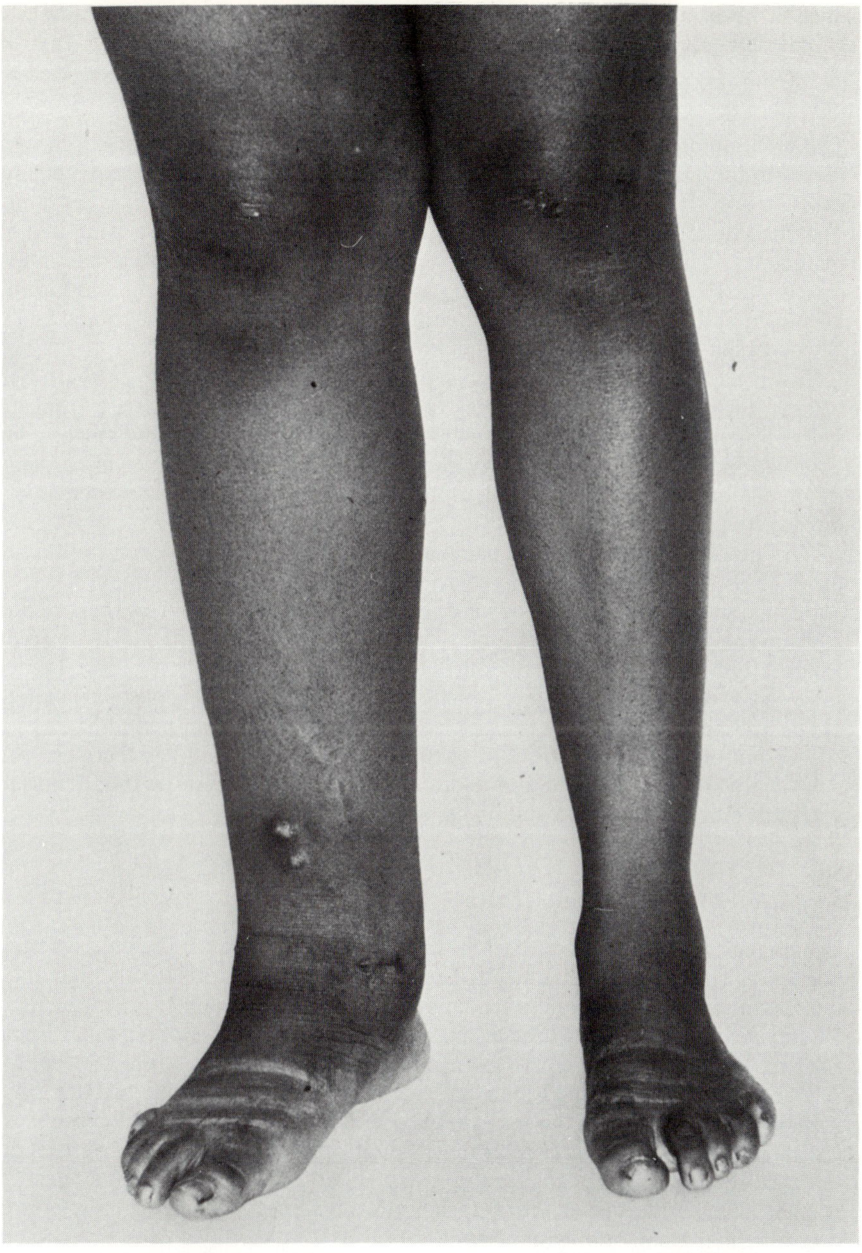

FIGURE 33-3 Untreated lymphedema precox is complicated by hyperkeratoses and skin thickening. Ankle ulcers are distinctly uncommon, in contrast to those seen in venous stasis problems.

Trauma

Occasionally there is a history of an acute precipitating factor followed shortly by the appearance of persistent lymphedema. Ankle sprains, direct blows, insect bites, minor infections, and a variety of other antecedent incidents have been observed. Kinmonth and associates reported that 17 of their 95 patients had a history of some such incident and postulated that once edema developed, a limb served by abnormal lymphatics might develop a cycle leading to a permanent lymphedema.[9]

Lymphangiosarcoma

This uncommon tumor arises from endothelium in a lymphedematous extremity and more often occurs in the upper arm following mastectomy, usually after enough years to assume cure of the breast lesion. It may occur in a lymphedematous leg, again usually after some years. It was described initially in 1918 by Kettle as a malignant endothelioma arising in a chronically edematous leg (hence Kettle's syndrome[23]) and later in 1948 by Stewart and Treves.[24] The 1957 review of 21 cases and the report of 5 additional ones by Hermann and Gruhn discussed the histologic similarity of lymphangiosarcoma and Kaposi's sarcoma but noted that the former usually occurs in women and the latter in men.[25]

It was earlier thought that lymphangiosarcoma did not occur in primary lymphedema, but Danese, Grishman, Oh, and Dreiling found 5 upper extremity and 14 lower extremity occurrences in patients with primary lymphedema. They noted that such "angiosarcomas have been observed in primary and secondary chronic lymphedema but never in cardiac, renal and cirrhotic edema, that is, in chronic lymphostatic and not in high flow edemas."[26] The reason is unknown.

The appearance of macular of papular bluish-red or purplish lesions in the extremity suggests the diagnosis. Long-term cures have been infrequent, whether treatment has been radical operation or radiation therapy. Woodward, Ivins, and Soule reviewed 163 reported cases, including 23 from the Mayo Clinic, and found there were only 2 long-term survivors among 24 nonmastectomy lymphedema patients. Both had undergone amputation.[27] Eby, Brennand, and Fine reviewed 114 collected cases and concluded that rapid subcutaneous extension along with lymphatic and hematogenous metastases led to death after a mean period of 19 months with little effect from operation, radiation, or chemotherapy.[28] Radiation has therefore been suggested as simpler therapy than amputation. Hermann's collective review in 1965 reported two apparent cures after radical operation and one after radiation therapy.[29]

LYMPHANGIOGRAPHY

Lymphangiography has never become as widely practiced or as useful as arteriography or phlebography. The technique is difficult. The complication rate is relatively high; the examination is unpleasant for the patient and often fails to provide information of practical clinical significance. Twenty years ago we learned the technique and made a number of lymphangiograms, but during the past 15 years we have employed it rarely.

The general plan of study for a new patient with edema of one or both extremities usually includes phlebography. If the patient has edematous legs and the phlebogram is abnormal and indicative of previous venous thrombosis, treatment is directed toward venous thrombosis without performance of lymphangiography, since it would be of academic interest only. Also if the edematous leg is associated with a normal phlebogram, lymphangiography is not done and nonoperative management of lymphedema is begun.

In the few instances in which severe swelling finally forces an attempt at operative relief, lymphangiography is done preoperatively to verify the diagnosis and postoperatively to obtain information about the result of the procedure.

Reduction of lymphedema prior to lymphangiography is accomplished by rest with the feet elevated, the frame of the bed being placed on 6-inch supports. The foot and leg are wrapped firmly with an elastic bandage from toes to knee, and this, with rest, is maintained for 48 hours. During this period a diuretic is administered twice daily to aid in removal of fluid.

Technique*

One or two drops of 10% aqueous solution of patent blue violet IV mixed with 5 mL of 1% lidocaine (Xylocaine) is injected intradermally into the first and second web spaces of the toes toward the dorsum of the foot, and gentle massage is performed in a proximal direction to speed the flow of the blue dye up the lymphatics.

Under 1% lidocaine local anesthesia a transverse skin incision is made on the dorsum of the foot, and the lymphatics containing the blue dye are found by gentle dissection. A ligature is passed to elevate one of these, and a special 27-gauge needle with attached polyethylene tubing is threaded into the lymphatic. Occasionally a 30-gauge needle must be used because of the unusually small size of the lymphatic vessels. It should be noted that with proximal ligation and gentle massage the lymphatics distend to 5 to 10 times their original diameter. A common mistake of the beginning lymphangiographer is to spend undue efforts in locating a "suitable" lymphatic when almost any vessel visualized directly will distend to accept the needle. A ligature is placed about the needle and lymphatic proximal to the needle's entrance into the lymphatic, after the needle tip has been carefully threaded into the lymphatic for 4 to 6 mm.

The radiopaque contrast material Ethiodol is slowly pumped into the lymphatic through the small needle with a lymphangiogram pump. A maximum of 6 to 8 mL is injected into the extremity at 9 to 12 lb/in^2 pressure, usually requiring a period of 45 to 120 minutes, and films are obtained which include not only the upper and lower leg but also the pelvis. These films are made during the procedure and at the conclusion of the injection. Later films are made at approximately 24 hours, although occasionally 2 to 6-hour postinjection films are made, depending on the speed of the contrast flow. Postoperatively, the extremity is kept elevated for 48 hours and the wound is kept clean and dry beneath an elastic bandage.

Complications

Minor complications involving wound infection and delayed wound healing occasionally occur and cause some discomfort. Lymphangitis may follow the injection. A few serious complications have been reported. Fairbairn, Juergens, and Spittell found that "16 fatalities related to the procedure occurred in 16,000 lymphangiographic examinations . . . generally related to pulmonary and less often to cerebral embolization."[17]

Koehler collected 16,501 lymphangiographies from the world literature, finding 18 deaths, 96 pulmonary infarctions, 27 lipoid pneumonias, and 75 other serious complications (1.3 percent).[31] O'Brien and associates in 1981 reported an increase in fluid volume of the extremity following the injection in 33 percent of 100 lymphangiograms, of which 12 percent did not return to the preexamination size, presumably because of inflammation or occlusion of the lymphatics by the injected Ethiodol. Their unit abandoned the examination in 1977 on the basis of excessive risk for the information obtained.[32] We virtually abandoned the procedure about the same time.

The recent development of safer and easier techniques to demonstrate the peripheral lymphatics are promising. Thus Partsch, Benzel-Hora, and Urbanek of Vienna demonstrated the opacification of quite peripheral lymphatics by the subepidermal injection of Iotasul (Schering AG, Berlin) in 32 patients.[33]

NONOPERATIVE TREATMENT OF LYMPHEDEMA

The vast majority of patients with lymphedema seen in the early stages can be managed perfectly well without operation. Although a few instances of lymphedema progress inexorably to elephantiasis, increasing knowledge and confidence in nonoperative management have decreased

*J. B. Kinmonth's detailed description of the technique of lymphangiography will be valuable to some readers.[30]

the number of neglected chronic extremities which do require operations. The statement that "little can be done [for] primary lymphedema"[18] is absolutely incorrect. While the limb may not be made 100 percent normal, the improvement which follows good management encourages both patient and doctor.

TABLE 33-7 NONOPERATIVE TREATMENT OF PRIMARY LYMPHEDEMA

1	Elevation—foot of bed raised 6 inches
2	External compression—elastic stocking, intermittent-compression unit
3	Diuretics
4	Avoidance of infection—foot hygiene (cleansing, antifungal agent); antibiotics early

The guiding principle in management of lymphedema initially is to rid the limb of as much edema as possible and then to teach the patient to maintain this. Alton Ochsner, in his pertinent comments on this in 1967, concluded that "the control of edema and the prevention of infection [prevent] the final elephantic process.[34] This appears to be perfectly true for most patients. Table 33-7 summarizes the program of nonoperative treatment.

Elevation of the Extremity

This is maintained as much as possible by sleeping in a bed whose frame is elevated 6 inches at the foot.

External Compression

A custom-fitted elastic stocking should be provided, which the patient should wear from the time of arising until the time of returning to bed. Since it is difficult for most people to wear a firmly supporting elastic stocking at the midthigh level, serious consideration should be given to prescribing the hose only to a level just below the knee, if that will control the problem. Most of our patients do not require thigh-length stockings. When such a stocking is needed, it should be prescribed to the high-thigh level, so that a firm panty girdle may be used to control swelling at the root of the thigh and overlap the more distally placed stocking. Alternatively, a leotard may be obtained, but its fitting is difficult. It is often wise for the patient to go to the factory for this.

There is available an alternating air-pressure device that is helpful for some patients. It milks or presses the edematous fluid out of the extremity toward the trunk.[35] This intermittent-pressure apparatus may be obtained as a hospital model (Figure 33-4) or a home model. Patients should be referred to the physical therapy department for a week or more of trial with the hospital model before purchasing the home model, since patient satisfaction with the intermittent-pressure device is variable. Some patients find it quite helpful.[36] It may be used twice daily or more often.

Diuretics

Because of the side effects of diuretics, their use should be intermittent rather than continuous. It is usually wise to begin management without resort to diuretics and add one only if necessary. Some patients find that a 2-day course bimonthly, weekly, or biweekly is necessary or that a 2- or 3-day course prior to the menstrual period is important. There are a number of drugs available. Furosemide (Lasix), 20 mg twice daily, is suitable. Diuretics are particularly useful if the patient is briefly hospitalized for control of edema and measurement for stockings.

Infection Control

Recurrent bouts of infection often occur in the lymphedematous extremity, and the patient should be carefully instructed in good hygiene and particularly in prevention of interdigital der-

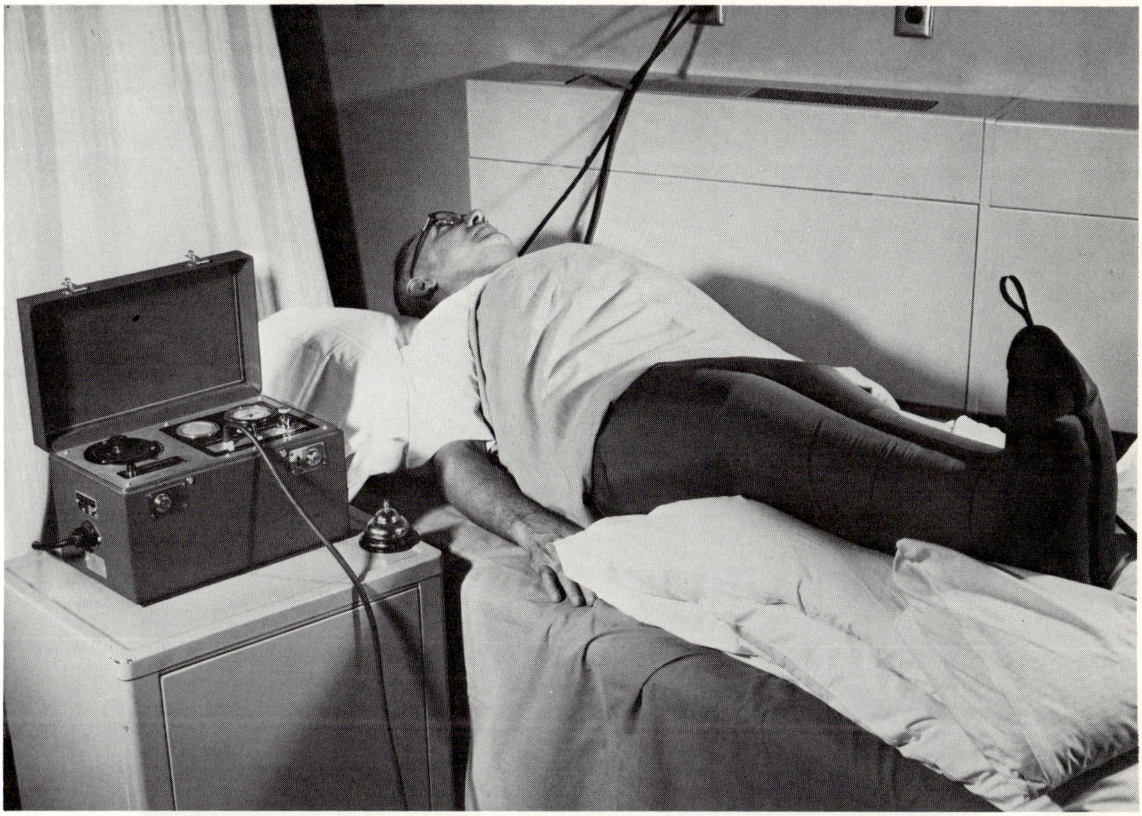

FIGURE 33-4 The Jobst intermittent-compression unit (milking machine) may be used several times a day to reduce edema of the extremities. (*Reproduced from* The Swollen Leg, *in the Current Problems of Surgery series, courtesy Year Book, 1973.*)

matitis (athlete's foot). Careful drying and powdering to prevent excessive moisture in interdigital spaces is important, and courses of tolnaftate (Tinactin), either prophylactic or as treatment, are effective. If actual infection occurs, general rest and rest of the part should occur immediately, along with administration of an antibiotic effective against the usual organism, *Streptococcus.*

SURGICAL TREATMENT OF LYMPHEDEMA

Most lymphedematous legs can be managed by nonoperative means, and cooperative patients whose treatment is begun prior to long-standing chronic swelling will ordinarily avoid the need for surgery. Thus, Wolfe and Kinmonth reported that only a small number of their 372 patients required operation.[16] My own experience is that 4 percent of patients have needed a surgical procedure.

Operation is done (1) to reduce the weighty bulk of a massively swollen limb, (2) to improve walking, (3) to allow ordinary clothes to be worn, and (4) to prevent frequent recurrent infections. The variety of surgical procedures which have been used and the continuing uncertainty as to which is the optimal one indicate failure to find a final solution to the problem.

Important preoperative measures are outlined in Table 33-8. Swelling may be reduced by the usual measures, to which a diuretic may be added for several days. Eradication of infection is obviously needed. Many of these patients harbor fungus infections and need 10 to 20 days of

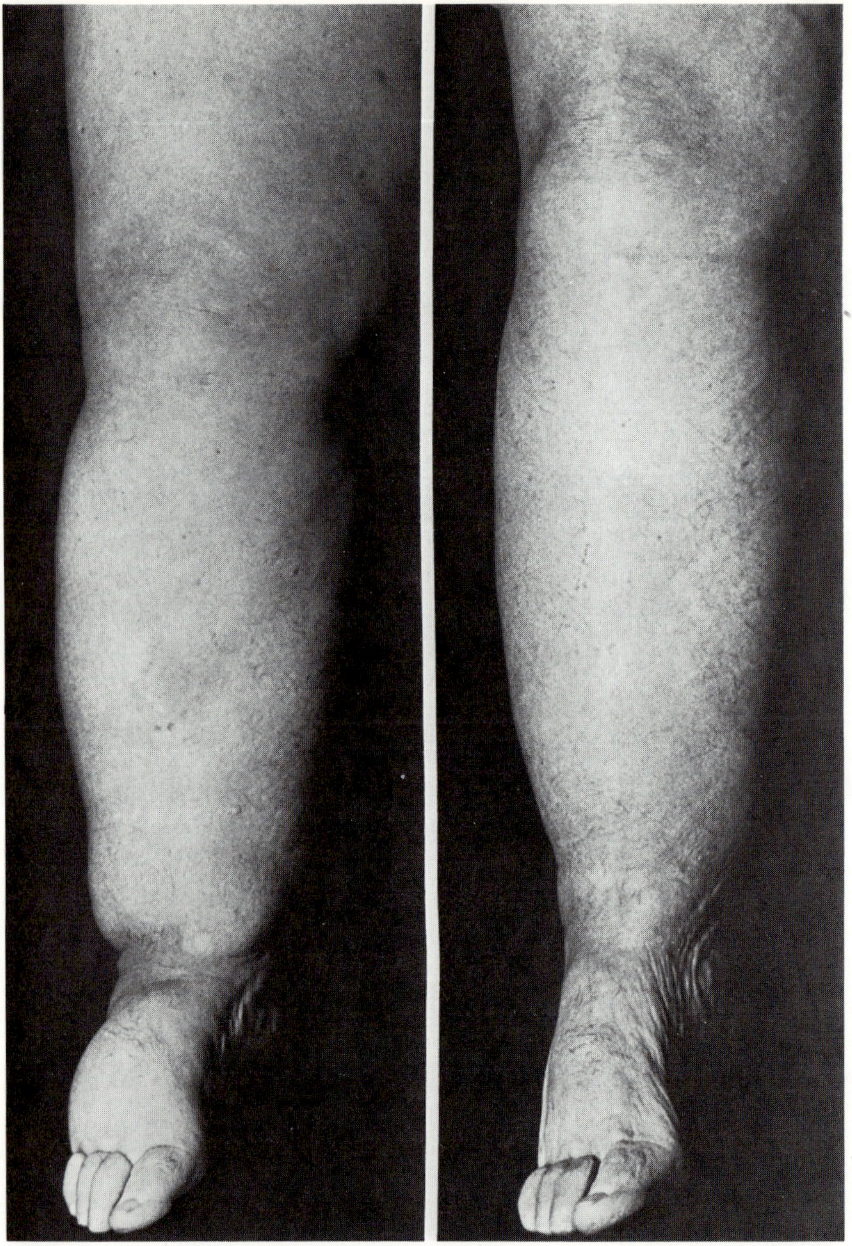

FIGURE 33-5 *Left,* severe lymphedema approaching elephantiasis prior to any form of treatment in a 40-year-old man. *Right,* following elevation and intermittent compression, there was immediate improvement which continued when the man became an outpatient.

tolnaftate therapy, as well as use of cotton in the interdigital spaces to prevent moisture between the toes. The entire skin is scrubbed for 5 minutes twice daily with chlorhexidine (Hibiclens) for 5 days before operation.

TABLE 33-8 PREOPERATIVE PREPARATION OF LYMPHEDEMATOUS EXTREMITY

1	Reduce swelling—elevation, external pressure, diuretics
2	Eradicate infection in tissues—rest, antibiotics, chlorhexidine scrubs
3	Control fungus infection of interdigital spaces—tolnaftate, cotton between digits

Operations may be classified as (1) excisional procedures to rid the limb of chronically edematous tissue and skin or (2) physiologic attempts to reconstitute or reconnect the lymphatics.

Excisional Procedures

Operations featuring excision of fascia, fat, and/or skin in various combinations have proved more reliable than other procedures to date. The Greek surgeon Kondoleon in 1912 removed strips of deep fascia, which by itself was useless. He later abandoned the procedure. In the same year Sir Havelock Charles described the excisional procedure that bears his name, which he used in India for secondary parasitic lymphedema of the lower extremities and genitalia. Sistrunk in 1918 combined Kondoleon's fascial strip excision with Charles's fat excision.[37,38] Homans in 1936 advised a two-stage excision of fat and fascia with primary closure of thinned flaps of skin and fat.[39] Since then a variety of modifications have been described, but all feature removing diseased fat along with its underlying fascia, exposing normal muscle, and covering this with skin either by the Homans method of excision of skin and fat with resuture of the remainder or by coverage with split-thickness grafts, as advised by Pratt.[5]

The 64 patients who had multiple excisional operations at the Mayo Clinic between 1936 and 1964 without mortality attest to the safety of these extensive and often bloody operations. Wound infections, skin flap necroses, and hematomas were frequent (44 percent of 135 operations).[17]

Charles's Excisional Operation The modern excisional procedure consists of removal of the boggy fat and fascia so that a muscle bed is prepared for split-thickness grafts, which may be taken from the involved extremity if the skin is not badly damaged (Figure 33-6). Principles are as follows:

1 The extremity is elevated to 30° upon a Zimmer rack to decrease venous bleeding. This prevents the need for a skeletal traction device for elevation. A proximal tourniquet decreases arterial blood loss.

2 Strips of skin are cut with the dermatome. These may be sutured together prior to their later placement, or as they are laid on. Alternatively, they may be cut from the excised block of skin and fat.[40]

3 The remaining deeper skin and the edematous fat and underlying fascia are excised so that normal muscle is laid bare over the entire leg, including the dorsum of the foot when necessary. The sole and sides of the foot are avoided. Areolar tissue should be left over the foot tendons. The original skin over the Achilles tendon is allowed to remain for its further protection. The common peroneal nerve over the proximal fibula is protected.

4 The tissues at the edges of excision are tailored to some extent to allow gradual transition to the grated area.

5 Careful hemostasis is accomplished before and after tourniquet release.

6 A pressure dressing is carefully applied.

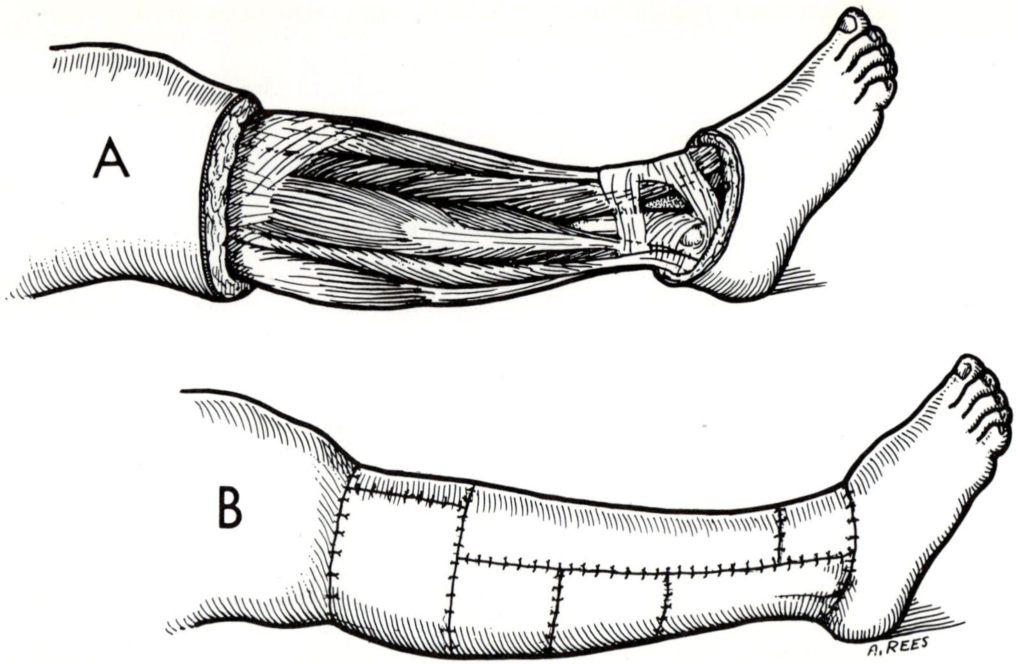

FIGURE 33-6 Severe lymphedema may be treated by excision of the waterlogged fat and thickened skin, followed by split-thickness skin grafts—the Charles operation. (*Reproduced from* The Swollen Leg, *in the Current Problems of Surgery series, courtesy Year Book, 1973.*)

Physiologic Operations

The rapid regeneration of lymphatics after surgical or accidental disruption long ago suggested the possibility of stimulating their regrowth by subcutaneous implantation of a variety of threads, including silk,[41] nylon,[42,43] rubber, and plastics.[44,45] None proved successful in regenerating lymphatics. Foley in 1955 found no further change after subcutaneous placement of sutures in 10 patients whose limbs had first been reduced in size by nonoperative measures.[46]

The observed improvements in the swelling are probably due to simultaneous adjuvant measures. Indeed, the effect of the elevation and wrapping which accompanies any operation on such a limb suggests that postoperative lymphangiograms are necessary to prove that any of the physiologic procedures is really effective. While normal lymphatics do rapidly regenerate, the mere placement of foreign bodies into boggy subcutaneous tissue should not be expected to do anything more than provoke a walling-off reaction to a foreign body, which is what occurs when threads and stents are implanted. Various grafts of fascia into muscle and skin-fat flaps to the trunk[47] have not proved worthwhile in the long run either, because lymphatic connections have failed.

Although the creation of tissue bridges to carry new lymphatics across obstructed areas have usually failed, there continue to be occasional successes such as the two described by Medgyesi in 1983. In each, a muscle-skin flap was transplanted to relieve postmastectomy edema of the arm.[48]

The physiologic *dermatoplasty* described by Noel Thompson in 1962 consisted of burial of a dermal flap into the deep muscles along the lateral and medial aspects of the extremity, to encourage lymphatic connections between the superficial and deep lymphatic systems (Figure 33-7)[49] In 1970 Thompson reported 79 cases and believed the results were better than obtained

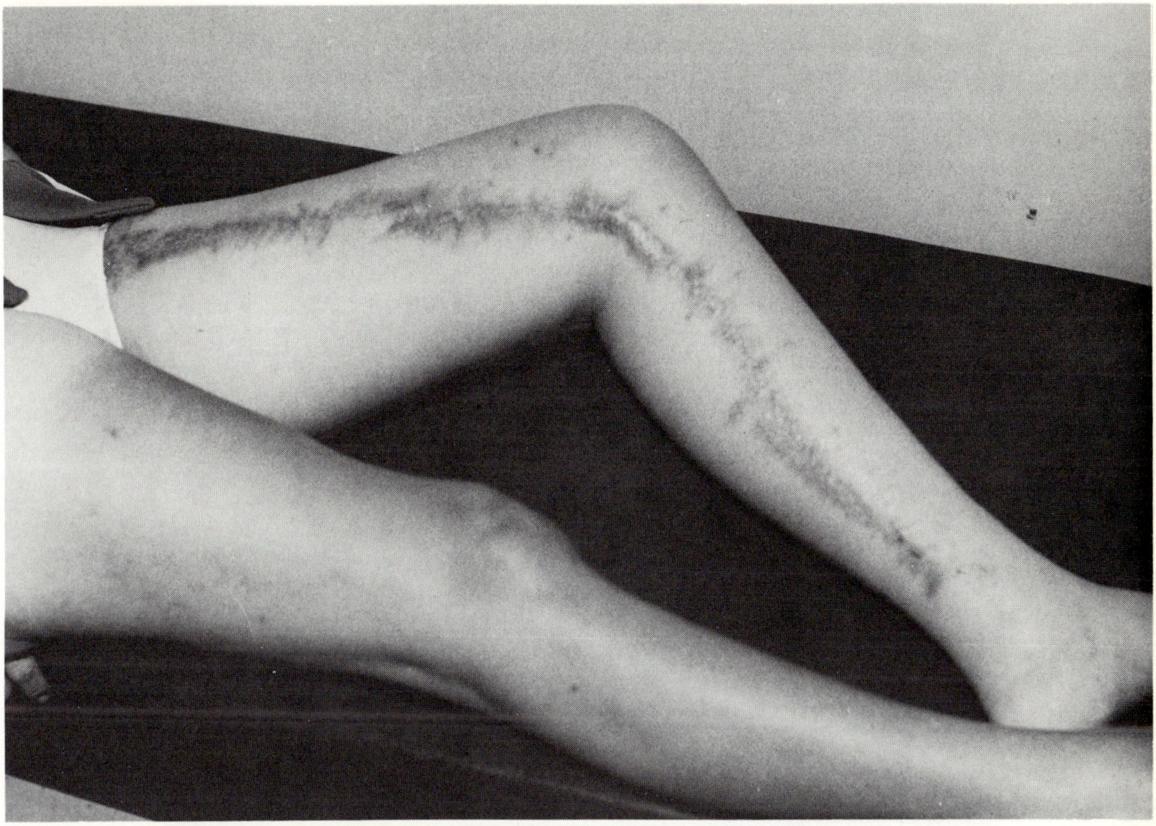

FIGURE 33-7 A medial scar 1 year following Noel Thompson's dermatoplasty.

by Charles's excision technique.[50] Tsadakas, Rigas, and Chrysanthakopoulos in 1970 modified the two-stage operation to a simple procedure and reported good results in 12 patients.[51]

Lymphangiographic confirmations of lymphatic connections have not been presented, and it is quite likely that the accompanying excision of fascia, fat, and skin accounts for the improvement. Our own recent experience with three patients is too limited to allow conclusions. All have appeared to benefit clinically. A lymphangiogram has been obtained postoperatively in one case, without evidence of lymphatic reconnection. Each patient's improvement has probably been due to the associated excision of fat and fascia rather than to any physiologic renewal of lymph vessels.

The physiologic operation of omentoplasty was described by Goldsmith, de los Santos, and Beattie in 1967.[52,53] Their study of the variations of the anatomy of the greater omentum led to the conclusion that it could be developed into a pedicle graft which, by tunneling, could be placed onto the fascia-denuded muscle of the thigh (or arm), where it was hoped new lymphatic connections would occur.

Animal experiments first showed that the omentum would transport Ethiodol into the retroperitoneal nodes following excisional division of the thigh lymphatics, and the results in four human legs and three arms were good over the 6- to 14-month follow-up periods. In one such patient the passage of blue dye from the thigh into the intraperitoneal omentum was demonstrated at a later secondary laparotomy.

It has been suggested that lymphatic connections do not persist through the omentum, yet the postoperative lymphangiogram in Figure 33-8 clearly shows patent connection 11 months after omentoplasty to the thigh in a patient whose improvement was objective as well as subjective. Despite concern that lack of absorption may hinder the result,[54] clinical experience has been promising in some patients. Further evaluation is clearly needed, and postoperative lymphangiograms are necessary to differentiate improvement due to the operation from that due to ancillary measures.

Goldsmith reported the results of omentoplasty in 22 patients (13 legs and 9 arms). Over the 7-year follow-up period there were 10 good, 4 fair, and 8 poor results. Frequent complications included two intestinal obstructions, five wound infections or hernias, and an embolus.[55] These complications parallel my experience with three transpositions and, taken along with their failure to relieve the edema (although lymphatic patency can be shown in some), suggest this to be a bad operation.

Goldsmith Omentoplasty

1 A midline longitudinal incision is made to allow mobilization of the omentum (Figure 33-9). This should be superior rather than inferior, because the required exposure is for careful dissection of the omentum off the colon and stomach.

FIGURE 33-8 Omentoplasty by Goldsmith's technique provides new pathways for passage of lymph from the leg into the abdominal cavity, bypassing the obstructed femoral lymph nodes. (*Reproduced from* The Swollen Leg, *in the Current Problems of Surgery series, courtesy Year Book, 1973.*)

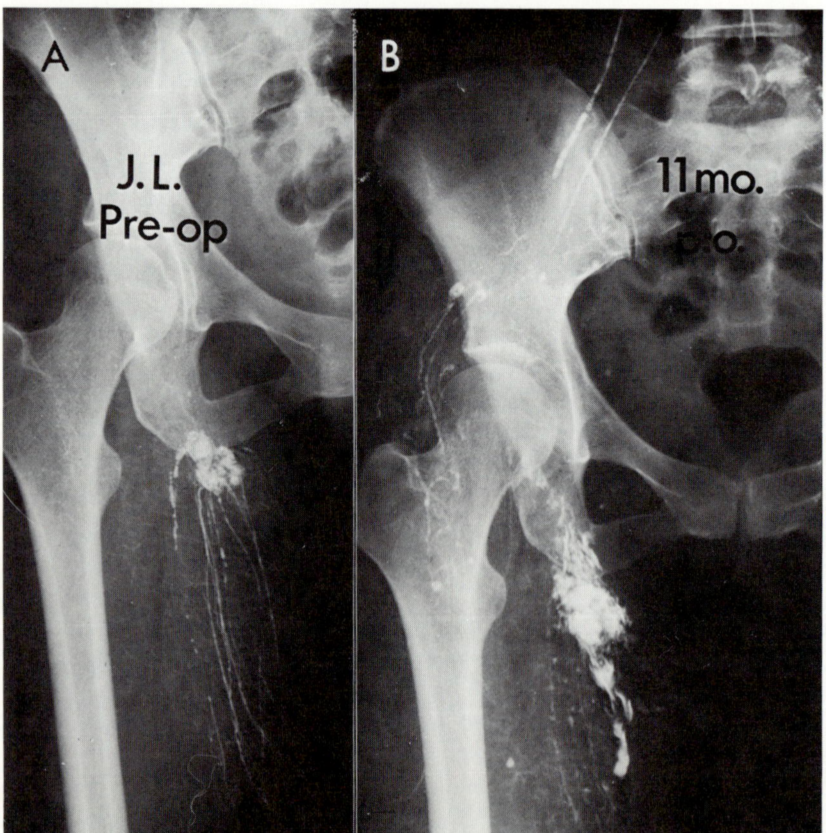

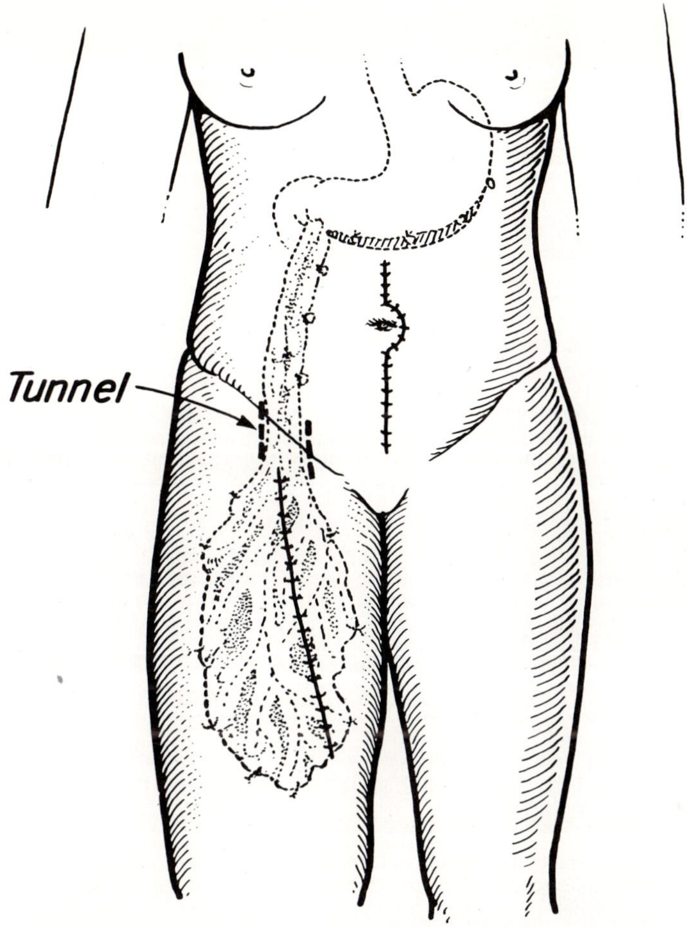

FIGURE 33-9 Omentoplasty. The omentum detached from the colon and greater curvature of the stomach is effected so that the omentum can be passed down and laid on the deep fascia of the upper thigh. (*Reproduced from* The Swollen Leg, *in the Current Problems of Surgery series, courtesy Year Book, 1973.*)

2 The omentum is detached from the half of the stomach away from the affected extremity, carrying with it the gastroepiploic vessels. It is detached from the colon in the nearby bloodless plane directly on the serosal surface of the bowel. The operator can check the omental length by laying it over the intended area on the thigh.

3 An incision is made along the anterior thigh, beginning 1 in below the inguinal ligament and extending to a point just above the patella. The edematous fibrotic fat and underlying fascia are removed to provide a muscle bed for the omentum. This extends laterally to the fascia lata, medially to the adductor longus, and proximally to the inguinal ligament. The skin flaps must be left sufficiently thick and vascularized to remain viable.

4 The omentum is oriented to prevent twisting and is passed out of the peritoneal cavity into the thigh via a tunnel overlying the iliac and femoral vessels. It is spread upon the denuded muscle of the thigh, and its edges are secured by interrupted absorbable sutures (Figure 33-10).

5 The soft tissues of the thigh are closed with interrupted sutures over indwelling suction drains.

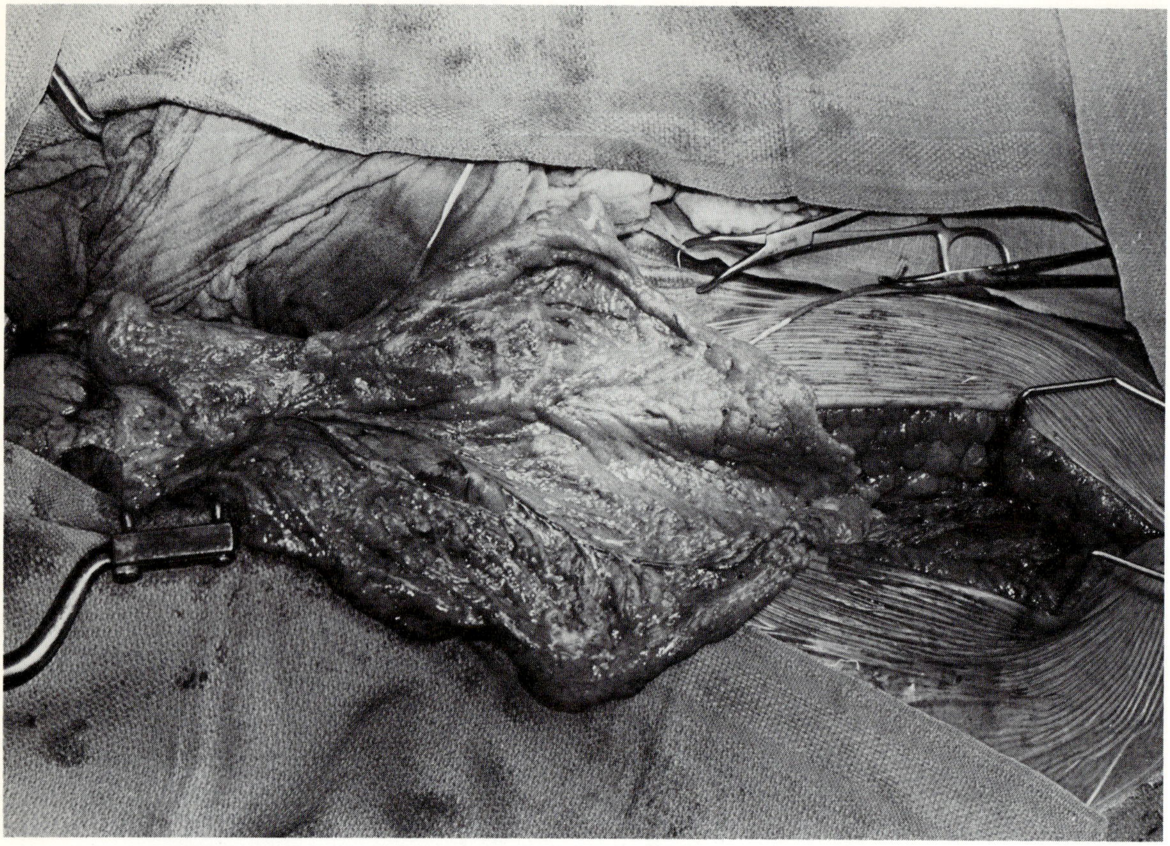

FIGURE 33-10 The semidetached omentum is tunneled through the groin and laid out on the anterior thigh. (*Reproduced from* The Swollen Leg, *in the Current Problems of Surgery series, courtesy Year Book, 1973.*)

Ileal Mesenteric Bridge Pugnaire in 1968 first reported the use of a mesenteric lymphatic bridge to cross obstructed iliac lymphatics.[56] In 1978 Kinmonth detailed the use of a mucosa-denuded isolated segment of ileum laid onto the retroperitoneal tissue in the iliac fossa to provide a lymphatic bridge across the obstructed pelvic lymphatics, showing patency in a postoperative lymphangiogram and mentioning two other successful cases.[57]

Lymphatic-to-Vein Anastomoses Experimental microsurgical anastomosis between lymph nodes and veins showed early promise, but the later patency rates were poor. O'Brien in 1976 reported 10 such operations upon patients but did not demonstrate late patency.[58] Degni devised a needle technique to insert a lymphatic within the lumen of a vein.[59] Fox, Montorsi, and Romagnoli in 1981 reported improvement, in terms of edema and patient comfort, in the majority of 20 cases done by this technique.[60] No lymphangiographic proof of success, however, has been offered following these operations.

Lumbar Sympathectomy Lumber sympathectomy is not useful.

SUMMARY

At present there is no complete surgical answer to the problem of lymphedema. The following principles appear to be sound: (1) Most patients do not require surgical procedures if they are managed properly. (2) Some type of excisional operation may be necessary for advanced cases, whereby the damaged skin and waterlogged fat are removed and covering is provided by either skin flaps or split-thickness grafts after the method of Charles. (3) Attempts to bridge obstructed lymphatics by omentoplasty and other techniques sometimes provide new pathways for lymphatic return. They are usually quantitatively insufficient to provide satisfactory clinical relief. (4) Anastomoses between lymphatics of lymph nodes and the venous system have not yet been proved successful by lymphangiograms, although clinical improvement often occurs due to adjuvant therapy. (5) All procedures must be followed with continued external elastic support.

REFERENCES

1 Rovner DR: The enigma of idiopathic cyclic edema. *Hosp Pract* 1972, 7:103.

2 Allen EV: Lymphedema of the extremities: Classification, etiology and differential diagnosis, a study of 300 cases. *Arch Int Med* 1934, 54:606.

3 Kinmonth JB, Rob CG, Simeone FA: *Vascular Surgery.* Williams & Wilkins, Baltimore, 1963.

4 Matas R: The surgical treatment of elephantiasis and elephantoid states dependent upon chronic obstruction of the lymphatic and venous channels. *Am J Trop Dis* 1913, 1:1.

5 Pratt GH: Surgical correction of lymphedema, with observations on use of electric dermatome. *JAMA* 1951, 257:1121.

6 Nonne MH: Elephantiasis congenita. *Dtsch Med Wchnschr* 1890, 16:1124.

7 Milroy WF: Chronic hereditary edema: Milroy's disease. *JAMA* 1928, 91:1172.

8 Ersek RA, Danese CA, Howard JM: Hereditary congenital lymphedema (Milroy's disease). *Surgery* 1966, 60:1098

9 Kinmonth JB, Tracey GD, Marsh JD: Primary lymphedema: Clinical and lymphangiographic studies of a series of 107 patients in which the lower limbs were affected. *Br J Surg* 1957, 45:1

10 Kinmonth JB: *The lymphatics: Surgery, Lymphography, and Disease of the Chyle and Lymph System.* E. Arnold, Baltimore, 1982.

11 Crockett DJ: Lymphatic anatomy and lymphedema. *Br J Plast Surg* 1965, 18:12.

12 Patterson RM, Ballard CL, Wasserman K, Mayerston HS: Lymphatic permeability to albumen. *Am J Physiol* 1958, 194:120.

13 Blocker TG Jr, Lewis SR, Smith JR, Dunton EF, Kirby EJ, Meyer, JV: Lymphodynamics. *Plast Reconst Surg* 1960, 25:337.

14 Yune HY, Klatte EC: Lymphography in lymphatic obstruction. *Radiology* 1969, 92:824.

15 Calnan J: Lymphoedema: The case for doubt. *Br J Plast Surg* 1968, 21:32.

16 Wolfe JH, Kinmonth JB: The prognosis of primary lymphedema of the lower limbs. *Arch Surg* 1981, 116:1157.

17 Fairbairn JF, Juergens JL, Spittel JA: *Peripheral Vascular Diseases.* 4th ed. Saunders, Philadelphia, 1972

18 de Rooe T: The value of lymphography in lymphedema. *Surg Gynecol Obstet* 1967, 124:755.

19 Gough MH: Primary lymphedema: Clinical and lymphangiographic studies. *Br J Surg* 1966, 53:917.

20 Schirger A, Harrison EG, Janes JM: Idiopathic lymphedema: Review of 131 cases. *JAMA* 1962, 182:14.

21 Kinmonth JB, Wolfe JHN: Lymph node fibrosis in primary lymphedema. *Ann R Coll Surg Eng* 1980, 62:344.

22 Stone EJ, Hugo NE: Lymphedema. *Surg Gynecol Obstet* 1972, 135:625.

23 Kettle EH: Tumors arising from endothelium. *Proc Soc Med (Sect Path)* 1918, 11:19.

24 Stewart FW, Treves N: Lymphangiosarcoma in postmastectomy lymphedema: A report of 6 cases in elephantiasis chirurgica. *Cancer* 1948, 1:64.

25 Hermann JB, Gruhn JG: Lymphangiosarcoma secondary to chronic lymphedema. *Surg Gynecol Obstet* 1957, 105:655.

26 Danese CA, Grishman E, Oh C, Dreiling DA: Malignant vascular tumors of the lymphedematous extremity. *Ann Surg* 1967, 166:245.

27 Woodward AH, Ivins JC, Soule EH: Lymphangiosarcoma arising in chronic lymphedematous extremities. *Cancer* 1972, 30:562,

28 Eby CS, Brennan MJ, Fine G: Lymphangiosarcoma: A lethal complication of chronic lymphedema: Report of two cases and review of the literature. *Arch Surg* 1957, 94:222.

29 Hermann JB: Lymphangiosarcoma of the chronically edematous extremity. *Surg Gynecol Obstet* 1965, 121:1107.

30 Kinmonth JB: Lymphography, 1977: A review of some technical points. *Lymphology* 1977, 10:102.

31 Koehler PR: Lymphography, Panel discussion: II. Complications and accidents, in Ruttiman A (ed): *Progress in Lymphology* Theim, Stuttgart, 1967, pp 306, 324.

32 O'Brien BM, Das SK, Franklin JD, Morrison WA: Effect of lymphangiography on lymphedema. *Plast Reconstr Surg* 1981, 68:922.

33 Partsch H, Wenzel-Hora BI, Urbanek A: Differential diagnosis of lymphedema after indirect lymphography with Iotasul. *Lymphology* 1983, 16:12.

34 Ochsner A: Discussion of Goldsmith HS, de los Santos R, Beattie EJ: Relief of chronic lymphedema by omental transposition. *Ann Surg* 1967, 166:584.

35 Brush BE, Wylie JH, Benison J: Some devices for management of lymphedema of the extremities. *Surg Clin North Am* 1959, 39:1493.

36 Schumaker HB Jr: Management of moderate lymphedema. *Arch Surg* 1981, 116:1097.

37 Sistrunk WE: Further experiences with the Kondoleon operation for elephantiasis. *JAMA* 1918, 71:800.

38 Sistrunk WE: Contribution to plastic surgery . . . the Kondoleon operation for elephantiasis. *Ann Surg* 1927, 85:185.

39 Homans J: The treatment of elephantiasis of the legs: A preliminary report. *N Engl J Med* 1963, 215:1099.

40 Gibson T, Tough TS: The surgical correction of clinical lymphoedema of the legs. *Br J Plast Surg* 1954, 7:195.

41 Handley WS: Lymphangioplasty: A new method for the relief of the brawn arm of breast cancer and for similar conditions of lymphatic oedema: Preliminary note. *Lancet* 1908, 1:783.

42 Ranshohoff JL: Surgical treatment of lymphedema. *Arch Surg* 1945, 50:296.

43 Zieman SA: Re-establishing lymph drainage for lymphoedema of the extremities. *J Int Coll Surg* 1951, 15:328.

44 Gorman JF, Navarre JR: Observation of lymphedema praecox and its management with lymphangioplasty. *Vasc Dis* 1965, 2:1.

45 Hogeman KE: Artificial subcutaneous channels in draining lymphoedema. *Acta Chir Scand* 1955, 110:154.

46 Foley WT: The medical management of lymphedema. *Mod Concepts Cardiovasc Dis* 1955, 24:255.

47 Wynn SK: Surgical approach to postmasectomy lymphedematous extremity. *Arch Surg* 1955, 70:418.

48 Medgyesi S: A successful operation for lymphoedema using a myocutaneous flap as a "wick." *Br J Plast Surg* 1983, 36:64.

49 Thompson N: Surgical treatment of chronic lymphoedema of the lower limb, with preliminary report of new operation. *Br Med J* 1962, 2:1566.

50 Thompson N: Buried dermal flap operation for chronic lymphedema of the extremities: Ten year survey of results in 79 cases. *Plast Reconstructr Surg* 1970, 45:541.

51 Tsadakas E, Rigas A, Chrysanthakopoulos S: New aspects in the surgical treatment of lymphedema of the extremities. *Surgery* 1970 68:419.

52 Goldsmith HS, de los Santos R, Beattie EJ: Relief of chronic lymphedema by omental transposition. *Ann Surg* 1967, 166:572.

53 Goldsmith HS, de los Santos R: Omental transposition in primary lymphedema. *Surg Gynecol Obstet* 1967, 125:607.

54 Nylander G, Tjernberg B: The lymphatics of the greater omentum: An experimental study in the dog. *Lymphology* 1969, 2:3.

55 Goldsmith HS: Long term evaluation of omental transposition for chronic lymphedema. *Ann Surg* 1974, 180:847.

56 Pugnaire M de R: Limfangioplastia mesenterica en el tratamiento de la elefantiasis de los membros inferiores. *Angiologica* 1968, 20:146.

57 Kinmonth JB, Hurst PA, Edwards JM, Rutt DL: Relief of lymph obstruction by use of a bridge of mesentery and ileum. *Br J Surg* 1978, 65:829.

58 O'Brien BMC: Replantation and reconstructive microvascular surgery. *Ann R Coll Surg* 1976, 58:171.

59 Degni M: New technique of lymphaticovenous anastomosis for the treatment of lymphedema. *J Cardiovasc Surg* (Torino) 1978, 19:577.

60 Fox U, Montorsi M, Romagnoli G: Microsurgical treatment of lymphedema of the limbs. *Int Surg* 1981, 66:53.

Invited Commentary

John E. Connolly, M.D.
Irvine, California

Lymphedema, while not a commonly encountered problem, continues to present a management challenge for the vascular surgeon. Congenital lymphatic lesions of both upper and lower extremities are rare and usually require surgical excision. More commonly the vascular surgeon has to deal with lymphedema coming on later in life. With the abandonment of more radical surgical procedures for carcinoma of the breast, these lesions are predominately of the lower extremity.

The most perplexing cases are of the primary, idiopathic variety rather than the secondary type usually associated with cancer or radiation damage to the lymphatic system. I agree wholeheartedly with the recommendation for conservative nonoperative treatment, particularly in the young female with idiopathic primary lymphedema. If Dr. Dale's principles are applied early and adhered to religiously by the patient, the problem can usually be reasonably controlled. In addition to the various theories of possible etiology listed by the author, I would like to add the possibility of subclinical infectious obstruction of the lymphatics as an acquired cause of insidious onset of lymphedema.

My personal experience with lymphangiography spans a 30 year period following the opportunity to work with Professor Kinmonth during the period that he was developing the technique, and it is more positive than Dr. Dale's. I think that the complications listed were seen during the development of the technique but are no longer encountered in experienced hands. One of the most helpful modifications has been performance of the study under fluoroscopic control, with the injection of dye stopped when it reaches the high periaortic lymph nodes. Some operators have become so experienced with the technique that they are able to identify the lymphatics on the dorsum of the foot even without the use of interdigital blue dye injection. Without experience or personal interest in the test, the average angiographer regards the procedure at best as tedious, so it behooves the vascular surgeon to seek out an experienced, interested radiographer in the community or even collaborate with one if necessary to facilitate good safe studies. By seeking out the interested experienced radiographer, I continue to use lymphangiography to confirm the diagnosis and help me in the proper planning of therapy.

Like Dr. Dale, I reserve surgical therapy for the rare case where conservative therapy has failed, remembering that the cosmetic result will be less than ideal whatever technique is employed. I have tried and discarded the passage of silk and nylon threads above and below the site of lymphatic obstruction, the use of omental flaps or pedicle ileum flaps, and operations based on transposition of skin or subcutaneous flaps. Likewise, I have found vein-to-lymphatic anastomosis in the groin to be useless. I agree that the best and only surgical treatment to be currently recommended is excision of all subcutaneous tissue down to muscle, with use of either the remaining skin flaps or split-thickness grafting if the native skin is not suitable.

34 THORACIC OUTLET COMPRESSION SYNDROME

Thoracic outlet compression syndrome (TOS) continues to be a diagnostic and management problem. Operations for its relief are the subject of debate, and their reported results are variable. These problems, along with the frequency of medicolegal disputes generated by them, concern primary care physicians as well as thoracic and vascular surgeons.

A few clinicians doubt the existence of the syndrome. Some do not believe there are any indications for surgical treatment; others, who once had advocated first-rib resection, currently have adopted a lesser operation on only the soft tissues. Finally, there are those who advocate first-rib resection by one or another approach. A few surgeons report remarkably high cure rates; others are less optimistic. Thus the problem is at once the source of disagreement and the cause of therapeutic disappointments.

Increasing experience with the results of operations for thoracic outlet syndrome caused me to review my management protocol in 1982 and to adhere to even stricter indications for operations. Every possible conservative nonoperative measure is used; operation has become a procedure of last resort.[1]

ILLUSTRATIVE CASE

A 51-year-old female had chronic pain in the left shoulder and neck radiating down the lateral arm following an automobile accident. Sixteen months later, despite various treatments, including shoulder girdle–strengthening exercises, there was no particular improvement. The left subclavian artery was occluded when the arm was elevated at arteriography (Figure 34-1). The arm pulse was absent in certain arm positions, and there was a bruit in the left supraclavicular space. Electromyographic examination was negative.

Transaxillary resection of the first rib was performed uneventfully. In the early postoperative period there was relief of all symptoms, and the result was classified as excellent. Ten months postoperatively the patient had recurrent pain in the left arm and hand.

Comment

The preoperative diagnoses included cervical arthritis, muscular strain, and several other soft tissue diagnoses. Eventually it was believed that the patient had a posttraumatic thoracic outlet syndrome despite the negative nerve conduction study. The complete relief which occurred in the early postoperative period suggested that her result should be classified as excellent, but the return of symptoms 10 months later changed her classification to good. The symptoms since then have not been severe, and secondary operation has not appeared advisable.

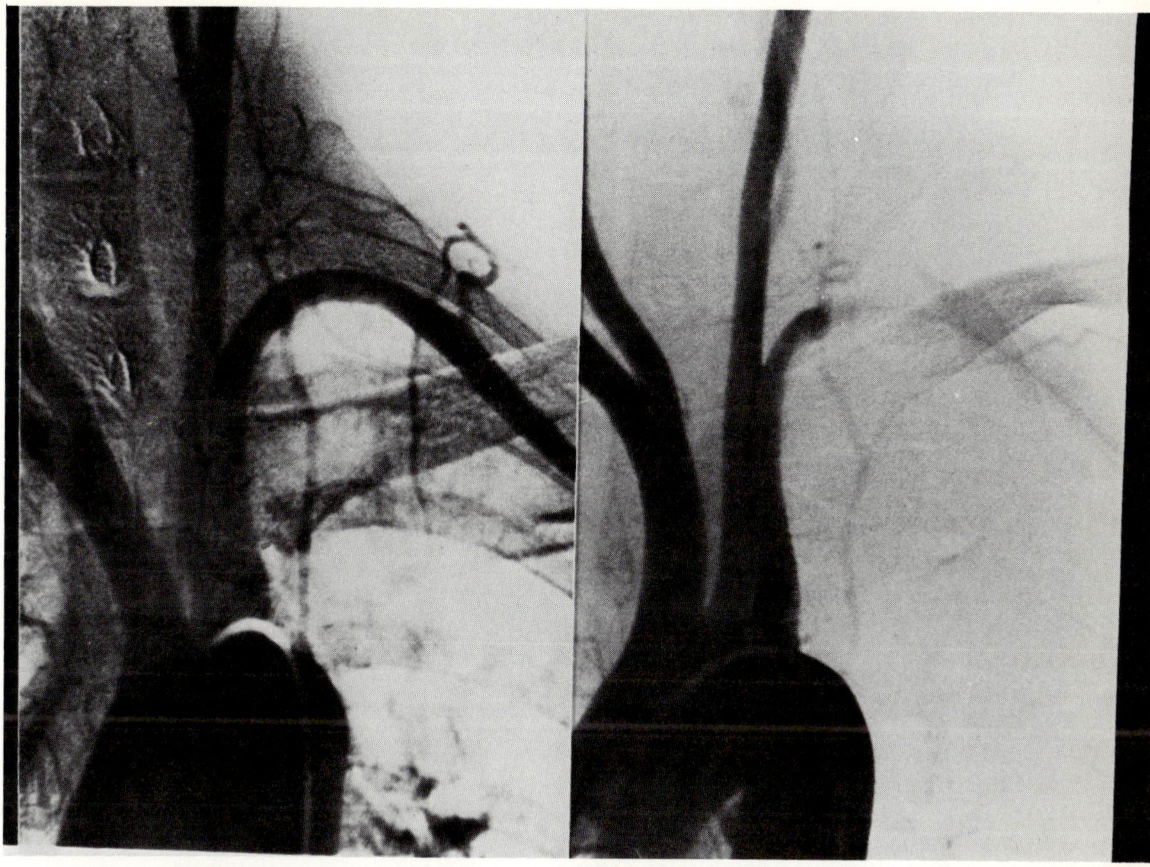

FIGURE 34-1 This two-position angiogram illustrates the normal curve of the patent subclavian artery with the arm at the side, *left,* and complete occlusion of the subclavian artery with the arm elevated, *right.*

DIAGNOSIS

The first problem in managing shoulder pain suggesting thoracic outlet syndrome is correct diagnosis. Gilliatt noted aptly that "clinical details do not establish a characteristic picture and objective confirmatory tests are also lacking."[2] Since there are no individual or combinations of signs or test which unequivocally make the diagnosis, it must be one of exclusion and clinical judgment. The existence of some form of pain is invariable. It is often vague, and the patient finds description difficult, since it is not localized to the shoulder or elbow; this may lead the inexperienced clinician to conclude that it is not real. Approximately 90 percent of patients have neurologic symptoms; 10 percent also have arterial or venous problems. Reports of a higher incidence of vascular problems[3] probably reflect a specific referral pattern.

Anterior chest pain may mimic angina pectoris and necessitate coronary arteriography for differentiation. Cervical arthritis and herniated discs may be differentiated by their response to traction or by myelography.

Important diagnostic questions are summarized in Table 34-1. In a minority of instances it is at once clear that the pain is organic, and in a few others the psychosomatic origin is obvious. Unfortunately, most patients with TOS have some degree of discomfort or pain with secondary overlapping psychosomatic symptoms due to its long continuation. The matter is often further complicated by a history of trauma and pending litigation, which often must be settled before the entire situation can be corrected or stabilized; however, it must be always remembered that more than one patient has been labeled a neurotic or malingerer who has been immediately relieved of symptoms by surgical decompression of the thoracic outlet.

TABLE 34-1 CLINICAL QUESTIONS REGARDING PAIN

1 Is it *organic,* psychosomatic, or a combination?
2 Is it *neurogenic or vascular?*
3 What is the *site of origin* (vertebral outlets, thoracic outlet, elbow, wrist)?

Pressure upon a nerve at either elbow or wrist tends to produce symptoms which are reflected proximally as well as distally. It should be particularly recalled that thoracic outlet syndrome and distal nerve compressions occasionally coexist, in which situation both should be surgically decompressed at the same time.[4]

Physical Examination This often is not particularly helpful. The pulse cutoff sign produced by elevation and external rotation of the upper extremity is not critical, since it is found in many completely asymptomatic patients. A more important finding is production of pain by elevation and external rotation.

Tenderness in the supraclavicular region is suggestive, as is a bruit. Peripheral sensory and motor dysfunction are unusual in Americans, who ordinarily seek medical advice prior to such a late stage of nerve pressure.

Arterial symptoms occur in approximately 5 percent of individuals because of ischemia or either thrombosis or embolism and occasionally Raynaud's syndrome.

Venous pressure either continuously or intermittently may cause edema, cyanosis, and development of collateral venous circulation around the shoulder girdle and adjacent chest wall. Subclinical edema may be noted by the patient whose ring becomes too tight, before the physician can actually demonstrate this by pressure or observation.

Adams, DeWeese, Mahoney, and Rob described a few patients with intermittent venous occlusion.[5] An unusual cause of this was the hypertrophy of the pectoralis major muscle in a man who repetitively lifted large sacks at work (Figure 34-2). Phlebography demonstrated axillary and subclavian vein patency at rest and occlusion during pectoral tightening (Figure 34-3).

OUTPATIENT MANAGEMENT

A flow sheet for management is shown in Figure 34-4. At the initial interview the clinical evaluation is followed by roentgenograms of the chest and neck to determine whether a cervical rib or first-rib anomaly is present. Cardiac studies may be indicated if there is any suggestion that the pain may be secondary to coronary arterial stenosis, since the pseudoangina of TOS sometimes reflects itself as anterior left chest pain.

If thoracic outlet nerve pressure appears to be the proper diagnosis, the patient is instructed in shoulder girdle–strengthening exercises (Table 34-2)[6] and asked to return after 3 weeks' use of these twice daily. During that time some form of tranquilizer or relaxant may be helpful. Patients who report aggravation of pain by the exercises are instructed to stop them at once. Whether exercise-induced increase in muscle tone benefits the patient or whether there is simply a spontaneous recession during the several-week period has never been clear.

After 3 weeks the patient may be improved, in which event further nonoperative management is clearly indicated. If the patient is not improved or is becoming worse, there is a trial of cervical halter traction on an outpatient basis for a week. Cervical traction should not benefit thoracic outlet syndrome but will temporarily, at least, relieve pressure on the nerve roots due to a protruded cervical disc or to pressure from arthritis. It is a therapeutic test as well as sometimes offering relief for those situations.

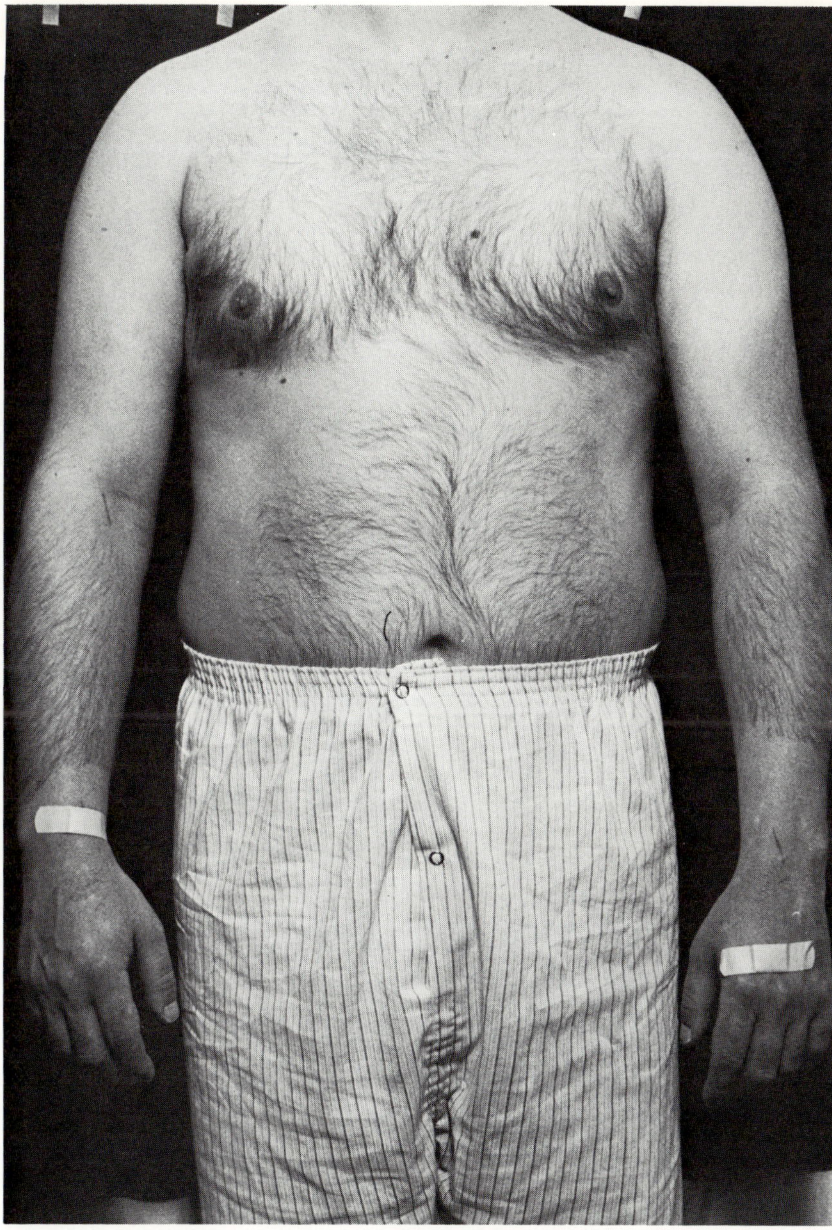

FIGURE 34-2 A heavily muscled male with intermittent axillary venous occlusion due to the overlying hypertrophied pectoralis major muscle resulting from his daily lifting at work.

If at the end of 4 to 6 weeks the patient retains symptoms severe enough to warrant operation, and particularly if opiate medication is being required, hospitalization is arranged for final testing and a decision regarding operation.

DIAGNOSTIC TESTS

A diagnosis which can be based upon objective signs or tests is often not possible in TOS. Certain procedures do have relative if not absolute values.

Chest and Neck X-rays

These may disclose a cervical rib (which exists in 10 percent of the population) or an anomaly of the first rib. Such a bony anomaly suggests two-position arteriograms to search for an arterial irregularity, dilatation, or even aneurysm, any of which at once suggests removal of the offending pressure.

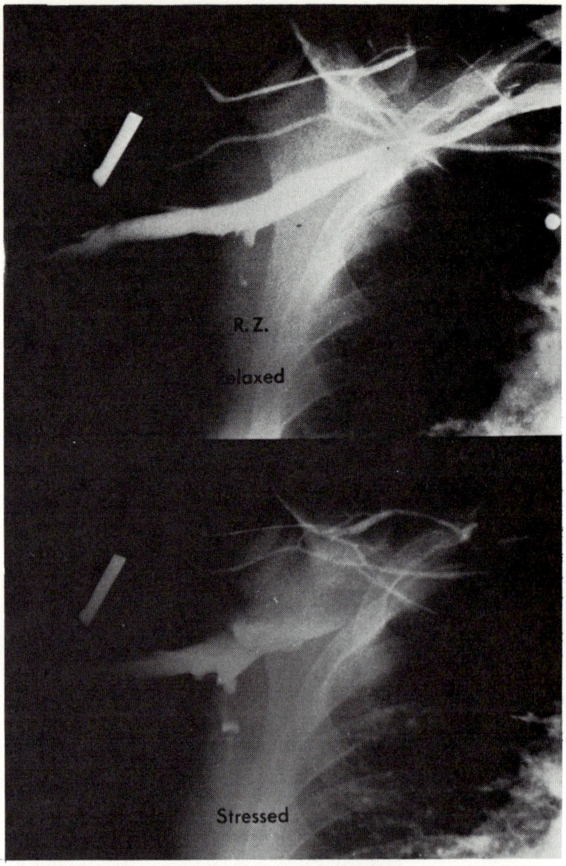

FIGURE 34-3 Intermittent occlusion of the axillary vein by the hypertrophied pectoralis major muscle. *Above,* the vein is patent during relaxation. *Below,* the vein is occluded by the taut muscle.

Arteriograms

Arteriograms are often unnecessary,[7] since only a minority of patients have abnormal findings.[8] Nevertheless, in that minority the arterial changes often are unsuspected and do suggest an operative rather than nonsurgical program to prevent continuing vascular damage. Two-position subclavian arteriograms (with the arm at the side and later elevated) are particularly apt to show arterial lesions in the presence of bony anomalies of the cervical or thoracic ribs (Figure 34-5).[4]

Phlebograms

Phlebograms have not been worthwhile and now are limited to those patients exhibiting edema or venous collateralization around the shoulder. They are mandatory for so-called effort thrombosis of the subclavian and axillary veins, this actually being an acute venous occlusion as a manifestation of TOS (Figure 34-6).

Venous Pressure Studies

Venous pressure studies are not useful in the absence of the aforementioned symptoms.

Nerve Conduction Studies

These are particularly worthwhile in detecting carpal tunnel syndrome, while the value of this examination in thoracic outlet nerve compresion is debatable. The study was reported to be of considerable diagnostic value by Urschel,[9] who cited 8400 examinations in 1 year and abnormal results in 8.5 percent. Stanton and associates similarly reported the value of this test, noting that all of their 28 patients had reversal of an abnormal test after operation.[10]

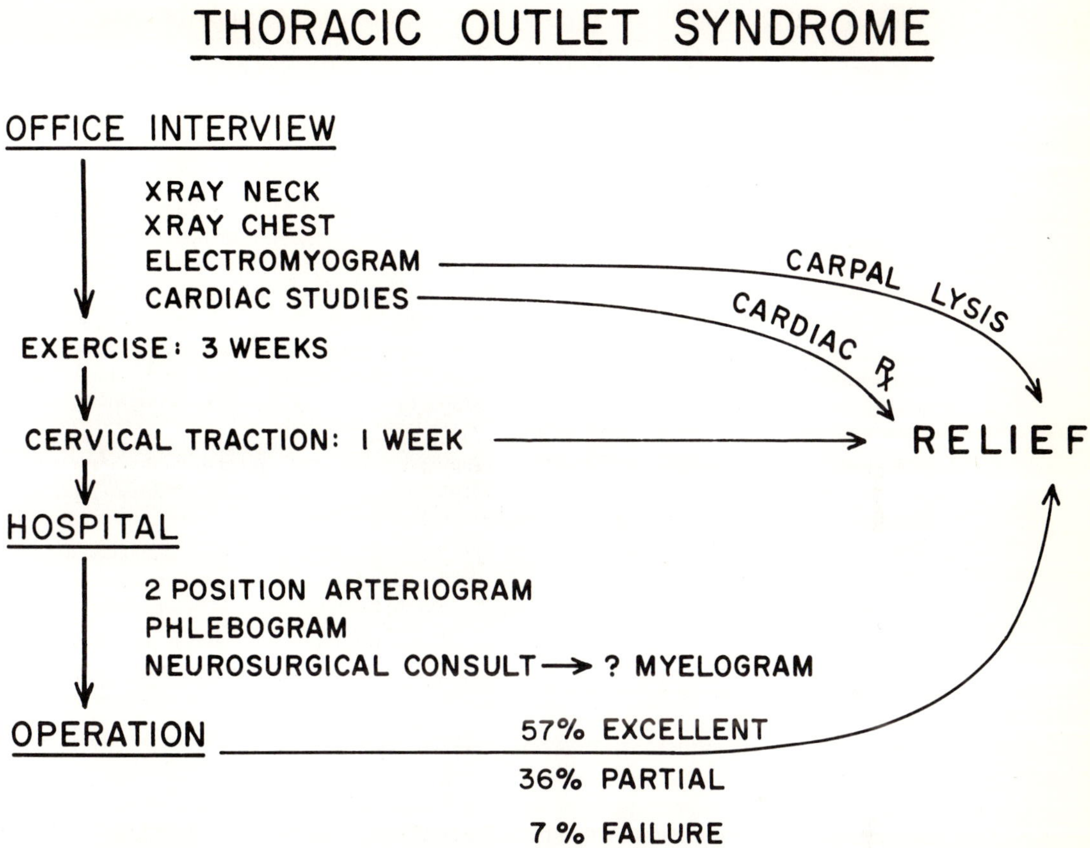

FIGURE 34-4 A clinical management flow diagram.

Others have not found the test as useful.[11,12] Cherington found no difference between 213 normal persons and 27 others with thoracic outlet syndrome and advised "caution in diagnosis . . . on the basis of ulnar nerve conduction velocity."[13] Even the advocates admit difficulties in reproducing their results. The issue was recently reexamined editorially[14] after a letter challenged the facts in the original publication, which the interested reader should examine.

An abnormal study in which the nerve conduction time is delayed may be worthwhile, but a normal study does not rule out relief of symptoms by operation. To reiterate, its chief value is in detecting carpel tunnel syndrome.

CT Scan

The role of the computerized tomography (CT) scan in the diagnostic protocol is not yet clear. One patient recently was saved a needless first-rib resection by discovery of a Pancoast tumor by this technique. The CT scan will show small rudimentary cervical ribs which are not apparent on either cervical spine films nor chest films. Whether this is associated with a high incidence of a cartilaginous attachment or a fibrous band is not yet known.

THE DECISION REGARDING OPERATION

Because of difficulties in diagnosis and a surprisingly large number of poor operative results, those patients with neurologic symptoms alone should have prolonged nonsurgical treatment,

TABLE 34-2 SHOULDER GIRDLE EXERCISES FOR THORACIC OUTLET SYNDROME

At the beginning, each exercise is done 10 times in succession twice a day. As the shoulders and neck gain strength, the number of times each exercise is done consecutively can be increased. The six exercises follow:

1 Stand erect with the arms at the sides, holding in each hand a 2-lb weight (sandbags—or bottles, jars, or sacks filled with sand). (*a*) Shrug the shoulders forward and upward. (*b*) Relax. (*c*) Shrug the shoulders backward and upward. (*d*) Relax. (*e*) Shrug the shoulders upward. (*f*) Relax and repeat.

2 Stand erect with the arms out straight from the sides at shoulder level; hold a 2-lb weight in each hand (palms should be down). (*a*) Raise the arms sideways and up until the backs of the hands meet above the head (keep elbows straight). (*b*) Relax and repeat. Note: As strength improves and exercises 1 and 2 become easier, weights should be made heavier; increase to 5-lb and later to 10 lb.

3 Stand facing a corner of the room with one hand on each wall, arms at shoulder level, palms forward, elbows bent, and abdominal muscles contracted. (*a*) Slowly let the upper part of the trunk lean forward, and press the chest into the corner. Inhale as the body leans forward. (*b*) Return to the original position by pushing out with the hands. Exhale with this movement.

4 Stand erect with the arms at the sides. (*a*) Bending the neck to the left, attempt to touch the left ear to the left shoulder without shrugging the shoulder. (*b*) Bending the neck to the right, attempt to touch the right ear to the right shoulder without shrugging the shoulder. (*c*) Relax and repeat.

5 Lie face down with the hands clasped behind the back. (*a*) Raise the head and chest from the floor as high as possible while pulling the shoulders backward and the chin in. Hold this position for a count of 3. Inhale as the chest is raised. (*b*) Exhale and return to the original position. (*c*) Repeat.

6 Lie down on the back with arms at the sides, with a rolled towel or small pillow under the upper part of the back between the shoulder blades and no pillow under the head. (*a*) Inhale slowly and raise the arms upward and backward overhead. (*b*) Exhale and lower the arms to the sides. (*c*) Repeat 5 to 20 times.

and operative decompression should be offered only as a last resort. As Jere Lord recently stated editorially, "conservatism . . . should be the order of the day."[15] Surgeons ordinarily emphasize the results of operative treatment and do not discuss the majority of patients whose symptoms are minor or who respond to nonoperative treatment. Stallworth in a recent letter reported operating on only 17 percent of 4140 patients who were studied, and McGough's group operated on only 8.3 percent of their 1200 treated patients.[7] My own operative rate during the past decade has been 26 percent of referred patients.

Operation indications are summarized in Table 34-3. Patients who have cervical ribs which are symptomatic in terms of either nerve pressure or vascular abnormalities should have the extra rib removed. The supraclavicular approach is preferable, but the cervical rib can be excised along with the first rib through the axilla.

At the same time, the question of a contralateral asymptomatic rib should be studied. If the other cervical rib is entirely asymptomatic, no question of its removal need arise. The question tightens a bit if there is no pain but there is evidence of subclavian arterial damage in the form of early dilatation or aneurysm formation, in which case second-stage removal of the rib on that side should be done to prevent continued arterial damage.

The second indication for thoracic outlet decompression is long-standing and continued pain due to pressure on the brachial plexus which cannot be relieved by nonoperative measures. The final indication consists of either venous or arterial lesions.

Factors which are relative indications for operation include electromyographic abnormalities and evidence of arterial compression. Relative contraindications include heavy muscling or obesity, where the technical difficulties can be expected to be severe; evidences of psychic instability;

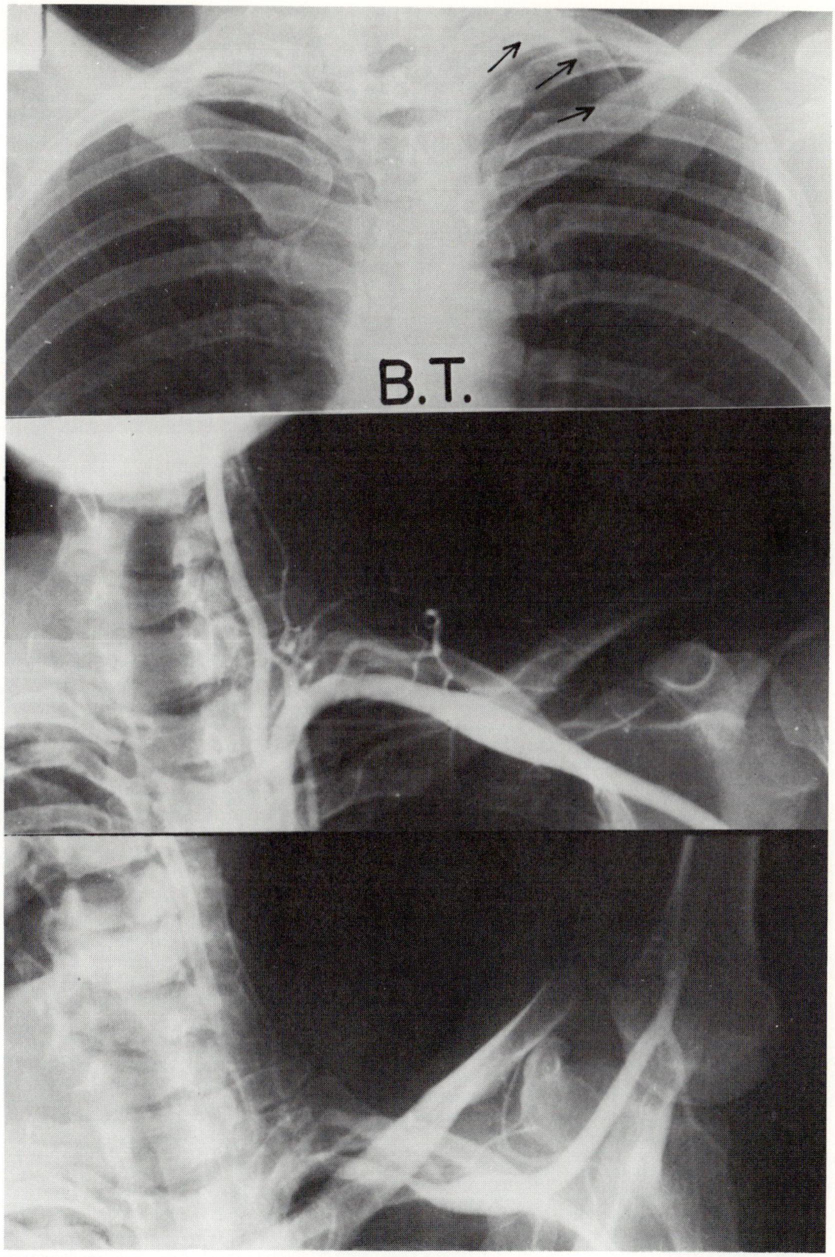

FIGURE 34-5 *Top,* the *arrows* outline the left cervical rib. *Middle,* the artery is patent with a poststenotic dilation with the arm dependent. *Bottom,* tight stenosis with poststenotic dilatation of the subclavian artery with the arm elevated.

and a history of trauma with litigation in the background. Sometimes it is possible to insist that the legal problem be settled prior to an operation, but usually there must be continuation and completion of medical treatment prior to the settlement.

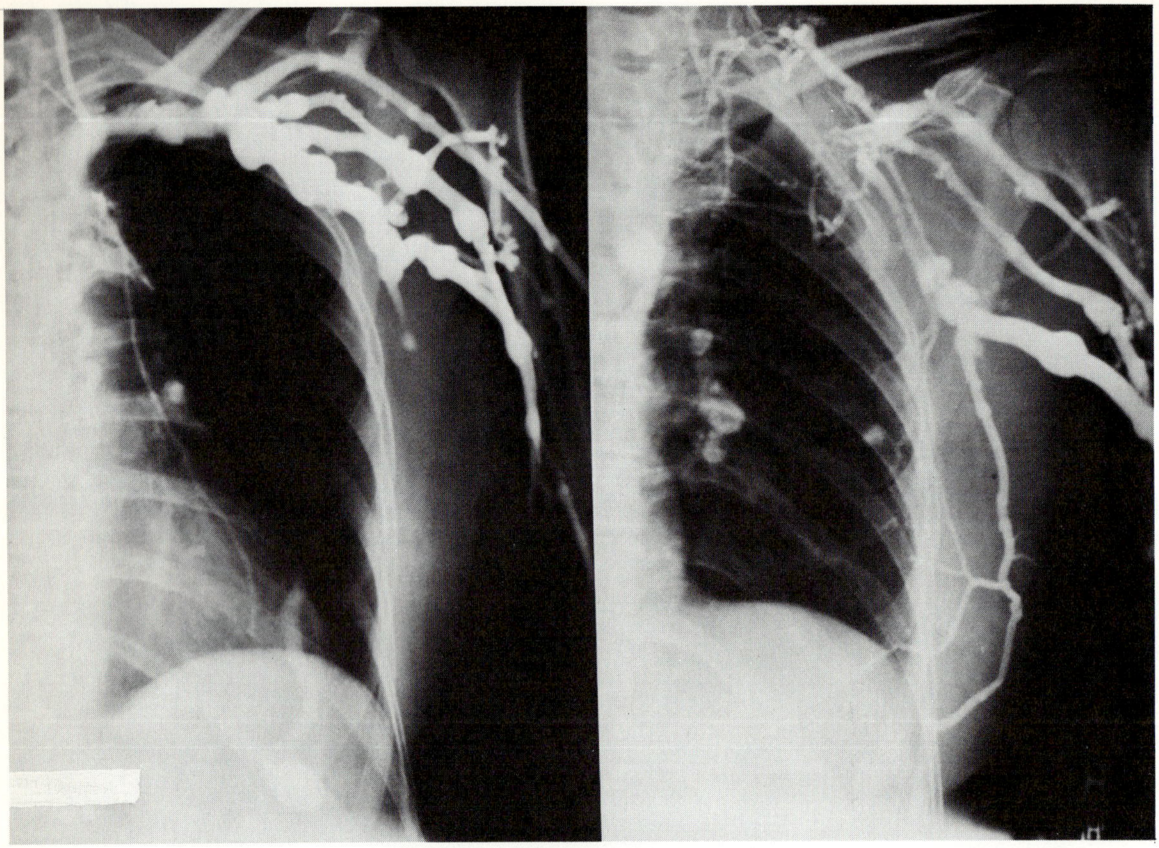

FIGURE 34-6 *Right,* deep venous occlusion of the subclavian-axillary vein in effort thrombosis. *Left,* recanalization later following intravenous heparin therapy.

THE CHOICE OF OPERATION

The history of operations for thoracic outlet syndrome includes many noted surgeons since Coote[16] in 1861 recorded an early attempt to remove the first rib. In 1905 John B. Murphy[17] of Chicago resected a cervical rib that had produced a subclavian aneurysm, and by 1916 William S. Halsted[18] was able to find records of 716 such patients.

Telford and Stopford[19] reported relief of vascular symptoms in six patients after resection of the first thoracic rib. The role of the anterior scalene muscle in neurovascular compression was developed further by Naffziger and Grant [20] and by Ochsner, Gage, and DeBakey in 1935.[21] Peet, Hendricksen, Anderson, and Martin in 1956 suggested that all of the compression syndromes might be termed thoracic outlet syndrome;[22] the name was later modified by Rob and Standeven to thoracic outlet compression syndrome.[23]

The substantial failure rate of division of the anterior scalene muscle alone led to efforts to achieve greater

TABLE 34-3 INDICATIONS FOR OPERATION

1 Pain: intractable, requires narcotics, or is associated with a cervical rib

2 Vascular problems
- Arterial
  - Aneurysm
  - Embolism
- Venous

decompression, such as the wider supraclavicular resection of McCleery, Kesterson, Kirtley, and Love[24] and the claviculectomy advocated by Rosati and Lord in 1961,[25] In 1962 Clagett again directed attention to resection of the first rib via the posterior approach.[26]

The modern transaxillary approach was described by David Roos in 1966.[27] This technique still is practiced by other experienced surgeons such as Kelly[28] and Urschel,[9] who believe that it allows decompression of the space without cutting muscle and that it produces few complications and good results.

From 1966 until recently I used the transaxillary approach as the procedure of choice for removal of the first rib along with severance of the scalene muscle. The mortality was zero and the complication rate was low. There always was concern with the deep circumscribed field of dissection that produced technical problems for even the experienced surgeon.

In 1982 I summarized the practices of other experienced surgeons (Table 34-4).[7,9,15,28–32] Martinez has developed a wide experience using the posterior parascapular route.[29] This modification of Clagett's old thoracoplasty approach[26] is not well known today, and at present most surgeons restrict its use to secondary procedures where the transaxillary approach was the original one. Munro suggests that if the posterior route is best for recurrences, it also may be preferable for the first-time operation.[33]

Thomas advised the anterior supraclavicular approach to the first rib, citing 91 percent good to excellent results and 7 percent failures among 38 operations.[34] He did note the delicate dissection necessary for this deep approach, which in my experience rules against it. Hempel, Rusher, Wheeler, Hunt, and Bukhari also prefer the supraclavicular approach, citing excellent results in 60 percent of 358 patients, good results in 37 percent, and a 2.5 percent failure rate.[30]

The infraclavicular route proposed by Nelson and Jensen[35] in 1970 was supported by Murphy, Piper, Kanar, and McAlexander in 1980[36] as a simple way to remove the anterior two thirds of the rib. Among 22 operations in 19 patients there were 16 excellent results, 4 good, and 2 failures.[36]

Stallworth, Quinn, and Aiken reported 194 operations among 1140 patients, 180 done by division of the soft tissues with good results in 96 percent; only 43 percent of the 14 patients

TABLE 34-4 RESULTS OF SERIES OF 100 OR MORE OPERATIONS FOR THORACIC OUTLET SYNDROME

Source, yr	No. of operations	Preferred operation	Results, % Excellent	Good	Failed
Urschel,[9] 1970	700	Transaxillary first rib	99%	0	1
Martinez,[29] 1978	350	Posterior first rib	85	15†	20
Kelly,[28] 1979	304	Transaxillary first rib	85	7	8
McGough, Pearce, Byrne,[7] 1979	113	Transaxillary first rib	80	13	7
Hempel, Rusher, Wheeler, Hunt, Bukhari,[30] 1981	433	Supraclavicular first rib	60	37	3
Stallworth, 1982‡	180	Resection of soft tissue	96	0	4
	14	First rib resection	43	0	57
Sanders,[31] 1982‡	239	Scalenectomy	85	8	7
	214	Transaxillary first rib	86	4	10
Roos,[32] 1982	566	Transaxillary first rib	89	11	11

*Only 9 recurrences among 700 operations.
†Residual symptoms.
‡Personal letter.

having resection of ribs were relieved. He concluded that "only on rare occasion is first rib resection indicated."[37]

Sanders, Monsour, Gerber, Adams, and Thompson in 1979 reported 239 scanlenectomies and 214 first-rib resections, whereby good to excellent results occurred in 85 percent and 86 percent, respectively, fair in 8 percent and 4 percent, poor in 7 percent and 10 percent, and recurrences in 17 percent and 16 percent.[11] These data suggest the lesser procedure. Sanders more recently reported that he now not only removes both the anterior and middle scalene muscles via the supraclavicular approach, but also resects the first rib through the same wound, finding this procedure satisfactory in 75 cases.[31]

Roos, who originally described the transaxillary approach, recently modified both his diagnostic considerations and his preference in operation, now proposing scalenectomy for the "upper root" syndrome while continuing to advocate transaxillary first-rib resection for the "lower root" syndrome.[32]

Among those with extensive experience, Urschel and Razzuk continue to advocate transaxillary resection of the first rib, reporting only 9 recurrences requiring a secondary operation among 700 patients. It is not clear what number of these successes had complete as opposed to partial relief.[38] Similarly, McGough, Pearce, and Byrne reported that this approach produced 93 percent good or excellent results and 7 percent failure among 113 patients.[7]

Thus, experienced surgeons still disagree on operative indications as well as details of technique, and there are other unpublished but frequent complaints of poor results from surgeons who do fewer such cases. Therefore, I have come to believe that in the absence of vascular complications or a bony anomaly such as a cervical rib, those patients with neurologic symptoms alone should have prolonged nonsurgical treatment and *operative decompression should be a last resort.*

When all measures fail and the last-resort operation must be undertaken to relieve intractable pain, I now perform resection (not simple severance) of the anterior scalene muscle. This relieves many patients at minimal risk. However, it should be understood clearly by patient and physician that some failures will occur and that some patients will require a secondary first-rib resection. Informed consent to the entire program along with understanding of possible complications is necesary.

Further recommendations include use of the supraclavicular route either for removal of a cervical rib or to repair a vascular problem and the posterior route for secondary procedures.

OPERATIVE TECHNIQUE

Details of techniques for thoracic outlet decompression by several routes are well-documented in other publications referenced herein and will not be repeated. Experience has led to delineation of some points which may be helpful and are therefore discussed below.

When the scalene muscle is resected via the supraclavicular route, the operator should remove a 2-cm segment of it rather than simply cut across it, to prevent reattachment to the adjacent brachial plexus (Figure 34-7). The phrenic nerve usually lies on the anterior surface of the anterior scalene muscle but may be buried within its substance and should be searched out and protected.

The subclavian artery lies directly behind the anterior scalene muscle. A branch may originate directly under the muscle, which is liable to damage at the time the muscle is cut.

The thoracic duct lies in the medial aspect of the field and should not ordinarily be visualized. If damaged in any way, it should be divided between ligatures.

Sometimes the cervical rib not only elevates the lower nerve roots but actually passes between cords of the brachial plexus. The gentlest-possible traction should be placed on the nerve roots,

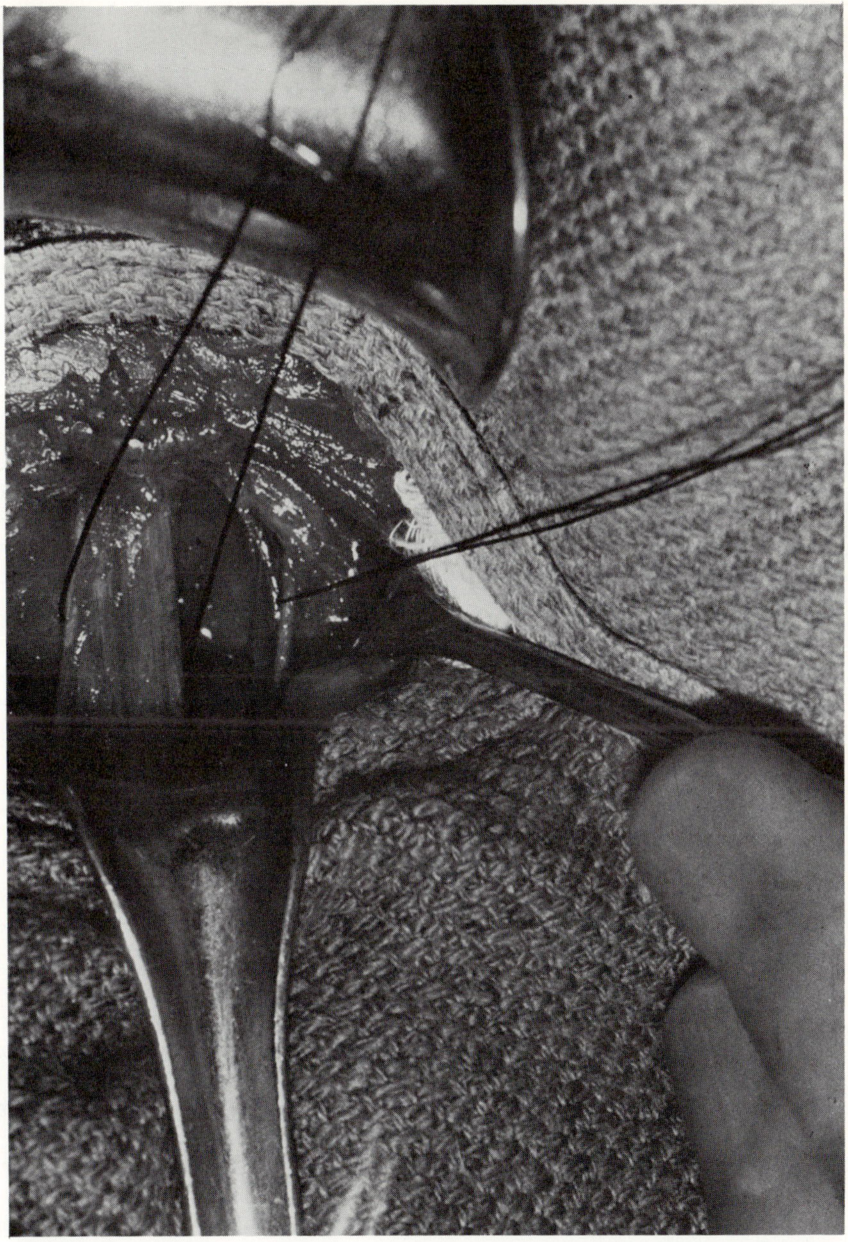

FIGURE 34-7 The anterior scalene muscle has been isolated and is ready for excision. The phrenic nerve is looped and retracted.

and cords should be constantly in mind and nothing divided until it is correctly identified (Figures 34-8 to 34-10).

A cervical rib may also be removed through the axilla along with the first rib (Figure 34-11).

The transaxillary approach demands proper placement of the patient on the operating table,

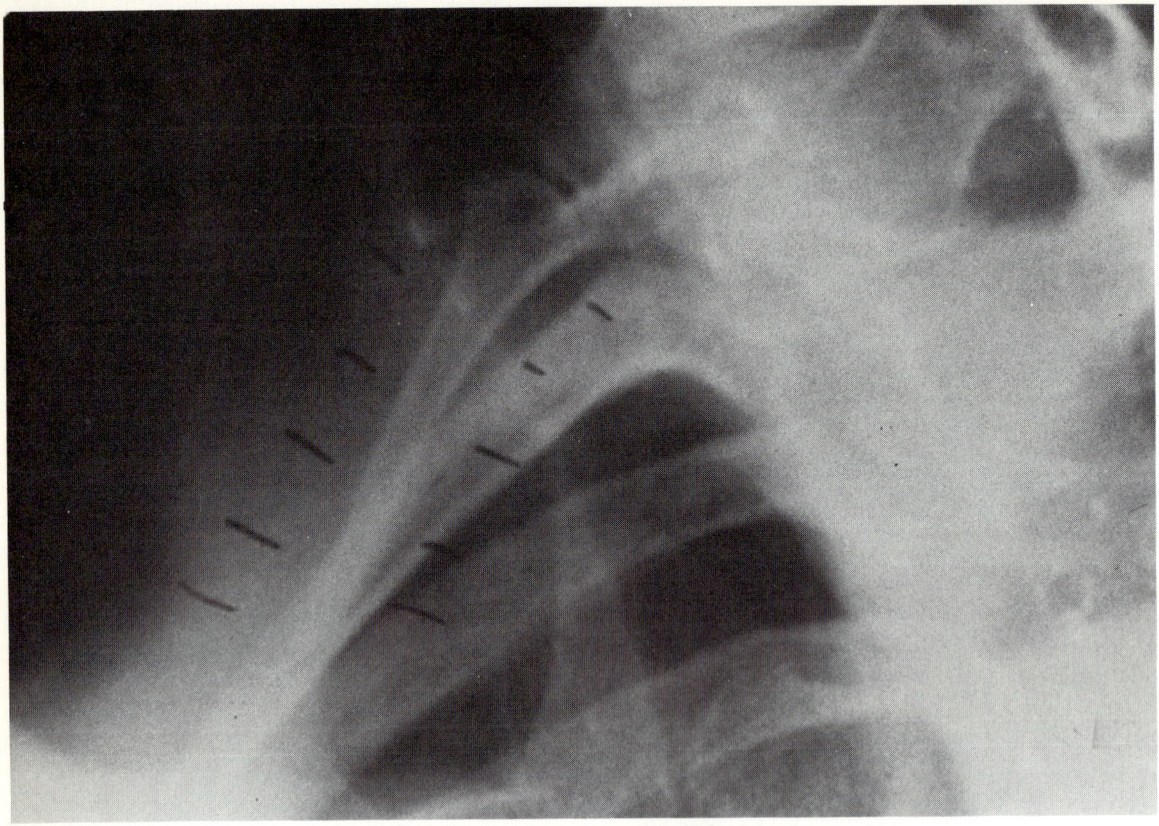

FIGURE 34-8 A long cervical rib outlined by *dashes.*

adequate lighting, and strong assistance to expose the operative field (Figure 34-12). The incision should be placed at the lower border of the axillary hairline because high placement leads into fat and lymph nodes, which causes needless bleeding. The intercostobrachial nerve crossing the field is a sensory nerve which if retracted without division usually produces painful neuritis. Despite some surgeons' advice to protect this, I intentionally divide it and advise the patient that an area of numbness on the medial aspect of the upper arm is preferable to a painful neuritis there. Division also facilitates exposure.

A variety of means of mechanical elevation of the shoulder girdle, including attachment of the arm to various poles and standards and to an orthopedic crank table, have been used without discovery of anything as efficient as a well-instructed assistant using a hammerlock upon the forearm, as originally described by Roos.[39] A strong assistant should pull firmly but without jerks, to avoid brachial plexus injury. He should be positioned comfortably so that the arms holding the forearm in a hammerlock are extended and the pull is produced by the large back muscles rather than the arms and forearms, which tire more easily (Figure 34-13). I request the supervisor prior to operation to assign a large muscular individual to furnish this traction, since a small person, even though well-intentioned, simply cannot hold open the axillary exposure as needed. A second assistant should also be available to relieve the first at the end of 10 minutes by the clock so that steady exposure can be maintained. Ordinarily, no more than 15 to 20 minutes of this exposure is needed. At that time both assistants may be discharged with thanks, to attend

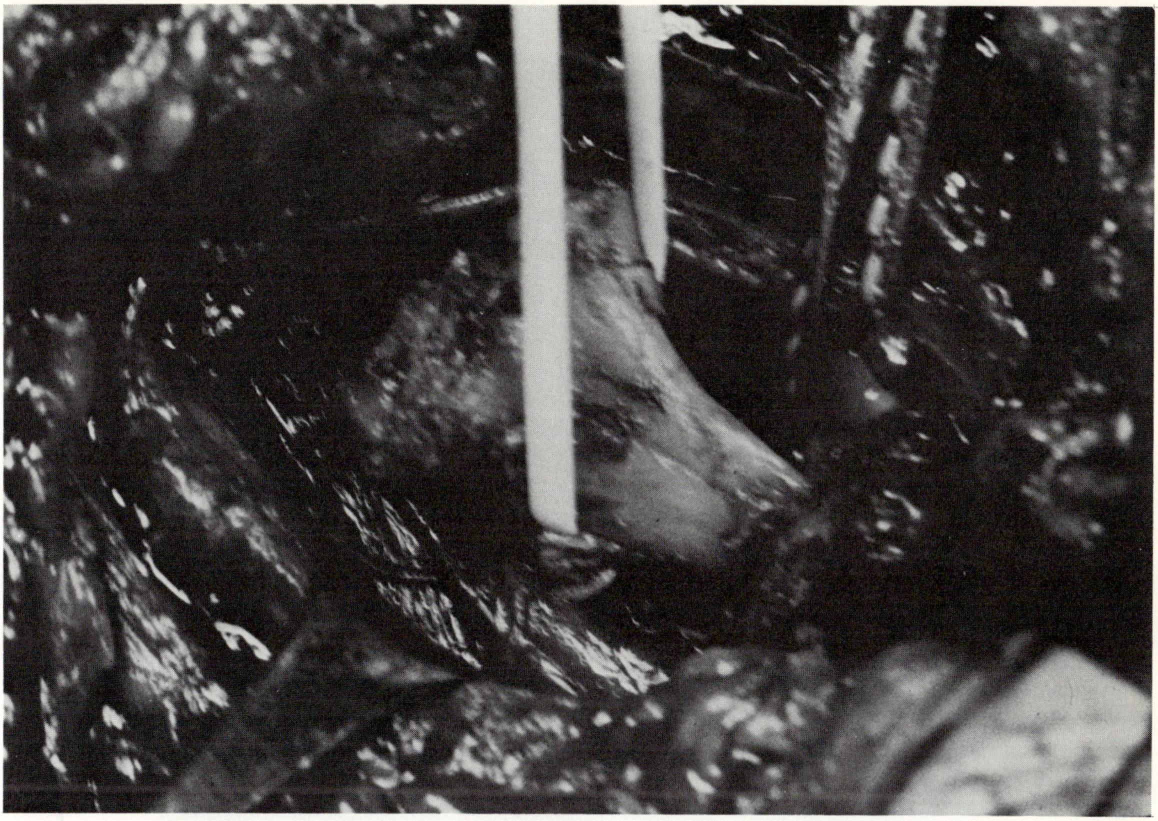

FIGURE 34-9 The long cervical rib has been resected and replaced in its bed for the photograph. The subclavian artery is looped inferiorly. Superior and left lie cords of the brachial plexus.

FIGURE 34-10 The excised cervical rib.

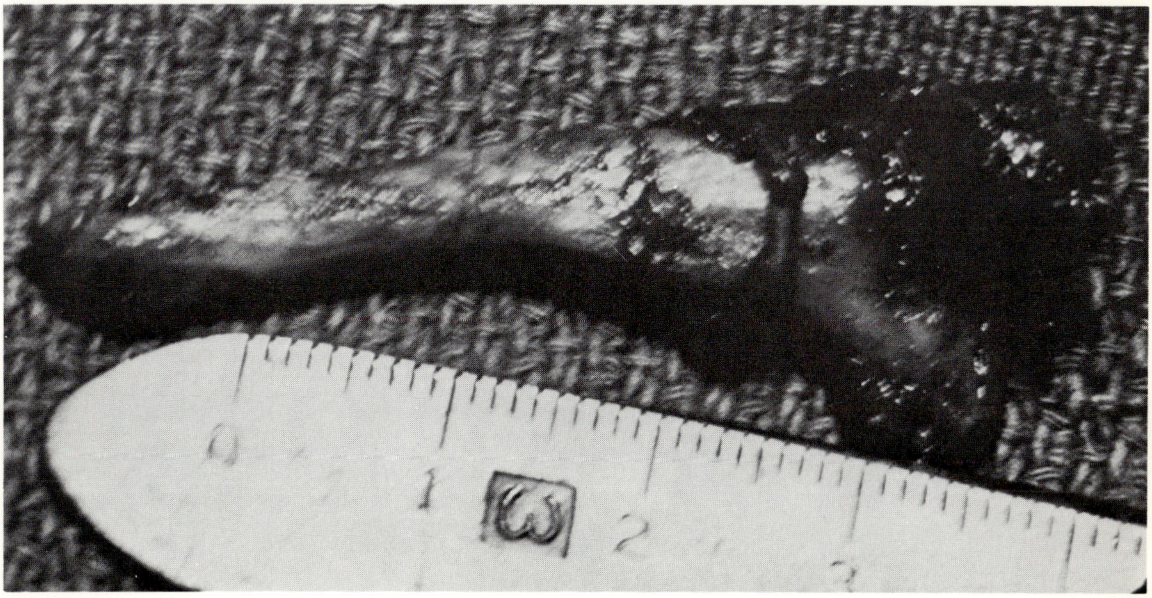

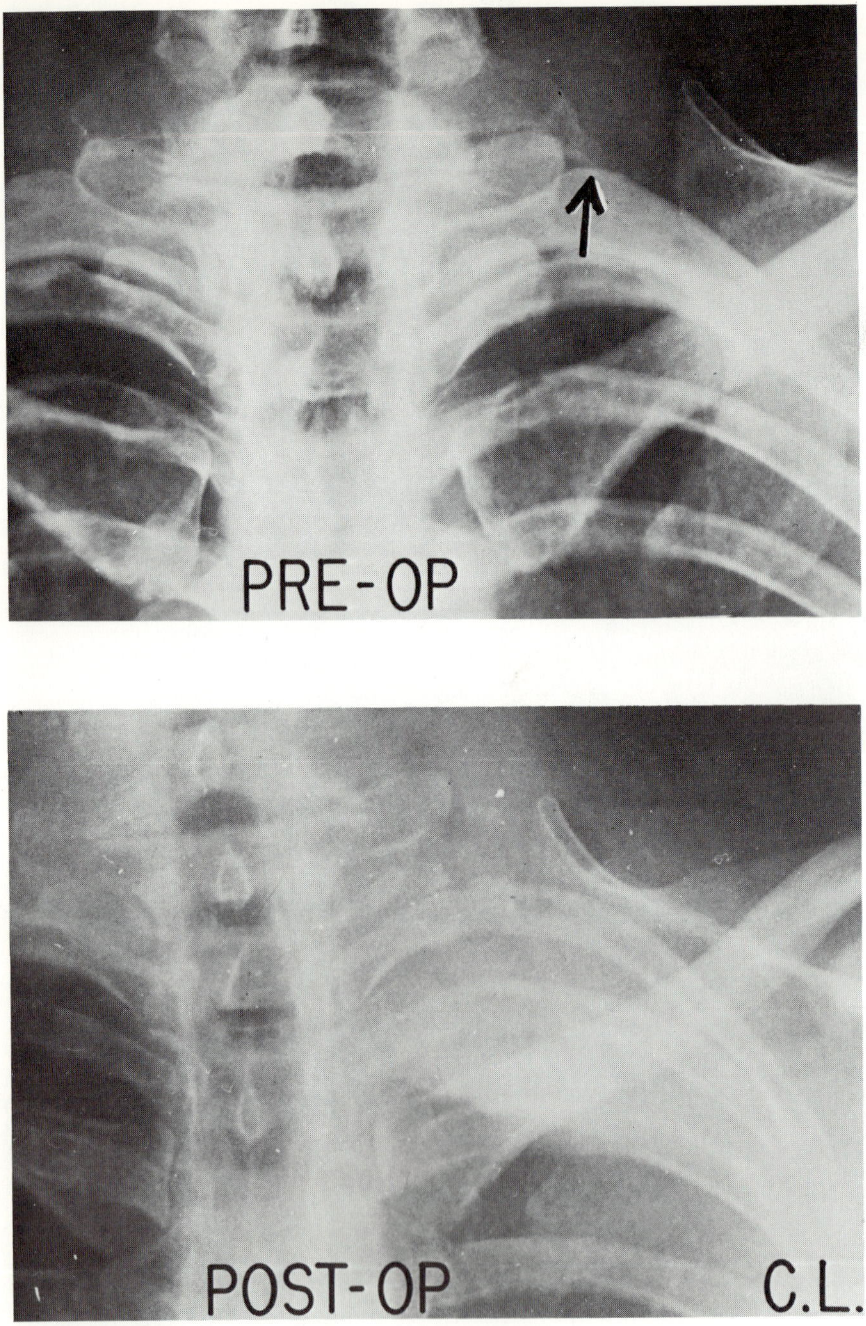

FIGURE 34-11 The cervical rib and first rib were both removed via the transaxillary approach.

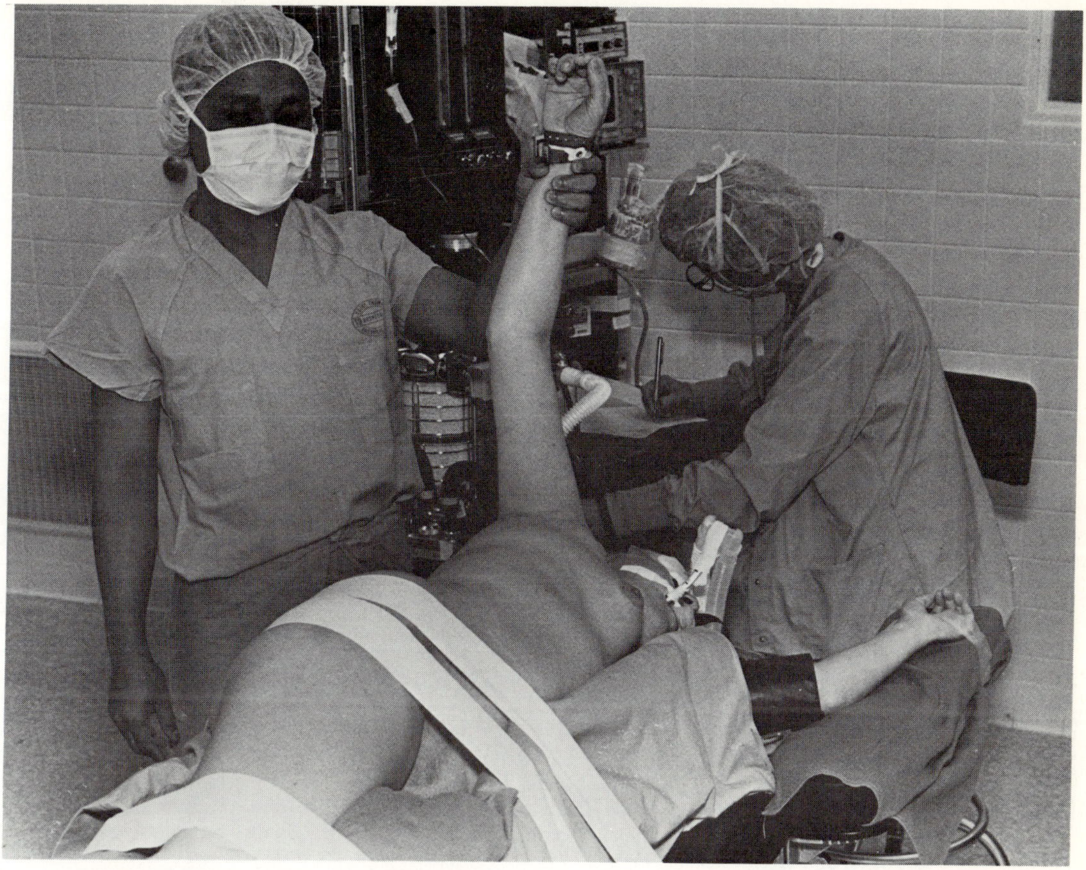

FIGURE 34-12 The position of the table with the arm free for retraction.

to other duties. Unless proper assistance and lighting are available, the transaxillary operation should not be attempted.

Dissection posteriorly and laterally should be limited, to avoid injury to the long thoracic nerve. This has occurred twice in my experience, with resultant winging of the scapula due to serratus denervation.

It is usually stated that extraperiosteal resection of the first rib should be performed. In my experience, corroborated by conversation with others, this guideline is followed only in theory; the procedure is difficult, and removal of the rib with or without periosteum is acceptable.

Frequently one is asked how much rib to remove? The usual answer is from the cartilage to the vertebral transverse process. This ideal is difficult to achieve posteriorly, even with needle-nose bone ronguers (Figure 34-14). The posterior limit is usually as far back as is consistent with safety to the brachial plexus. Clearly this is variable.

Finally, the surgeon must search for a pleural opening prior to closure and remove air by suction tube if necessary. Absolute hemostasis must be obtained in the wound prior to its closure.

David Roos's 12 "essentials and safeguards" are important points for anyone performing this operation.[32] I follow all of his recommendations except restrictions of use of the shoulder. This is apt to result in prolonged shoulder immobility. There has been as yet no comparative study

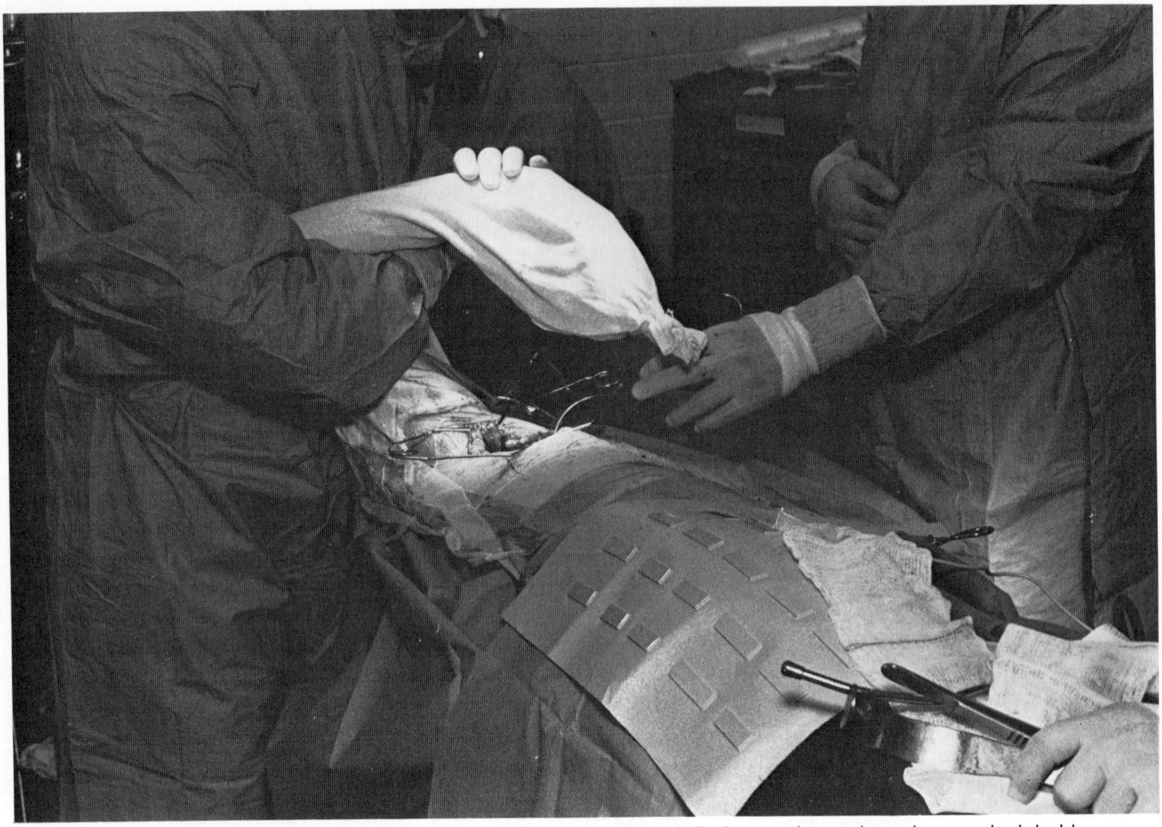

FIGURE 34-13 An assistant elevates the shoulder girdle by traction, using a hammerlock hold upon the wrist and forearm.

of whether early motion or delayed motion is better, but I prefer to enlist the help of the physical therapist beginning the day following surgery.

VASCULAR COMPLICATIONS OF THORACIC OUTLET SYNDROME

Vascular lesions occur in about 10 percent of patients with thoracic outlet syndrome—5 percent arterial and 5 percent venous. The arterial problem usually requires operation, while the venous one does not.

Arterial Constant pressure upon the subclavian artery by bone, a fibrous band, or a muscle sometimes produces poststenotic dilatation, which may continue to form an aneurysm, thrombosis, or embolism. Figure 34-15 shows almost complete occlusion of the subclavian artery with the arm abducted and elevated. This produced thrombosis with embolism requiring an autogenous vein bypass in this patient. The first rib and scalene muscle were simultaneously resected. Approximately 5 percent of patients with thoracic outlet syndrome have such arterial problems, which force operative relief.

Venous Occasional instances of acute occlusion of the subclavian-axillary veins cause congestion with edema, pain, and cyanosis. The syndrome has been termed *effort thrombosis* and *Paget-Schroetter Syndrome* and represents an acute manifestation of thoracic outlet syndrome.

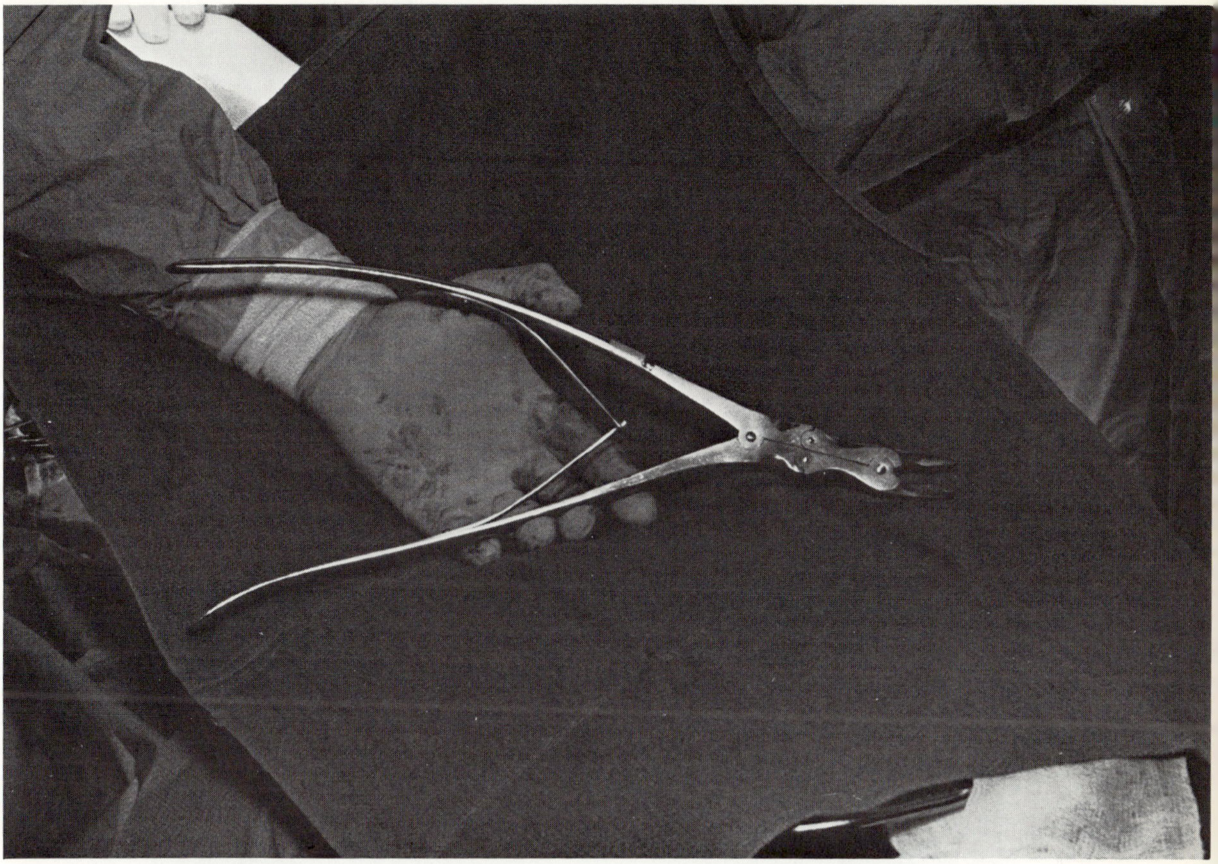

FIGURE 34-14 Needle-nose long rib ronguers. *(Reprinted courtesy of Codman, Boston.)*

Alternative treatment lies between heparinization, enzyme resolution, and venous thrombectomy. Since the well-know tendency of all deep venous thrombosis is toward later patency via internal recanalization, there is a reasonable rationale to select either enzyme resolution or heparinization rather than immediate venous thrombectomy. Occasionally, operative removal of a clot may be indicated because of an extremely severe and widespread venous thrombosis which produces secondary arterial ischemia and thus does not allow the longer time necessary for non-operative resolution by drugs. In general, however, the results of drug therapy have been equal to those of venous thrombectomy in the large veins of the pelvis and thigh as well as those around the shoulder girdle, so operation is indicated only occasionally in clinical situations where arterial ischemia has complicated the situation. At the time of writing, my own experience with enzyme therapy is limited and includes the unhappy development of pulmonary embolism in one instance, whereas standard treatment by continuous intravenous heparinization has been safe and effective, so the latter continues as the bench-mark therapy. Thus treated, the acute deep venous occlusion seen in Figure 34-6 was recanalized completely several months later.

In recent years I have treated three professional baseball pitchers with acute subclavian-axillary venous thrombosis. One had immediate heparinization, the second had delayed heparinization beginning 10 days after the incident, and the third had heparinization after pulmonary embolism due to intravenous streptokinase. In each incidence there was clinical resolution with phlebographic demonstration of recanalization, essentially complete in two and partial in the

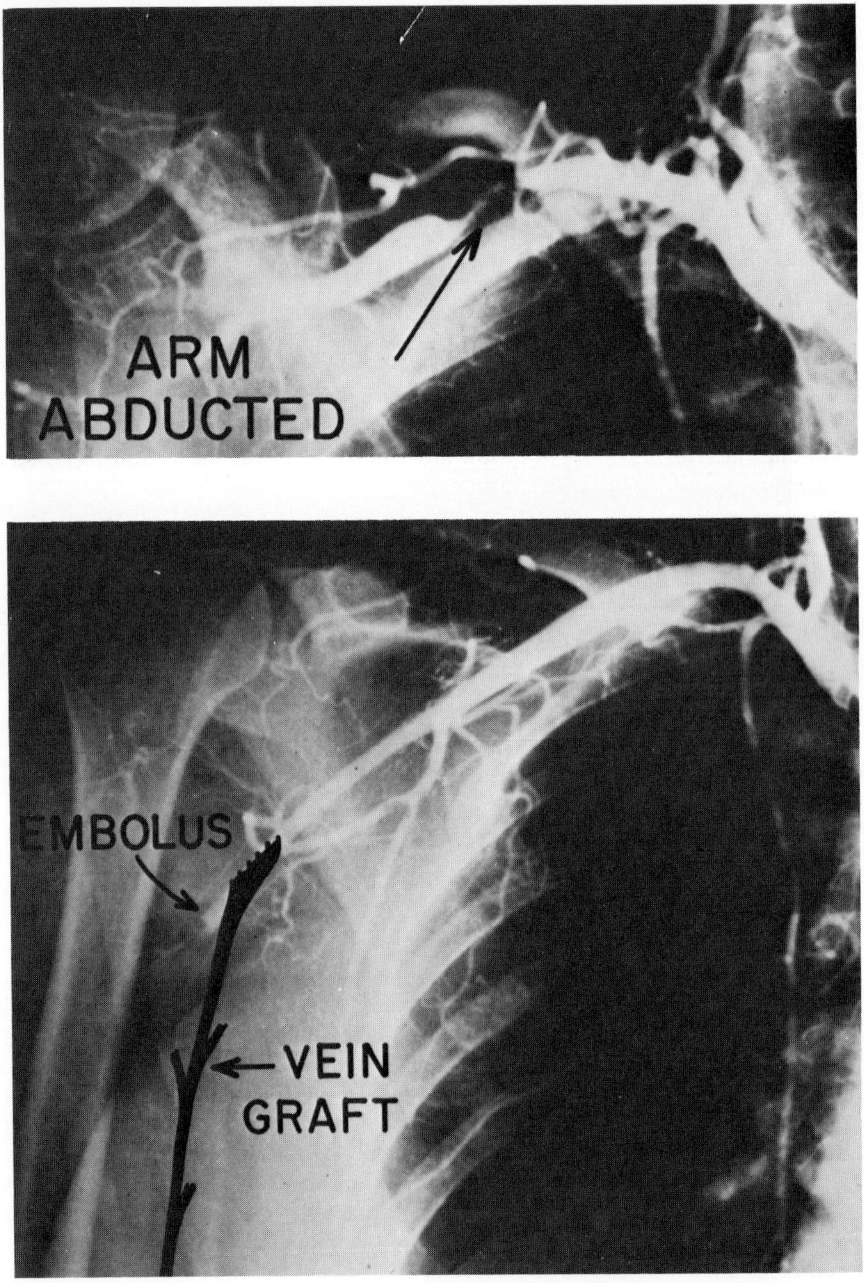

FIGURE 34-15 Arterial stenosis with brachial thrombotic occlusion and later embolism. *Above,* tight arterial stenosis is apparent with the arm abducted. *Below,* the first rib and scalene muscle have been removed, and the brachial artery occlusion has been bypassed by a saphenous vein graft.

third. This small experience does suggest nonoperative therapy, particularly since earlier thrombectomies of the subclavian veins had poor functional results for athletes.

INJURY OF THE BRACHIAL PLEXUS

Several years ago the occurrence of complete paralysis of the upper extremity following a transaxillary resection of the first rib alerted me to this severe complication. Inquiry locally revealed another such case, also with complete recovery. However, another patient in a distant part of Tennessee did not achieve complete relief and later brought suit for alleged damages, which were settled for a considerable sum. Since then a considerable number of professional liability suits have come to my attention in several other states.

Illustrative Case

A 43-year-old woman with a 3-month history of pain and paresthesia of the arm and hand had a prominent supraclavicular space with an underlying bruit. The radial pulse was diminished, although arteriography did not show any abnormality. Roentgenograms showed no bony anomaly. The electromyogram was normal.

On March 15, 1979, the left first rib was resected via the transaxillary approach. No unusual intraoperative features were noted.

Postoperatively the patient was unable to move the entire upper extremity. Three days later there was some improvement that slowly continued. The neurologic diagnosis was diffuse left brachial plexus injury.

Physical therapy encouraged muscular return and prevented joint contractures. Five weeks following the operation, finger flexion and wrist dorsiflexion were possible but still abnormal. Ten weeks after the operation there was strong dorsiflexion of the wrist and other evidence of complete return of function. Four months following operation, there was a complete return of all neurologic function, the preoperative pain had been relieved, and the patient no longer needed medication.

Comment No member of the surgical team could remember any jerk or sudden motion by the arm holder or any other unusual intraoperative maneuver.

National Inquiry

During the June 1980 meeting of the International Cardiovascular Society, it was learned from a query of the audience (estimated at 800) that similar complications were known to approximately 30 surgeons present.[40] In an effort to learn more concerning this severe neurologic complication of the first-rib operation, a questionnaire regarding upper extremity paralysis or weakness following transaxillary resection of the first rib for thoracic outlet syndrome was mailed to the 920 members of the International Cardiovascular Society in April 1981. The 351 replies constituted 38 percent of the queries. Ninety-two responding surgeons stated that they did not perform the operation. Among the 259 surgeons who performed the operation, there were 125 (48 percent who had never personally observed such a neurologic complication among their own patients or those of their associates. The yearly experience rate of these fortunate surgeons varied from 1 to 30, with an average of 5.6 such operations yearly. The 134 surgeons (52 percent of responders) reporting personal or observed neurologic complications indicated an average operation rate of 10 per year. Only eight surgeons averaged more than two cases monthly; the procedure was an uncommon one for most.

Complete postoperative paralysis was reported 102 times (33 personal cases and 69 observed); 22 patients had failed to achieve complete return of function during the follow-up period, ranging from a few months to many years. There were an additional 171 instances of partial neurologic deficit (60 personal cases and 111 observed), with 30 instances of failure of complete recovery of function. While percentage values cannot be stated accurately, it is apparent that neurologic complications have been more frequent than generally recognized, particularly in view of their gravity.

Responses to the questionnaires reported several other complications, including an injury to the subclavian artery with hemorrhage and intraoperative cardiac arrest. Another instance of subclavian artery injury required ligation with later reconstruction.

Survey of the English-language literature at that time did not disclose any reports of brachial plexus injury with arm paralysis, although there was one suggestion that this might occur. Perhaps the devastating effect of this complication has discouraged publication. It must be recognized now, however, that brachial plexus injury may occur even when the utmost care is taken to prevent direct trauma or excessive traction and is a risk of every transaxillary operation. It is not known whether it is more likely to occur in the heavily muscled patient, where more traction is necessary, or in the smaller patient, where the same pull may be excessive. It is not clear whether any particular method of traction, such as attachment to an overhead rack or frame, is more or less dangerous than the manual pull with a hammerlock on the forearm.

The long-term outlook for brachial plexus injuries is variable. Some 80 percent of the patients described herein recovered competely, while the remaining 20 percent had incomplete return of function. Hoffer, Braun, Hsu, Mitani, and Temes recently discussed their experiences with 133 such patients (none, however, due to first-rib resection) and noted that completely recovered patients showed some return of function prior to 3 months, with improvement continuing for as long as 15 months. Clinical examination provided as much information as did either myelography or electromyography. Early and continued stretching exercises, day and night positioning orthoses, and determined follow-up care constituted the optimal treatment program. Hoffer recommended that reconstructive tendon and muscle operations be delayed for 2 years to allow the functional return to plateau.[41]

Professional liability claims following permanent neurologic deficit after thoracic outlet operations have become commonplace. The National Association of Insurance Commissioners summarized a $3\frac{1}{2}$-year study, from 1975 to 1978, of 71,782 claims, 546 of which involved thoracic surgeons. Twenty-one percent of the thoracic claims were related to operations for thoracic outlet syndrome. Since the occurrence of a brachial plexus injury is presently unpredictable, patients should be warned of this possibility during the process of obtaining informed consent.

Secondary Procedures

Attempts at operative relief of recurrent symptoms by secondary procedures usually are based upon removal of regenerated bony structures, lysis of bands or adhesions which were "missed" previously, or placement of fat pads adjacent to the nerves to prevent new adhesions. Whether the benefit from this fat transfer is a hope or a reality is not clear.

Sessions recently discussed secondary procedures in the light of his own 28 cases.[42] Whether his optimism is justified remains to be seen. The increased risks versus the lesser results persuade me to approach a secondary procedure with great reluctance or to refer such patients to a pain center or to a distant authority. If operation is done, the posterior route should be considered, since it affords good exposure through unscarred tissues.

Overview

Retrospective study of my own experience along with the reports of others suggests a cautious approach to surgical treatment, especially for the indication of pain without objective findings. Table 34-5 summarizes the results of 76 recent consecutive cases. The statistics are similar to those published earlier.[4] Combining the "excellent" (no remaining symptoms) group of 55 percent with the "good" (some residual symptoms) group indicates benefit for 90 percent of patients,

TABLE 34-5 RESULTS OF 76 OPERATIONS FOR THORACIC OUTLET SYNDROME

	Results		
	Excellent	Good	Failure
Transaxillary first-rib resection			
Alone	28	17	6
With clavicle resection	2	0	0
With cervical rib resection	5	3	0
With carpal ligament repair	4	2	1
Resection of cervical rib and scalene muscle	1	5	0
Scalenectomy alone	2	0	0
Total	42 (55%)	27 (35%)	7 (9%)

while the others are absolute failures. These results parallel the experiences of most surgeons across the land, rather than the optimistic reports of several widely recognized authorities who state that practically all patients can be relieved.

This difference has been the source of many private conversations as well as published discussions. It has been debated that the technique is too demanding for most surgeons,[43] that the operator must be a technician who refers complainers to sympathetic paramedical personnel, or that reoperation will solve the problem.[42] None of these discussions have resolved the controversy surrounding thoracic outlet compression syndrome today. Despite all our presentations, meetings, and symposiums the diagnosis often remains doubtful and treatment often fails. A final case report illustrates these problems.

Illustrative Case A 29-year-old female with right-upper-extremity pain and paresthesia in January 1971 was started on shoulder girdle exercises, which failed to relieve her symptoms. Her long and complicated ensuing history is summarized below.

February 1971: excision of the right cervical rib and scalenectomy (surgeon *A*)

May 1972: transaxillary resection of the right first rib and carpal tunnel release (surgeon *A*)

August 1972: left carpal tunnel release (surgeon *A*)

December 1972: left transaxillary resection of the first rib (surgeon *A*)

September 1973: transplantation of the right ulnar nerve (surgeon *B*)

November 1973: implantation of electrodes on the brachial plexus (surgeon *B*)

December 1973: removal of the electrodes from the brachial pletius (surgeon *B*)

April 1974: initial psychiatric consultation

May 1974: manipulation of the shoulder (surgeon *C*)

May 1974: secondary carpal tunnel release (surgeon *D*)

August 1974: right thoracic sympathectomy (surgeon *E*)

July 1977: tertiary bilateral carpal tunnel release (surgeon *D*)

Ocober 1981: the patient was wearing bilateral ventral wrist splints, stating that all her symptoms were now relieved

Final Comment Ten years, 11 operations, five surgeons! *Res ipsa loquitur.*

REFERENCES

1 Dale WA: Thoracic outlet compression syndrome: Critique in 1982. *Arch Surg* 1982, 117:1437–45.
2 Gilliatt RW: Thoracic outlet compression syndrome. *Br Med J* 1976, 1:1274–75.
3 Parry E: The thoracic outlet compression syndrome. *Aust NZ J Surg* 1981, 52:84–91.
4 Dale WA, Lewis MR: Management of thoracic outlet syndrome. *Ann Surg* 1975, 151:575–85.
5 Adams JT, DeWeese JA, Mahoney EB, Rob CG: Intermittent subclavian vein obstruction without thrombosis. *Surgery* 1968, 63:147–65.
6 Fairbairn JF, Juergens JL, Spittell JA: *Peripheral Vascular Diseases.* Saunders, Philadelphia, 1972, p 473.
7 McGough EC, Pearce MB, Byrne JP: Management of thoracic outlet syndrome. *J Thorac Cardiovasc Surg* 1979, 77:169–73.
8 Sadler TR, Rainer WG, Wombley G: Thoracic outlet compression: Application of positional arteriographic and nerve conduction studies. *Am J Surg* 1975, 130:704–5.
9 Urschel HC: Discussion of McGough EC, Pearce, MB, Byrne, JP: Management of thoracic outlet syndrome. *J Thorac Cardiovasc Surg* 1979, 77:169–73.
10 Stanton PE, McClusky DA, Richards HD, Lamis PA: Thoracic outlet syndrome: A comprehensive evaluation. *South Med J* 1978, 71:1070–73.
11 Sanders RJ, Monsour JW, Gerber WF, Adams WR, Thompson N: Scalenectomy versus first rib resection for treatment of thoracic outlet syndrome. *Surgery* 1979, 85:109–21.
12 Glassenberg M: The thoracic outlet syndrome: An assessment of 20 cases with regard to new clinical and electromyographic findings. *Angiology* 1981, 32:18.
13 Cherington M: Ulnar conduction velocity in thoracic outlet syndrome. *N Engl J Med* 1976, 274:1185.
14 Relman AS: Responsibilities of authorship: Where does the buck stop *N Engl J Med* 1984, 310:1048.
15 Lord JW Jr: Thoracic outlet syndromes: Real or imaginary? *NY State J Med* 1981, 81:1488.
16 Coote H: Exostosis of the seventh cervical vertebra surrounded by blood vessels and nerves. *Lancet* 1861, 1:360.
17 Murphy JB: Case of cervical rib with symptoms resembling subclavian aneurysm. *Ann Surg* 1905, 42:399.
18 Halsted WS: An experimental study of circumscribed dilation of an artery immediately distal to a partially occluding band and its bearing on the dilation of the subclavian artery observed in certain cases of cervica rib. *J Exp Med* 1916, 24:271.
19 Telford ED, Stopford JSB: The vascular complications of the cervical rib. *Br J Surg* 1937, 18:559.
20 Naffziger HC, Grant WT: Neuritis of the brachial plexus mechanical in origin: The scalenus anticus syndrome. *Surg Gynecol Obstet* 1938, 67:711.
21 Ochsner A, Gage M, DeBakey M: Scalenus anticus (Naffziger) syndrome. *Am J Surg* 1935, 28:669.
22 Peet RM, Hendrickensen JD, Anderson TP, Martin G: Thoracic outlet syndrome. *Proc Staff Mtg Mayo Clinic* 1956, 31:281.
23 Rob CG, Standeven A: Arterial occlusion complicating thoracic compression syndrome. *Br Med J* 1958, 2:1709–12.
24 McCleery RS, Kesterson JE, Kirtley JA, Love RB: Subclavius and anterior scalene muscle compression as a cause of intermittent obstruction of subclavian vein: *Ann Surg* 1951, 133:588–602.
25 Rosati LM, Lord JW: *Neurovascular Compression Syndromes of the Shoulder Girdle.* Grune & Stratton, New York, 1961.
26 Clagett OT: Presidential address: Research and prosearch. *J Thorac Cardiovasc Surg* 1962, 44:153–66.
27 Roos DB: Transaxillary approach for first rib resection to relieve thoracic outlet syndrome. *Ann Surg* 1966, 164:354–58.
28 Kelly TR: Thoracic outlet syndrome: Current concepts of treatment. *Ann Surg* 1979, 190:657–62.
29 Martinez NS: Posterior first rib resection for total thoracic outlet syndrome decompression. *Contemp Surg* 1979, 15:13–21.
30 Hempel GK, Rusher AH Jr, Wheeler CG, Hunt DG, Bukhari, HI: Supraclavicular resection of the first rib for thoracic outlet syndrome. *Am J Surg* 1981, 141:213–15.
31 Sanders, RJ: Letter, May 1982.
32 Roos D: The place for scalenectomy and first-rib resection in thoracic outlet syndrome. *Surgery* 1982, 92:1077–85.
33 Munro DD: Discussion of Urschel HC, Razzuk MA, Alber JE, Wood RE, Paulson DL: Reoperation for recurrent thoracic outlet syndrome. *Ann Thor Surg* 1976, 21:19–25.
34 Thomas GI: Discussion of McGough EC, Pearce MB, Byrne JP: Management of thoracic outlet syndrome. *J Thorac Cardiovasc Surg* 1979, 77:169–73.

35 Nelson RH, Jensen CB: Anterior approach for excision of first rib: Surgical technique. *Ann Thorac Surg* 1970, 9:30–35.
36 Murphy TO, Piper CA, Kanar EA, McAlexander RA: Subclavicular approach to first rib resection. *Am J Surg* 1980, 139:634–36.
37 Stallworth JM, Quinn GJ, Aiken AF: Is rib resection necessary for relief of thoracic outlet syndrome? *Ann Surg* 1977, 185:581–92.
38 Urschel HC, Razzuk MA: Management of the thoracic outlet syndrome. *N Engl J Med* 1972, 286:1140–43.
39 Roos DB: Transaxillary approach for first rib resection to relieve thoracic outlet syndrome. *Ann Surg* 1966, 163:354–58.
40 Dale WA: Discussion of Glover JL, Worth RM, Bendick PJ, Hall PV, Markand OM: Evoked responses in the diagnosis of thoracic outlet syndrome. *Surgery* 1981, 89:86–93.
41 Hoffer HM, Braun R, Hsu J, Mitani M, Temes K: Functional recovery and orthopedic management of brachial plexus palsies. *JAMA* 1981, 246:1467–70.
42 Sessions RT: Recurrent thoracic outlet syndrome: Causes and treatment. *South Med J* 1981, 75:1453–61.
43 Brantigan CO; Discussion of Dale WA: Thoracic outlet compression syndrome: Critique in 1982. *Arch Surg* 1982, 117:1437–45.

Invited Commentary

David B. Roos, M.D.
Denver, Colorado

This is a scholarly overview of complex problems of TOS and is backed by personal experience. My own opinions and experience agree in many aspects and vary in others.

In all patients evaluated for thoracic outlet syndrome, the surgeon must carefully consider problems that may mimic or coexist with TOS, such as cervical arthritis and sprain injury, shoulder tendinitis and capsulitis, cubital tunnel syndrome of the ulnar nerve at the elbow, and carpal tunnel syndrome at the wrist. It is necessary to become adept at diagnosing these problems in order to understand the clinical picture and explain the reasonable limitations anticipated if surgical treatment of the outlet syndrome seems advisable. If other problems are overlooked, the patient will have unexpected residual symptoms, everyone will be disappointed, and the operation will be considered ineffective.

The common reliance on radial pulse changes with the arm elevated (hyperabduction test) or with the head turned with the hand in the *lap* (Adson's test) unfortunately persists in the literature and in clinical practice as the most commonly relied upon means of diagnosis of TOS. As 65 to 92 percent of normal asyptomatic people show such positional pulse alterations,[1,2] these tests are of no diagnostic importance and have led to numerous inappropriate operations with poor results. When the patient's symptoms fail to respond, the operation is condemned as being ineffective when, in fact, the diagnosis was incorrect and the operation should not have been performed.

I agree that the emotional and neurotic tendencies seen in many TOS patients may be more the *result* of the symptoms and the frustrations that develop from failure to obtain an accurate diagnosis and effective treatment than the actual *cause* of the symptoms, as some physicians claim. The emotions and personality often improve dramatically after effective surgical treatment is finally achieved.

Again I agree with the assessment of the limited role of ulnar nerve conduction times in the diagnosis of TOS. I have found nerve conduction time study results to be normal in some severe cases of carpal tunnel and ulnar nerve entrapment at the elbow, which responded well to surgical decompression when the *clinical* diagnosis seemed clear. Thus, nerve conduction studies seem to be of value in these various nerve entrapments only when they clearly are abnormal. Normal results cannot be used to rule out these syndromes!

The most accurate and least expensive means of detecting cervical ribs, which a surgeon must know about before operating on any patient for TOS, is obtainment of anterior-posterior and both oblique x-ray views of the cervical spine. These, plus a routine chest film, are all the radiologic studies needed for preoperative evaluation of the great majority of TOS patients. More elaborate and expensive studies are rarely indicated.

A cervical rib can be removed from either the supraclavicular, parascapular, or transaxillary approach. However, I have seen several patients who obtained poor results from removal of the cervical rib only, through a supraclavicular approach, and later required transaxillary removal of the first thoracic rib before good relief was achieved. Therefore, I feel the first rib should always be removed initially along with the cervical rib, through the transaxillary approach, for the best result.

In variance with the author, I believe that if the upper nerves of the brachial plexus, C5, C6, and C7, are the apparent causes of the severe symptoms, the *entire* anterior scalene muscle should be resected (total anterior scalenectomy) to remove all the anomalous contacts of this muscle with these specific nerves,[3] rather than merely relaxation of the muscle by removal of a 2-cm segment. This latter procedure was advocated by Adson in 1947[4] and fell into disfavor because of inconsistent long-term results.[5] In reoperating on many patients who had this procedure, I always found extensive scar tissue formation, with reattachment of the divided anterior scalene muscle, and impressive anomalies in the thoracic outlet of the upper two-thirds of the muscle affecting the upper nerves of the brachial plexus. Only by total removal of the first rib for lower plexus nerve involvement, or the entire anterior scalene muscle for upper nerve involvement, did the patients ultimately obtain relief.

Regarding the technique of the transaxillary operation, elevating the arm is simple with the arm lock as described, and a hard pull by the assistant is never required in thin patients and should be brief in obese or heavily muscled patients. Every time the surgeon pauses to change instruments, the assistant should release the arm to relieve tension on the brachial plexus, and to conserve his or her own strength. If the arm-lock procedure is properly performed, the assistant should feel no fatigue after the case is completed, and no plexus palsy should ensue. A sustained hard pull on the plexus is probably more damaging than a sudden jerk of the arm, as the microscopic vessels of the plexus are stretched closed with a sustained pull, thus depriving the oxygen-sensitive nerve tissue of all blood supply at the capillary level. Therefore, frequent release of the pull on the plexus is required, to permit refilling of the microvasculature of these major nerves. With this technique of gentle and intermittent arm elevation in use, no case of brachial plexus palsy has occurred in my series of 1600 cases. I quite agree that the transaxillary operation should not be attempted without proper assistance, lighting, and instruments.

Finally, I do lightly restrict the patient's shoulder use and motion postoperatively to minimize pain, muscle spasm, and medication, but I have the patient slowly abduct the involved arm by pulling the hand upward with the other hand over the head twice daily. This seems to be all that is required to maintain normal joint mobility, and joint stiffness has been little problem with this simple routine in my experience. Most physical therapists are too vigorous with these patients postoperatively and overdo exercises for joint mobility, to the patient's great distress and possible increase of recurrent symptoms.

COMMENTARY REFERENCES

1 Gilroy J, Mayer JS: Compression of the subclavian artery as a cause of ischemic brachial neuropathy. *Brain* 1963, 86:733–746.

2 Wright IS: The neruovascular syndrome produced by hyperabduction of the arms. *Am Heart J* 1945, 29:1–19.
3 Roos DB: The place for scalenectomy and first rib resection in thoracic outlet syndrome. *Surgery* 1982, 92:1077–1085.
4 Adson, AW: Surgical treatment for symptoms produced by cervical ribs and the scalenus anticus muscle. *Surg Gynecol Obstet* 1947, 85:687–700.
5 Clagett OT: Presidential address: Research and prosearch. *J Thorac Cardiovasc Surg* 1962, 44:153–166.

INDEX